MODERN
PSYCHIATRIC
TREATMENT

MODERN PSYCHIATRIC TREATMENT

THOMAS P. DETRE, MD, FAPA

Professor of Psychiatry
Department of Psychiatry, Yale University School of Medicine
Psychiatrist-in-Chief, Yale-New Haven Hospital

and

HENRY G. JARECKI, MD

Assistant Clinical Professor of Psychiatry
Department of Psychiatry, Yale University School of Medicine
Attending Psychiatrist, Yale-New Haven Hospital

Philadelphia & Toronto
J. B. LIPPINCOTT COMPANY

Preface

THE ADVANCES MADE over the past two decades in the medical management of mental disorders have prompted us to write this synopsis of psychiatric treatment. Modeled after the handbooks that have long proved their usefulness in other medical specialties, it emphasizes differential diagnosis and practical recommendations and avoids speculations about etiology that are of no proved relevance to patient care.

Because pharmacotherapy constitutes most of what is modern and effective in contemporary psychiatry, and empathy and common sense—psychotherapy's most essential ingredients—cannot in our opinion be conveyed by the printed page, we discuss drug treatment in greater detail than we do psychotherapy. The controlled studies currently available document only the overall efficacy of somatic treatments, however, and not any step-by-step treatment approach. It is therefore acknowledged that the detailed recommendations provided herein are based on uncontrolled case reports and our own clinical observations. In moving from history and clinical examination to diagnosis and thence to treatment, we rely largely on the diagnostic criteria embodied in the American Psychiatric Association's Diagnostic and Statistical Manual (DSM-II; see Table 50), though in some instances we have found it useful to modify them in the light of treatment experiences.

Certain innovations in format deserve a few words of explanation. For one, the text is peppered with parenthesized references to the pertinent authors and dates, a convention that may prove an interruption to reading at first. This stylistic decision derives from our own impatience in having to look up superscripted references and our pleasure at recognizing familiar names; we hope the reader will learn to pass over those in which he has no interest. In addition to the references selected to support or give a citation for a specific point, we have included monographs and review articles that provide access to further information. In some sections, we have italicized certain key words in order to help the reader locate and summarize topics he is looking for. Finally, to spare him the bewilderment of distinguishing among charts, tables, plates, diagrams, figures, and illustrations, we have labeled all departures from the text itself as Tables.

The views we express have developed within our academic and professional setting, and it is to this community and the many people in it that we owe an unparalleled opportunity to learn and observe. In the first line are our patients, who have not only conscientiously and faithfully reported their experiences but have constantly justified our belief in man's ability to face adversity with courage and dignity. Boris Astrachan, MD, Gary Tucker, MD, and Eugene Eliasoph, ACSW, by unstintingly assuming major portions of our clinical and teaching duties at Yale-New Haven Hospital and at Psychiatric Associates, respectively, have permitted us a leisure to write without which this work could not have been completed.

Our opinions cannot be considered to represent those of our professional community or even those of our own Department or Medical School, which, thanks to the leadership of Doctor Fredrik C. Redlich (formerly our Chairman and currently our Dean), operates in an intellectual climate that encourages maximal curiosity and permits the expression of controversial views. Frank disagreement with much of what we say has not prevented Doctors Redlich, Stephen Fleck, Theodore Lidz, and George Mahl from permitting us to draw on their wide fund of information by discussing particular chapters with them. Doctors Philip Bondy, William Collins, Charles Cook, José Delgado, Jack Green, Nicholas Greene, Paul Greengard, Walter Herrmann, Marc Hollender, Gerald Klatskin, Paul Lavietes, Howard Levitin, Murdoch Ritchie, Burt Rosner, Albert Solnit, and the late Nicholas Giarman generously reviewed sections in their particular specialties. Our collaborators in the chapter on childhood illnesses, Doctors Gilbert Glaser, Jonathan Pincus, and Sally Provence, and our contributor to the chapter on psychopharmacology, Professor Erik Jacobsen, provided stimulation and advice on other aspects of the book as well.

We wish to express our appreciation for permission to reprint data on cognitive changes in early schizophrenia to Doctors Andrew McGhie and James Chapman; on clinical features of the antisocial personality to Dr. Hervey Cleckley; on the identification of potential delinquents to Doctors Sheldon and Eleanor Glueck; on the relationship between impotence and aging to the Indiana University

Institute for Sex Research; on alcoholism to the National Council on Alcoholism; on the identification of drug abuse in students to the American Pharmaceutical Association; on the sleep habits of children to Dr. Louise Ames; on childhood development to Dr. Stella Chess; on a ten-question mental status examination to Dr. Robert Kahn; on delirium to Doctors Fred Plum and Jerome Posner; on the relationship between spike discharges and age to Dr. Frederic Gibbs and his collaborators; and on urine testing for psychotropic agents to Doctors Fred and Irene Forrest.

For gathering literature, helping to create some of the tables, and reviewing some of the sections, we gratefully acknowledge the assistance of Carol Anderson, Beverly Eliasoph, and Nea Norton, and of Doctors Robert Becker, Malcolm Bowers, Eugene A. Brody, John Colbert, Arthur Greenspan, Martin Harrow, Jonathan Himmelhoch, David Kupfer, and David Musto. The reader's thanks—if not always our own—should go to Gloria Jarecki, Ron Riddle, and Jean Savage, who, with judicious blue pencils, shears, and indefatigable questioning, did what was possible to translate our manuscript from the original Austro-Hungarian in the name of readability.

Ever since our friend, Lee Gordon, first encouraged us to write this book, Jack Benson has accompanied us through nocturnal vigils without complaint as its able coordinator, with a devotion and concentration that deserve an exceptional expression of gratitude. Florence Osborne's many years of transforming hieroglyphics into handsome copy have greatly eased our task, as have Joan Aaboe's typing skills and Lee Baldwin's preparation and coordination of the final manuscript. Walter Kahoe and the late Carter Harrison offered many valuable suggestions and exerted the coercive maneuvers necessary to speed our work with an urbanity and a kindness that have made them palatable and assured its completion.

THOMAS DETRE, MD
HENRY JARECKI, MD

New Haven, Connecticut
March 15, 1971

Contents

3

CHAPTER TWO:

EXAMINATION, DISPOSITION, AND MANAGEMENT

TREATMENT OF PARTICULAR SYNDROMES
INTRODUCTION TO CHAPTERS THREE TO TWELVE

CHAPTER THREE: SCHIZOPHRENIC DISORDERS

CHAPTER FOUR: AFFECTIVE DISORDERS

CHAPTER NINE:
DRUG DEPENDENCE, ADDICTION, AND ABUSE

CHAPTER TEN: # PSYCHIATRIC ILLNESS IN CHILDHOOD

CHAPTER ELEVEN: ORGANIC BRAIN SYNDROMES

CHAPTER TWELVE: THE PSYCHIATRIST AS CONSULTANT

CHAPTER THIRTEEN: PSYCHOTHERAPY

CHAPTER FOURTEEN: PSYCHOTROPIC AGENTS

CHAPTER FIFTEEN: CONVULSIVE THERAPIES

CHAPTER SIXTEEN: SOME SPECIAL TECHNIQUES

List of Tables

MODERN
PSYCHIATRIC
TREATMENT

CHAPTER
ONE

The Assessment of the Patient

IF THE CLINICAL PSYCHIATRIST OF 1900 were to spend a day in the consulting room of his modern counterpart, he would find much to surprise and puzzle him. He might first notice that most patients come of their own accord and that their symptoms and behavior are quite different from those he is accustomed to treating. As he heard some of them complain of overweight, stomach pain, or marital discord, he might feel embarrassed, glad that it is his colleague and not he who must tactfully explain that they have wandered into the wrong office. His embarrassment would likely turn to perplexity, however, as he watched his colleague proceed to interview these obviously nonpsychiatric patients. Many of the diagnostic labels he heard in the course of his visit would be unfamiliar to him; and even those he recognized might seem misapplied. After a while, he might begin to cast anxious glances at the door, hoping to see a familiar face—a "dilapidated" hebephrenic, a grandiose luetic, or a mute catatonic—but in all likelihood he would look in vain. He would undoubtedly be struck by his colleague's way of talking with patients, but even if he considered its informality lacking in delicacy, he would be impressed by its frankness and above all its optimistic tone. As he noticed how many new tests and drugs today's physician has at his command, and how well the patients respond, he might feel more than a twinge of envy. Perhaps he would be consoled as he learned how many of these opportunities pose special problems that back in his own time he had had no need to face.

FACTORS THAT HAVE CHANGED THE PRACTICE OF PSYCHIATRY

Innumerable factors account for the changes that have taken place. Increasing industrialization and a higher standard of living have both permitted and necessitated the development of modern tools in medicine and public health. Many of the infectious, metabolic, and nutritional deficiency diseases that once caused encephalopathies have today been virtually eliminated, and most of those that remain can be treated before their effects become irreversible. Advances in chemotherapy and pathophysiology have vastly improved the care of patients with medical and surgical illnesses; as a result, once-common psychiatric complications like febrile delirium are now rare, while a host of new ones—like postcardiotomy psychoses or cortisone psychoses—present new riddles for research.

More sensitive diagnostic tools have made it possible to identify and treat many illnesses that cause psychological symptoms before such symptoms appear, and to distinguish between certain illnesses that, though they look deceivingly alike, have divergent causes and need different treatment programs. For example, the adolescent girl with dramatic fits of temper whose electroencephalogram shows her to be suffering from temporal lobe epilepsy can now be neatly extracted from that ragbag of riddles once called "hysteria" and offered specific treatment. And, if her disorder is treated before her family and friends start to berate and then ignore her, she may not develop the psychological disturbances that result from an environment's negative response.

While the newly developed investigative tools have made it necessary to revise some of our thinking about mental illnesses, the introduction of *effective treatment methods* has forced even more radical changes. For example, physicians of earlier times were so sure that schizophrenic illness was incurable that they revised the diagnosis if the patient got well. Ever since phenothiazines were introduced, however, innumerable patients with symptoms indistinguishable from those of their incurable nineteenth-century counterparts have recovered (Fleishman 1968, Kramer 1969). Indeed, one recent well-controlled study showed that over half of a group of patients whose symptoms seemed to define them as schizophrenic were free of symptoms after six weeks of phenothiazine administration (NIMH 1964).

Today's patient also differs from yesterday's because he is usually *seen by a psychiatrist far earlier* in the course of his illness. Today's industrialized society requires more participation and a greater degree of conformity and predictability from its members than did the largely agricultural society of the past. As a result, the socially aberrant individual becomes both harder to tolerate and easier to identify. In addition, psychiatry has become an increasingly important medical specialty and is assuming new roles in the community at large. Both psychiatrists and those who consult them are afforded greater respect than they were half a century ago, when physicians, patients, and relatives alike considered psychiatric treatment embarrassing, esoteric, nonmedical, custodial, and futile (Rootman 1969). Still another reason for change is the increasing willingness of *medical insurance* organizations to pay some of the costs, so that the patient need no longer be totally incapacitated before coming for treatment or totally impoverished thereafter. All these factors have helped to develop a salutary cycle: timely referrals improve the average patient's outcome; the improved outcome enhances public acceptance; and the resultant community support encourages early referrals (Statistical Bull 1969).

Yet, even though a patient who is referred when his illness is just beginning may be easier to treat and more apt to recover, he may also be *harder to diagnose*. In the past, by the time the patient came to the psychiatrist, his illness was usually so advanced that his need for treatment was obvious, and his symptoms so well-defined that they were easy to categorize. Because the patient's presenting symptoms were usually so bizarre and disruptive that they engaged all his family's attention, yesterday's clinician heard little of the patient's earliest symptoms. As a result, he could gauge his patient's illness only by its most advanced symptoms, and in constructing diagnostic categories used these symptoms as criteria. While these categories sufficed for their time, they are of little help today, when it is no longer so important to classify advanced illness as to assign the proper diagnosis to a patient in the early stages of his illness. That patients are nowadays seen and treated as promptly as they are leads to other diagnostic problems, for early treatment may prevent their disorder's true character from surfacing. If, for example, a patient becomes anxious or phobic and is treated with antidepressants, these symptoms may recede so rapidly that neither he nor the physician will realize that they were in fact precursors of the depression the patient would have developed had he not been treated. Should a patient of this kind become sick at some future time, he may neglect to mention his previous symptoms or may describe them in such a way that it is hard to suspect that his previous illness was an incipient depression. Early treatment can thus dilute the value of the previous history and produce diagnostic problems.

The increasing *use of psychopharmacologic agents by the general practitioner* has also changed the clinical pictures seen by the specialist. Many patients who, 15 years ago, would have been referred directly to a psychiatrist are now successfully treated with medications by their family doctor, and thus not seen by a psychiatrist at all. He will, on the other hand, see many patients who, though treated with psychotropic agents, have shown little improvement or, conversely, apparently become worse. If a patient 'with anxiety is given a phenothiazine and soon thereafter complains of restlessness and internal disquiet, the treating physician may be hard put to decide whether the discomfort results from the drug or the illness and refer him to a psychiatrist for a more specialized evaluation. Similarly, if the patient is given an antidepressant and some 10 to 14 days later becomes confused and agitated for two or three days, he may be sent to a psychiatrist in the belief that he is getting worse when in reality such symptoms are often the precursors of improvement.

Today's psychiatrist may even see people whose need for treatment is questionable. For example, he may see an individual whose symptoms are so exceptionally mild or whose reasons for coming so unusual that he may be at a loss to determine whether he is seeing someone whose illness is just beginning or whether the community's sanguine view of psychiatric treatment has in this case led an individual who is not ill at all to hope that a psychiatrist is better equipped than a friend, parent, or minister to advise him about his life. The distinction is made even harder because today the mentally ill look less "sick" than their counterparts of a generation ago, for they are generally not only better nourished and physically healthier but likely to have received treatment from their family doctor and derived some measure of benefit from it.

A PSYCHOBIOLOGIC APPROACH

The preceding comments suggest why the information reported by psychiatrists in the past regarding the symptoms, distribution, course, prognosis, and treatment of mental illnesses is of little practical value today. The chapters that follow are, in part, a distillate of contemporary literature, so presented as to help the clinician recognize and study the symptoms of mental illnesses as they appear in our time and treat them with the tools now available. Today's clinician must identify not only those illnesses that are grave or far advanced, but also those that are mild or just beginning. He must know how they look and how they change as time or treatment affect them for better or worse. This chapter suggests some criteria for assessing the nature, severity, and progression of the clinical syndromes that the psychiatrist is most likely to see and, in so doing, provides guidelines for choosing a rational treatment plan and evaluating its results.

THE CONCEPT OF HEALTH AND ILLNESS IN PSYCHIATRY

Before discussing treatment, however, we must first try to define "illness." Two circular and equally unsatisfactory alternatives exist, the first being to define illness as a state that needs treatment, the second to define it as the absence of health. The second has created some special problems in psychiatry, for the term "mental health" is used to designate not only the absence of mental illness but also some idealized state of comfort, maturity, and creativity to which all men aspire but no man achieves.

Mental health has often been equated with "normality," but this merely begs the question, for there is no greater agreement on defining "normality" than there is on defining "mental health." The term, as Redlich (1952) points out, has several meanings, and it is useful to distinguish between the statistical, the adaptive, and the pattern norm. That the *statistical* norm is inadequate is obvious, for even though phobias of some kind are as ubiquitous as dental caries, they are also as patently pathological. Exclusive use of the *adaptational* standard of normality also has serious limitations, for equating conformity and the acceptance of cultural mores with normality stifles creativity, protest, and progress. Some of these limitations can be avoided by using the concept of the *pattern* norm, which labels as normal any object that functions according to its inherent design (King 1945). When this concept is translated into social and psychiatric terms, it labels that individual as "normal" who—whatever his peculiar ways—has worked out a livable adjustment with himself and his surroundings. By making the individual's social interaction one of normality's standards, this definition acknowledges that man is a social being who cannot be judged outside a social context. This idea of a social context must not be carried too far, however, or it will end in labeling a person as mentally ill simply because he pursues an unusual life style. Thus, the community's view of the individual must be balanced against that person's own judgment of his social and individual functioning. How comfortable and competent is he at getting along with himself, his friends, his co-workers, and his family? How well and how vigorously does he pursue his occupation, initiate goal-directed action, and create something new and worthwhile for himself and.

for others? Answers to such questions may help us approach with clearer vision the decision about a given individual's state of health or illness, especially if they are based not on a single moment in time but on the individual's development, and compare the way he functions at present with the way he has functioned in the past.

True objectivity can of course never be achieved, for the judgment inevitably depends on the observer's ability to understand and empathize with the patient's behavior and the motives that underlie it. This "empathizability," which Jaspers (1959) called *Einfuehlbarkeit,* is a crucial determinant in diagnosis, for the more a person's behavior or motives conform to the observer's, the less likely it is that he will be considered mentally ill.

Despite the vagueness and subjectivity of the criteria by which normality or illness is defined, the physician's need to communicate with his colleagues and to develop a conceptual framework in which to work has led him to assign diagnostic labels to particular types of behavior or groups of symptoms (Strömgren 1969). Just as in other specialties (Fletcher 1952, Garland 1960), however, even those clinicians who use the same criteria agree only slightly more than half the time on what label to apply to any given patient (Babigian 1965, Beck, 1962a, b, Sandifer 1964). And even if it were possible to achieve greater nosologic conformity, the labels would be useful only to the extent that they made it easier to predict how a patient would behave or how his illness would progress and could be used as standards for measuring the effectiveness of different approaches to treatment.

All too few of the current diagnostic categories meet this criterion of utility, however. In large measure, this is because so little is known about the etiology or pathogenesis of mental illnesses that it is a matter of seeing not diseases at all but only behavior or collections of symptoms (Cohen 1943). The difficulty is not that the cause of most psychiatric illnesses is unknown, for this is true of a host of other medical illnesses, but that most other illnesses exhibit a few symptoms that are so clearly unique that they permit the disease to be labeled or show some signs that are objective enough to be measured, even if this is no more than a change in some biologic function that the affected organ system normally performs.

THE NONSPECIFICITY OF SYMPTOMS

It is not that causal relationships can never be suspected in psychiatric disorders, but only that this is rare (Dalén 1969). Occasionally, an event such as a head injury or an intoxication so immediately precedes a behavioral syndrome that the connection appears obvious. Even in these situations, however, it cannot be said that the preceding event is the syndrome's only cause, for a single causative factor in different persons, or even in the same person at different times under different conditions, can lead to the most diverse clinical pictures; and diverse causative factors can lead to nearly identical syndromes. Encephalitis, head injury, or a catastrophic family situation can lead to disturbances in thinking that appear identical, yet each of these conditions can also lead to many other symptoms. A psychomotor seizure disorder can as easily manifest itself in thinking of the type seen in schizophrenia as it can in a conversion symptom; it can even appear as one and then shift to the other, or show both kinds of symptoms at the same time. Thus, a valid diagnosis cannot be based on the patient's symptoms alone.

Even when the patient's history and the development of his symptoms permit a specific diagnosis to be made, the clinical picture inevitably undergoes modifications so that at any given time it is a complex mixture of different orders of symptoms (Marrazzi 1962). The *primary* disturbances seen in schizophrenia, for example, are often disordered sleep, overattention to stimuli, and perplexity. During this state, the patient is fearful and uncomfortable, and factors within him move to counteract his sense of disorganization; this and the sleep loss then cause new symptoms. These *secondary* disturbances may take many forms: delusional ideas may help the patient "explain" why he is being bombarded by stimuli and what these stimuli mean (Sarvis 1962); social withdrawal, diminished motility, rigidity, or the monotonously manneristic repetition of certain movements may diminish his sensory input (McGhie 1961); his sleep loss may cause dreamlike imagery to occur even while he is awake (Berger 1962, Bliss 1959). When, as a consequence of these primary and secondary disturbances, he withdraws from normal social interaction or (as through hospitalization) is withdrawn from it by others, his isolation and social deprivation result in *tertiary* disturbances, such as inattentiveness to social stimuli or ineptitude in social situations (Venables 1964). Since all these symptoms may overlap, the clinical picture represents the vector of innumerable psychobiologic forces.

THE RELATIONSHIP BETWEEN AGE AND SYMPTOMS

The nonspecificity of symptoms is further demonstrated by the fact that a given illness tends to exhibit different symptoms in persons of different ages, and to manifest one set of symptoms early in a patient's life and another set at a later time (Ruesch 1964). Moreover, syndromes with quite diverse causes or courses often show certain similarities in patients of like age.

Focal activity in the EEG, for example, which in early childhood is typically seen in the occipital regions, usually disappears with the passage of time or "migrates" into the temporal lobe (Gibbs 1953).

The incidence of each of the many types of spike discharges varies significantly from one age group to the next (Gibbs 1963) (see Table 27).

The symptoms and psychodynamics of younger schizophrenic patients tend to resemble each other and to differ from those of older schizophrenic patients (Nathan 1964).

Comparable brain lesions more frequently and more markedly impair the functioning of older than of younger patients (Smith 1964); affective disorders that arise in younger persons are more likely to have been provoked by external factors than those that arise in older ones (Morozova 1963).

Younger persons and others whose biologic reactivity for one reason or another is heightened generally react to stress in a diffuse and anxious fashion, while middle-aged persons tend to develop more clearly differentiated symptoms and to become depressed.

Moreover, whatever their nature, the syndromes seen in youth usually arise, progress, and remit more quickly than those that occur in older persons (Kramer 1963).

The relationship between age and symptoms is particularly obvious in affective disorders and, in the section describing them, we have outlined the different ways in which depressions appear at different times in an individual's life (see p. 169). This outline is, however, with minor modifications, equally applicable to other syndromes.

DEFINITION OF PSYCHIATRIC ILLNESS

Having explored some of the difficulties inherent in the problem, let us continue our quest for a definition of mental illness. Although few physicians would define the term in quite the same manner, they would agree that those persons whom most people would consider mentally ill have one feature in common: their social functioning is impaired. When a person becomes ill, his social functioning suffers; the sicker he becomes, the more it deteriorates; and as he recovers, his social functioning returns. For these reasons, we consider an individual to have a psychiatric illness only when we see evidence of *social dysfunctioning* coupled with symptoms of *psychological and biologic discomfort,* and believe that the dysfunctioning and discomfort are *caused by disturbances in the mechanisms that regulate mood and cognition.*

We emphasize disturbed social functioning as a criterion of mental illness for three reasons. First, impairments in social functioning are observable and need not be inferred. Second, since it is easier to say what a person must do in order to function and survive in a social setting than to say what he needs to achieve mental health, it is easier to find a yardstick with which to measure an individual's social functioning than it is to find one with which to measure his mental health. Third, since the term *social dysfunctioning* implies only that an individual has failed to meet certain minimal standards and not that he has failed to achieve some maximal goal, it is not meant to be contrasted with the superlative or idealized state implied by the term *mental health.*

Admittedly, this view leaves unresolved many of the questions inherent in defining who is and who is not mentally ill. Some physicians believe that anyone who is uncomfortable or behaves in an unusual or rigid manner is entitled to a psychiatric diagnosis even if his social functioning is unimpaired. Such traits are relatively common, however, and we have chosen to exclude such individuals from our definition in the belief that including them all would so broaden the concept of psychiatric illness as to render it meaningless. In this sense, our definition encompasses the lowest common denominator of agreement: it includes all those persons whose symptoms are so pronounced that almost any observer would agree they are mentally ill, but excludes, for example, the socially competent person with a "character neurosis" whose "illness" some clinicians would dispute.

SOCIAL DYSFUNCTIONING

Determinants of Social Functioning

A person's social functioning is the result of the complex interplay between his biologic equipment, his early experience and training, and the events in his current situation.

The *biologic equipment* with which a person is born is the substrate on which all subsequent influences act. It has been shown that the patterns of one individual's physiologic responsivity differ from those of another, that these differences may be demonstrated from the first day of life (Freedman 1963, Grossman 1957, Richmond 1955), and that they correlate with behavioral characteristics observable in later life. Yet, while this equipment profoundly affects the way the individual will deal with the world (Scarr 1966, Walter 1960), both his equipment and his behavior in turn are modified by innumerable environmental factors, biologic and psychosocial as well. The first and in some ways the most important psychosocial factors are the responses he evokes from the sociofamilial environment in which he is reared (Escalona 1965, Schaffer 1964)—the setting in which he first observes how others behave and has an opportunity to learn what values they and the culture around them hold. The environment's responses are also determined by a number of factors over which he has no control, such as his sex, his conformance to standards of physical attractiveness, and the values, interests, and behavioral patterns that prevail in the social class, culture, subculture, and family in which he is reared.

Environmental factors mesh with the biologic to determine the nature, temporal sequence, and effect of an individual's *early experience and training* (Clarke 1968, Eassom 1966). That these experiences are important for a person's subsequent functioning is self-evident, but which of their features are critical is a subject of controversy (Hunt 1965, Wolff 1970). The *timing* of such experiences certainly affects their impact. Scott (1962) extends his finding that animals can be socialized more rapidly at a given period in early life to postulate the existence of *critical periods* during which particular skills are learned best. Within certain limits, the more an individual is emotionally aroused during the period in which a particular skill is usually acquired, the more likely he is to master it. Moreover, once the period has passed, the likelihood of his acquiring the skill and the ease with which he can do so will diminish. Indeed, some skills, if not acquired at the right time, may remain impaired, thereby creating a barrier to further steps in learning (Green 1964, Harlow 1965).

It is widely believed that conflicting desires or erroneous views that develop during childhood can lead an individual to experience certain later events as stressful and can affect the way he deals with them to such an extent that he develops a psychological disorder. Yet, while *conflicts and stresses* are operative in many persons who are mentally ill, they are also so common in persons who are not that we can hardly assume that any life difficulty that precedes a mental illness precipitates it. Simple day-to-day living involves an almost constant barrage of troubles: deaths and separations involving friends and relatives; financial, educational, residential, and occupational changes and reverses (Hall 1966, Maddison 1968, Munro 1965, 1969); physically stressful and traumatizing events; and events that require an individual to establish new interpersonal relationships (Imboden 1963). From a clinical standpoint, most persons react to such troubling experiences only briefly and sur- vive them well (Bourne 1967, Chodoff 1964). Those who do not are often assumed to have had certain underlying conflicts that prevented them from doing so; but even when we understand these conflicts and are able to pinpoint which of the individual's experi- ences are most likely to have triggered his upset, we cannot with any degree of precision explain why he became ill or why his ill- ness takes the particular form that it does, nor can we predict how, when, or whether his symptoms will develop, progress, or recede (Badgley 1964, Murphy 1962).

An individual's adaptational deficiencies determine *which* events are most likely to disturb him and color his symptoms if he falls ill. If he encounters a situation that requires him to react in a way he cannot, he is likely to become anxious or confused. The more urgent and prolonged the demand and the more poorly developed the bio- logic capacities or social skills that he would need in order to re- spond adequately, the more severe his discomfort is likely to be. More- over, once illness develops, those social skills that were most poorly developed and in which he was least competent before becoming ill are usually the ones that become impaired first. A boy who is the only Negro in a school may not learn how to socialize because he is ostracized. Another's development may be hampered because a protracted illness delays his entering school or because a seizure disorder disrupts the integrity of his experience during these years. Yet whatever the cause, an individual whose development is inter- rupted at the time he enters school may, even in later years, be- come anxious in situations that require him to show skill and comfort in peer relationships, and if he develops an illness, his incompetence in relationships of this kind is likely to be its first and most obvious feature.

Measures of Social Dysfunctioning

In general, an individual's social functioning may be measured by assessing his competence in pursuing his *occupation,* in relating to his *family,* and in transacting with his *peers* (Ruesch 1968, 1969). A person may be said to be functioning well, and almost certainly *not* to be mentally ill, if he is holding *a job* that is commensurate with his skills and interests and, within the limits of his situation, permits him to earn what he needs to live more or less like those around him; if he spends time with his *family*, enjoys their company, is enjoyed by them, permits them to be economically interdependent with him, makes decisions with them, permits and encourages them to transact with persons outside the family, handles family crises adequately and is willing and able, at least temporarily, to assume the role of another family member if that person is absent or becomes ill; and if he is able to interact with his *peers* in a way that both he and they enjoy, trust them without being gullible, and distinguish those who are closest to him from others more distant.

These three areas of social functioning overlap in so many ways that it is not always possible to consider each separately. A woman's care of her family is often her sole occupation, and most of a man's peer relationships may be connected with his job. Nevertheless, it is usually possible to estimate an individual's functioning in each of these areas, and a physician's estimates usually correlate well with those of the patient's family, friends, and employers.

The foregoing criteria should not be considered absolute. By no means do we intend to suggest that a person who does not perform in this manner is socially inadequate, and far less to suggest that he is mentally ill. An individual may be unemployed because of a disabling physical illness; because he is so poor that it is more profitable to accept social welfare benefits, or so wealthy that he can devote all his time to leisure activities; or because of an ideologic conviction or artistic talent that leads him to pursue an occupation without economic return. Thus, even though the failure to work is a form of social dysfunctioning, it cannot in itself be considered evidence of mental illness unless it is based on a disorder of mood or cognition.

The minimal standards of social functioning must be defined negatively. An individual may be said to conform to them when he does not burden those around him more than they can tolerate and when he avoids activities that endanger his continued social existence. Naturally, these minimal standards vary from one culture and subculture to the next; depend on an individual's intellectual equipment, training, and experience; and are different for children, the aged, and the physically ill. In using the measures of social functioning to determine whether an individual is mentally ill, however, it is not so important to determine whether he satisfies the minimal standards as it is to determine whether his social functioning has declined or otherwise changed. It is one thing when the son of a farmer sells produce from door to door, but it is far different when the intellectually promising son of a college professor drops out of graduate school to sell brushes or magazines. The proper utilization of these parameters often requires a *longitudinal evaluation* of the individual's life; his performance in each of the social areas must be compared not only with certain minimal standards applicable to others of his skills, culture, training, and experience, but also with his own previous highest level of functioning.

The Development of Social Dysfunctioning

Most people respond to stress by becoming anxious or depressed for a brief time and recover without any change in their personality or competence. Sometimes the return to homeostasis occurs spontaneously, sometimes the affected individual utilizes one of the traditional nonmedical coping mechanisms: crying it out, cursing, talking to a friend, or acquiring a new suit, hairdo, or romance. When the stress is severe or prolonged, when the individual's stress responses are inadequate, or when the relationship between the two is disproportionate, social dysfunctioning ensues (Arsenian 1968). At this time, the interrelationships between the organism, its biologic response, and its environment can cyclically perpetuate or worsen the disturbance, and the patient's difficulty is no longer a transient response to stress but an "illness" (Dohrenwend 1969, Phillips 1966, Steinberg 1968).

The longer such a self-perpetuating cycle continues, the more likely it is that the patient will incorporate the maladaptive symptoms into his life style. When a patient who is being bombarded by perceptual stimuli develops a delusional system, his unusual experiences start to make more sense to him, and his anxiety and perplexity diminish. Initially, his delusional interpretation may help him adapt to his difficulties, but, since his bizarre ideas will soon isolate him from others to such an extent that they result in his social bankruptcy, it makes little sense to consider delusions adaptive. Similarly, even though the husband of a woman who develops a phobia may initially pay more attention to her, his solicitude usually gives way to irritation after a few weeks or months; even when it does not, his attentions may so gratify her that she becomes a hermit.

The length of the interval between the emergence of the first symptoms and the beginning of treatment depends both on the speed with which the illness progresses and on the extent to which its symptoms are compatible with the patient's continuing social adjustment (Zusman 1966). A rapidly progressing illness is likely to receive treatment more promptly than one in which the changes, being more subtle, more gradual, and more difficult to identify, are easier for the family to adapt to or ignore. Most clinicians are familiar with those situations in which a completely senile grandparent is surrounded by relatives who have not only failed to notice his progressive dementia but stoutly deny it. Patients of whom little is demanded may remain sick without treatment much longer than those whose work, family, or social position demands a certain level of performance. Thus, while the speed with which an individual's illness progresses and his social functioning declines depends on the illness itself and on such factors as his age, maturation, and psychological organization, the compatibility of his symptoms with his current adjustment depends as much or more on such apparently extraneous factors as his occupation, social class, and family structure (Hollingshead 1958, Walsh 1969).

THE SOCIAL IMPACT OF ILLNESS

In general, a patient's family and associates respond to his illness according to their own personalities and experiences and in congruence with the sociocultural setting's expectations. Nonetheless, some illnesses seem to evoke fairly typical responses. These characteristic responses are worth mentioning not only because they can give some clues to the patient's diagnosis, but also because knowledge of what to expect helps us to moderate the discomfort caused by the interaction between the patient and his environment.

A *depressed* patient, for example, tends to make those around him feel so burdened and frustrated that they become angry and anxious to avoid being with him. These feelings will in turn make them feel guilty and, at least for a time, act more solicitous toward him until they finally view themselves as fraudulent and become even more frustrated. A *manic* patient, too, will initially cause his friends and relatives to feel guilty. Since they can at the outset see merit in some of his plans and suggestions, they may berate themselves for being too conservative. The patient's tactlessness and grandiosity soon irritate them, however: considering his behavior intentional, they become furious at his display of poor judgment and his obliviousness to social embarrassment. When a manic patient is hospitalized, both patients and staff are likely to welcome his enthusiasm and good humor and greet him with great friendliness—at least for the first few hours—but he soon begins to annoy everyone around him with his incessant plans and chatter. After that, his only supporters are the disorganized schizophrenics, who, perhaps because they have so much difficulty in making sense out of what is going on about them, seem especially attracted to the manic's apparent sense of direction and his ability to reduce the complexities of the environment to monochromatic judgments about other people's motives.

The disability of a patient with *conversion symptoms* seems so implausible that those around him tend to disbelieve and distrust most of what he says and does. Some people view his behavior as manipulative and want to control him, and, failing in this, become angry with him. A patient with an *antisocial personality* often impresses others as so charming and attractive that, letting hope triumph over experience, they trust him and repeatedly permit him to betray them.

The environment is rarely angry with the *schizophrenic* patient —at least when his illness begins. The usual response tends rather to be a certain degree of anxiety and fearfulness and a sense of eeriness. Such patients seem interesting to their families and physicians, perhaps because the things they say are so unexpected, candid, and complex. Yet, when the patient's recovery is long delayed and it becomes clear that his verbal productions will remain incomprehensible riddles, the fascination gives way to more pressing business, and the patient is shunted to an attic or hospital by his unnerved relatives or to a chronic ward by his physician. The young chronic schizophrenic patient's apparent lucidity may cause those around him to view his aimlessness and disorganization as insufficient motivation, and, especially if he at one time showed promise of achievement, to become monotonously exhortational in futile efforts to help him return to his previous path. Older ambulatory chronic schizophrenics or those whose intellectual or creative skills are limited are more likely simply to be ostracized by family and friends as odd and undesirable.

Many patients have in common a special intuitive sense, rather like an antenna, the effectiveness of which can be gauged only by the environment's response. Although a patient is best able to intuit and interact with another person's feelings when issues are involved with which he is himself concerned, this ability becomes most noticeable when it is tuned in to traits and conflicts that the other usually hides. The behavior of the confidence man, who satisfies his own avarice by discerning and promising to satisfy his victim's, illustrates the *psychopath*'s use of an antenna. The *manic*'s antenna attunes him to his vis-à-vis's pretentiousness, self-aggrandizement, and dissatisfaction with the way he organizes his affairs. Since most people feel uncomfortable about having such characteristics and prefer not to talk about them, they become irritated by the attention that the manic pays to them. The eerie discomfort that many people experience in the company of a *schizophrenic* may be traced to their feeling that his antenna is attuned to their most primitive impulses and that he pays as close attention to these as he does to their manifest actions or statements.

In some cases, the patient seems so relaxed and the *relatives* so excited that at first the clinician may think that they need treatment more than he does, or that they are the cause of his illness, only to find out their excitement arose from their concern about the patient's illness and social pathology and abated as soon as treatment was assured. Their initial reactions should not be ignored, however, for they are useful indices of their characteristic way of responding to stress.

THE SYMPTOMS OF ILLNESS

Although our definition of mental illness as a form of social dysfunctioning makes it possible to measure the severity of the patient's illness by measuring the extent to which it impairs his social functioning, it is not always easy to decide whether a patient's social functioning is impaired and, when it is, whether the impairment 1/ derives from a currently active disorder of mood and cognition, 2/ is traceable to unusual features of the patient's environment, or 3/ is a remnant of a past illness. The character and severity of the patient's social dysfunctioning depend on so many external factors that its delineation alone is of little help in assigning a specific diagnostic label or predicting the illness' progress. Fortunately, other criteria, such as the nature and severity of the patient's psychological and biologic symptoms, also differ from one illness to the next; so they, too, can be used to distinguish one illness from others and to determine its stage, severity, and progress.

PSYCHOLOGICAL SYMPTOMS AS INDEXES OF THE SEVERITY OF ILLNESS

No matter what the illness, we may assume that the patient is getting worse when preexisting limitations in his adaptational style become more severe or his *previous personality problems become more pronounced.* Regardless of whether he is becoming depressed, schizophrenic, obsessional, or organic, an individual whose personality has always been passive-dependent, compulsive, or anti-social tends to become even more so as he gets sicker. Again we may suspect that an illness is progressing when the patient's *symptoms become more numerous or more bizarre,* especially when they *increasingly govern his behavior.* A paranoid patient may believe that new pursuers have been assigned to his trail or that the devices with which he is being tortured are more complex or dangerous than they were; a patient whose phobia was initially limited to subway travel may start to fear other forms of transportation until he is finally too fearful to venture out of his house; a schizophrenic who has kept his delusions and hallucinations to himself for years may start to talk about them and accuse his associates of causing them. Careful observation of the way an individual's symptoms develop during one episode of illness may be helpful in assessing symptoms in a future episode. When a patient's last episode of manic decompensation was ushered in by mildly psychopathic behavior, such as inappropriate and unnecessary lies or petty thefts, the *return of the previously prodromal behavior* is a warning signal that a new round of illness is about to begin.

INDEXES OF BIOLOGIC DYSFUNCTIONING

These criteria—the impairments in the patient's social skills, the nature of his social impact, the changes in his psychological symptoms, and the measure that reflects them all: the individual's overall social functioning—help the clinician to gauge the severity and progress of the illness. They are of limited value, however, because innumerable *extraneous influences* can cause them to fluctuate and because so many *cultural, psychological,* and *constitutional factors* determine the way an individual translates his subjective experience into social behavior: each individual's behavior is inevitably unique. Furthermore, both *patient and family distort* their description of the events that preceded the referral for reasons that range from guilt to selfishness and include the deleterious effect the illness may have had on the patient's capacity to understand his situation accurately or describe it comprehensibly.

Another set of observable indexes that vary with the severity of the illness and can be used to assess it are those that measure *biologic functions.* These include observations of the patient's sleep-wakefulness cycles, temperature, blood pressure, respiration, appetite, and sexual activity. By calling these measures biologic, we do not imply that the behavioral symptoms that eventuate in social dysfunctioning are not. Of course, there is no way to determine whether behavioral symptoms are caused by one set of mechanisms and biologic symptoms by another, or whether a single mechanism gives rise to both. Nevertheless, even though clinical observations show numerous interrelationships between the occurrence of aberrant behavior and biologic symptoms, both tradition and the insolubility of the age-old, brain-mind problem lead us to distinguish between the behavioral indexes mentioned earlier and the biologic listed below.

Sleep Patterns

For numerous reasons, measurements of sleep patterns are among the most promising tools uncovered in the search for biologic correlates of mental illness. In the first place, changed sleep patterns are found in the majority of mental illnesses. In addition, the speed and manner in which these changes take place generally parallel the development of the illness. Furthermore, the nature of the sleep disturbance is often related to the nature of the illness. Finally, factors that deleteriously affect an individual's behavior during the time he is awake, such as stress, drugs, or excessive or insufficient sensory stimulation, also lead to sleep disturbances; and factors that interfere with an individual's sleep, such as experimental sleep deprivation or interdream awakening, also affect his waking behavior, mood, and thinking. It is of particular interest for both theory and therapy that most drugs that affect mood and cognition appear to affect sleep and dreaming as well, while most of those that affect an individual's sleep also affect his behavior while he is awake.

THE RELATIONSHIP BETWEEN SLEEP AND CONSCIOUSNESS

Recent findings regarding attention, perception, cognition, and dreaming may help to explain these clinical observations, for it appears increasingly likely that the functions performed during wakefulness are so closely intermeshed with those involved in sleep that the two states cannot easily be considered separately (Hilgard 1969). One parameter that both sleep and wakefulness have in common is alertness. In some ways, the two appear to be no more than partially separated and partially overlapping areas on a *continuum of alertness*. This continuum is measured largely by an individual's arousability, that is, his ability to respond to the stimuli of his environment. On the behavioral level, his responses consist of discriminating these stimuli, responding to them, or awakening. On the biologic level, his response to arousal includes changes in his EEG pattern, called desynchronization: an increase in the frequency of the waves and a decrease in their amplitude. Since arousability is the measure of the alertness continuum, a relatively precise measure of alertness can be obtained by determining the intensity and relevance that an afferent stimulus must have to arouse a person sufficiently to discriminate it or to produce the characteristic electrocortical arousal response (Lindsley 1960).

The alertness continuum, on which some aspects of both sleep and wakefulness lie, ranges from *coma* to *hyperexcitability*. Coma is measurable by so complete a loss of perceptual contact with the environment that not even the most intense or significant stimuli are perceived or lead to electrocortical arousal; hyperexcitability, by so complete an openness to perceptual stimuli that even the subtlest are perceived and the least significant considered meaningful.

Seen in these terms, *normal waking consciousness* may be defined as that part of the continuum in which the intensity or relevance required of a stimulus in order that it be perceived approximates that which the average individual is likely to encounter in his normal waking experience. This level of consciousness is thus consistent with an individual's behavioral efficiency or capacity to engage in adaptive social behavior. When a person is awake and moderately attentive, both external and internal stimuli are experienced in a selective fashion: the relevant are noted and the irrelevant are not; the objects considered worthy of thought are perceived, while the background in which they appear is ignored. In this manner, a meaningful, constant, and stable perceptual matrix is maintained (Oswald 1962). To some extent, the individual appears to choose the content and direction of his attention and thought. Yet his ability to attend to external stimuli and so to direct his thoughts as to engage in mental tasks independent of his immediate environment depends on his maintaining the readiness to perceive and perhaps to process the stimuli of his perceptual field.

This readiness of the cortex to perceive stimuli during wakefulness is often termed *cortical vigilance* by observers of psychological events. The neurophysiologist is more likely to term it a *general state of arousal* (Moruzzi 1949). The condition appears to depend on a continuous flow of nonspecific excitation from the brainstem reticular formation to the cortex via the *ascending reticular activating system* (ARAS). When, in this stage of waking, strong or novel afferent stimuli signals are presented, the individual's "readiness" to perceive and process information increases, and he demonstrates what may be termed an arousal response. Behaviorally, this is a state of heightened cortical vigilance in which increased attention is paid to environmental stimuli. Electrocortically, the EEG desynchronizes even further: the amplitude of the waves becomes even lower and their frequency even greater. This further heightening of cortical vigilance or arousal appears to depend also on another flow of nonspecific stimuli via the *diffuse thalamic projection system* (DTPS), which has its origins in the nonspecific nuclei of the thalamus and interlocks with the ARAS. Thus, the ARAS mechanisms maintain the general excitability of the cortex over a long period, while the activity of the DTPS increases it during briefer periods of specific requirements. Together they provide a gross and fine adjustment, as it were, of cortical vigilance or the state of alertness (Lindsley 1960).

Although our knowledge of the complex interrelationships of these mechanisms with others that help determine consciousness and behavior is still fragmentary, it appears that the alertness continuum, delimited by coma and hyperexcitability, includes not only the various stages of sleep and wakefulness but, with some modifications, those of dreaming sleep as well. Even the *neural mechanisms* that regulate these seemingly disparate activities appear to be interrelated (Jouvet 1963, Othmer 1969, Rossi 1963) and to affect and be affected by a large number of other feedback mechanisms. The significance of *autonomic and neurohumoral activity* on these mechanisms, for example is suggested by the sensitivity of the pontine reticular formation to adrenergic and cholinergic agents (Courville 1962). More detailed information regarding the mechanisms that determine the maintenance of normal consciousness may be found in a number of reviews (Gellhorn 1963, 1968, Hernandez-Péon 1964, Jouvet 1969, Kales 1969, Kleitman 1963, Lindsley 1960, Oswald 1962, Snyder 1963).

While the investigations on which the foregoing account is based lend a new perspective to the study of mental activity and mental illness, observations derived from them are by no means sufficient to explain how, in health or illness, that unique internal experience of the human being known as *consciousness* correlates with the observable activity known as *behavior*. Obviously, such investigations do not explain how or why a person becomes mentally ill any better than those that focus on the psychological mechanisms alone. Moreover, they neither exclude nor contradict psychodynamic formulations of mental mechanisms; some even show that events, memories, or attitudes that make people anxious are likely to affect their cognitive functioning, and that this can occur whether they are mentally ill or not (Agnew 1963, Callaway 1953). Animal experiments have even demonstrated that sustained sensory overstimulation or deprivation can affect the normal maturation of the arousal mechanisms to such an extent that predictable, permanent, and measurable malfunctioning in this system ensues and, with it, major behavioral disturbances are seen (Heron 1964, Lindsley 1964).

The intricacy of the relationship between the biologic and the environmental determinants of behavior may shed some light on the fact that it is impossible to determine an illness' etiology solely by observing its symptoms. The view that symptoms are largely an end-product of a complex mind-brain interaction helps to explain why a single etiologic factor can present itself in so many symptomatic variations and why so many different factors underlie clinically indistinguishable syndromes.

SLEEP-WAKEFULNESS CYCLES AND MENTAL ACTIVITY

To think of mental activity in both the sleeping and the waking state in a unified fashion is made more plausible by *developmental studies* that suggest that an individual's brain, EEG pattern, mental functioning, and sleep-wakefulness regulation mature in an orderly and interrelated manner. In the newborn, long periods of sleep alternate with brief periods of wakefulness at regular, frequent intervals. As children become older, they progressively sleep less, and the intervals between one period of sleep and the next become longer (Parmalee 1961, Roffwarg 1964). By the time they are two years old, their sleep consists of an afternoon nap and an extended period of nocturnal sleep. While afternoon naps are habitual even with adults in some cultures, children in the United States and Northern Europe usually abandon them around the age of three or four. Thereafter, their nocturnal sleep continues to diminish, and by the time they are around 15, their sleep patterns are those of the adult (Ames 1964) (see Table 20).

The gradual maturation of sleep and wakefulness patterns correlates with that of mental functioning and is mirrored to some extent by changes in the EEG (Bartoshuk 1964). The characteristic alpha rhythm does not appear in a persistent manner before the age of three to four months. The first patterns show a rather low frequency of 3 to 4 cycles per second (cps), which gradually increases over a 10 to 15 year period until, during puberty, it reaches the adult frequency range of 9 to 12 cps (Lindsley 1960). Thus, adult sleep and EEG patterns are achieved at about the same time that an individual achieves adult intellectual functioning.

The close relationship between the mechanisms that regulate consciousness and waking behavior and those that regulate sleep may account for the clinical observation that disturbances in waking functions are almost invariably coupled with sleep disorders. Indeed, it is reasonable to assume that observations of a patient's sleep disturbance not only measure the mechanisms that underlie sleep, but simultaneously measure some part of those that underlie normal consciousness, thinking, mood, and behavior.

It may appear paradoxical to draw conclusions about an individual's waking behavior by observing his sleep, but this approach has the added advantage that sleep patterns, being less complex and less subject to sociocultural distortion, are both easier to elicit and simpler to quantify. Since sleep is generally considered desirable, most people regard questions about it as psychologically neutral and answer them as accurately as they can. Even patients who are reluctant to talk about other things are usually willing to describe their sleep, and this is even more true when their sleep is disturbed. Furthermore, since sleep patterns are more dependent on physiologic needs than on individual and cultural variations, and since they can be measured in units of time, it has been possible to establish quantitative and qualitative norms for individuals of given age groups with which a patient's sleep patterns can be compared (Ames 1964, Feinberg 1968, Kahn 1969, McGhie 1962, Tune 1969, Webb 1963, Weiss 1962).

During the course of each day, the normal adult travels along the continuum of consciousness at a relatively fixed rate. Typically, whatever the season, climate, or level of his physical activity (Lewis 1961), he spends about a third of his time asleep. He falls asleep within a half hour of going to bed and, during the time that he is asleep, passes with regularity through certain stages of sleep that can be distinguished by assessing his arousability and observing his EEG (Dement 1957, Kales 1969, Loomis 1937, Williams 1964). About a quarter of his sleeping time is occupied by episodes of REM, or dreaming sleep, that start about an hour after he falls asleep, last about 20 minutes, and recur every 90 minutes or so. These episodes are characterized by rapid eye movements (REM) and a typical EEG pattern and are considered the time of dreaming because subjects awakened during such periods are more likely to report that they have been dreaming than those awakened during REM-free intervals (Aserinsky 1953, 1955a,b). After a person has slept 5½ to 8 hours (McGhie 1962), he awakens and during the next 15 to 30 minutes becomes more alert and attentive to his environment. He maintains his alertness with fluctuations (Haider 1964, Patrushev 1964) for another 15 to 18 hours, then becomes drowsy, falls asleep again, and continues his path through the spectrum of consciousness.

Sleep norms are so widely accepted that most people are able to classify themselves as "good" or "poor" sleepers, and their own judgments can usually be confirmed by observation. Even in the absence of mental illness, poor sleepers differ from those who sleep well. As a group, their level of arousal during sleep and in the presleep period is higher, their Minnesota Multiphasic Personality Inventory (MMPI) scores are higher in the psychopathologic direction, and their scores on the Cornell Medical Index suggest more psychosomatic and emotional disturbances (Monroe 1967).

THE RELATIONSHIP BETWEEN SLEEP DISORDER AND MENTAL ILLNESS

Although no comprehensive understanding of the relationships between sleep and mental illness has yet been achieved, much can be learned about an individual's illness by exploring his sleep patterns (Luce 1966). At present, only some of the more significant parameters are known, and not all are practical enough to use for clinical purposes. Some studies, for example, suggest that the amount or proportion of time that an individual spends in each stage of sleep can be correlated with his clinical diagnosis, but the instrumentation required to determine the stages of sleep is so complex that such studies are at present limited to research settings (Diaz-Guerrero 1946, Feinberg 1965, Hartmann 1965, Kales 1969, Lairy 1965, Oswald 1963, Rechtschaffen 1963, Snyder 1968, Zung 1964).

Therefore, in discussing the relationship between sleep disorder and mental illness, we shall consider only those measures of sleep that the clinician—by his own observation and by the patient's reports—can determine with relative ease: the duration of sleep, its quality, the time at which it occurs or, more significantly, does not occur, and the nature and frequency of reported dreams. These factors change measurably as an individual becomes ill and gradually return to their previous state as he becomes well. Since the manner and speed of change correlate with the nature and severity of the patient's illness, precise information concerning the patient's sleep patterns helps the clinician to

1/ assess the severity of an individual's illness at the time he is first seen,
2/ map its progress, and
3/ anticipate its course;
4/ distinguish certain illnesses from others,
5/ determine the optimal treatment program, and
6/ gauge the program's effectiveness.

While a full discussion of sleep disorders would cover both sleep loss and hypersomnia and detail the wide variety of physical and mental disorders in which such disturbances may take place, the discussion that follows is limited largely to the sleep loss seen in neuroses, schizophrenias, and depression. The extreme increase in sleep found in the depressed phase of manic-depressive disease, in narcolepsy, and in a number of other medical illnesses, will be discussed further in Chapters 4, 11, and 12.

CAUSES AND CONSEQUENCES OF SLEEP LOSS

It is often hard to know exactly why an individual's sleep is disturbed, since most factors that cause sleep loss—drugs, illness, danger, or upsetting events—also affect his psychological state. Even if the event that causes the sleep loss does not disturb the individual's psychological state directly—as in experimental sleep deprivation —it will do so indirectly, for, regardless of its cause, sleep loss has deleterious psychological consequences of its own. Indeed, the *consequences of sleep loss* are at times so severe that they can be mistaken for its cause. Although many of these consequences have long been known (Patrick 1896), current studies on the effects of experimental sleep deprivation are helping to define them in even greater detail. The effects include fatigue, dysattention, waxing and waning of consciousness, disorientation, impairment of perceptual-motor performance, and hallucinatory and delusional episodes (Cohen 1961, Kollar 1969, Luby 1960, Pasnau 1968, Tyler 1955, Williams 1959). Sleep deprivation can also be followed by centrencephalic seizures and abnormal EEG patterns even in subjects who have never had them before (Bennett 1963, Rodin 1962).

Whether the symptoms of an illness are hyperalertness and anxiety, as in schizophrenia (see p. 109), or sadness and guilt, as in depressions (see p. 162), the associated sleep disturbance can in turn lead to a marked decline in the patient's state of arousal (Ax 1961) and to secondary symptoms similar to those seen in the sleep deprivation experiments (Berger 1962). The greater the nightly sleep loss and the longer the sleep disturbance lasts, the more drowsy and disoriented the patient becomes. Indeed, almost any patient who loses at least three hours of sleep a night for three to six months, or does not sleep at all for a period of three days or more, experiences slowed thinking, motor retardation, dysmnesia, and some degree of confusion in addition to whatever other symptoms he may have. Symptoms and signs secondary to sleep loss appear so "organic" that the differential diagnosis between "functional" and "organic" syndromes is sometimes difficult (see p. 114); this factor can even make one functional illness associated with severe sleep loss hard to distinguish from another.

The extent to which sleep loss can cause such symptoms depends on a number of other factors. The more isolated a patient was before his illness began, the more isolated he becomes as the illness progresses, the less structured or more stressful his environment, the poorer his physical health or nutritional state, and the more advanced his age, the more likely it is that he will become confused and disoriented after losing some sleep, and the less sleep he must lose for this to occur. Furthermore, when, in an effort to relieve his sleep disturbance, an individual takes barbiturates, minor tranquilizers, or alcohol—agents that by themselves can lead to disorientation, dysmnesia, and drowsiness—it may be difficult to determine whether his confusion is caused by the drugs or the sleep loss (see p. 292).

For purposes of schematization, sleep disturbances characterized by sleep loss may be divided into *difficulty falling asleep* (DFA) and *early morning awakening* (EMA) (see Table 1). This dichotomization is, of course, an intentional oversimplification, and it might be more accurate to distinguish those sleep difficulties that occur in the first hours after falling asleep from those that occur thereafter. Thus, sleep continuity disturbances (SCD) in the early part of the night may be related to DFA, and those that occur toward morning to EMA.

Sleep disorder may begin gradually. Its first signs may be no more than an occasional brief episode of nocturnal awakening, the sense of having slept poorly or too little, awakening without feeling rested, or the increased occurrence of unpleasant dreams. A person whose sleep disturbance is mild may compensate for his sleep loss by taking a nap on the following day. If he has EMA, he may go to bed earlier the following evening; if he has DFA, he may sleep longer

TABLE 1. *Classification of Sleep Disorders*

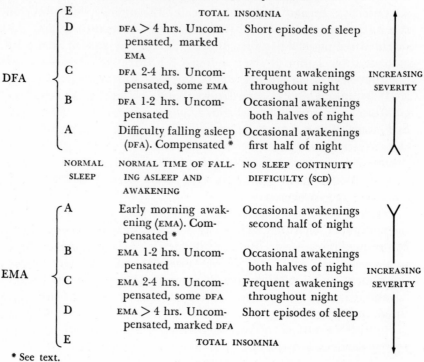

	E		TOTAL INSOMNIA	
	D	DFA > 4 hrs. Uncompensated, marked EMA	Short episodes of sleep	
DFA	C	DFA 2-4 hrs. Uncompensated, some EMA	Frequent awakenings throughout night	INCREASING SEVERITY
	B	DFA 1-2 hrs. Uncompensated	Occasional awakenings both halves of night	
	A	Difficulty falling asleep (DFA). Compensated *	Occasional awakenings first half of night	
	NORMAL SLEEP	NORMAL TIME OF FALLING ASLEEP AND AWAKENING	NO SLEEP CONTINUITY DIFFICULTY (SCD)	
	A	Early morning awakening (EMA). Compensated *	Occasional awakenings second half of night	
	B	EMA 1-2 hrs. Uncompensated	Occasional awakenings both halves of night	
EMA	C	EMA 2-4 hrs. Uncompensated, some DFA	Frequent awakenings throughout night	INCREASING SEVERITY
	D	EMA > 4 hrs. Uncompensated, marked DFA	Short episodes of sleep	
	E		TOTAL INSOMNIA	

* See text.

in the morning. Yet, regardless of how the psychiatric patient's sleep disturbance begins, it may, as his illness progresses, advance along steps of increasing severity and admixture to the common endpoint of total insomnia.

CHANGES IN DREAM PATTERNS ASSOCIATED WITH PSYCHIATRIC ILLNESSES

As an illness progresses, the patient reports changes in the form, content, and quantity of his dreams. While these changes offer some clues to the course of the illness, they are by no means as useful a measure as the duration of the patient's sleep or the time of night in which his difficulty in sleeping occurs. One reason for the unreliability of dream observations is that it is hard to know whether the individual has really experienced a change in the amount that he *dreams* or only the amount he *recalls*. Even among people who are not mentally ill, some naturally recall fewer dreams than others. Interestingly, the distinction between dream-recallers and dream-nonrecallers is even reflected in the fact that the EEG patterns of the two groups show slight differences. That nonrecallers seem to spend as much time engaged in REM activity as do the dream-recallers and that they are less prone to recall dreams even when awakened during REM activity raises some questions about the assumption that REM time may be uniformly equated with dream time (Goodenough 1959). Indeed, some recent studies have shown that people tend to recall dreams that occur during REM periods only if they awaken during their course or are awakened immediately thereafter, and that most of the dreams that an individual remembers after awaking from a full night's sleep are ones that took place during non-REM periods (Goodenough 1965). Despite these problems in distinguishing between dreaming and dream recalling, changes in the frequency of dreaming (as measured by the patient's report) often parallel changes in REM activity. For example, individuals who take CNS depressants not only report that they dream less, but may also be shown to have diminished REM time (Freeman 1965, Gresham 1963, Oswald 1968).

Whatever the reason, increased dreaming or increased dream recall, both individuals who are anxious and those who are becoming mentally ill report that they *dream more* than they did before. Reports of increased dream activity are particularly common in the acute phase of an anxiety neurosis and the prodromal phase of a schizophrenic or depressive syndrome. Initially, only the *frequency* and *length* of the reported dreams increase, while their *content* remains fairly neutral. As the illness progresses and the patient reports that he is dreaming even more, the dream content changes as well. His dreams first become more vivid, then include more and more figures and events of his past, until finally these themes come to dominate the entire dream. In some cases, these memories will have lain dormant for so many years that the patient expresses surprise at being able to recall them at all. While the first of these more vivid or more frequent dreams have a fairly nonsymbolic, undistorted, and matter-of-fact quality, they are later described as nightmares (Bastos 1964). The events in the dream appear dangerous or seem to have a special or symbolic meaning. The further progress of the patient's dreaming may be of diagnostic significance. Just before the full-blown psychosis develops, the patient whose anxiety state is a forerunner of psychotic depression usually reports a complete cessation of dreaming, while the one whose anxiety state precedes a schizophrenic illness reports a dramatic increase in dreaming.

Dream changes of this nature usually go hand in hand with

sleep disturbances, but can also occur in patients who seem to sleep fairly well, in which case they may be the first or only symptom of illness. Such changes are of particular importance in evaluating the depressed adolescent or the patient who takes excessive amounts of sedatives, for his sleep pattern is often equivocal, and his desire to manage his difficulties independently may lead him to tell the physician little or even to misinform him, but will not usually prevent him from describing his dream pattern. Indeed, a patient's report that his dreaming has ceased entirely is sometimes the first or only clue that he is taking unauthorized hypnotics, that his mood disorder is deepening, or that he is increasingly preoccupied with thoughts about suicide.

A SCHEMATIZATION OF SLEEP DISORDERS ASSOCIATED
WITH PSYCHIATRIC ILLNESS

Table 2 outlines in a highly schematic fashion some relationships that have been observed between sleep and mental disorders. To some extent, it is based on a distinction we make between two general patterns of illness, which, for want of better names, we call Types A and B. In *Type A* disorders, exemplified by acute schizophrenic illnesses, manic episodes, and atypical depressions, both the behavioral symptoms and the concomitant sleep disturbances tend to arise, progress, and remit relatively quickly; the most striking clinical features are anxiety and excitement; the patients, at least at the time of their first episode, are usually under the age of 30; and the earliest and most obvious type of sleep disturbance is DFA. In *Type B* illnesses, exemplified by the typical depressive episode, both illness and sleep disturbance develop and recede more slowly; the most striking clinical features are sadness and psychomotor retardation; the patients are usually over the age of 40; and the earliest and most obvious type of sleep disturbance is EMA (Hinton 1963, Johns 1970, Kupfer 1969). This dichotomization spells out only a trend, of course; patients over 40 can become manic, those under 30 can show typical depressions, depressions can arise quickly or schizophrenias slowly. The distinction indicates only that those features found in each group tend to cluster together, not that they must.

Deciding whether a given patient's illness belongs to Type A or B, however, is of particular value when the illness is severe enough to require somatic treatment. Type A illnesses—in which the sleep disturbance progresses rapidly and is of the DFA variety—often show symptomatic improvement when treated with sedatives or tranquilizers; those of Type B, in which the sleep disturbance arises slowly and is of the EMA variety, tend to respond to antidepressants. Conversely, when antidepressants are given to patients with Type A illness, DFA, agitation, and anxiety may become worse, while the use of sedatives or certain tranquilizers (such as chlorpromazine [Thorazine]) in Type B illnesses tends after some time to intensify the depressive pattern (see p. 539).

Table 2 shows how a history of the patient's sleep disturbance makes it possible to distinguish between certain similar looking syndromes. For example, the difficulty in distinguishing between a manic episode and an acute catatonic excitement can often be overcome by determining the speed with which the insomnia has progressed, for the manic's insomnia tends to progress more slowly than the catatonic's (Kupfer 1970). Similarly, when a patient who has been anxious or mildly depressed starts to experience EMA and gradually loses more and more sleep, the clinician—even if the anxiety or depression followed an understandably upsetting event, like a death in the family—should be alert to the possibility that the patient is developing a mood disorder that, without biologic treatment, will last for some time.

Table 2 also depicts the way in which the progression of a patient's illness is reflected in the progression of his sleep disturbance. It shows that an individual's sleep loss increases as his illness becomes more severe, and lists some general observations made earlier relating the frequency and content of dreams reported by the patient to the severity of his illness. In particular, it helps the clinician identify that phase of illness we have labeled *Stage D,* in which the patient's impulse control is diminished to the point that he may become suicidal or violent. This table also illustrates what we describe on pages 54 and 94 as the *rollback phenomenon:* as the illness remits, it progressively recapitulates, albeit in reverse order, many of the stages and symptoms that were seen during the time it developed. Thus, both the progression and remission of a mental illness are reflected in changes of sleep and dream patterns. Since there is some regularity to the sequence in which these patterns change, longitudinal observation of the patient's sleep permits us to make an informed guess about the illness' future, determine whether the patient is getting better or worse, and in this manner draw some conclusions about the effects of the treatment being offered.

Such observations are often a more reliable measure of a patient's clinical course than his own estimate of progress (Zung

TABLE 2. *Schematization of Sleep Disorders Associated with Psychiatric Illness*

ILLNESS, & APPROX TIME STAGES A TO E	ASSOCIATED SYMPTOMS	STAGE OF SLEEP DISORDERS†	
		STAGE A	STAGE B
	Dreams *	Increased "meaning-ful" dreaming	Nightmares
Organic delirium, excited type 3-5 da	Mood	Elation, moroseness, irritability, bewilderment	Increasing lability, irritability
	Activity	Restlessness, talkativeness	Overactivity that appears purposive
Acute catatonic schizophrenia 1-3 wk	Dreams	Increased dreaming	"Meaningful" dreams
	Mood	Expansiveness, elation	Mild depression
	Activity	Hyperactivity	Mild hyperactivity
Acute undifferentiated schizophrenia 3-6 wk	Dreams	Increased dreaming	"Meaningful" dreams
	Mood	Increasing lability———————————————	
	Activity	Variable, gradual increase with fluctuations	
Manic-depressive disease, manic phase 6-12 wk	Dreams	Insufficient data———————————————	
	Mood	Good	Elevated
	Activity	Moderate increase	Great increase
Neurotic disorders		While neurotic symptoms also progress in a charac insomnia.———————————————————————————	
Manic-depressive disease, depressed phase 6-12 wk		Hypersomnia is more common than insomnia. The may or may not show diurnality. The patient's logic, particularly when, even for brief periods, a	
Depressive & paranoid disorders in older persons 3-6 mo	Dreams	Increased	Early-life dreams
	Mood	Depression shows diurnality: better in evening———	
	Activity	Fluctuating	Fluctuating with decrease
Depressive disorders in younger patients 1-3 mo		Similar to above but with less retardation and diurnality, and more impulsivity	

* As reported by patient.   † See Table 1.

TABLE 2. *(Continued)*

STAGE OF SLEEP DISORDERS †

STAGE C	*Danger Stage* STAGE D	*Total Insomnia* STAGE E	TYPE OF SLEEP DISTURBANCE
Hypnagogic hallucinations	Olfactory and auditory hallucinations	Vivid visual hallucinations (in scenes or extended sequences of hypnoidal imagery)	
and suspiciousness ———————————————————————→			DFA and EMA
Purposeless activity	Constant, usually purposeless, activity	Purposeless thrashing, rubbing, trembling, muttering or screaming, sudden outbursts of violence	
Nightmares	Hypnagogic hallucinations	Hallucinations	
Moderate depression	Severe depression	World destruction fantasies	DFA
Moderate hyperactivity	Severe hyperactivity with bizarre acts	Immobility or diffuse excitement	
Nightmares	Hypnagogic hallucinations	Hallucinations	
————————————————————————————————————→			DFA
————————————————————————————————————→			
————————————————————————————————————→			
Euphoria	Increased euphoria	Euphoric tone with depressed content	
Socially inappropriate hyperactivity which though purposeful does not pursue a single goal for long	Constant activity, some of which is purposeful, though directed to shifting goals	Constant, usually purposeless, activity	DFA and EMA
eristic manner (see p. 237), only those preceding psychosis lead to total ————————————————→			Either DFA or EMA at onset; illnesses that are prodromal to depression show EMA after 6-8 weeks, regardless of how they begin
attern of dream changes is similar to that seen in other depressions. Mood ehavior becomes increasingly negatistic. His hypoactivity looks charactero- ood social facade can be maintained. ———————————————————→			Hypersomnia, sometimes with day/night reversal EMA or DFA
Nightmares	Decreased dreaming ——→ Organized paranoid delusions common when course is protracted	Dream cessation	EMA
May be decreased or increased	Agitation	Retardation	
			DFA and EMA

1965). For example, a patient whose depression is responsive to drugs will almost surely sleep better within a few days of their administration. Despite this improvement in sleep, he is likely to persevere in his recital of despair and discomfort for some days thereafter, and thereby confuse the physician. Yet, since we know that the return of sleep usually signals the imminent return of daytime comfort and that many illnesses that proceed to remission do so on the same amount of drugs as that which restores sleep, it is unnecessary to increase the medications of a patient whose sleep is improving unless his symptoms continue for some time thereafter. Conversely, even if a patient who has recovered from a mental illness reports himself to be "feeling well," one should suspect him of relapsing if his sleep deteriorates again (Kupfer 1967)—especially if his sleep disturbance or even his dream content is similar to the one that preceded the earlier episode. When the sleep disorder recurs soon after the patient's drug dosage has been reduced, it indicates that the current pharmacologic treatment is inadequate and that the previous dosage was terminated prematurely. The *sleep pattern of a relapse* usually starts with good nights alternating with bad, progresses until the bad outnumber the good, and finally reaches the point at which the patient has no good nights at all. The patient's reports about his dreams are similarly instructive. When, for example, a depressed patient has reported nightmares for some time and then suddenly stops dreaming entirely, we must suspect that his illness has reached the ominous Stage D previously described. Similarly, even though nightmares are sometimes prodromal to more severe decompensation, Table 2 illustrates that their reappearance following the dream cessation typical of Stage D may be a manifestation of the rollback phenomenon and thus a welcome sign of amelioration.

The patient's sleep pattern is also a better *predictor of his ability to cope* with new or stressful situations, such as meeting social obligations or taking on a new job, than his judgment or the doctor's intuition. If he has been sleeping well, he will probably handle such situations fairly well; if his sleep has been poor or becomes poor immediately beforehand, he is less likely to cope with them satisfactorily and likely to become even more troubled by his failure to do so.

SOME EXCEPTIONS TO THE SCHEMATIZATION

This schematization describes some very general trends that we have observed in our efforts to correlate disordered sleep and behavior. In outlining the continuum along which many illnesses progress, we do not intend to suggest that each mental illness is marked by only one type of sleep disturbance and that this remains constant throughout its course. Even if an individual's sleep disturbance was easy to classify as EMA or DFA at the time that his illness began, he is likely to add the other as his illness becomes more severe. Moreover, in some illnesses both kinds of sleep disturbances may be seen from the outset; or the pattern may convert from one type to the other. Schizophrenic episodes with depressive features are typical examples of illnesses in which DFA and EMA coexist from the outset. Especially in the later stages of illness, when both patterns are likely to be present, it may be necessary to obtain a detailed account of the way the sleep disturbance developed.

The progression of sleep disturbance outlined in Table 2 is more relevant to illnesses that are still active than to those that have become chronic. No matter how severely a patient's illness disables him, his sleep usually improves somewhat with the passage of time, in part perhaps because fewer demands are made of the chronically ill. Chronic schizophrenic patients kept in the back wards of a state hospital, for example, tend to sleep relatively well until they are subjected to stress, at which time their original sleep difficulties return. This *reactivation of sleep disorder* is particularly apparent if a patient is subjected to an all-out rehabilitation program in which constant and intensive social, familial, and medical pressure is exerted on him to learn how to function independently and to leave the hospital. On the other hand, the improvement in sleep that follows a *diminution of demands* is not restricted to the chronically ill. Even patients who are in the throes of an acute mental illness sleep better once they are relieved of external pressures. An important practical conclusion may be drawn from this observation: that the clinician should not in a burst of undue optimism discharge from the hospital every patient whose sleep and behavior improve dramatically immediately after entering, for the improvement in such cases may be due only to the relief that the patient experiences from being hospitalized, and tends to be short lived.

The assessment of the patient's sleep pattern, and thus of his illness, is especially difficult when he *is taking barbiturates, alcohol, or other agents that help induce sleep.* When such agents are used, the typical sleep disturbances may be absent, and the patient may report only that he awakens for brief intervals throughout the night or has fewer dreams. In the absence of the typical sleep disorder, we must rely even more on the patient's history and description of how his other symptoms developed. It is indeed so difficult to assess the patient's illness until he has stopped taking such drugs that if he cannot be trusted to do this by himself, it may be necessary to hospitalize him.

Other Biologic Indexes

Biologic indexes other than sleep-wakefulness regulation also change in the course of most mental illnesses, but few are as useful (Dykman 1968). Quantifiable measures of autonomic nervous system functioning, like *blood pressure,* have not yet been validated; others, like *pupillary reactivity* (Hakarem 1964, Lowenstein 1964, Rubin 1964, 1968), require instruments too complex to permit routine measurement. Such relatively valid measures as the experienced sense of *energy level* and the feeling of *well-being,* on the other hand, cannot be quantified; and many theoretically quantifiable measures—*eating, sexual behavior,* and what the patient reports about them—arise from so complex a mixture of biologic and cultural determinants that, even though some segments of the underlying drives may be measurable, their expression is almost impossible to standardize or validate, especially because the patient often explains the way he feels and acts as if it were a logical consequence of his experiences and interpersonal relationships. Such explanations need not be accepted at face value, however. For example, a patient may report that he is impotent because he and his wife are at odds when in reality they got along famously until his sexual interest diminished; had been fighting for years before he became impotent; or continue to scrap even after his potency returns.

One of the few yardsticks of *autonomic function* that is of operational value is the patient's *blood pressure,* which tends to mirror his level of excitement. This measure is of particular value in catatonic states, for the extent and rapidity of the rise in systolic pressure yield important clues to the patient's condition. When the rise is steep, one may assume that he is in severe inner turmoil and has a potential for violence that might be overlooked if one were gauging him by his tensely inhibited exterior alone.

Even though it is not a quantifiable measure, the validity of *anhedonia,* the lack of a state of pleasant feeling, as an important index cannot be denied. So closely associated with *anergia* that the patient may perceive the two as a single phenomenon, it is the first symptom to appear (and the last to remit) in many emotional disorders. Differential diagnostic questions arise, however, because tiredness, easy fatigability, or simply "not feeling well" occur in innumerable medical illnesses. Thus the patient may be exposed to repeated medical workups before being referred to a psychiatrist, either as a last resort or because more specific psychiatric symptoms have developed in the interim.

Appetite is recognized as a measure of well-being and its absence as a sign of illness, but it is subjective and thus not directly measurable. However, by determining the amount of food an individual consumes and the way his weight changes, one can obtain important clues to his psychological state. Caloric and weight norms exist, but their upper and lower limits vary so widely that only gross deviations distinguish the well person from the ill. The qualitative assessment of eating patterns is especially difficult because the meaning of food and food habits depends so greatly on the patient's culture (Kaufman 1959). Nearly every civilization or subculture has its own view of the significance of food and eating: Mediterranean cultures tend to overemphasize and Anglo-Saxon cultures to deemphasize them. Nevertheless, changed eating patterns often correlate with changes in health.

Patients who eat too much or too little may see a physician only when *1/* their eating habits do not satisfy their nutritional requirements, *2/* these habits or their weight have undergone a relatively recent and rapid change, *3/* other causes have been ruled out, *4/* they ask to see a psychiatrist, or *5/* they have psychological symptoms that suggest that the disturbed eating habits may have an emotional source. While many of the obese patients seen by psychiatrists have minor or major psychological difficulties throughout their lives, overeating is rarely an early symptom of severe mental illness. Conversely, patients who have always weighed little seem to have no greater incidence of psychological difficulties than others, but anorexia of recent onset is a fairly common symptom of acute mental illness and most particularly of depressions. It often appears with the onset of sleep disturbance or shortly thereafter, and subsides as the patient recovers. When patients with acute schizophrenic episodes are treated with drugs, their sleep and appetite return concomitantly, while the improvement in appetite of depressed patients usually lags a few steps behind that in sleep. In both cases, improvements in the patient's energy level and sense of well-being tend to lag even further behind, and to remain abnormal until after his sleep and appetite are fully restored.

Many patients gain weight after an acute schizophrenic illness. In some instances, the gain may be due to the effect of the *drugs* they are taking, for both phenothiazines and reserpine tend to produce an extremely hearty appetite, especially for sweets. Such increases in weight, however, were also observed in the era before these drugs were introduced, though at that time they were more likely to signify that the illness was *becoming chronic*. Even today, one must become concerned that the patient is unlikely ever to recover fully if he overeats, gains weight, and is in addition increasingly apathetic, especially if his overeating continues after the drugs are reduced or withdrawn.

Sexual Behavior and Illness

An investigation of the patient's sexual drive and interest and the way he expresses them offers additional diagnostic pointers. Even though the cultural mores tend to hinder their accurate determination, sexual drives are so universal that changes in the *frequency, duration,* and *functional success* of the various components of sexual behavior are often a direct expression of a person's state of health. However, because sexual behavior is a uniquely intricate composite of biologic and cultural factors and because cultural taboos interfere with its investigation, there are no statistically controlled studies of the way an individual's sexual behavior changes while he is becoming mentally ill. For this reason, it is possible to give only the most general of impressions concerning the relationship between illness and sexual behavior.

Illnesses in the anxiety or DFA continuum tend to be accompanied by progressively increasing sexual desire or activity, but from Stage D (Table 2) on, the patient retains only his desire and is unable to pursue traditional mating patterns. Since social competence is a *conditio sine qua non* for traditional sexual behavior, it is not surprising that the social impairments of the schizophrenic and the manic become manifest in their sexual behavior. Although sexual drive and fantasies often increase in the *acute phase of schizophrenia,* such patients usually find any kind of intimacy disturbing. This and their tendency to interpret sexual feelings in a delusional way affect their sexual behavior. Many schizophrenic patients masturbate a good deal in order to dampen their anxiety; sexual contact with another person is, however, likely to lead to panic. The undifferentiated character of the heightened sexual drive often releases bisexual appetites, a process that, in traditionally reared patients, can lead to a state of self-derogation, projection, and fearfulness, which is often termed "homosexual panic" as if it were a discrete syndrome. Patients with *chronic schizophrenia,* who tend to disregard traditional social modes and to whom heterosexual outlets are usually closed, often engage in socially indiscreet or flagrantly obvious homosexual behavior and, even more frequently, masturbate in public, especially when they are in anxiety-provoking situations.

The *manic* patient usually has an increased sexual appetite that is connected with his general hyperactivity, elation, talkativeness, candor, and social inappropriateness. His contacts are many and fleeting, and he "loves" them all. His sexual behavior appears promiscuous—even when it is not—because he readily tells anyone who will listen all the details of his sexual encounters and then adds a few more for their shock value. During *withdrawal from* CNS *depressants,* the patient's sexual desire increases, but the discomfort of his other symptoms makes sexual relations difficult. Persons taking *amphetamines and cocaine* also experience an increase in sexual desire and activity, but these agents usually delay or even altogether inhibit ejaculation and orgasm.

Sexual interest and activity generally diminish in patients whose illnesses show features of depression and anergia, such as depressive and phobic syndromes, "burned-out" schizophrenias, chronic brain syndromes, or CNS depressant addictions. Women who suffer from one of these disorders tend to become frigid; men to become or remain impotent. Genital-oral contact or other sexual practices that demand little physical exertion can sometimes still arouse sexual interest, and some depressed patients even increase their sexual activity in a desperate effort to obtain pleasure. While this may lead to both promiscuity and perversion, these are usually short-lived, because the patient generally discovers that he does not enjoy them either and in addition feels guilty thereafter. Some individuals are given psychiatric diagnoses solely because of their *deviant sexual interests or habits.* Undeniably, it is difficult to empathize with perversions that forego all pretense of an interpersonal relationship, such as fetishism, exhibitionism, necrophilia, or the like. But that does not make it legitimate to assign labels that imply illness to individuals whose interests or practices do not impair their social effectiveness, are of long standing, are part of their way of life, and are not associated with any other signs of mental illness (see Chap. 8).

The Patterns of Change in the Biologic Indexes

Many of the changes in biologic functions show a common progression. The usual combination is a general decrease in the patient's sense of well-being, energy level, sexual interest and activity, appetite, and sleep; but in some illnesses the patterns are less uniform. In manic illnesses, elevated mood and increased drive and energy level are often coupled with insomnia. In the depressive phase of manic-depressive illnesses, diminished drive and energy are often associated with hypersomnia and overeating.

Circadian Rhythms and the Assessment of Illness

Certain cyclical physiologic events known as circadian rhythms or biological clocks also appear to affect the patient's sleep-wakefulness patterns, energy level, sense of well-being, appetite, and sexual interest (Mills 1966, Richter 1965, Sollberger 1965, 1970). Twenty-four-hour cycles of increase and decrease in productivity are so common that the average human being can describe the time of day at which he functions best by labeling himself a "day" or a "night" person. The association of menstrual periods with weight gain, fluid retention, changes in sexual interest, and heightened irritability may demonstrate a four-to-six-week cycle. The regularity with which REM sleep appears every 60 to 90 minutes during the night may stem from the activity of one of the briefer biologic clocks (Aserinsky 1955a,b, Globus 1969, Hartmann 1968). The daily occurrence of heightened plasma and urinary corticoid levels in the morning hours (Migeon 1956) may represent the functioning of intermediate or 24-hour clocks. Such a 24-hour biological clock may be responsible for symptoms like early morning awakening, the subsequent anxious wakefulness, and the "feeling worse in the morning" that some depressed patients report.

The concept that biologic rhythms can affect psychological functioning is useful in assessing a patient's symptoms from several standpoints. The recognition that mood may be subject to diurnal fluctuations makes it obvious that patients must be seen at different times of the day if their symptoms are to be accurately gauged. Thus morning interviews are especially important when depressed patients are being considered for hospitalization or discharge, as they typically feel better as evening approaches. Conversely, morning evaluations alone may be inadequate and misleading in organic syndromes, particularly those secondary to cardiac failure and cerebrovascular insufficiency. Indeed, the nightly deterioration of the cardiac patient's behavior is so typical and can be so severe that it has aptly been called "sundown madness." The relationship between biologic rhythms and psychological functioning is also reflected in the moodiness and difficulty in sleeping that many women experience during their menstrual periods (Kopell 1969, Moos 1969, Reynolds 1969, Smith 1969). This tendency may be accentuated in patients with emotional disorders: preexisting symptoms may become more intense, symptoms that had waned may briefly recur, and new symptoms may emerge (Mandell 1967, Torghele 1957). Changes of this kind need not be routinely interpreted then as evidence of further deterioration. Nevertheless, that the impact of biologic rhythms or any other stress *can* lead to new symptoms shows how precarious the organism's balance is. Rhythmic fluctuations in mood that occur after an illness has remitted may thus indicate a continuing, albeit subclinical, disease process.

The converse relationship also obtains: both illness and treatment can affect the biologic rhythms. Disorders of the brain or the administration of hormones, sedatives, or tranquilizers may give rise to periodic phenomena that manifest themselves in symptoms of various kinds (DuBois 1959, Richter 1965) or, on the other hand, obliterate normal periodic activity (Bridges 1966, Krieger 1966, 1967). Typical examples of the latter are the diminution of REM time following the administration of CNS depressants and the prolonged amenorrhea that can occur not only as a symptom in a number of psychotic illnesses but as a result of the administration of a wide variety of psychopharmacologic agents (Chap. 14).

PATTERNS OF DECOMPENSATION AND REMISSION

Since disturbances in the patient's mood, activity level, sleep, and other biologic functions progress in measurable increments as the illness develops, the progression of a patient's illness can usually be assessed by sequential observations of these functions. Although each of the patient's symptoms may have a timetable of its own, symptoms tend to progress in concert, and the resulting constellation defines the stage of the illness. Table 2 presents a five-stage scale by which some of the more common syndromes may be assessed and illustrates that the stages of illness occur in a fairly regular and predictable sequence. Though this table includes the end stages to which some psychotic illnesses progress, we do not suggest that all untreated mental illnesses must proceed this far, for the majority proceed only to one of the earlier stages and remit without reaching Stages D or E. The stage to which an illness progresses correlates only with the severity of the clinical picture, not with the individual's potential for recovery: a patient whose illness has proceeded to Stage E may recover completely, and one whose illness has proceeded only to one of the earlier stages may become chronically ill.

Just as the course of decompensation proceeds with a certain regularity, so does the course of the patient's remission. Indeed, remission and decompensation have so many features in common that careful observation of the way the patient becomes ill permits the clinician to make some educated guesses about the speed and manner in which he will get well. The length of time an illness takes to remit is proportionate to the length of time it has lasted, and the length of each stage of decompensation has a counterpart in each stage of remission. Even in the treated patient, in whom the total recovery time may be shorter than in the untreated, longstanding illnesses remit more slowly than those of recent origin. In addition to this *temporal rollback* phenomenon, *symptomatic rollback* is often observed as well. For example, if an illness begins with occasional anxiety attacks that are superseded some weeks later by depressive symptoms which then become progressively more severe until after several months the patient develops total insomnia and confusion, the symptoms tend, as the condition improves, to remit in reverse order, the confusion and insomnia diminishing first, and the depressed mood next. After the depression lifts, the patient may again experience anxiety attacks for several weeks, until finally these symptoms, too, disappear.

THE INDICATIONS FOR TREATMENT

This chapter began with a brief discussion of constitutional and developmental factors that mesh with a patient's current life situation to determine the nature of his biologic and social dysfunction. This was followed by the suggestion that the assessment of a patient's social, psychological, and biologic dysfunctioning makes it possible to measure the severity of his illness and to predict its course. These criteria of severity will help the clinician to distinguish situations in which treatment is *mandatory* from those in which it is *elective,* or even *contraindicated.* This distinction is important because many forms of treatment have deleterious or even dangerous side effects, and the potential benefits of treatment have to be weighed against its cost and inconvenience. The physician who seeks to avoid messianism will restrict his recommendations for treatment to those situations in which current or impending symptoms are likely to produce greater discomfort, dysfunction, or danger than the treatment form proposed to relieve them and will consider the indications absolute only when an individual's illness

1/ may weaken his impulse control,
2/ manifests itself in catastrophic social dysfunctioning, or
3/ is marked by major disturbances in biologic functions, and when
4/ one or more of these factors are persistent in time or progressive in severity.

IMPAIRED IMPULSE CONTROL

Although aggressive, antisocial, self-damaging, or suicidal behavior is not pathognomonic of any specific set of illnesses (Cohen 1969, Stürup 1968), it is most frequent in individuals who are suffering from depressions (Schipkowensky 1968, Toolan 1962), paranoid syndromes (Shepherd 1961), postpartum psychoses, and catatonic excitements, or are under the influence of CNS depressants and stimulants (Lachman 1969). The observation that impulse control may also be disturbed in patients with brain damage is of particular significance in the elderly, and may account for the fact that the likelihood of an individual's committing suicide increases with age, even to the degree of being more common in the seventies than in the sixties (Vital Statistics 1959). Organic brain disorders can also account for excessive impulsivity in children: a high percentage of aggressive, delinquent, and even homicidal children have been shown to be suffering from some kind of brain dysfunction (Bender 1959). The potential for violence must be viewed with particular concern in patients who stem from a family or subculture in which such behavior is commonplace. Similarly, whatever the patient's diagnosis, a family history of suicide entitles him to an even closer degree of supervision and protection than one would otherwise offer him, for it demonstrates that radical gestures of this kind are a part of the family tradition and in addition suggests a depressive predisposition.

Impulsive behavior seems particularly common at times of *hormonal change:* puberty, premenstrual and postpartum periods (Tonks 1968), and the onset of menopause. *Adolescents* are especially difficult to evaluate (Masterson 1967, 1968), for even those

who never before or after exhibit signs of illness occasionally behave in an impulsive or antisocial manner. Emotional turmoil is
not so overriding an aspect of adolescence, however, as to justify
the much-used label of "normative psychosis": indeed, most adolescents who show major degrees of impulsivity are, and often remain, mentally ill (Masterson 1967, 1968, Offer 1965). What makes
the assessment even more difficult is that drinking episodes, school
difficulties, car thefts, or (in the case of girls) sexual promiscuity
may be the first and, for some time, the only visible sign that
the adolescent is becoming mentally ill. The possibility is often
overlooked in adolescents who were sullen, rebellious, and negativistic even before their delinquency began. All too often, their
new difficulties are considered no more than an outgrowth or ex-
aggeration of the old, when in fact they herald the onset of illness
(Hamilton 1959). The adolescent's impulsivity is not limited to
antisocial behavior, however. Between the ages of 15 and 19, the
suicide rate is so high (3.1/100,000) and the death rate from other
causes so low that it is the fifth most frequent cause of death
(Bakwin 1957). In college and university students, suicide ranks
second only to accidents (Parrish 1956, 1957, Raphael 1937, Ross
1969).

Some patients have both homicidal and suicidal impulses. Patients with postpartum psychoses, for example, often think about
killing their children (Resnick 1969), especially the youngest,
and those who do so often make a serious suicide attempt thereafter. Patients with paranoid syndromes also may commit both
murder and suicide, particularly if they are morbidly jealous, and
even more so when their disorder is precipitated or accompanied
by addiction to alcohol or other sedative and hypnotic drugs (Shepherd 1961). Socially isolated psychotic patients sometimes resort
to violence when an external force threatens to disrupt their protective adjustment. If, for example, a patient is bizarre, withdrawn, and able to remain at home only because his family tailors
all its activities to suit his delusional ideas, efforts to mobilize him
or remove him from his environment by enlisting medical assistance may prompt him to murder, suicide, or both.

SUICIDAL DANGER

Some physicians automatically consider anyone who seriously con-
templates suicide to be mentally ill. This simplifies the evaluative
task, for it relieves the physician of the responsibility of finding

other evidence of mental illness with which to support his opinion. Since, at least in this culture, most people who commit suicide have other psychiatric symptoms as well, it is statistically safe to take this position. Nevertheless, suicides are also known among individuals who have shown no psychiatric symptoms prior to their deaths and have demonstrated so much judgment and wisdom in arranging their final affairs that calling them mentally ill stretches the label out of recognizable shape. Circumstances of this kind are not unusual among patients with severe, painful, and obviously incurable medical illnesses. Our point is not that the physician can stand aside when he sees a rational person who is intent on suicide, but only that the decision to intervene in such situations is more likely to be based on humanitarian and ethical considerations than on evidence that the patient is mentally ill.

Because an individual who threatens or attempts suicide can mobilize a good deal of emotional support from his environment and even effect environmental changes of which he would otherwise be incapable (Rubenstein 1958), some patients use threats of this kind as the stakes in a game of "dependency brinkmanship": whenever they want to achieve a particular end or avoid a demand, they threaten to kill themselves. While this game is often effective, it cannot usually be played for long: eventually, the patients' families, friends, and even their therapists ignore their distress. The difficulty in distinguishing between serious and manipulative suicidal threats may immobilize a patient's therapist and make it hard for him to handle the situation correctly. Since ignoring such threats may increase the patient's sense of isolation (Stengel 1962) and provoke him to suicide, while overresponding to them may encourage their repetition and destroy the therapist's effectiveness, it may in such cases be best to ask a colleague to see the patient and render an independent opinion (Litman 1964).

Some suicide attempts, especially those that fail, are called "gestures," as if to indicate that they are innocuous. Such attempts should not be ignored, however, for even those that are conscious manipulations can backfire, and anyone who uses a gesture of this kind to get what he wants demonstrates thereby that he is unable to find better ways of coping with his problems or mobilizing support. The need for special caution is underscored by the fact that persons who have previously attempted suicide are almost 35 times likelier to die as a result of suicide than those who have never made such an attempt (Ettlinger 1964, Pokorny 1966). Moreover, while the second attempt most commonly occurs within three months of the first, the risk is in reality lifelong. Indeed, from a statistical standpoint, one out of every 10 patients who makes a suicide attempt serious enough to be brought to medical attention will, within 10 years of the initial, unsuccessful attempt, make another that succeeds (Ettlinger 1964, Schneider 1954). For these reasons, it is safest to take seriously all suicide gestures, attempts, and threats (Delong 1961, Robins 1959, Tuckman 1960) until both the dynamic roots and the potential dangers are better understood (Watkins 1969, Wilkins 1967).

While the layman often gauges the extent of the danger in terms of his own assessment of the patient's reality situation, the only clinically significant factor is the patient's view of his situation. Certain motives and attitudes toward life are particularly common in patients who succeed in committing suicide:

1/ The patient's subjective discomfort, depression, and anguish are so unbearable that, like the cancer patient with intractable pain, he prefers suicide to continued suffering. In protracted illnesses, both physical and mental, the patient's certainty—justified or not— that he will suffer as long as he lives may persuade him that suicide is desirable. Such concerns are common in patients with *physical illnesses,* and in fact are the most frequent precipitating factor of successful suicide (Pokorny 1966).

2/ The patient is subject to delusions or auditory hallucinations that urge him to suicide or give him reasons for dying. His self-hatred and self-derogation are sometimes delusionally elaborated into such beliefs as that the only way he can expiate his sins or deficiencies is to kill himself or that his family would be better off without him (Singer 1969). In more fragmented forms of depression, just as in some catatonias, patients sometimes believe that their death will *save the world* from misery or destruction.

3/ The patient feels that his life position is untenable, that there is no further use in discussing his problems with anyone, and that he has *no important and meaningful relationship* with any other human being (Farberow 1961, Fawcett 1969, Krauss 1968, Wilson 1968). Views of this kind are not uncommon after death, divorce, dispute, or circumstances have separated an individual from a relationship that was important to him. Most people cope with a loss of this kind by engaging in compensatory mechanisms that blunt the edge of sadness. Mourning rituals and the fuss connected with funeral, legal, or living arrangements usually provide helpful distractions to an individual who has sustained a loss, at least for a while. He may thereafter make efforts to establish a similarly meaningful relationship by becoming involved in a friendship or romance, or try to develop a new interest in life through organizational activities, an upsurge of religious interest, or the like. If the individual is unable to find a substitute, or, having found one, discovers it to be unsatisfactory, his sense of isolation and abandonment may increase even further and cause him to consider suicide preferable to the emptiness, meaninglessness, and despair that his current existence entails. Thus, the greater the difficulty in replacing a lost relationship, the greater the suicidal danger. Suicide attempts are, for example, common in *homosexuals* who have just been abandoned by a partner with whom they had had an intense relationship, particularly if their social position is so sensitive that they cannot conduct too vigorous a search for a new partner. Individuals who are poorly equipped to tolerate separation are also more likely to react poorly to the loss of an important figure: suicide attempts are said to be particularly common in individuals who have been either overprotected by their parents or deprived of them at an early age (Bruhn 1962, Dorpat 1965, Tuckman 1966, Walton 1958).

4/ The patient feels depressed and decides to commit suicide as soon as he can find a convenient and painless opportunity. In some cases, however, his illness progresses so rapidly that he loses the initiative, energy, and organizational ability needed to carry out his plan, while retaining his intention of doing so. As his depression lifts, and his retardation diminishes, he may regain the initiative and energy that suicide requires and, if he finds the opportunity to do so before he improves sufficiently to abandon his plan, may indeed succeed in committing suicide. This kind of sequence is another example of the *rollback phenomenon,* and explains why it is especially important that close surveillance of the patient not be discontinued as soon as he starts to look better. Indeed, during the initial phase of improvement, he may be in even greater danger than he was at the peak of his illness.

Certain demographic factors are also relevant in assessing the probability that a patient will commit suicide. *Women* make three times as many attempts as men but succeed one third as often (Lester 1969); *Caucasians* commit suicide more frequently than Negroes; *older* persons more than younger, the *unmarried* more than the married, *lawyers* and *doctors* (especially psychiatrists) (Blachly 1968, Simon 1968) more than those in other occupations; and *residents of urban areas* more than those of rural ones (Blachly 1963, Ettlinger 1964, Vital Statistics 1959).

Although the risk of suicide is greatest for the depressed patient (Murphy 1969, Pitts 1964) and the young catatonic (Balser 1959), no diagnostic category is immune from this danger, not even the antisocial personality disorder or the seemingly innocuous organic syndrome. It is, therefore, of utmost importance to determine the patient's level of comfort, both by attending to his reports of his subjective experience and by inquiring about his sleep and appetite. The latter inquiries seem particularly helpful, for patients who sleep and eat well are rarely in sufficient discomfort to commit suicide (Otto 1964, Rosen 1970).

The foregoing rule does not apply, however, to *patients who are taking narcotics, alcohol, or other* CNS *depressants* (see Chap. 9), for these generally mask most of the classical symptoms that would make the severity of the patient's depression obvious, such as sleep disturbance or a sense of despair, and the only symptoms, if any, that remain are severe hypochondriasis and somatic delusions (Dorfman 1961). The suicidal risk in these so-called *"masked"* or *"smiling" depressions* should be considered to have increased even further when the patient's sleep or appetite suddenly deteriorates or his drug intake increases abruptly. The use of alcohol and other CNS depressants in the course of a depression is particularly dangerous not only because they impair the individual's judgment and impulse control but also because long-term drug use can cause or intensify a depressive syndrome (Detre 1966). If, as often the case, a patient appears to feel good or even somewhat euphoric after making a suicide attempt with a CNS depressant, the physician may think that the attempt has in some way helped the patient, whether by permitting him to expiate his guilt, providing him with an affirmative answer to the implied question whether he is worthy of living, or helping him to achieve some practical goal. Such theories cannot be confirmed in all cases, however: the euphoria may in fact be no more than the neurophysiologic consequence of abrupt drug withdrawal and, if seen as a sign of improvement, may lead to an incautious decision such as premature release from the hospital.

CATASTROPHIC SOCIAL DYSFUNCTIONING

Although behavior that is considered catastrophic in one environment will not necessarily be regarded in the same way in another, every culture has certain taboos that must not be transgressed and certain demands that must be fulfilled. Whatever the cultural milieu may be, a single item of disturbed behavior is rarely the only evidence of illness; and conversely, no brief period of normal behavior can be considered evidence of health. Even when a patient is able to maintain his social facade during a medical consultation, assessment of his employment history, family life, and interpersonal relationships may show a very different and often far more accurate picture.

Since information about the patient's *work performance* is less liable to subjective interpretation and distortion than descriptions of family life or interpersonal relationships, it often provides a more valid and quantifiable measure of social functioning than the patient's own estimate. In general, the faster a patient's illness progresses and the more complex his occupation, the more rapid his occupational decline. *Illnesses of rapid onset,* like acute schizophrenic psychoses and acute brain syndromes, usually render the patient diffusely incompetent at his work within days or weeks. The work performance of patients who have *illnesses that develop more slowly,* such as depressions and chronic brain syndromes, deteriorates over a longer period, and the protracted course permits numerous compensatory efforts. At the time a patient first becomes depressed, for example, he may have difficulty in concentrating and in remembering things relating to his work. His decreased effectiveness meshes with his self-denigration, and he may try to compensate for his impaired performance by lengthening his working hours or taking his work home. As the depression continues, he may start to see his tasks as insurmountable, begin to leave work early, and, some weeks later, ask for simpler work or look for a new and less demanding job. Finally, he may consider it futile and upsetting to work at all. The housewife's course is similar: at first her habits become increasingly sloppy, and the meals she prepares skimpy and unimaginative. Next, she tries to compensate by working constantly and making great efforts to regiment her family's behavior so that she can cope with it. Finally, she neglects the safety and cleanliness of her children and stops cooking altogether.

THE "NEED" FOR TREATMENT

When a person's psychological discomfort endangers his life or that of others, or paralyzes his social functioning, treatment is mandatory; when his life is in no danger and his social functioning relatively intact, it is not. Among the individuals who fall into the latter group, some are so dissatisfied with themselves that they ask no questions before seeking psychological help. Others first ask whether they "need" treatment or whether it will help them. Since there are no objective criteria to distinguish between individuals for whom treatment is desirable but not mandatory and those who are unlikely to benefit from it, and since most reports of treatment results are at variance with one another, the answer the patient gets depends upon whom he asks.

In defining "need," physicians are usually more influenced by the particular definition of mental health and normality that they accept and the particular school of psychotherapy to which they adhere than they are by empirical evidence. Some believe that even a person who is "obviously healthy" would benefit from the increased self-understanding that a psychotherapeutic enounter can offer and that he too would thus "need" treatment. We have no quarrel with the first part of the proposition, for, as we shall suggest later (see p. 520), there are good reasons to believe that the better integrated a patient is at the beginning of treatment, the more he is likely to learn from it. We question, however, whether need and benefit can be equated in this manner and, sharing Szasz's (1961) concern that too many situations formerly regarded as life problems are now inaccurately labeled as illnesses, find no contradiction in telling a patient that we think treatment will help him even though he does not by any means "need" it.

Though we doubt Szasz's view that most of the disorders referred for psychiatric attention lie outside the province of treatable illness, we would agree that there are situations in which treatment is *contraindicated* (Chapman 1960, Whitaker 1969). If a patient is offered psychotherapy before he is convinced that he needs it, he may find it so disagreeable that he will, even at a later time, refuse to see a psychiatrist. Another may enter treatment only to avoid facing an unpleasant reality, to postpone an inevitable but troublesome decision, or even to embarrass or irritate his family (see also p. 253). Finally, when a patient's need for treatment is marginal, we consider the fact that, despite all the advances cited above, cultural attitudes still discriminate against the mentally ill and weigh our inclination to suggest treatment against the possibility that this recommendation alone may ever after have a deleterious effect on the patient's insurability, employability, and right to be heard as an equal within his family and community.

REFERENCES

Agnew, N., and Agnew, M.: Drive level effects on tasks of narrow and broad attention, Quart J Exp Psychol *15*:58-62, 1963.

Ames, L. B.: Sleep and dreams in childhood, *in* Harms, E., ed.: Problems of Sleep and Dreams in Children, vol. 2, New York: Macmillan, 1964, pp. 6-29.

Arsenian, J.: Life cycle factors in mental illness: Biosocial theory with implications for prevention, Ment Hyg *52*:19-26, 1968.

Aserinsky, E., and Kleitman, N.: Regularly occurring periods of eye motility, and concomitant phenomena, during sleep, Science *118*:273-274, 1953.

———: Two types of ocular motility occurring in sleep, J Appl Physiol *8*:1-10, 1955a.

———: A motility cycle in sleeping infants as manifested by ocular and gross bodily activity, J Appl Physiol *8*:11-18, 1955b.

Ax, A., and Luby, E. D.: Autonomic responses to sleep deprivation, Arch Gen Psychiat (Chicago) *4*:55-59, 1961.

Babigian, H. M., *et al.*: Diagnostic consistency and change in a follow-up study of 1215 patients, Amer J Psychiat *121*: 895-901, 1965.

Badgley, T., *et al.*: Characteristics of the schizophrenic decompensation, Arch Gen Psychiat (Chicago) *10*:138-142, 1964.

Bakwin, H.: Suicide in children and adolescents, J Pediat *50*:749-769, 1957.

Balser, B. H., and Masterson, J. F.: Suicide in adolescents, Amer J Psychiat *116*:400-404, 1959.

Bartoshuk, A. K., and Tennant, J. M.: Human neonatal EEG correlates of sleep-wakefulness and neural maturation, J Psychiat Res *2*:73-83, 1964.

Bastos, O.: Dream activity in depressive states, Evolut Psychiat (Paris) *28*:101-127, 1964.

Beck, A. T.: Reliability of psychiatric diagnoses: (1) A critique of systematic studies, Amer J Psychiat *119*:210-216, 1962a.

Beck, A. T., *et al.*: Reliability of psychiatric diagnoses: (2) Study of consistency of clinical judgments and ratings, Amer J Psychiat *119*:351-357, 1962b.

Bender, L.: Children and adolescents who have killed, Amer J Psychiat *116*: 510-513, 1959.

Bennett, D. R.: Sleep deprivation and major motor convulsions, Neurology *13*: 953-958, 1963.

Berger, R. J., and Oswald, I.: Effects of sleep deprivation on behaviour, subsequent sleep and dreaming, Brit J Psychiat *108*:457-465, 1962.

Blachly, P. H., Disher, W., and Roduner, G.: Suicide by physicians, Bull Suicidology, Dec. 1968, pp. 1-18.

Blachly, P. H., Osterud, H. T., and Josslin, R.: Suicide in professional groups, New Eng J Med *268*:1278-1282, 1963.

Bliss, E. L., Clark, L. D., and West, C. D.: Studies in sleep deprivation: Relationship to schizophrenia, Arch Neurol Psychiat *81*:348-359, 1959.

Bourne, P. G., Rose, R. M., and Mason, J. W.: Urinary 17-OHCS levels, Arch Gen Psychiat (Chicago) *17*:104-110, 1967.

Bridges, P. K., and Jones, M. T.: Diurnal rhythm of plasma cortisol concentration in depression, Brit J Psychiat *112*:1257-1261, 1966.

Bruhn, J. G.: Broken homes among attempted suicides and psychiatric outpatients: A comparative study, Brit J Psychiat *108*:772-779, 1962.

Callaway, E., III, and Thompson, S. V.: Sympathetic activity and perception: An approach to the relationships between autonomic activity and personality, Psychosom Med *15*:443-355, 1953.

Chapman, A. H.: Psychiatrogenic illness, Amer J Psychiat *116*:873-877, 1960.

Chodoff, P., Friedman, S. B., and Hamburg, D. A.: Stress, defenses and coping behavior: Observations in parents of children with malignant disease, Amer J Psychiat *120*:743-749, 1964.

Clarke, A. D. B.: Learning and human development, Brit J Psychiat *114*:1061-1077, 1968.

Cohen, B. D., Grisell, J. L., and Ax, A. F.: The effects of voluntary sleep loss on psychological and physiological functions, Proc III World Cong Psychiat, vol. 2, 1961, pp. 986-991.

Cohen, E.: Self-assault in psychiatric evaluation: Proposed clinical classification, Arch Gen Psychiat (Chicago) *21*:64-71, 1969.

Cohen, H.: The nature, purpose, and methods of diagnosis, Lancet *244*:23-25, 1943.

Courville, J., Walsh, J., and Cordeau, J. P.: Functional organization of the brainstem reticular formation and sensory input, Science *138*:973-975, 1962.

Dalén, P.: Causal explanations in psychiatry: Critique of some current concepts, Brit J Psychiat *115*:129-137, 1969.

Delong, W. B., and Robins, E.: The communication of suicidal intent prior to psychiatric hospitalization: A study of 87 patients, Amer J Psychiat *117*:695-705, 1961.

Dement, W., and Kleitman, N.: Cyclic variations in EEG during sleep and their relation to eye movements, body motility, and dreaming, Electroenceph Clin Neurophysiol *9*:663-690, 1957.

Detre, T.: Sleep disorder and psychosis, Canad Psychiat Ass J *2* (Spec Suppl):169-177, 1966.

Diaz-Guerrero, R., Gottlieb, J. S., and Knott, J. R.: The sleep of patients with manic-depressive psychosis depressive type, Psychosom Med *8*:399-404, 1946.

Dohrenwend, B. P., and Dohrenwend, B. S.: Social Status and Psychological Disorder: A Causal Inquiry, New York: Wiley, 1969.

Dorfman, W.: Masked depression, Dis Nerv Syst *22*:41-45, 1961.

Dorpat, T. L., Jackson, J. K., and Ripley, H. S.: Broken homes and attempted and completed suicide, Arch Gen Psychiat (Chicago) *12*:213-216, 1965.

DuBois, F. S.: Rhythms, cycles and periods in health and disease, Amer J Psychiat *116*:114-119, 1959.

Dykman, R. A., et al.: Autonomic responses in psychiatric patients, Ann NY Acad Sci *147*:237-303, 1968.

Eassom, W. M.: Psychopathological environmental reaction to congenital defect, J Nerv Ment Dis *142*:453-459, 1966.

Escalona, S. K.: Some determinants of individual differences, Trans NY Acad Sci *27*:802-816, 1965.

Ettlinger, R. W.: Suicides in a group of patients who had previously attempted suicide, Acta Psychiat Scand *40*:363-378, 1964.

Farberow, N. L., and Shneidman, E. S., eds.: The Cry for Help, New York: McGraw-Hill, 1961.

Fawcett, J., Leff, M., and Bunney, W. E.: Suicide: Clues from interpersonal communication, Arch Gen Psychiat (Chicago) *21*:129-137, 1969.

Feinberg, I.: Ontogenesis of human sleep and the relationship of sleep variables to intellectual function in the aged, Compr Psychiat *9*:138-147, 1968.

Feinberg, I., Koresko, R. L., and Gottlieb, F.: Further observations on electrophysiological sleep patterns in schizophrenia, Compr Psychiat *6*:21-24, 1965.

Fleishman, M.: Will the real third revolution please stand up?, Amer J Psychiat *124*:1260-1262, 1968.

Fletcher, C. M.: The clinical diagnosis of pulmonary emphysema—an experimental study, Proc Roy Soc Med *45*:577-584, 1952.

Freedman, D. G.: Inheritance of behavior in infants, Science *140*:196-198, 1963.

Freeman, F. R., Agnew, H. W., Jr., and Williams, R. L.: An electroencephalographic study of the effects of meprobamate on human sleep, Clin Pharmacol Ther *6*:172-176, 1965.

Garland, L. H.: The problem of observer error, Bull NY Acad Med *36*:570-584, 1960.

Gellhorn, E.: Central nervous system tuning and its implications for neuropsychiatry, J Nerv Ment Dis *147*:148-162, 1968.

Gellhorn, E., and Loofbourrow, G. N.: Emotions and Emotional Disorders: A Neurophysiological Study, New York: Hoeber, 1963.

Gibbs, F. A., and Gibbs, E. L.: Changes in epileptic foci with age, Electroenceph Clin Neurophysiol *4* (Suppl):233-234, 1953.

Gibbs, F. A., Rich, C. L., and Gibbs, E. L.: Psychomotor variant type of seizure discharge, Neurology *13*:991-998, 1963.

Globus, G. G., Gardner, R., and Williams, T. A.: Relation of sleep onset to rapid eye movement sleep, Arch Gen Psychiat (Chicago) *21*:151-154, 1969.

Goodenough, D. R., et al.: Comparison of "dreamers" and "nondreamers": Eye movements, electroencephalograms and the recall of dreams, J Abnorm Psychol *59*:295-302, 1959.

————: Dream reporting following abrupt and gradual awakenings from different types of sleep, J Personality Soc Psychol *2*:170-179, 1965.

Green, P. C., and Gordon, M.: Maternal deprivation: Its influences on visual exploration in infant monkeys, Science *145*:292-294, 1964.

Gresham, S. C., Webb, W. B., and Williams, R. L.: Alcohol and caffeine: Effect on inferred visual dreaming, Science *140*:1226-1227, 1963.

Grossman, H. J., and Greenberg, N. H.: Psychosomatic differentiation in infancy

1. Autonomic activity in the newborn, Psychosom Med *19*:293-306, 1957.

Haider, M., Spong, P., and Lindsley, D. B.: Attention, vigilance and cortical evoked potentials in humans, Science *145*: 180-182, 1964.

Hakarem, G., Sutton, S., and Zubin, J.: Pupillary reactions to light in schizophrenic patients and normals, Ann NY Acad Sci *105*:820-831, 1964.

Hall, P.: Some clinical aspects of moving house as an apparent precipitant of psychiatric symptoms, J Psychosom Res *10*:59-70, 1966.

Hamilton, M., and White, J. M.: Clinical syndromes in depressive states, Brit J Psychiat *105*:985-998, 1959.

Harlow, H. F., and Harlow, M. K.: The effect of rearing conditions on behavior, Int J Psychiat *1*:43-51, 1965.

Hartmann, E.: The D-State: A review and discussion of studies on the physiologic state concomitant with dreaming, New Eng J Med *273*:30-35, 87-92, 1965.

————: The 90-minute sleep-dream cycle, Arch Gen Psychiat (Chicago) *18*:280-286, 1968.

Hernandez-Péon, R.: Psychiatric implications of neurophysiological research, Bull Menninger Clin *28*:165-185, 1964.

Heron, W., and Anchel, H.: Synchronous sensory bombardment of young rats: Effects on the electroencephalogram, Science *145*:946-947, 1964.

Hilgard, E. R.: Altered states of awareness, J Nerv Ment Dis *149*:68-79, 1969.

Hinton, J. M.: Patterns of insomnia in depressive states, J Neurol Neurosurg Psychiat *26*:184-189, 1963.

Hollingshead, A. B., and Redlich, F. C.: Social Class and Mental Illness: A Community Study, New York: Wiley, 1958.

Hunt, J. McV.: Traditional personality theory in the light of recent evidence, Amer Sci *53*:80-96, 1965.

Imboden, J. B., Canter, A., and Cluff, L.: Separation experiences and health records in a group of normal adults, Psychosom Med *25*:433-440, 1963.

Jaspers, K.: Allgemeine Psychopathologie, Berlin: Springer, 1959.

Johns, M. W., *et al.*: Sleep habits in male medical and surgical patients, Brit Med J *2*:509-512, 1970.

Jouvet, M.: Biogenic amines and the states of sleep, Science *163*:32-41, 1969.

Jouvet, M., and Jouvet, D.: A study of the neurophysiological mechanisms of dreaming, *in* Hernandez-Péon, R., ed.: Physiological Basis of Mental Activity, (Suppl 24), Amsterdam: Elsevier, 1963, pp. 133-157.

Kahn, E., and Fisher, C.: Sleep characteristics of the normal aged male, J Nerv Ment Dis *148*:447-494, 1969.

Kales, A., ed.: Sleep, Physiology and Pathology: A Symposium, Philadelphia: Lippincott, 1969.

Kaufman, W.: Some emotional uses of foods, Conn Med *23*:158-163, 1959.

King, C. D.: The meaning of normal, Yale J Biol Med *17*:493-501, 1945.

Kleitman, N.: Sleep and Wakefulness, Chicago: Univ Chicago Press, 1963.

Kollar, E. J., *et al.*: Psychological, psychophysiological, and biochemical correlates of prolonged sleep deprivation, Amer J Psychiat *126*:488-497, 1969.

Kopell, B. S., *et al.*: Variations in some measures of arousal during the menstrual cycle, J Nerv Ment Dis *148*:180-187, 1969.

Kramer, M.: Collection and utilization of statistical data from psychiatric facilities in the United States of America, Bull WHO *29*:491-510, 1963.

————: Statistics of mental disorders in the United States: Current status, some urgent needs and suggested solutions, read before the Royal Statistical Society, March 19, 1969.

Krauss, H. H., and Krauss, B. J.: Cross-cultural study of the thwarting-disorientation theory of suicide, J Abnorm Psychol *73*:353-357, 1968.

Krieger, D. T., and Krieger, H. P.: Circadian variation of the plasma 17-hydroxycorticosteroids in central nervous system disease, J Clin Endocr *26*:929-940, 1966.

————: Circadian pattern of plasma 17-hydroxycorticosteroid: Alteration by anticholinergic agents, Science *155*:1421-1422, 1967.

Kupfer, D. J., Detre, T., and Harrow, M.: Relationship between sleep disorders and symptomatology, Arch Gen Psychiat (Chicago) *17*:710-716, 1967.

Kupfer, D. J., Harrow, M., and Detre, T.: Sleep patterns and psychopathology, Acta Psychiat Scand *45*:75-89, 1969.

Kupfer, D. J., *et al.*: Sleep disturbance in acute schizophrenic patients, Amer J Psychiat, *126*:1213-1223, 1970.

Lachman, J. H., and Cravens, J. M.: Murderers—before and after, Ment Hlth Dig *1*:23-24, 1969.

Lairy, G. C., *et al.*: Recording of night sleep during periods of delusion, Electroenceph Clin Neurophysiol *18*:96-97, 1965.

Lester, D.: Suicidal behavior in men and women, Ment Hyg *53*:340-345, 1969.

Lewis, H. E.: Sleep patterns on polar expeditions, *in* Wolstenholme, G. E. E., and O'Connor, M., eds.: CIBA Foundation

Symposium on the Nature of Sleep, Boston: Little, 1961, pp. 322-328.

Lindsley, D. B.: Attention, counsciousness, sleep, and wakefulness, *in* Field, J., Magoun, H. W., and Hall, V. E., eds.: Handbook of Physiology, vol. 3, Amer Physiol Soc, 1960, pp. 1553-1593.

Lindsley, D. B., *et al.:* Diurnal activity, behavior and EEG responses in visually deprived monkeys, Ann NY Acad Sci *117:* 564-587, 1964.

Litman, R. E.: Immobilization response to suicidal behavior, Arch Gen Psychiat (Chicago) *11:*282-285, 1964.

Loomis, A. L., Harvey, E. N., and Hobart, G. A.: Cerebral states during sleep, as studied by human brain potentials, J Exp Psychol *21:*127-144, 1937.

Lowenstein, O., and Lowenfeld, I. E.: The sleep-waking cycle and pupillary activity, Ann NY Acad Sci *117:*142-156, 1964.

Luby, E. D., *et al.:* Sleep deprivation: Effects on behavior, thinking, motor performance, and biological energy transfer systems, Psychosom Med *22:*182-192, 1960.

Luce, G. G., and Segal, J.: Sleep, New York: Coward, 1966.

Maddison, D., and Viola, A.: Health of widows in the year following bereavement, J Psychosom Res *12:*297-306, 1968.

Mandell, A. J., and Mandell, M. P.: Suicide and the menstrual cycle, JAMA *200:*792-793, 1967.

Marrazzi, A. S., Hart, E. R., and Ray, O. S.: Cerebral homeostasis, dysfunction, and psychosis, Recent Advances Biol Psychiat *5:*309-320, 1962.

Masterson, J. F., Jr.: The Psychiatric Dilemma of Adolescence, Boston: Little, 1967.

——:Psychiatric significance of adolescent turmoil, Amer J Psychiat *124:*1549-1554, 1968.

McGhie, A., and Chapman, J.: Disorders of attention and perception in early schizophrenia, Brit J Med Psychol *34:*103-116, 1961.

McGhie, A., and Russell, S. M.: The subjective assessment of normal sleep patterns, Brit J Psychiat *108:*642-654, 1962.

Migeon, C. J., *et al.:* Diurnal variation of plasma levels and urinary excretion of 17-hydroxycorticosteroids in normal subjects, night workers and blind subjects, J Clin Endocr *16:*622-633, 1956.

Mills, J. N.: Human circadian rhythms, Physiol Rev *46:*128-171, 1966.

Monroe, L. J.: Psychological and physiological differences between good and poor sleepers, J Abnorm Psychol *72:*255-264, 1967.

Moos, R. H., *et al.:* Fluctuations in symptoms and moods during the menstrual cycle, J Psychosom Res *13:*37-44, 1969.

Morozova, T. N., and Shumskii, N. G.: Endogenous depressions and external factors, Zh Nevropat Psikhiat *63:*33-38, 1963.

Moruzzi, G., and Magoun, H. W.: Brainstem reticular formation and activation of the EEG, Electroenceph Clin Neurophysiol *1:*455-473, 1949.

Munro, A.: Childhood parent-loss in a psychiatrically normal population, Brit J Prev Soc Med *19:*69-79, 1965.

Munro, A., and Griffiths, A. B.: Some psychiatric non-sequelae of childhood bereavement, Brit J Psychiat *115:*305-311, 1969.

Murphy, G. E.: Recognition of suicidal risk, Southern Med J *62:*723-728, 1969.

Murphy, G. E., *et al.:* Stress, sickness and psychiatric disorder in a "normal" population: Study of 101 young women, J Nerv Ment Dis *134:*228-236, 1962.

Nathan, R. J.: Age of patient and diagnosis of schizophrenia, Arch Gen Psychiat (Chicago) *11:*185-191, 1964.

National Institute of Mental Health (Collaborative Study Group): Phenothiazine treatment in acute schizophrenia: Effectiveness, Arch Gen Psychiat (Chicago) *10:*246-261, 1964.

Offer, D., Sabshin, M., and Marcus, D.: Clinical evaluation of normal adolescents, Amer J Psychiat *121:*864-872, 1965.

Oswald, I.: Sleeping and Waking: Physiology and Psychology, Amsterdam, Elsevier, 1962.

——:Drugs and Sleep, Pharmacol Rev *20:*273-303, 1968.

Oswald, I., *et al.:* Melancholia and barbiturates: Controlled EEG, body and eye movement study of sleep, Brit J Psychiat *109:*66-78, 1963.

Othmer, E., Hayden, M. P., and Segelbaum, R.: Encephalic cycles during sleep and wakefulness in humans: A 24-hour pattern, Science *164:*447-449, 1969.

Otto, U.: Changes in the behaviour of children and adolescents preceding suicidal attempts, Acta Psychiat Scand *40:*386-400, 1964.

Parmalee, A. H., Jr.: Sleep patterns in infancy: A study of one infant from birth to eight months of age, Acta Paediat Scand *50:*160-170, 1961.

Parrish, H. M.: Causes of death among college students—A study of 209 deaths at Yale University, 1920-1955, Public Health Rep *71:*1081-1085, 1956.

——: Epidemiology of suicide among college students, Yale J Biol Med *29:*585-595, 1957.

Pasnau, R. O., *et al.:* Psychological effects of 205 hours of sleep deprivation, Arch

Gen Psychiat (Chicago) *18:*496-505, 1968.

Patrick, G. W. T., and Gilbert, J. A.: On the effects of loss of sleep, Psychol Rev *3:*469-483, 1896.

Patrushev, V. I., and Zhukov, V. G.: Cognition: On the physiology of attention, Soviet Psychol Psychiat 2(4):40-44, 1964.

Phillips, L.: Social competence, the process-reactive distinction, and the nature of mental disorder, Proc Amer Psychopath Ass *54:*471-481, 1966.

Pitts, F. N., Jr., and Winokur, G.: Affective disorder, III: Diagnostic correlates and incidence of suicide, J Nerv Ment Dis *139:*176-181, 1964.

Pokorny, A. D.: Follow-up study of 618 suicidal patients, Amer J Psychiat *122:* 1109-1116, 1966.

Raphael, T., Power, S. H., and Berridge, W. L.: The question of suicide as a problem in college mental hygiene, Amer J Orthopsychiat *7:*1-14, 1937.

Rechtschaffen, A.: Nocturnal sleep of narcoleptics, Electroenceph Clin Neurophysiol *15:*599-609, 1963.

Redlich, F. C.: The concept of normality, Amer J Psychother *6:*551-569, 1952.

Resnick, P. J.: Child murder by parents: A psychiatric review of filicide, Amer J Psychiat *126:*325-334, 1969.

Reynolds, E.: Variations of mood and recall in the menstrual cycle, J Psychosom Res *13:*163-166, 1969.

Richmond, J. B., and Lustman, S. L.: Autonomic function in the neonate: 1. Implications for psychosomatic theory, Psychosom Med *17:*269-275, 1955.

Richter, C. P.: Biological Clocks in Medicine and Psychiatry, Springfield (Ill): Thomas, 1965.

Robins, E., *et al.:* Communication of suicidal intent: Study of 134 consecutive cases of successful (completed) suicide, Amer J Psychiat *115:*724-733, 1959.

Rodin, E. A., Luby, E. D., and Gottlieb, J. S.: The electroencephalogram during prolonged experimental sleep deprivation, Electroenceph Clin Neurophysiol *14:*544-551, 1962.

Roffwarg, H., Dement, W., and Fisher, C.: Preliminary observations of sleep-dream patterns in neonates, infants, children, and adults, *in* Harms, E., ed.: Problems of Sleep and Dreams in Children, vol. 2, New York: Macmillan, 1964, pp. 60-72.

Rootman, I., and Lafave, G.: Are popular attitudes toward the mentally ill changing?, Amer J Psychiat *126:*261-265, 1969.

Rosen, D. H.: The serious suicide attempt: Epidemiological and follow-up study of 886 patients, Amer J Psychiat *127:*764-770, 1970.

Ross, M.: Suicide among college students, Amer J Psychiat *126:*220-225, 1969.

Rossi, G. F.: Sleep inducing mechanisms in the brainstem, *in* Hernandez-Péon, R., ed.: The Physiological Basis of Mental Activity, (Suppl 24), Amsterdam: Elsevier, 1963, pp. 113-132.

Rubenstein, R., Moses, R., and Lidz, T.: On attempted suicide, Arch Neurol (Chicago) *79:*103-112, 1958.

Rubin, L. S.: Autonomic dysfunction as a concomitant of neurotic behavior, J Nerv Ment Dis *138:*558-574, 1964.

Rubin, L. S., and Barry, T. J.: Autonomic fatigue in psychoses, J Nerv Ment Dis *147:*211-222, 1968.

Ruesch, J.: Assessment of social disability, Arch Gen Psychiat (Chicago) *21:* 655-664, 1969.

Ruesch, J., and Brodsky, C. M.: Concept of social disability, Arch Gen Psychiat (Chicago) *19:*394-403, 1968.

Ruesch, J., Brodsky, C. M., and Fisher, A.: Psychiatric Care: Psychiatry Simplified for Therapeutic Action, New York: Grune, 1964.

Sandifer, M. G., Jr., Pettus, C., and Quade, D.: A study of psychiatric diagnosis, J Nerv Ment Dis *139:*350-356, 1964.

Sarvis, M. A.: Paranoid reactions: Perceptual distortion as an etiological agent, Arch Gen Psychiat (Chicago) *6:*157-162, 1962.

Scarr, S.: The origins of individual differences in adjective check list scores, J Consult Psychol *30:*354-357 (No. 4), 1966.

Schaffer, H. R., and Emerson, P. E.: Patterns of response to physical contact in early human development, J Child Psychol Psychiat *5:*1-13, 1964.

Schipkowensky, N.: Affective disorders: Cyclophrenia and murder, *in* deReuck, A. V. S., and Porter, R., eds.: The Mentally Abnormal Offender, Ciba Foundation Symposium, Boston: Little, 1968.

Schneider, P. B.: La Tentative de Suicide: Étude Statistique, Clinique, Psychologique et Catamnestique, Neuchâtel: Delachaux & Niestle, 1954.

Scott, J. P.: Critical periods in behavioral development, Science *138:*949:958, 1962.

Shepherd, M.: Morbid jealousy: Some clinical and social aspects of a psychiatric symptom, Brit J Psychiat *107:*687-753, 1961.

Simon, W., and Lumry, G. K.: Suicide among physician-patients, J Nerv Ment Dis *147:*105-112, 1968.

Singer, R. G., and Blumenthal, I. J.: Suicide clues in psychotic patients, Ment Hyg *53:*346-350, 1969.

Smith, A.: Changing effects of frontal

lesions in man, J Neurol Neurosurg Psychiat 27:511-515, 1964.

Smith, S. L., and Sauder, C.: Food cravings, depression, and premenstrual problems, Psychosom Med 31:281-287, 1969.

Snyder, F.: The new biology of dreaming, Arch Gen Psychiat (Chicago) 8:381-391, 1963.

——: Electrographic studies of sleep in depression, in Kline, N. S., and Laska, E., eds.: Computers and Electronic Devices in Psychiatry, New York: Grune, 1968.

Sollberger, A.: Biological Rhythm Research, Amsterdam: Elsevier, 1965.

——: Biological rhythm research, to be published in Gadamer, H. G., and Vogler, P., eds.: Neue Anthropologie, Stuttgart: Thieme, 1970.

Statistical Bulletin: Recent trends in hospitalization and disability from mental disorders, Statist Bull 50:4-6, 1969.

Steinberg, H. R., and Durell, J.: Stressful social situation as a precipitant of schizophrenic symptoms: An epidemiological study, Brit J Psychiat 114:1097-1105, 1968.

Stengel, E.: Recent research into suicide and attempted suicide, Amer J Psychiat 118:725-727, 1962.

Strömgren, E.: Uses and abuses of concepts in psychiatry, Amer J Psychiat 126:777-788, 1969.

Stürup, G. K.: "Will this man be dangerous?," in deReuck, A. V. S., and Porter, R., eds.: The Mentally Abnormal Offender, Ciba Foundation Symposium, Boston: Little, 1968.

Szasz, T.: The Myth of Mental Illness, New York: Harper, 1961.

Tonks, C. M., Rack, P. H., and Rose, M. J.: Attempted suicide and the menstrual cycle, J Psychosom Res 11:319-323, 1968.

Toolan, J. M.: Suicide and suicidal attempts in children and adolescents, Amer J Psychiat 118:719-724, 1962.

Torghele, J. R.: Premenstrual tension in psychotic women, J Lancet 77:163-170, 1957.

Tuckman, J., Kleiner, R. J., and Lavell, M.: Credibility of suicide notes, Amer J Psychiat 116:1104-1106, 1960.

Tuckman, J., Youngman, W. F., and Leifer, B.: Suicide and family disorganization, Int J Soc Psychiat 12:187-191, 1966.

Tune, G. S.: Sleep and wakefulness in 509 normal human adults, Brit J Med Psychol 42:75-80, 1969.

Tyler, D. B.: Psychological changes during experimental sleep deprivation, Dis Nerv Syst 16:293-299, 1955.

Venables, P. H.: Input dysfunction in schizophrenia, in Maher, B. A., ed.: Progress in Experimental Personality Research, vol. 1, New York: Acad Press, 1964.

Vital Statistics—Special Reports: Suicide-Death rates for selected causes by age, color, and sex: United States and each state, 1949-51, vol. 49, no. 61, US Dept HEW, Natl Office of Vital Statistics, 1959.

Walsh, D.: Social class and mental illness in Dublin, Brit J Psychiat 115:1151-1161, 1969.

Walter, W. G.: Where vital things happen, Amer J Psychiat 116:673-694, 1960.

Walton, H. J.: Suicidal behaviour in depressive illness: A study of aetiological factors in suicide, Brit J Psychiat 104:884-891, 1958.

Watkins, C., Gilbert, J. E., and Bass, W.: Persistent suicidal patient, Amer J Psychiat 125:1590-1593, 1969.

Webb, W. B., and Stone, W.: A note on the sleep responses of young college adults, Percept Motor Skills 16:162, 1963.

Weiss, H. R., Kasinoff, B. H., and Bailey, M. A.: An exploration of reported sleep disturbance, J Nerv Ment Dis 134:528-534, 1962.

Whitaker, C. A., and Miller, M. H.: Re-evaluation of "Psychic Help" when divorce impends, Amer J Psychiat 126:611-618, 1969.

Wilkins, J.: Suicidal behavior, Amer Sociol Rev 32:286-298, 1967.

Williams, H. L., Lubin, A., and Goodnow, J. J.: Impaired performance with acute sleep loss, Psychol Monogr 73:1-26, 1959.

Williams, H. L., et al.: Responses to auditory stimulation, sleep loss and EEG stages of sleep, Electroenceph Clin Neurophysiol 16:269-279, 1964.

Wilson, G. C.: Suicide in psychiatric patients who have received hospital treatment, Amer J Psychiat 125:752-757, 1968.

Wolff, P. H.: "Critical periods" in human cognitive development, Hosp Pract 5:77-87 (No. 11), 1970.

Zung, W. W. K.: A self-rating depression scale, Arch Gen Psychiat (Chicago) 12:63-70, 1965.

Zung, W. W. K., Wilson, W. P., and Dodson, W. E.: Effect of depressive disorders on sleep EEG responses, Arch Gen Psychiat (Chicago) 10:439-445, 1964.

Zusman, J.: Sociology and mental illness: Some neglected implications for treatment, Arch Gen Psychiat (Chicago) 15:635-648, 1966.

CHAPTER TWO

Examination, Disposition, and Management

THE INITIAL EVALUATION

THE PSYCHIATRIC INTERVIEW

CENTRAL TO THE COMPREHENSIVE DIAGNOSTIC STUDY are a chronological review of the present illness, an evaluation of the patient's current physical and mental status, and a history of past medical and psychiatric illness in both patient and family. To be of value, a history of the present illness must focus not only on the patient's symptoms but on the manner and rapidity of their development. Just when did the patient last feel "like himself"? What were his earliest symptoms, and how quickly did these evolve into the current ones? And what event, if any, constituted "the last straw"—that finally impelled the patient or his family to seek medical attention (Smith 1963, Whitmer, 1959)?

If the patient has a *previous psychiatric history*, a detailed description of his earlier symptoms and treatment should be obtained. This information is often of diagnostic, prognostic, and therapeutic import, particularly in phobic neuroses, depressive syndromes, schizophrenias, and other illnesses that have a recurring or cyclical course. It is important to ask whether there is a *family history of psychiatric disorder*, but the facts may be hard to come by. The stigma attached to mental illness may prevent both patient and family from knowing the truth or, if they know it, from talking about it. Affirmative answers must also be interpreted with caution, for almost anyone with a large enough family will have had some mentally-ill relative. Even though too little is known of the genetic aspects of mental illness to permit drawing a meaningful conclusion in the individual case, it is established that certain illnesses occur more frequently among relatives of patients with like disorders than in the general population, and the incidence increases with the closeness of the kinship (Essen-Möller 1955, 1963, Kallman 1959,

Parker 1964, Perris 1966, Rainer 1966, Reich 1969, Shields 1962, Winokur 1965). Such information can be of value even in disorders without a clearly established genetic basis. Learning that an anxious or phobic patient's mother or sister had once suffered a depression and that it had been relieved by a particular antidepressant might not only provide the clinician with an additional impetus to administer an antidepressant, but might even suggest the one to try first.

In Chapter 1, we stressed the importance of obtaining clear information about the patient's biologic and social functioning. In gathering the *biologic* data, special attention is paid to sleep, appetite, energy level, and sexual interest and activity. In learning about the patient's *social functioning,* all aspects—interpersonal, familial, and occupational—must be explored. The simplest approach is often the most fruitful: the patient is first asked to describe his previous day in detail, and only then asked more specific questions concerning each of the areas in question.

TABLE 3. *Sleep Questionnaire*

1. How do you usually sleep? Have you noticed any recent changes in your sleep? If so, what kind? Since when?

2. At what time do you go to bed nowadays? Is this earlier than it used to be? Later? If so, since when has this been happening?

3. How long does it take you to fall asleep once you get to bed? Has it always taken that long? If not, since when has this been happening?

4. Do you awaken during the night? If so, how often and at what time(s)? More in the beginning of the night or more toward morning? How long do you stay awake? When did you last sleep through the whole night?

5. At what time do you have to get up in the morning? What time do you usually wake up? How do you feel when you awaken? Do you know right away that you're no longer asleep? Do you get out of bed as soon as you wake up? Is this pattern the way it's always been? If not, how was it before and when did it change?

6. Do you take naps during the day? How long? How often? Is this your usual pattern? If not, when did this change?

7. Do you dream? If so, how often? Is this the same as it's always been? If not, when did it change?

8. What do you dream about? Do you dream about people or events of the present or of the past? Do you have nightmares? How often? Do you ever confuse your dreams with your waking state? Is all of this your usual pattern? If not, when did it change?

9. Do you take anything to help you sleep? If so, what? Since when? Do you take any alcohol between dinner and bedtime? Have you always? If not, since when have you done so? Have you needed more alcohol or medication to help you sleep recently? Since when?

10. What time did you go to bed last night? Did you take anything to help you sleep? How long did it take you to fall asleep? Did you wake up during the night? At what time(s)? How long did it take you to fall asleep again? At what time did you awaken this morning? Did you get right up? If not, at what time did you get up? Did you dream last night? What about? Was it pleasant? Did you take a nap today? If so, at what time(s)? For how long?

Questions about the patient's *sleep* should be as precise as possible (see Table 3). At what time did he use to go to bed, fall asleep, and arise in the morning, and at what time does he do so now? Did he and does he now awaken during the night? Did he and does he dream, and if so, what about? How and over what period of time did any of these factors change? Questions of this kind will elicit more data than a vague "Have you had trouble sleeping?" particularly because most people fail to report disturbances that they consider minor or think they understand. The clinician should not be misled, however, by the patient's explanations for sleep changes. He may, for example, attribute difficulty in falling asleep to a newly developed desire to watch the "Late Late Show" on television or to read novels in bed; or believe that his nocturnal awakening is caused by "noise in the street," or "getting hungry during the night," when it is in fact symptomatic of his illness. Patients who have just had an operation or given birth may believe that their sleep difficulties arise from the "new routine" of the hospital, postoperative pain, or "getting up to feed the baby." That these explanations are often given in good faith by patients whose streets have become no noisier and whose babies slumber in peace highlights the all-too-human tendency to explain puzzling or troubling events in a reasonable way. Such rationalizing may reassure the patient at the price of confusing the physician, for the person who overlooks or rationalizes his sleep difficulty will in all likelihood be unable to tell just when it first appeared. Thorough questioning will often reveal that his sleep was disturbed long before he developed what he views as his earliest symptoms; in some cases, even before the events to which he attributes his illness.

INITIAL INTERVIEW WITH THE FAMILY

Family interviews are indicated when the patient is too disturbed or retarded to provide a clear history or there is some other reason to question the reliability of his report. They are also useful when the patient denies or does not recognize that he needs psychiatric attention, for without such discussions, one may be unable to determine just why he has come. Relatives often ask to speak with the doctor alone, but rarely object to joint interviews once they understand that excluding the patient can disturb his relationship to the doctor, whereas frank discussion in his presence is unlikely to harm him. The relatives' opinions on *why* the patient became ill may be of less importance at this point than their account of his social behavior and the development of his symptoms. Even when the patient is coherent and candid, the comments of those who live with him are likely to broaden the clinician's understanding of his symptoms.

Both the tone and the content of such meetings can be used to obtain an overview of the family's interactional pattern. The way they address themselves to the issues that arise and their modes of relating to each other and making decisions can help the therapist to gauge their ability and preparedness to offer the patient emotional support and to collaborate in his treatment. Who decided that the consultation was needed? Who initiated contact with the psychiatrist? Was the family doctor involved? How was the decision communicated to the others? If the patient did not make the decision, how was he informed of it? Who expects to assume the financial responsibility? Who opens the discussion and how? Who waits for permission before speaking frankly, and who gives it? How ready are the family members to air their "secrets" before a stranger or even before each other? Who becomes uncomfortable when candid talk is required? Who interrupts whom, and who keeps quiet when interrupted? How much do the family members trust each other, and how much do they trust the doctor? Which of them elicit the therapist's trust and empathy? The answers to these questions may well highlight major problem areas, but it is important that the clinician refrain from commenting on family dynamics. The purpose of the first interview is to obtain information—not to advise, criticize, or interpret. The physician who ignores this rule is more likely to compound than relieve the family's guilt and anxiety (Fleck 1963) and will thus have a harder time finding out what is really going on.

When information about the patient's occupational functioning is required, it is often useful to ask the patient for his permission to speak with his employer. Here the physician can learn how well or how poorly the patient completes his tasks, how this compares with the past, how he reacts to his work, fellow employees, and supervisor, and in what way the work situation is likely to be either stressful or supportive. Discretion is required in deciding whom and what to ask, however, for an excessively broad inquiry may adversely affect the patient's future employability and social acceptability.

How much the physician is likely to learn in the interview situation depends largely on the transactional climate he creates. Patients are generally accustomed to having their doctors ask direct questions, and the more matter-of-fact the inquiries are, the easier they will be to answer. Naturally, if a patient is unusually timid or reluctant, he may first need to be put at ease by tactfully phrased, indirect, or hypothetical questions, and it may even be necessary to steer him away from especially troubling areas, but eventually his ability to discuss even embarrassing material must be put to the test.

The process of data-gathering elicits more than "facts": it offers valuable insights into the patient's and family's transactional modes and provides the interviewer with an opportunity to develop some feelings of his own about them. By exploring these further, the physician will broaden his understanding of the setting in which the illness takes place and the role that the patient and family expect him to play. In this manner he develops a "feel" for the patient that, despite its indefinableness, is as crucial in psychiatry as in any medical specialty and distinguishes the talented craftsman from the competent technician.

Other Sources of Information

A complete evaluation may require certain specialized tests and techniques. A *psychological examination* may help in gauging such variables as intellectual functioning, depression, impulse control, and fantasy material, but the tests available have numerous limitations, and their accuracy and applicability depend largely on the competence and training of the individual who administers them. Such tests are of greatest value when sequential measures of intellectual competence or impairment are required, as in the case of the patient suffering from a brain disease that proceeds so slowly that it might otherwise be imperceptible (Gilbert 1969). Organic brain syndromes, moreover, tend to resemble or mesh with retarded depressions; thus a baseline measure of the patient's intellectual and affective status is necessary in order to judge his further course (see p. 404). Tests for comparing a child's development with that of his peers may also be valuable (see Chap. 10).

The value of psychological tests does not lie in the findings alone, however. That such tests are popularly believed to be "objective" causes patients and families to accept recommendations based on them, when they would reject an "unsubstantiated" impression. Those that purport to measure an individual's intellectual capacity may help dissuade him or, more frequently, his relatives from unrealistic expectations. An "objective" assessment of the potential hazards may even serve to reassure the physician, as in the case of the sullen, rebellious adolescent whose symptoms may look like manifestations of an antisocial personality but whose tests indicate that he is suffering from a depression, or in the case of other potentially impulsive patients who insist on having outpatient care. An additional value of psychological tests is that patients who are uncommunicative or consider their fantasies objectionable will sometimes express their forbidden thoughts more easily within the structured, formal framework of testing than in the clinical interview. The test situation thus serves as a useful aid in communication, for it permits and even encourages projection and allows the patient to believe, if he so chooses, that his underlying affective state is not being explored. The traditional test situation, moreover, does not demand the kind of informal interpersonal encounter that only fosters anxiety and odd, inappropriate behavior in socially awkward patients. It can thus be used to measure optimal intellectual performance in a way that would otherwise be impossible. In some situations, however, it is desirable to measure the patient's performance under stress or unusual circumstances. *Interview techniques,* in which the patient is placed under psychological stress or given a stimulant, sedative, or hallucinogen (see Chap. 16), for example, can unveil disorders of impulse, mood, or thought that would otherwise be hard to discern.

The importance of a thorough knowledge of the patient's current *medical status* and past *medical history* is underscored by the ubiquitous imprecision of psychiatric diagnoses (Herridge 1960). As we have emphasized, no psychological symptom, either alone or in combination with others, is pathognomonic of any particular mental illness. Physical illnesses and their treatment may lead to mental symptoms (Maguire 1968; see Table 4), and patients with mental disorders may complain only of physical symptoms. Since the very concept of a distinction between physical and mental illness is but a crude convenience for classification, a treatment-oriented diagnostic workup cannot operate on the assumption that it is ever possible to tell whether the patient's symptoms are "organic" or "functional." Above all, it must always be kept in mind that a psychiatric illness and its treatment can affect and be affected by the patient's physical condition (Johnson 1968).

TABLE 4. *Some Syndromes with Demonstrable Organic Findings in Which Anxiety Attacks May Occur*

Cerebral arteriosclerosis	Hyperthyroidism
Cocaine and amphetamine abuse	Paroxysmal tachycardia
Coronary insufficiency	Pheochromocytoma
Hyperinsulinism	Psychomotor epilepsy
Withdrawal from CNS depressants	

In the course of the examination, the patient should be asked routinely whether he is taking *medications,* and if so, what kind, for what reason, for how long a period of time, and who prescribed them. If the patient takes narcotics, sedatives, or alcohol, it is important to find out whether this started before or only after he fell ill. Surprisingly, the patient often has no idea what he is taking, having simply asked his family doctor for "something for sleep" or used a friend's or relative's leftover medication; in such cases the physician should talk to the prescribing physician or dispensing pharmacist or, if this is of no avail, ask to inspect the drug in question. Women should be asked when their *last menstrual period* occurred, both because knowing that a patient is premenstrual at the time of the initial examination helps put her symptoms into clearer perspective and because many disorders first appear at the time of the menopause.

Some years hence, the value of the *electroencephalogram* may become so firmly established that it will be a routine part of every initial examination. At present, however, the expense of this examination, the difficulty in arranging it, and the scarcity of experts to evaluate it restrict its use to patients with a known or suspected organic brain syndrome (Table 5). Occasionally, a concealed or in-

TABLE 5. *Some Indications for* EEG *Study*

Seizures	Fainting spells
Prior history of EEG abnormalities	Intellectual performance inconsistent
Brief and intermittent symptoms of almost any kind	with previous achievement
	Frequent or persistent headache
Lapses in awareness	Visual hallucinations
Confusional episodes, especially in the evening or when watching television	Enuresis or encopresis

significant EEG abnormality can be clarified by the use of repeated examinations, nonstandard leads, or activation techniques, such as hyperventilation, sleep, photic stimulation, or the administration of drugs (see Chap. 11).

In addition to the laboratory studies required to complete the diagnostic workup, a special group of tests and examinations should be ordered when somatic treatment is being considered. A hematocrit, white blood count and differential, alkaline phosphatase, serum glutamic oxaloacetic transaminase (SGOT), and (especially in older people) an electrocardiogram should be obtained routinely before treatment begins in order to safeguard the patient against unnoticed and unchecked hematologic, hepatic, and cardiac complications. If abnormal findings are obtained only *after* a patient has been given a drug and there are no baseline values with which to compare them, it may be impossible to assess their significance or to determine whether the risk of continued administration is greater than that of discontinuing drug treatment and thereby jeopardizing the patient's recovery.

Much of the necessary information regarding the patient's past and present medical condition can be obtained from his *family doctor*. Patients rarely object to collaboration of this kind and indeed often turn to their family doctors for additional advice or support, even while seeing a psychiatrist. The more information the family doctor is given, the better equipped he will be to reassure the patient about his condition, to support the psychiatrist's recommendations, and to call attention to medical and psychosocial factors that may not have been considered in the initial assessment. Parenthetically, we might note that such communication, a rule in all other medical specialties, has the additional advantage of helping bridge the gap that psychiatry's long-standing devotion to secrecy and arcane ritual has created between itself and the general medical community (Garber 1963).

DISPOSITION

If the initial examination reveals that treatment is indicated, the next step is to decide what kind it should be, who should provide it, and where. If the examining physician is not a psychiatrist, he must choose between referring the patient to a psychiatrist and managing the patient's care by himself, possibly with a psychiatrist's assistance. Since the advent of the newer psychopharmacologic agents, more and more physicians in other specialties are providing ambulatory psychiatric treatment. Some offer their patients nothing beyond psychotropic agents; others provide them with psychotherapy; while still others direct the patient's drug treatment, but delegate the psychotherapeutic aspect of treatment to a nonmedical therapist or a specialized community agency. Such plans are often successful as many patients accept, and some even prefer, having their treatment directed by their family physician.

Whether or not the doctor is a psychiatrist, he should offer his services only on his own terms and refuse compromises that might undermine the establishment of a proper treatment relationship. If, for example, a family doctor feels that a psychiatric consultation is mandatory, but the patient or family simply refuses, he should not allow himself to be coerced into taking on more responsibility than he considers prudent. Tact, skill, and perseverance will usually overcome the family's reluctance; when, however, the patient's condition is too critical to permit protracted attempts at persuasion, as in the case of patients with destructive or suicidal tendencies, the family doctor must explain that he does not plan to abandon the patient, but will limit his services to making arrangements for specialized treatment.

THE "SPECIAL" CASE

The psychiatrist, too, may be subjected to coercion and may need to be equally firm. This approach is especially relevant when he is asked to treat a socially prominent community member or a professional colleague (Franklin 1965). Without close self-scrutiny, the therapist may become paralyzed, either because he identifies with the patient or because he is afraid of making an error that would reflect on his competence or endanger his professional reputation. Naturally, the more bizarre the symptoms and the more overtly they are displayed, the less likely the therapist is to identify with the patient and the easier it is for him to be firm (Alexander 1954).

All too often, the therapist is asked to engage in a corrupt contract. The family may ask to have the examination take place without the patient's knowledge in such an unlikely or unprofessional setting as a cocktail or dinner party. The patient may want to swear the psychiatrist to secrecy about such threatening issues as suicide plans. If hospitalization is needed, he or his family may try to mitigate the ensuing social embarrassment by asking that it take place in another city or state. This request alone is understandable and need not be denied, but it is often coupled with the request that the local psychiatrist or family doctor remain in charge, and this is impossible without interfering with the work of the physician who has the actual responsibility for the patient's care. Physicians, especially, are apt to make unusual requests or ignore their professional training when it comes to the illness of a family member. Most psychiatrists are familiar with that uncomfortable situation in which a colleague asks for advice about someone who is identified only as an "interesting patient," but turns out to be the questioner's own wife or child. The treatment of physicians or their families is further complicated and in some ways corrupted by their tendency to "adjust" the dosage or substitute an "equivalent" drug. In an emergency, they may even refrain from calling the psychiatrist as

TABLE 6. *75 Consecutive "Chief Complaints" as Transcribed by Psychiatrists in a General Hospital Emergency Room*

Drunk, fighting with police.

Confusion.

Nervous, delusional, voices.

"I felt tired and sad all the time."

"My husband is no good."

Swallowed a number of Seconal capsules.

"Detectives are tailing me and have put waves over my head." Has been drinking heavily.

Pain in the head, nervous, mixed up.

"I am nervous, and I'm afraid; sometimes I don't know where I am or who I am."

Dizziness, "stomach pain."

Drinking, nervous, seeing ants.

Can't stop drinking, depressed, suicide 'gesture.'

"Forgetful, losing my sight, nervous."

Lightheaded, nervous.

"I can no longer go on. I'm depressed and nervous."

Can't manage her anymore.

Depression.

Repeated attempted suicide today.

Temper tantrums, breaking furniture, threatening grandmother.

Attacks of weakness, nervousness, chest pain.

Depression, attempted to gas himself.

"I can't breathe and my heart skips."

"I want a rest."

"I am going to kill myself."

Hearing voices, suspicious.

Threatened to kill himself.

Pain in heart.

"My heart beats too fast."

"Something is wrong with my son in California."

"I can't work and my state unemployment funds are running out."

Tension, trouble controlling anger.

"Spell"—paralysis of legs.

Deep slashes on both wrists; a man failed to phone her; drinking.

Feeling tired and strange.

Hearing voices—anxious.

"My legs are weak and I am upset."

Brought in by force by parents after throwing dishes.

Delusional and disorganized.

Blackouts—dizzy spells.

Wife is concerned that he might harm her.

Hears voices that want to take away her "illegal" baby.

Tried to kill his sister and himself.

Recent seizure, dizzy.

Fear of killing brother-in-law.

Wants prescription for medication.

Has been hearing voices, says house is wired, and has been violent.

Attacks of difficulty in breathing.

Nervousness and fear of a nervous breakdown.

Pain in throat and difficulty with breathing.

Drinking excessively, unpleasant toward family.

Upset because his wife is leaving him.

Inability to speak.

"My son no like me any more."

"I have chest pains."

"I want to stop my pregnancy and maybe kill myself."

"I was spasming again."

Blackout spell.

Difficulty breathing.

Abdominal pain.

"Am I crazy or not?"

"What different buildings you all have here in Ireland."

"Who am I?"

"I'd like to know if I can work."

"I'm scared."

Dizziness, pains in shoulder, difficulty in sleeping.

"I'm lonesome."

"Can I go to work?"

Fear of blackouts.

"People are putting things in my mind."

"I need psychiatric help, but don't want it." Quit school.

"I need help. I've been drinking."

Feels faint, can't sleep, sees bugs, can't control bladder.

Tried to hang herself while drunk.

"They are trying to kill me."

"Everything I do turns out wrong."

---

instructed because they "understand" the pressures under which "we doctors" operate.

In such situations, the flexibility that is usually helpful in a therapeutic relationship may in actuality be harmful. Accordingly, it is wise to give instructions that are so precise as to allow little room for maneuvering or independent action. All prescriptions should be in writing and should be filled by a pharmacist rather than from samples. If consultation with another psychiatrist seems advisable, it should be initiated by the physician in charge or in any case discussed with him in advance: informal consultations, in which another physician is asked to "just take a look" at the patient, should be discouraged. If the patient or family ignore these instructions, the psychiatrist should inform them that he will interpret further behavior of this kind to mean that they are dissatisfied with him and are asking him to withdraw from the case.

The Psychiatric Emergency

When the patient's clinical condition is so severe that immediate treatment is mandatory, the niceties of evaluation become irrelevant. Among the most common psychiatric emergencies are *1/* alcoholic intoxication, *2/* acute schizophrenic episode, *3/* psychotic depression, and *4/* acute situational reaction expressed either in histrionic behavior or in anxiety (Errera 1963). Table 6, which lists the complaints heard by psychiatrists in a general hospital emergency room over a one-month period (Jarecki: unpublished data), illustrates how varied the patient's, the family's, or the community's complaints may be and how frequently the request for treatment is made by someone acting on the patient's behalf.

Families rarely consult a physician or an outside agency on an emergency basis unless the patient's behavior frightens or embarrasses them. For example, if an alcoholic habitually becomes violent while drinking, his family is likely to be used to such episodes and unlikely to ask for medical assistance. If, however, the same individual calmly states that he is being persecuted by Russian spies, his family might well become fearful enough to ask for help. Once family members become frightened, they react to the patient in a way that intensifies all his own fears of becoming "crazy," so that he feels and acts even worse. By the time the patient is seen, his family may be asking for more than his treatment: they may want him removed from their midst (Langsley 1968). The more chaotic or protracted the situation, the more likely it is that the physician will be confronted with the double challenge of establishing a relationship between himself and the patient and of reestablishing communication between the patient and his family.

The physician's role in an emergency is above all to ensure safety for all concerned. Sometimes this may entail simply keeping the patient under observation, with or without medication, until his most acute symptoms subside; at other times, hospitalization will be called for. When the patient's condition is grave and all efforts to reason with him have failed, it may become necessary to give him medications in order to implement any decisions for his disposition and treatment.

THE TREATMENT SETTING

If the situation requires that the patient's environment be changed, numerous alternatives are possible: full-time hospitalization, day or night hospitalization, or placement in a halfway house, foster home, or residential treatment setting. The patient may be advised to stay home from work, work outside the home, take a vacation, visit relatives, have a relative stay with him, or engage a full-time or visiting nurse or homemaker. Whenever there is any question about the patient's judgment or his ability to control his impulses, obligations to the patient must be balanced against those to the family and the community. Two decades ago, when security-oriented hospitalization was the rule, these obligations could be met simultaneously. Since then it has become more common to treat patients at home, in general hospitals, and in open wards; and the desire to treat patients humanely often takes precedence over considerations of security. This advance is not without its pitfalls, for the less carefully a patient is supervised, the more opportunity he will have to attempt suicide or behave impulsively in other ways (Lewis 1962). Thus the desire to unfetter the patient must be coupled with more careful attention to his potential impulsivity: the physician must make himself more available to the patient and his family and be willing and prepared to act quickly when necessary.

Since more liberal custodial practices may increase the incidence of malpractice suits, it is fortunate that the courts have increasingly come to understand that the short-term risks of carefully weighed outpatient treatment are more than counterbalanced by the long-term disadvantages of routine custodial care, and that hospitalizing a patient offers no guarantee against suicide (Perr 1965). Legal immunity does not, however, ease the psychiatrist's constant dilemma: hospitalizing a patient disrupts his day-to-day activities, reputation, self-image, and self-reliance, while failing to hospitalize him may endanger either his life or that of others.

Outpatient Care

Since illness constricts an individual's freedom and one of the major goals of treatment is to increase a patient's ability to govern his life, outpatient care is preferable whenever it does not endanger his life, health or reputation, or the continuity and adequacy of his medical care. In general, even if he is experiencing considerable subjective discomfort, a patient may be considered a good candidate for outpatient care if he functions with reasonable social effectiveness; sleeps at least five or six hours a night; eats enough to prevent major weight loss; shows no indications of severe perceptual disturbances, delusional thinking, or suicidal preoccupation; understands the physician's recommendations and is able and willing to follow them. Some of these criteria may be superfluous when the patient's family is able to provide sufficient supervision during the critical period, or when he can be seen by the physician or even by a visiting nurse every day. Not all patients who meet these criteria should be treated as outpatients, however, for some require treatment programs so specialized or complex that a hospital setting is needed to carry them out. Outpatient treatment, in any case, is an experiment, not a commitment: if the patient's condition deteriorates, his collaboration proves insufficient, or his safety is for any other reason in doubt, hospitalization may still become necessary.

Hospitalization

When the patient is too ill to care for himself and has neither relatives nor friends who can supervise him, help implement the medical recommendations, and provide the information the physician needs to evaluate his condition, hospitalization is inevitable. In addition, when a patient has been ill for so long that both he and his relatives are exhausted, hospitalization is usually the most humane course for all concerned. If he is unable to satisfy even the minimal requirements of family life or feels guilty about the difficulties he causes those around him, he is likely to find hospitalization a welcome relief. Other purposes of hospitalization are listed in Table 7.

If full-time psychiatric hospitalization is required, three alternatives may be considered: public mental hospitals, general hospitals, and private psychiatric hospitals. In recent years, comprehensive community mental health centers, which may combine the features of all three, have also become available in many localities (APA 1964, Knight 1964, Redlich 1966). The current fashion of heaping opprobrium on the *public mental hospital* is often misplaced. In-

TABLE 7. *The Purposes of Hospitalization*

1. Protective-custodial
   a. Safeguarding the patient's life and reputation
   b. Safeguarding the community from the patient's behavior
   c. Removing the patient from a noxious environment

2. Diagnostic
   a. Closer observation
   b. Availability of specialized procedures

3. Therapeutic
   a. Motivation of the patient and family to
      (1) accept and support therapy
      (2) make necessary life changes
   b. Pharmacotherapy
      (1) Administration of medication schedules too complex to be carried out at home
      (2) Rapid initiation of potentially toxic medication schedules that require careful observation
      (3) Assurance that confused or uncooperative patients take the prescribed medications
   c. Social-familial
      (1) Social rehabilitation, group therapy meetings, group living experience, exposure to therapeutic community, assumption of social responsibilities in hospital setting
      (2) Relief of intrafamilial tensions so that exploration of critical relationships and issues can proceed without emergence of family crises
   d. Special therapy not possible outside the hospital (convulsive or prolonged sleep treatments or even concomitant observation and treatment of the patient and key relative or relatives)

creasingly, these facilities are being modernized, decentralized, and adequately staffed. Even when operated in the more traditional manner, however, the public mental hospital may not be so harmful as it is often painted. If the patient requires a good deal of environmental structure, is unable to tolerate too insistent a demand that he get well, or is suffering from an illness that is either so advanced or so self-limited that the therapeutic setting is of little moment, it may be as good as, or even better than, other facilities. Furthermore, when the family's economic means are limited, the physician must decide whether the potential advantages of a private or general hospital outweigh the resultant financial hardship. At times, the expense of hospitalization becomes just one additional obstacle in the way of the patient's rehabilitation and remains so long after his discharge.

The use of *psychiatric wards in general hospitals* has markedly increased as private and public health insurance plans have started to recognize the economic feasibility of short-term hospitalization for mental illnesses (Avnet 1962, Blue Cross 1964, 1965). Such facilities are of particular value when a medical illness complicates diagnosis or treatment, and (like the community mental health center) usually have the further advantage of being close to the patient's home. This proximity makes it possible for his friends and family to visit him frequently, thereby decreasing his social isolation and permitting him to maintain what ties he had before falling ill. It makes it easier for the physican to hold family meetings at regular intervals and enables the patient to visit his home or resume his work before leaving the hospital for good. Such trial visits are especially useful in planning discharge, for they make it possible to monitor and assess any difficulties the patient may encounter on returning to his former surroundings. Further in favor of the general hospital is that it is more likely to be viewed as an "old friend," free of the stigma attached to the traditional mental hospital. In this climate, there is less resistance to the recommendation of hospital care, referrals are more prompt, illnesses are detected earlier, catastrophic emergencies can be avoided, and patients can be readmitted before serious relapses occur (Detre 1963).

Private psychiatric hospitals usually have a far higher ratio of staff to patients than the public mental hospitals and can provide certain comforts unobtainable elsewhere. Those oriented toward a particular type of program, such as the long-term treatment of adolescents or the withdrawal of drugs or alcohol, may have unique advantages in the individual case.

Even under the most ideal conditions, psychiatric hospitalization has many *disadvantages*. Although its impact alone can sometimes persuade a patient to take his illness more seriously, it is also likely to tarnish his self-image and obstruct his ability to regain self-confidence. Efforts to minimize or ignore the stigma attached to psychiatric hospitalization have not erased it: it remains a reality that affects not only the patient's view of himself but also his educational and occupational prospects, and can compromise his family and community position. In addition, the values and norms of a mental hospital's subculture are so unusual that extended exposure to them often impairs the patient's ability to understand or relate to the outside world. In many mental hospitals, a "cult of psyche" prevails; extensive introspection is the order of the day; and discussions that focus on the participants' symptoms and untutored interpretations replace conventional social intercourse. Such a milieu, in which deviant social patterns are the norm, can hinder an individual's extramural adjustment (Talbot 1964). After months or years of frankly discussing sexual interests and practices, marital problems, and unhappy childhood memories with fellow patients, the individual may find it difficult to adjust to a world in which such topics are avoided rather than emphasized. Furthermore, since hospitalization can teach a receptive patient what threats and symptoms are most likely to require readmission, it entails the danger of promoting a life pattern in which repeated confinements are used to escape uncomfortable situations and secure a vacation from everyday stresses.

Many of the illnesses that arise in the larger community cannot be treated optimally in the regressive vacuum of a full-time hospital. When the patient's condition may benefit from the reestablishment of traditional social contact or his family is available only part-time, it may be preferable to utilize a *day hospital,* which provides organized activities and medical supervision during the day, but permits the patient to return home every evening, or a *night hospital,* which provides medical supervision and a respite from nocturnal discomfort, isolation, or loneliness, but permits the patient to leave during the day to pursue school, work, or home activities (Moll 1961, Odenheimer 1965). When family contact or some equivalent support is needed, it may be advantageous to place the patient in a foster home or to involve his family in a home care program (Pasamanick 1964). When the development of competence in peer-group relationships seems a paramount treatment issue, halfway houses (Clark 1960, Huseth 1961, Raush 1968), boarding schools, or —when the patient's condition requires even closer supervision—residential treatment settings may be indicated (Fleck 1962).

TREATMENT PLANNING

Psychotherapy or Somatic Therapy?

As in all medical illnesses, the choice of the treatment plan should be based on what is known of the speed, effectiveness, durability, safety, and feasibility of a given treatment in a given illness (APA 1967). Many clinicians believe that the major choice is between psychotherapy or somatic therapy, but there is no evidence that either of the two schismatized modalities is superior in all illnesses (Heilbrunn 1964). Moreover, since most illnesses are of unclear etiology, are multidetermined, and have multiple consequences, it is usually inefficient to rely on any one treatment form alone (Fessel 1964). A combination of treatment programs is thus preferable in most cases, and it may even be necessary to use several kinds of psychotherapy or somatic therapy together. A general rule for determining the best combination may be derived from the principles outlined in Chapter 1: the nature of the precipitating event, the patient's premorbid functioning, and his transactions with the doctor will reflect his deficiencies in social skills and suggest what kind of psychotherapy is indicated, whereas the length and magnitude of his stress response will suggest the nature and amount of somatic treatment required.

Psychotherapy as such does not refer to any specific way of interacting with a patient. It is a generic term that covers a multitude of activities and relationships. Used broadly, it includes all contact between patient and therapist intended to be helpful to the patient's psychological functioning. In this sense, "the only doctor who can continue his work without using some form of psychotherapy is the one who confines himself to the study of the dead" (Hopkins 1956). The choice, then, of whether to administer somatic therapies *or* psychotherapy is artificial: the only real treatment possibilities are psychotherapy *with* or psychotherapy *without* concomitant somatic therapies. It is generally agreed that the length, frequency, setting, or content of the interviews, the duration of the entire treatment process, and the concurrent use or avoidance of somatic therapies affect the prognosis, but there is little agreement on how best to combine these factors in any given situation. Since there are no controlled studies concerning this question, most physicians choose the ingredients of the psychotherapeutic encounter by relying on one or another of the numerous theoretical frameworks, making whatever modifications their personal experiences have led them to adopt. A further discussion of these issues may be found in Chapter 13.

Psychotherapy alone may suffice for the "minor" psychiatric syndromes, by which we mean disorders in which

1/ the patient's troubled feelings are a greater source of difficulty than his aberrant behavior;

2/ his aberrant behavior, when it exists, either excludes destructive or self-damaging acts or is limited to indirect or symbolic expression of these;

3/ he retains an adequate level of social functioning, even in the face of considerable subjective discomfort;

4/ his comfort and his adaptation to his disabilities is likely to be enhanced by an exploration of the nature, meaning, and roots of his life style and characteristic responses to psychological stress; and

5/ his symptoms are unlikely to respond to any somatic therapy.

In the "major" psychiatric syndromes, however, it is usually necessary to offer a combination of *psychotherapy and somatic therapy*,
the term "major" serving to distinguish disorders in which

> 1/ the patient's discomfort or social dysfunctioning is so massive
> that his pursuit of life goals is at a total standstill;
> 2/ his behavior is or appears likely to become overtly destructive
> toward himself or others; or
> 3/ his psychological problems are coupled with severe distur-
> bances of sleep, appetite, or other biologic functions.

Psychotherapeutic interventions in the major syndromes should include such supportive measures as advising the patient about work,
assisting him with his life plans, and teaching him what he needs to
know about his illness. Since an individual who has suffered from a
cognitive or affective disturbance for some time is likely to have experienced profound and deleterious changes in his life outlook and
adaptive mechanisms, exploratory or reconstructive psychotherapy is
often valuable; but it should not be initiated until the acute symptoms subside. The more severe the patient's distress, the more likely
he is to find the traditional insight-oriented psychotherapeutic relationship alien and irrelevant to his immediate needs. He may
misunderstand it entirely, worry about what is "expected" of him,
believe that excessive demands are being made on him, or feel
guilty that he is not "producing" adequately.

In many ways, somatic therapy can substantially aid the psychotherapeutic relationship (Grinspoon 1961). By relieving some of
the patient's symptoms, it permits him to develop confidence in
the physician, to concentrate on something beyond his most immediate symptoms, and to discuss anxiety-provoking issues, thus
facilitating the establishment of a straightforward, informative, and
meaningful doctor-patient relationship. If, for example, a patient
reacts to the loss of an important friend by becoming agitated, retarded, or suspicious, his symptoms may place him beyond the reach
of psychotherapeutic help. The intensity of his grief may well stem
from the fact that the current loss recapitulates a bereavement he
sustained during his childhood, but such roots will probably remain
hidden until he is comfortable enough to engage in an exploration
of his feelings. Similarly, if a psychiatric illness has caused a patient
to withdraw from social contact for so long a time that he has
become socially inept, the social stimulation and retraining that his
rehabilitation requires will be of little benefit until his underlying

illness has been modified by somatic therapies. Indeed, our estimate of the patient's accessibility to psychotherapy is a key factor in our decisions about the use, nature, and even the dosage of somatic treatment: the less accessible the patient is to a psychotherapeutic relationship, the greater his need for somatic treatment.

The Impact of Attitudes on Treatment

The use and effectiveness of somatic therapies are influenced by the attitudes held by the patient, family, and doctor (Klerman 1963, Sarwer-Foner 1961, Sheard 1963). Some physicians are reluctant to use somatic therapies because they are unfamiliar with them. Others resist out of a deep-seated loyalty to a particular view of the etiology of mental illnesses or to an alternate way of treating them (Detre 1960). Still others doubt the effectiveness of somatic therapies or are unduly apprehensive about their potential dangers. These attitudes, reminiscent of the skepticism that half a century ago greeted the introduction of psychodynamic psychiatry, may greatly affect the outcome of treatment. When the physician couples his doubts with excessive caution, he may set in motion a self-fulfilling prophecy: fearing their toxic effects, he may give drugs in such low doses or for so brief a time that they can have little effect, and his original reservations about their value are "confirmed."

The treatment process is often complicated by the preferences of the patient or his family: some patients want to be given medications or shock treatments and object to psychological explorations of any kind; others prefer or even insist on discussing their life situations at length and strenuously oppose somatic treatment. *Objections to psychological treatment* can stem from many sources: the patient may fear being confronted with real or imagined inadequacies; foresee great distress in having to discuss intimate matters; harbor a generalized distrust of his environment, a specific distrust of the doctor, or both; be fearful of relating his secret thoughts or actions, lest he be censured or urged to change; or feel that his "real" self, revealed, would turn out to be malevolent, weak, or "insane." *Opposition to somatic therapy,* on the other hand, often stems from the wish to deny that the patient is ill. Some patients and families tend to view the prescription of a drug as more convincing confirmation of illness or "insanity" than even the most aberrant behavior and take it as proof that the patient is "incurable" or genetically tainted.

The preference for one form of treatment over another seems in some cases to be almost a moral issue. Quite apart from those who object on religious grounds, some families regard pill-taking as a sign of weakness; others find it acceptable to have a physical illness or to use medications, but disdain any need to talk to someone. The distortions and misinterpretations of the environment that derive from the patient's illness may also color his view of treatment. He may believe that the purpose of a psychotherapeutic discussion is to hypnotize him, make him immoral, or prove that he is to blame; he may believe that a drug is addictive or even poisonous, that his illness is so severe or his depression so well founded that treatment is futile, or that the cost of the treatment will ruin his family.

Discussing his treatment preference with the patient can clarify his attitude toward his illness and his life. Such discussion, which must seek the motives behind the patient's preferences, is often essential before treatment begins, not only because it sheds light on the individual's dynamics, but also because the patient's collaboration can hinge upon its outcome. Nevertheless, the physician alone must make the final decision. Catering to the concerns and preferences of the patient and family may do no more than nourish their difficulty in accepting the idea of treatment and confirm their view that mental illnesses are quite unlike other illnesses and psychiatric therapies unlike other medical treatments.

When treatment is mandatory and the patient is considered incapable of making a rational decision, the doctor and the family must be prepared to ensure proper treatment. If discussion and persuasion do not suffice, hospitalization—even involuntary hospitalization—may be required. A firm posture regarding such decisions is as likely to reassure a patient as it is to offend him. Protracted discussions and bargaining tend only to increase his panic and his distrust of the doctor, especially if he realizes that, even in his disorganized state, he is able to control his physician and prevent him from assuming authority and responsibility.

THE CONTINUATION OF TREATMENT

Throughout the course of treatment, repeated assessments of the patient's condition are required in order to ascertain the effect of the measures employed and to decide when and how they must be modified. The discussion that follows focuses primarily on the evaluation of overall functioning and the management of drug treatment, for these issues permit generalizations applicable to most

TABLE 8. *Patient's Reporting Chart*

Month _____   Name of Patient _____

Day	Sleep (Quality and Hours)	Weight	Appetite	Medications	Menstrual Period (+ or 0)	Mood

THIS CHART SHOULD BE BROUGHT TO THE OFFICE ON EACH VISIT.

TABLE 9. *Instructions for Completing "Patient's Reporting Chart"*

In filling out the "Patient's Reporting Chart," please note the following:

1. Sleep: Write down each morning the quality of the previous night's sleep, that is, "good," "restless," "poor," and note daytime naps as well. In addition, state the hours of sleep. If you went to bed at 9 PM, slept till 3 AM, awakened for 45 minutes and slept until 7 AM, write: 9-3, 3:45-7.

2. Weight: You should weigh yourself each morning before breakfast. A small bathroom scale is satisfactory for this purpose.

3. Appetite: Write "good," "moderate," or "bad," comparing it with your appetite when you are feeling well.

4. Medications: Write in each medication taken each day. You should know the names of the medications you are taking and the dosages. Your druggist has been instructed to write this information on the prescription bottle. You should check to see that he has done so.

5. Menstrual Period: If you are now having a menstrual period, write "+." If not, write "0."

6. Mood: Your mood each day should be recorded. In addition, if you find that it fluctuates or that it is better in the morning, after- noon, or evening, you should mention this.

A sample line might look like this:

Day	Sleep (Quality and Hours)	Weight	Appetite	Medications	Menstrual Period (+ or 0)	Mood
26 *	Restless 10-2 Nightmare 2:30-6:30 Aft. nap 1-3	142	Poor at lunch, better at dinner	Telavon, 50 mg, 9, 2, 9 Aquasil, 5 mg, 10, 4, 8 Silicol, 50 mg, 9 PM	+	Good until sister's visit in AM, crying in afternoon, better at dinnertime

* In this entry, the "Sleep" column refers to the night of the 25-26th and the day of the 26th, while the remaining columns refer to the day of the 26th.

patients. Issues of psychodynamic assessment and psychotherapeutic management vary from case to case and are discussed more fully in Chapter 13.

ONGOING EVALUATION OF OVERALL FUNCTIONING

Patients who are or have been seriously ill or who are taking psychotropic agents must be seen at regular intervals by a physician, even if a nonmedical therapist is conducting the psychotherapeutic aspect of their treatment. Precise reports concerning the patient's *sleep, appetite,* and *mood* must be obtained at each followup interview. To ensure that the patient and his family pay close attention to these factors, we provide a chart on which they are instructed to record their observations (Tables 8 and 9).

If anything about the patient suggests that he may have *aggressive or suicidal impulses,* he should be asked about them directly. Frank questions usually elicit more information than subtle or devious ones. Candid discussions encourage the patient to describe his aggressive or suicidal ideas as alien symptoms that he need not defend, rather than as facets of his self-image. In general, the same may be said for delusions and hallucinations, which, when treated matter-of-factly, are often reported in such terms as: "Here's another one of those strange ideas I keep getting." When a physician inquires about the patient's life situation, he ought not to be satisfied with a statement that "things are going pretty well," but must explore in some detail the patient's *occupational, social, and recreational activities.* Continuing contact with the family or employer may make it possible to assess factors of which the patient may not be fully aware, such as increased psychomotor activity or socially inappropriate behavior. If there is any question about the patient's reliability, it will be useful to have a relative accompany him to the office and spend at least a few minutes talking with the two together.

DRUG MANAGEMENT

Safeguards in Drug Therapy

The difficulties inherent in administering drugs underscore the importance of providing the patient with close personal attention. While the patient is acutely ill, he should be seen several times a week; daily telephone calls are often helpful adjuncts to the office visits. The physician can provide immeasurable psychological sup-

TABLE 10. *Instructions for Treatment*

Name of Patient _____   Date _____

| Day | Medication | | | Hours at which to take medication |
	Name	Dose	Color	

Call me at any time of day or night should *any* questions arise.
☐ Awaken   ☐ Do not awaken patient to give medications after 9 PM
Someone should be with the patient   ☐ at all times   ☐ until _____
☐ Blurring of vision and dryness of mouth   ☐ drowsiness *may* occur.
☐ Fill out chart given you.   ☐ Go to laboratory for ordered tests.

Call me at _____   at _____
                    (time)   (telephone number)

See me again on _____ , _____ 19 ____ at _____

Since you are now taking medications, it is important that you understand their use, as well as the occasional problems that may arise. In the first three or four days of use, you may notice some drowsiness. This will disappear gradually during the first week. A few patients may have other side effects as well, which may include skin rashes, blurred vision, dry mouth, muscle spasms, and restlessness. These side effects are not common or dangerous, but should be reported immediately. They do not mean that the use of the medicine must be stopped; frequently, a small adjustment will again provide comfort.

During the course of your treatment, adjustments will probably be made in your medications to suit your own needs. Thus, when your dose is raised or lowered, your medication changed, or different medications are added, it need not mean that your situation is getting better or worse; it is merely an adjustment in medication directed to your particular needs at a given time.

It is important that you take the medications regularly and at the times prescribed. The effects of these medications mount up; therefore, you should not decide to discontinue taking them because you are "feeling good." Changing or discontinuing medications should be done only by your physician. If you or your family have any questions about the use of the medications, they should be discussed with the doctor. Decisions about medications require medical training and experience and should not be taken lightly.

You should show this chart to someone who is living with you so that they will know what medications you are taking and in what amounts. Keep the medicine out of the hands of children because they are more sensitive to them, and adult doses can have serious consequences.

Should you consult your family physician or any other doctor during this time, you should immediately tell him what medications you are taking. Your pharmacist has been instructed to label the bottles so that you will know exactly the names and the dosages of the medications that you are taking.

port and optimal safety by being available 24 hours a day and making it clear to patient and family that he not only permits but insists that they contact him whenever questions or problems arise.

Because the drugs used in psychiatric disorders are manufactured in such variety that no physician may be familiar with them all, Tables 34-41, which list doses and forms for each of the most commonly used drugs, have been assembled for the reader's convenience.* The pharmacist should be routinely instructed to label each bottle with the drug name and dosage, so that the patient will know what medicines he is taking and be able to discuss them sensibly. Although the ingredients of an unlabeled pill can usually be determined by comparing it with the photographs in the current *Physicians' Desk Reference* (PDR*) or calling the patient's pharmacist, things are far simpler when the bottle is labeled or the patient is able to describe his medications by names and amounts, rather than sizes and colors. Since many patients with psychiatric illnesses are either constantly or episodically confused, the physician's directions must be clear and simple enough for the patient or a responsible relative to follow. We have found it useful to give patients written instructions regarding their treatment regimen (see Table 10) and often insist that a relative read them as well.

Patients who are given drugs should be told of the side effects they may experience (Tables 34-41). While patients occasionally misuse this information and report symptoms they do not in fact have, we have been far more impressed by the advantages of their knowing what to expect. The better informed the patient is, the more likely he is to report side effects quickly and accurately and the less likely he is to become so frightened by some harmless side effect or so disgruntled at not having been forewarned that he stops taking what was prescribed.

The Assessment of Side Effects

In the course of the follow-up interview, it is important to determine whether the patient is taking his medications as prescribed (see p. 98) and what side effects, if any, they are producing. A side effects questionnaire that we administer (or have the patient administer to himself), both before treatment begins and at each visit thereafter, is shown in Table 11. Laboratory tests are necessary at regular intervals until the patient's response to the drugs is established. The most commonly reported side effects—mild drowsi-

* See pages 551 to 573.

TABLE 11. *Side Effects Questionnaire*

NAME   DATE

	Yes	No	Physician's Comments
1. Apathy			
2. Drowsiness			
3. Stiffness or rigidity of muscles in legs or arms			
4. Tremors or "shakes"			
5. Difficulty in swallowing			
6. Spasms of neck or tongue			
7. Restlessness, inability to be still			
8. Poor memory			
9. Dizziness			
10. Seizures			
11. Loss of coordination			
12. Fainting spells			
13. Blurred vision			
14. Headache			
15. Nervousness			
16. Nausea or vomiting			
17. Diarrhea			
18. Constipation			
19. Dry mouth and throat			
20. Increased salivation			
21. Nasal congestion (stuffiness)			
22. Rapid weight gain			
23. Skin rash			
24. Jaundice (yellow discoloration of skin or eyes)			
25. Difficulty in starting urination			
26. Frequent urge to urinate			
27. Unable to urinate			
28. Lack of energy			
29. Irregularity or absence of menstrual period			
30. Swelling of breasts			
31. Fluid discharge from breast			
32. Difficulty in concentration			
33. Rapid or pounding heart beat			
34. Sweating			
5. Edema (swelling of legs)			
6. Unsteady gait			
7. Slurred speech			
8. Painful sores in mouth			
9. Always hungry			

ness, dry mouth, blurred vision, weight gain, and motor restlessness—
are fairly innocuous and do not necessitate discontinuing drugs.
Individuals who have such symptoms need only be reassured that
they are in no danger and given whatever relief is available. Dryness of the mouth or throat may respond well to lozenges, saline
gargles, or chewing gum. Blurred vision caused by drug-induced
accommodation disturbance can usually be relieved by prescribing
+0.5 to +1.5 diopter spectacles or clip-ons. If the patient reports
episodes of dizziness or faintness, he should be tested for orthostatic
hypotension, which, if mild, may require nothing beyond caution
while arising from a recumbent position; if such episodes are severe,
however, further measures may be required (see p. 584). If a
patient displays dystonia, restlessness, or increased motor activity,
or complains of feeling "jittery" or "jumpy inside," it is possible
to determine whether his symptoms are manifestations of drug-
induced parkinsonism by injecting diphenhydramine (Benadryl)
50 mg in 10 cc of saline intravenously. If this relieves the symptoms,
his discomfort is probably drug-induced and can be relieved by
adding antiparkinsonian agents to the previous medication schedule
(see p. 581). If nausea, sore throat, or other signs suggestive of
hepatic or hematologic complications are present, more vigorous
efforts are required to establish their cause. Since even side effects
that seem innocuous can be important danger signals, the physician
must be familiar with their significance and know what studies and
countermeasures may be needed in each case. A more detailed discussion of the hazards and side effects of drug treatment will be
found in Chapter 14.

Duration of Drug Treatment

Decisions concerning the proper time for decreasing the patient's
drug dosage, withdrawing him from drugs entirely, diminishing
the frequency of visits, or terminating his treatment are hampered
by the paucity of research studies concerning these questions. There
are not even objective criteria for distinguishing between patients
who can eventually stop taking drugs and those who should take
them permanently. The guidelines proposed below are for this
reason based more on empirical observations and what we view as
common sense than on controlled studies.

Two related observations that we have found helpful in deciding
on the timing and feasibility of drug discontinuation are that 1/ illnesses tend to remit in much the same manner as they arose and
2/ recurrences tend to follow the pattern shown in a prior episode of

illness. Thus an illness that has arisen quickly is likely to recede quickly and, if it recurs, is likely to do so with the same rapidity that characterized previous episodes. Acute catatonic episodes—in which the interval between the first symptoms and total decompensation may be no longer than two to six weeks—often remit within a month or two. But if they recur, they may become florid so quickly that the patient's judgment and impulse control are lost within a few days. The converse is true of illnesses that arise slowly. Depressive syndromes, which commonly progress for a number of months before becoming severe enough to require hospitalization or treatment, usually take several months to remit; those that recur tend to reappear so slowly that the patient's judgment, insight, and impulse control remain unimpaired long enough to permit him to recognize that something is wrong and to consult a physician before things get completely out of hand. From the standpoint of protecting the patient against an immediate relapse, then, it is safer to lower the dosage of a catatonic patient soon after his symptoms subside than it is to manage a depressed patient in this way. From the standpoint of the dangers to which the patient is exposed if he should relapse, however, the catatonic is in greater jeopardy.

The likelihood that the patient will remain in *contact with a physician* is a further consideration in deciding when it is safe to decrease his drug dosage. Thus, if a patient whose illness arose rapidly wishes to have his drugs discontinued soon after his symptoms subside, the physician should accede only if the patient's behavior while ill was not dangerous and his current behavior and attitude suggest that he will probably remain in treatment. If, on the other hand, a patient whose illness arose slowly wishes to discontinue drug use, it is best to advise him to wait until he has been feeling well for a number of months. No rigid position is required in this situation, however, especially if the patient has established a positive relationship with the doctor and has learned how to recognize an imminent relapse. Even if he were to have a relapse after his drugs have been stopped, he is likely to resume treatment rapidly enough to avoid danger. The question of when it is safe to decrease the patient's drugs presumes, of course, that it is desirable to do so, and the foregoing comments apply chiefly to patients whose illnesses are self-limited or have not relapsed repeatedly. As discussed on page 142, it may sometimes be preferable to continue a patient on drugs indefinitely or to increase the drug dosage even after the presenting symptoms subside.

The amount of *intercurrent stress* to which the patient is exposed is also relevant in deciding whether or when to reduce his drugs. During a particularly stressful period, such as leaving the hospital, taking on a new job, or reentering school, medications should not be reduced nor should any treatment change be undertaken that could possibly confuse the patient, add to his discomfort, or be seen as a threat to the continuation of the therapeutic relationship. Multiple changes can also be confusing to the physician: if a patient's symptoms return soon after his drugs have been changed and he is simultaneously in the midst of a new or stressful life situation, it is difficult to determine whether the change in drugs or the new stress is responsible.

When a patient says he feels worse soon after his drug dosage is decreased, it may mean either that the reduction was premature and his illness is relapsing or that he is experiencing a transient drug withdrawal effect. Since relapses following medication reduction require that the previous dose levels be reinstituted and maintained, while withdrawal effects require only a more gradual reduction schedule, the distinction between the two is of practical significance. In general, this distinction can be based on the nature and temporal development of the symptoms that arise. The symptoms of a relapse are likely to be those of the original illness, while those of the withdrawal syndrome will vary with the nature of the agent withdrawn. The withdrawal of barbiturates, meprobamate, benzodiazepines, or other "minor" tranquilizers (see Table 35), for example, tends to cause anxiety, restlessness, insomnia, tremor, and EEG changes. Occasionally, a confusional syndrome or even a convulsion may occur. Phenothiazine or antidepressant withdrawal may also cause some anxiety or restlessness, but its most characteristic feature is gastrointestinal distress, such as nausea, vomiting, diarrhea, and abdominal cramps (Bennett 1961, Kramer 1961). The timing of the symptoms is also relevant for the distinction: withdrawal symptoms appear within the first few days, almost never appear after a lapse of 10 days, and usually disappear within a week or 10 days; symptoms of relapse tend not to occur in the first week or so (during which time the patient may even feel better) and usually last until the former level of drugs is reinstituted. In some cases, the new symptoms indicate neither relapse nor withdrawal effects, but rather that the patient fears that the reduction is a prelude to termination and finds complaining about his symptoms the only acceptable way of expressing his desire to continue the relationship.

When adequate *follow-up facilities* for psychopharmacologic management are available, dose reduction can be closely titrated to the patient's clinical improvement; when not, it is usually safest to maintain patients on high dose levels for longer periods of time. The patient who is seen twice weekly by the same physician can usually be placed on a more rapid reduction schedule than the one who attends a large outpatient clinic at four-to-six-week intervals. If a patient lives far from the facility where his medications are adjusted, he will need some kind of medical supervision between visits, but this can usually be provided by his family physician.

Premature Discontinuation of Drug Treatment

Whether a patient stops taking his drugs independently or with the agreement of his physician, subsequent events may show the decision to have been based on false optimism. Occasionally, a patient runs out of medicines or must stop using them temporarily because of an intercurrent illness or projected surgery. As the drug's cumulative dampening effect lifts, he may find that he feels even better than he did while he was taking them and refuse to take them again. While the rate at which drugs like phenothiazines or antidepressants are excreted is so slow that most patients remain free of marked symptoms for a week or more after they stop taking them, some relapse within hours or days. Periods of withdrawal lasting longer than one week are therefore especially dangerous for schizophrenic patients whose symptoms have disappeared on phenothiazines, but whose disease process is still active. Even if the patient's disease process is quiescent, and he initially tolerates drug withdrawal quite well, he is quite likely to relapse whenever the process becomes active again. Indeed, if a patient has had several recurrences, each of which responded only to drugs, he will in all likelihood become psychotic again without them and should take them indefinitely (Bernstein 1966, Gantz 1965, Garfield 1966).

Drugs are sometimes withdrawn for "psychological" reasons: to encourage the patient, restore his confidence in himself and his future, or increase his motivation to stand on his own feet. While withdrawal can indeed have this beneficial effect, the good feelings often last no more than a few days or weeks. That a patient has acquired insight into the sources of his psychological discomfort is another inadequate reason for reducing or withdrawing his drugs, for the change in the drug regimen may dispel the insight he has gained, cause his earlier symptoms to return, and make him once more inaccessible to a meaningful psychotherapeutic encounter.

Discontinuation of drugs against medical advice is one of the most common causes of relapse. In some cases, the decision represents *the first symptom of a relapsing psychosis* and stems from the specific loss of insight associated with it. In other cases, the patient feels that the use of drugs *diminishes his image* in his own eyes or those of his family; he may be trying to prove that he is no longer (or perhaps never was) ill or a weakling. He may be troubled by side effects such as *daytime drowsiness* or an *unusually large weight gain*. At times, the patient's feelings can be assuaged by pointing out that his objections have some validity but that even dependency and obesity are better than overt psychosis.

The patient's family plays a large role in determining whether he will remain in treatment and continue to take his medications. Some families encourage the patient to stop treatment as soon as he expresses any interest in doing so. The most unfortunate thing about this kind of encouragement is that many patients talk about wanting to stop solely in order to find out whether they have their family's permission to continue. Unauthorized drug discontinuation, of course, is not unique to mental patients. Efforts to *deny* illness, to *test* the interest of doctors or families, or to *escape* to a hospital can also occur in nonpsychiatric disorders. Indeed, the schizophrenic who, at times of family crisis, stops taking his drugs in order to "get away from it all," has much in common with the diabetic who responds to family conflict by relaxing his diet or discontinuing his insulin, and thus becoming acidotic enough to warrant hospitalization. *False economy* may also be a factor; both patient and family,. in their concern about the considerable expense of the drugs and the visits required to regulate them, may ignore the far greater cost of relapse. Sometimes the patient simply cannot believe that a pill can help prevent a breakdown. Still others, noticing their discomfort when they withdraw, become concerned that they will become addicted and ignore the physician's assurance that phenothiazine or antidepressant withdrawal leads only to the mild, rare, and transient withdrawal symptoms mentioned above but not to craving or other signs typical of opiate, sedative, or alcohol addiction.

The rapport between the doctor and patient appears to be the single most important factor in determining whether the patient will continue to take what is prescribed. Such rapport is most tenuous, however, in those patients who need the drugs most and must be reinforced in such cases with regularly scheduled follow-up visits. Moreover, from the time he is first given drugs, the patient must be taught enough about his illness and about the risks inherent in abrupt, unsupervised drug withdrawal to understand and accept the necessity of taking drugs for as long as recommended.

In some cases, the patient reports that he is no longer taking the drugs as prescribed; in others, he alleges he is continuing though he has in fact stopped. Either way, the doctor may have to propose *termination of treatment* or, if the patient's condition warrants it, *hospitalization*. Patients who show any signs of withdrawal (such as increasing tension, irritability, or recrudescence of symptoms), who have too many pills left over at the end of the week, or who have in the past surreptitiously discontinued their drugs should from time to time be subjected to a urine test (see Table 43). These tests, which are simple office procedures using standard, easily obtained laboratory equipment and reagents (Caffey 1963, Forrest 1961), detect virtually all clinically useful phenothiazine compounds as well as certain structurally related compounds, such as imipramine (Tofranil). False positive reactions can occur, but are very rare. The FPN or Universal test can detect and measure the intake of a wide variety of drugs, but because of individual differences in the pattern of phenothiazine excretion (Huang 1961), may not be valid at doses below 70 mg per day (Posner 1963) and may thus be unsuitable for detecting the discontinuation of drugs like fluphenazine (Prolixin) or trifluoperazine (Stelazine) that are generally given in far lower doses.

Questions Regarding Long-term Drug Treatment

Maintenance drug treatment is often of value for patients with recurrent psychotic reactions, but it is only one of the factors involved in keeping them well. Numerous studies have documented the importance of *sociocultural and economic factors* (Hollingshead 1958, Malzberg 1958), and there is general agreement that the patient is most likely to avoid rehospitalization if his *family situation is stable* (Ødegard 1960, Sherman 1964), his *illness is brief,* and he is *able to support himself.* Indeed, whatever salutary effects a drug has on an individual's long-term prognosis are likely to derive in largest measure from its role in setting the stage for the operation of those social factors that have a beneficial influence on his long-term adjustment.

Although the dangers of relapsing mental illness seem far greater than those of maintenance drug treatment, there is increasing evidence that long-term drug use is not without hazards. Persistent dyskinesias and irreversible eye changes, for example, have been reported after prolonged administration of certain phenothiazines, and it is not unlikely that the number and kind of deleterious effects reported will continue to rise as these drugs are used for longer and longer periods of time in more and more patients (see p. 589). Further discussion of maintenance drug treatment will be found on pages 138 and 177.

THE TERMINATION OF TREATMENT

When a patient whose treatment was elective or whose illness was minor decides to terminate treatment, the physician has neither reason nor (in most cases) opportunity to do anything but accede. He may suggest but should by no means require that termination be postponed until the patient's motives for raising the issue have been explored and its pros and cons discussed. Indeed, when a patient who exhibits little or no social impairment asks for help with a relatively benign symptom or a recently encountered life problem and after several sessions finds his discomfort is relieved, the physician who advises him to engage in a protracted course of reconstructive psychotherapy may be likened to the haberdasher who cannot rest content with selling a tie but must add a suit and a raincoat to match. There is one sobering difference, however: the man who enters the clothing store generally feels sure that he knows more about the condition of his wardrobe than any overzealous salesman could, while the recovered patient's sales resistance may be understandably weak in the face of the lurking psychological dangers that an overzealous therapist can portray. The patient as a result may come to fear that leaving treatment without first working through his problems will cause all his previous difficulties to return and a host of new ones to appear.

The situation is different if the patient makes an explicit and spontaneous request for help in changing his life style, but the decision to proceed or to terminate should be his rather than the therapist's. Indeed, when the patient in elective treatment insists that the physician make the decision, the first order of business may be to help the patient define his problem sufficiently to make the decision for himself.

Such latitude is not appropriate, however, for patients who have just recovered from a psychotic episode or whose illnesses are known to be chronic and relapsing. Under these circumstances, the physician must be most direct in expressing his disapproval of termination and may even need to explain that a patient's safety and well-being often depend on his ability to permit the doctor's judgment to be the determining factor in the decision. By and large, the decision in such cases rests more on the physician's knowledge and inferences about the natural history of the particular patient's disorder than it does on such factors as the patient's increased understanding of his life situation or an external improvement in his environment.

From the standpoint of natural history, some mental illnesses resemble acute infections or nutritional deficiency states, in that they are marked by *single, nonrepetitive episodes* and that treatment can end when the patient's symptoms subside, his functioning is restored, and there is no further evidence or suspicion of a continuing disease process. Others are more like diabetes or rheumatoid arthritis in that they have a *long course punctuated by clinical or subclinical exacerbations* and require the patient to have a continuing relationship with some physician who will remain "in charge," and be available for questions, emergencies, and the evaluation of any changes that might require intervention. Such patients may not need to be seen for months or years at a time if their symptoms are quiescent, but they should never be terminated. Somewhere between these two extremes lie the patients who, though they have had more than one episode of illness in their lives, tend to recover quite fully between them and to have long periods during which they are, for all practical purposes, symptom-free. Such patients ought neither be terminated nor held over for a long engagement; it is usually enough for them to know where to turn when symptoms recur.

The decision to terminate is on both sides based more often on feelings than on facts. The longer the physician and patient have been meeting, the more likely they are to want to remain together. Conversely, their desire to put their relationship into some kind of goal-oriented framework may cause them to view even a slight improvement as a significant step toward recovery and an indication to terminate. Such optimism can make the patient feel better for a time, but will not prevent a chronic, relapsing illness from remaining so. Some physicians find it hard to face the fact that many diseases do not remit permanently, however they are treated, and, much like a person who refuses to acknowledge the presence of an offensive guest at a social gathering, virtually deny its existence. Hope, wishful or magical thinking, and indignation over his disability may also be reasons for the patient's desire to terminate. Continued treatment may serve to remind him of the cloud under which he feels he must live. He may interpret continued therapy to mean that decompensation is possible at any time and think that being ineligible for formal discharge demonstrates that he is incurable and destined for permanent institutionalization.

The criteria used to decide whether the patient with a non-relapsing illness is ready to terminate or the patient with a chronically relapsing illness can tolerate longer intervals between visits are the same as the criteria used to decide whether a patient needs treatment in the first place. Thus, until the patient's symptoms no longer interfere with his comfort, his social functioning has improved, and his isolation has decreased, it is unsound to propose discontinuing the meetings or lengthening the intervals between them.

Before the patient's ties to the therapist can be loosened or severed, he must also be *educated* about his illness and treatment. He should be able to recognize the signs of incipient trouble early enough to take appropriate countermeasures while he still has enough insight to do so. He must know what countermeasures he can take: calling his doctor, regulating his sleeping habits and food intake, and even initiating or increasing his drug intake until he can reach his physician. He must be taught how important it is to seek consultation early in the course of a relapse and whenever he changes his residence to contact a local physician to whom he can turn for treatment (Astrachan 1968).

These lessons are best learned in the context of a sustained interpersonal relationship that, in addition, can serve as an important vehicle for an *increase in the patient's self-knowledge*. In our experience, the doctor-patient relationship that seeks only to unravel the psychodynamic determinants of the patient's symptoms is of less benefit for the psychotic patient than the one that emphasizes reality-testing, helps him to appreciate his impact on others, and offers him a setting in which he can acknowledge and express his feelings in a socially acceptable manner. Which kind of learning is of greater benefit is a moot point (see p. 515). Nevertheless, the establishment of the kind of relationship in which this can take place seems to promote the patient's adherence to medical recommendations even after his termination and is an important feature of most successful psychotherapeutic encounters.

The close relationship that usually develops between patient and doctor, especially when the illness is prolonged, can promote certain other problems that must be resolved before termination can take place. The longer the patient's treatment has lasted and the stronger his emotional tie to the physician, the more important it is that he *see the relationship realistically* by the time he terminates. He should understand why he came to treatment and why he can leave and must have assurance that he may return if the need arises. In addition, he must have found adequate substitutes for the therapeutic relationship, have learned how to use them as sources of gratification, and know how to find others when these no longer suffice.

In some cases, the resolution of the patient's emotional ties to the doctor remains a problem even after all other criteria for termination are met. That this can occur even when the patient himself has proposed termination may seem paradoxical, but is not too surprising, for the issues surrounding separation are problems central to life itself. From birth to death, from the earliest frustrations through each new step toward maturation and independence, separations are inevitable, and an individual's ability to handle the discomfort they cause is a good measure of his maturity and psychological well-being. Indeed, when termination appears too difficult or (particularly after a prolonged relationship) too easy, the therapist should bear in mind the possibility that a new siege of symptoms is about to ensue.

The severity of a patient's termination anxiety depends only in part on the nature of the clinical problem. Fully as important are his characterologic style and the extent of his involvement with persons or events quite unrelated to his treatment. Profound depression, regressive behavior, and even psychotic decompensation are not at all uncommon in patients whose treatment course has been relatively smooth, but for whom the doctor-patient relationship has become a way of life. When the patient's distress endangers his life or when the therapist's relationship with the patient has become so entangled that he is no longer in a position to remain objective, it may be best to ask a colleague to see the patient and to get his advice on how—or whether—to proceed with the termination. In some cases, it may even be necessary to transfer him to another therapist, in the hope that the less charged atmosphere of a new treatment relationship will make it possible for the patient to resolve the problems of termination.

REFERENCES

Alexander, L.: The commitment and suicide of King Ludwig II of Bavaria, Amer J Psychiat *111*:100-107, 1954.

APA: The Community Mental Health Center: An analysis of existing models, APA, Dept Ment Health, AMA, 1964.

——: Position statement on question of adequacy of treatment, Official Actions, Amer J Psychiat *123*:1458-1461, 1967.

Astrachan, B. M., and Detre, T. P.: Post-hospital treatment of the psychotic patient, Compr Psychiat *9*:71-80, 1968.

Avnet, H. H.: Psychiatric Insurance: Financing Short-term Ambulatory Treatment, New York, Group Health Insurance, 1962.

Bennett, J. L., and Kooi, K. A.: Five phenothiazine derivatives: Evaluation and toxicity studies, Arch Gen Psychiat (Chicago) *4*:413-418, 1961.

Bernstein, A. E. H., and Mason, P.: Effects of phenothiazine discontinuation in patients compensated from acute psychosis, J Mount Sinai Hosp NY *33*:131-139, 1966.

Blue Cross Reports: New directions toward community mental health, Blue Cross Reports 2:1-18, 1964.

——: Use of inpatient hospital services for mental illness under Blue Cross coverage, Blue Cross Reports *3*:1-16, 1965.

Caffey, E. M., *et al.*: Phenothiazine excretion in chronic schizophrenics, Amer J Psychiat *120*:578-582, 1963.

Clark, D. H., and Cooper, L. W.: Psychiatric halfway hostel: Cambridge experiment, Lancet *1*:588-590, 1960.

Detre, T. P.: Countertransference problems arising from the use of drugs in the psychotherapeutic management of psychotic patients, *in* Sarwer-Foner, G. J., ed.: The Dynamics of Psychiatric Drug Therapy, Springfield (Ill): Thomas, 1960, pp. 335-351.

Detre, T. P., Kessler, D. R., and Jarecki, H. G.: The role of the general hospital in modern community psychiatry, Amer J Orthopsychiat 33:690-700, 1963.

Errera, P., Wyshak, G., and Jarecki, H. G.: Psychiatric care in a general hospital emergency room, Arch Gen Psychiat (Chicago) *9*:105-112, 1963.

Essen-Möller, E.: The calculation of morbid risk in parents of index cases, as applied to a family sample of schizo-phrenics, Acta Genet (Basel) *5*:334-342, 1955.

——: Über die Schizophreniehäufigkeit bei Müttern von Schizophrenen, Schweiz Arch Neurol Psychiat *91*:260-266, 1963.

Fessel, W. J.: Interaction of multiple determinants of schizophrenia: A tentative synthesis and review, Arch Gen Psychiat (Chicago) *11*:1-17, 1964.

Fleck, S.: Residential treatment of young schizophrenics, Conn Med *26*:369-376, 1962.

——: Psychiatric hospitalization as a family experience, Acta Psychiat Scand *39* (Suppl 169):1-24, 1963.

Forrest, F. M., Forrest, I. S., and Mason, A. S.: Review of rapid urine color tests, Amer J Psychiat *118*:300-307, 1961.

Franklin, R. W., Goolishian, H. A., and White, R. B.: Psychological hazards involved in treatment of medical colleagues: A further report, Dis Nerv Syst *26*:731-734, 1965.

Gantz, R. S., and Birkett, D. P.: Phenothiazine reduction as a cause of rehospitalization, Arch Gen Psychiat (Chicago) *12*:586-588, 1965.

Garber, R. S.: What do other M.D.s think of psychiatrists?, SKF Psychiatric Reporter *6*:16-20, 1963.

Garfield, S. L.: Withdrawal of ataractic medication in schizophrenic patients, Dis Nerv Sys *27*:321-325, 1966.

Gilbert, J.: Clinical Psychological Tests in Psychiatric and Medical Practice, Springfield (Ill): Thomas, 1969.

Grinspoon, L., and Greenblatt, M.: Pharmacotherapy combined with other treatment methods, Proc III World Cong Psychiat *3*:453-458, 1961.

Heilbrunn, G.: Objectivity in psychiatry, Compr Psychiat *5*:219-231, 1964.

Herridge, C. F.: Physical disorders in psychiatric illness: A study of 209 consecutive admissions, Lancet *2*:949-951, 1960.

Hollingshead, A. B., and Redlich, F. C.: Social Class and Mental Illness: A Community Study, New York: Wiley, 1958.

Hopkins, P.: Psychotherapy in general practice, Lancet *2*:71-74, 1956.

Huang, C. L., and Kurland, A. A.: A quantitative study of chlorpromazine and its sulfoxides in the urine of psychotic patients, Amer J Psychiat *118*:428-437, 1961.

Huseth, B.: What is a halfway house?

Functions and types, Ment Hygiene *45:* 116-121, 1961.

Jarecki, H. G.: Unpublished data, gathered in Emergency Room of Yale-New Haven Hospital in January, 1961.

Johnson, D. A. W.: Evaluation of routine physical examination in psychiatric cases, Practitioner *200:*686-691, 1968.

Kallman, F. J.: The genetics of mental illness, *in* Arieti, Silvano, ed.: American Handbook of Psychiatry, vol 1, New York: Basic, 1959, pp. 175-196.

Klerman, G. L.: Assessing the influence of the hospital milieu upon the effectiveness of psychiatric drug therapy: Problems of conceptualization and of research methodology, J Nerv Ment Dis *137:*143-154, 1963.

Knight, J., and Davis, W.: *In* Rome, H. P., ed.: Manual for the Comprehensive Community Mental Health Clinic, Springfield (Ill): Thomas, 1964.

Kramer, J. C., Klein, D. F., and Fink, M.: Withdrawal symptoms following discontinuation of imipramine therapy, Amer J Psychiat *118:*549-550, 1961.

Langsley, D. G.: Family crisis therapy. Results and implications, Fam Proc *7:* 145-158, 1968.

Lewis, A. B., and Kohl, R. N.: The risk and prevention of abscondence from an open psychiatric unit, Compr Psychiat *3:* 302-308, 1962.

Maguire, G. P., and Granville-Grossman, K. L.: Physical illness in psychiatric patients, Brit J Psychiat *115:*1365-1369, 1968.

Malzberg, B.: Cohort Studies of Mental Disease in New York State, 1943-1949, New York, Nat Assoc Ment Health, 1958.

Moll, A. E.: Night and day psychiatric treatment units in a general hospital, *in* Linn, L., ed.: Frontiers in General Hospital Psychiatry, New York: Internat Univ Press, 1961, pp. 111-144.

Ødegard, O.: A statistical study of factors influencing discharge from psychiatric hospitals, Brit J Psychiat *106:*1124-1133, 1960.

Odenheimer, J. F.: Day hospital as an alternative to the psychiatric ward, Arch Gen Psychiat (Chicago) *13:*46-53, 1965.

Parker, N.: Close identification in twins discordant for obsessional neurosis, Brit J Psychiat *110:*496-504, 1964.

Pasamanick, B., *et al.:* Home vs hospital care for schizophrenics, JAMA *187:*177-181, 1964.

PDR: Physicians' Desk Reference to Pharmaceutical Specialties and Biologicals, Oradell (NJ): Medical Economics Inc.

Perr, I. N.: Liability of hospital and psychiatrist in suicide, Amer J Psychiat *122:* 631-638, 1965.

Perris, C.: Study of bipolar (manic-depressive) and unipolar recurrent depressive psychoses, Acta Psychiat Scand Suppl *194:*197-198, 1966.

Posner, H. S., and Levine, J.: Inability to validate the urinary FPN test for phenothiazine drugs: Suggestions as to the cause of the discrepancy, J Nerv Ment Dis *136:*591-593, 1963.

Rainer, J. D.: The contributions of Franz Josef Kallman to the genetics of schizophrenia, Behav Sci *2:*413-437, 1966.

Raush, H. L., with Raush, C. L.: The Halfway House Movement. A Search for Sanity, New York: Appleton, 1968.

Redlich, F. C., *et al.:* Connecticut Mental Health Center: Joint venture of state and university in community psychiatry, Conn Med *30:*656-662, 1966.

Reich, T., Clayton, P. J., and Winokur, G.: Family history studies: V. The genetics of mania, Amer J Psychiat *125:*1358-1368, 1969.

Sarwer-Foner, G. J., and Kerenyi, A. B.: Accumulated experience with transference and counter-transference aspects of the psychotropic drugs, 1953-1960, *in* Rothlin, E., ed.: Neuro-psychopharmacology, vol 2, Amsterdam: Elsevier, 1961, pp. 385-391.

Sheard, M. H.: The influence of doctor's attitude on the patient's response to antidepressant medication, J Nerv Ment Dis *136:*555-560, 1963.

Sherman, L. J., *et al.:* Prognosis in schizophrenia: Follow-up study of 588 patients, Arch Gen Psychiat (Chicago) *10:* 123-130, 1964.

Shields, J.: Monozygotic Twins Brought Up Apart and Brought Up Together, London: Oxford, 1962.

Smith, K., Pumphrey, M. W., and Hall, J. C.: The "last straw": The decisive incident resulting in the request for hospitalization in 100 schizophrenic patients, Amer J Psychiat *120:*228-233, 1963.

Talbot, E., Miller, S. C., and White, R. B.: Some antitherapeutic side effects of hospitalization and psychotherapy, Psychiatry *27:*170-176, 1964.

Whitmer, C. A., and Conover, C. G.: A study of critical incidents in the hospitalization of the mentally ill, Soc Work *4:*89-94, 1959.

Winokur, G., and Pitts, F. N., Jr.: Affective disorder VI: A family history study of prevalence, sex difference and possible genetic factors, J Psychiat Res *3:*113-123, 1965.

Treatment of Particular Syndromes

INTRODUCTION TO CHAPTERS 3 TO 12

THE PREVIOUS CHAPTERS HAVE DESCRIBED *some of the general characteristics and clinical criteria by which psychiatric disorders can
be judged and treated. The following chapters discuss these topics
in reference to particular clinical syndromes. Taken individually,
they seek to provide practical guidelines for treatment; taken together, they question many of the dichotomizations on which current
diagnostic concepts rest, such as the distinction between neurotic
and psychotic, organic and functional, reactive and process, endogenous and exogenous, and acute and chronic.* *

In order to choose among the various treatment possibilities
and predict the probable outcome, the physician needs criteria that
help him determine the meaning of the patient's disturbed thinking,
mood, and behavior. Are the disturbances simply normal variants
of human experience? Do they represent one of the more or less
clearly defined psychiatric syndromes, and, if so, which one? Are
they the sequel or the precursor of another disorder? Or, despite
masquerading as psychiatric, are they in fact attributable to a medical or surgical illness and, thus, not exclusively the psychiatrist's
concern?

As we shall show, current diagnostic criteria are often insufficient
for answering these questions. This is not surprising, for any heuristically intended effort to divide the broad spectrum of psychological
difficulties into discrete, well-defined syndromes must of necessity
make artificial distinctions. For practical reasons, our chapter head-
ings are based on the classification system currently used in psychiatry (Table 50). This system has the flaw of defining each
syndrome in terms of no more than two or three of such features
as the pathological findings, the personality type of the patient,
the current symptom cluster, the leading symptoms, the social effects,

* For page references, see Index.

or the patient's age (Pokorny 1965). In assessing the value of a particular treatment, however, each of these factors and a host of others must be taken into account in order to specify the nature of the illness in question.

Chapters 3 through 12 describe at some length those treatment measures we have found most effective. Our confidence in these recommendations, however, is tempered by the knowledge that many syndromes remit or change their course even without treatment and that treatment plans other than those we propose have also been reported effective. The prime difficulty in comparing one treatment plan with another stems from the fact that most published reports about treatment results limit themselves to the statement: this was the illness, this the treatment, and this the outcome. Far too few define the natural course of a given illness or compare its response to several different treatment programs. Were more of these studies available, it would at least be possible to know what odds, averages, and outcome would need to be surpassed in order to justify a preference for one treatment over another.

The multiplicity of the criteria used to define a successful outcome adds to the problems inherent in comparing treatment plans. One study measures treatment results by the diminution of symptoms or even of a single symptom like excitability; another, in terms of release from the hospital or return to work. Still other studies consider treatment successful only if it achieves more ambitious goals, such as the restoration of the premorbid personality, "insight," creativity, or improvement beyond the premorbid state. Although these disparities make it hard to assess the many reports that are published each month, it would be unrealistic to expect such data to be uniform, for the goals of treatment must vary with the severity of the syndrome. One measure of effectiveness may suffice for treatment given chronic schizophrenics on a violent ward, another for that given enuretic children, and a third for the treatment of artists troubled by blocked creativity.

Chapters 3 to 12 therefore present treatment recommendations against the backdrop of the available information on each illness' prognosis, both with and without treatment, but it is important that the reader bear the paucity of these data in mind. For the sake of economy, the clinical chapters discuss the recommended treatment measures only in relationship to the illness being described. A more detailed account of these techniques and of their indications, rationale, method of administration, complications, and hazards is presented in Chapters 13 to 16.

CHAPTER
THREE

Schizophrenic Disorders

Kraepelin's (1899) use of the term *dementia praecox* to refer to certain mental disorders that he considered related to each other and distinguishable as a group from other psychoses marks an important milestone in clinical psychiatry. This achievement was confirmed and expanded some years later by Bleuler (1911), who proposed that these illnesses be called *schizophrenias* in order to avoid the implication that dementia was inevitable and emphasize what he saw as their most characteristic feature: the splitting, or fragmentation, of the patient's psychic functions. Bleuler considered the fundamental symptoms to consist of disturbances of *association* and *affectivity,* morbid *ambivalence,* a predilection for *fantasy,* and a withdrawal from reality that he called *autism.* Recognizing that patients showing these basic or primary symptoms commonly had numerous other symptoms as well and that the clinical pictures were thus quite varied, he proposed a classification system for schizophrenic disorders that, in large measure, has survived to this day. The identification of the entire group of disorders and their subclassification into *paranoid, catatonic, hebephrenic,* and *simple* types gave a semblance of order to what had been chaos and, playing on man's age-old fantasy that he can control what he can name, encouraged physicians to feel that they might be able to influence these disorders. In addition, it offered some criteria by which to predict the course and outcome of the patient's illness.

The diagnostic label had the faults of its virtues, however, for the enthusiasm with which it was accepted obscured the unresolved question of whether the many clinical pictures called schizophrenia are really a single disease. The possibility that schizophrenia is in fact an aggregate of different diseases, which share a number of psychological symptoms, is at any rate hard to rebut. Some disorders labeled schizophrenic remit spontaneously, while others do not. Some respond well to phenothiazines, while others do not. Some arise in the context of emotional stress, some in the wake of an organic brain syndrome (Davison 1966), some in families in which other members show an identical disorder (Fischer 1969, Heston 1966, Kallmann 1964, Kringlen 1967, Pollin 1969, Reisby 1967 Shields 1967), and some in patients for whom none of these factors is operative (Wender 1969).

The problems of diagnosis and definition have indeed become so complex that the label of schizophrenia is sometimes used to refer to disorders that do not at any time in their course meet the original diagnostic criteria. It is thus not at all unusual for two clinicians to agree completely about a given patient's symptoms or course without being able to agree on whether or not he is "really" schizophrenic. The diagnostic definitions of the past are thus of less value today than they were when first proposed. Patients now come for treatment much earlier than they used to and show symptoms quite unlike those of the classical descriptions (Brill 1965, Klaf 1961). The development of effective treatment measures has made it even more urgent that new diagnostic criteria be found. If such criteria are to be of maximum value, however, they must be applicable early in the course of illness, for the more rapidly the patient's illness is diagnosed and treated, the greater the chance of avoiding a chronic course.

The difficulty inherent in early diagnosis is not essentially different from that hindering diagnosis even in far advanced cases: *there is no symptom or symptom complex that appears in every schizophrenic episode and in no other disease.* Thus, even though it has long been recognized that there is something very unusual about the schizophrenic's manner of thinking, this *something* has been hard to define. Much interest has been aroused therefore by recent studies that have made use of the statements of schizophrenic patients who were examined so early in the course of their illness that they had not yet lost the ability to communicate or forgotten their initial symptoms. The patient's own description of his subjective experience can thus be used to try to determine just how it feels to think and perceive in a schizophrenic way (Chapman 1966, MacDonald 1960, McGhie 1961). According to these reports, the schizophrenic's cognitive mode can be identified fairly easily, sometimes even before any other symptoms are exhibited.

THE SCHIZOPHRENIFORM COGNITIVE MODE (SCM)

Unlike the normal person, who responds selectively to the innumerable stimuli that impinge on his perceptual field and focuses largely on those most relevant to the task at hand, the schizophrenic is open and vulnerable to stimuli of all kinds—so much so that he has been aptly described as being "at the mercy of his environment" (Chapman 1966). Some patients are aware of this process and complain of feeling forced to attend to irrelevant details; others are not and consider many or all of their experiences highly significant —even those they would otherwise have viewed as neutral or commonplace. What the schizophrenic hears may seem louder, and what he sees may seem brighter than it did in the past. Most patients report that their thinking speeds up, some that it slows down or fluctuates. Sometimes the patient feels blocked in his thinking; at other times he feels compelled to pursue the same thought processes over and over again. He may find it hard to distinguish between external and internal stimuli (Stafford-Clark 1958) or to separate

---

TABLE 12. *Cognitive Changes Reported by Patients in the Earliest Stages of Schizophrenia*

It's as if I am too wide awake. Everything seems to go through me. I just can't shut things out. I let all the sounds come in that are there.

There is a brightness and clarity of outline of things around me.

My concentration is very poor. I jump from one thing to another.

I try to read even a paragraph in a book but it takes me ages because each bit I read starts me thinking in ten different directions at once.

You might think about something, let's say that ashtray and just think, oh! yes, that's for putting my cigarette in, but I would think of it and then I would think of a dozen different things connected with it at the same time.

I am attending to everything at once and as a result I do not really attend to anything.

I don't like dividing my attention at any time because it leads to confusion and I don't know where I am or who I am.

Often the silliest little things that are going on seem to interest me. That's not even true, they don't interest me, but I find myself attending to them and wasting a lot of time this way.

Noises all seem to be louder to me than they were before. It's as if someone had turned up the volume . . . I notice it most with background noises—you know what I mean, noises that are always around you but you don't notice them. Now they seem to be just as loud and sometimes louder than the main noises that are going on.

Colors seem to be brighter now, almost as if they are luminous. Everything's brighter and louder and noisier.

When people are talking I have to think what the words mean. I have to pay all my attention to people when they are speaking or I get all mixed up and don't understand them. If there are three or four people talking at one time I can't take it in. If it is just one person who is speaking that's not so bad, but if others join in, then I can't pick it up at all. It's just words in the air unless you can figure it out from their faces. I can concentrate quite well on what people are saying if they talk simply. It's when they go on into long sentences that I lose the meanings.

Everything I see is split up. It's like a photograph that's torn in bits and put together again.

figure from ground in the sense of distinguishing the relevant objects from the rest of the perceptual field (Matussek 1952). His attention is without direction and thus universal, his perception and thinking are overinclusive (Cameron 1938, Payne 1962), and he is unable to inhibit or selectively direct or control his thought processes (Fleck 1953). Bombarded by stimuli and unable to determine their significance or source, he can no longer maintain a meaningful, constant, and stable perceptual matrix and develops a changed understanding of his surroundings and his relationship to them.

Many attempts have been made to explain these superficially disparate cognitive changes. One currently useful concept ascribes them to the defective functioning of a "central filter," by which is meant that mechanism or set of mechanisms that screens out irrelevant stimuli and thus promotes the most efficient processing of incoming

---

TABLE 12. *Cognitive Changes Reported by Patients in the Earliest Stages of Schizophrenia* (continued)

I have to put things together in my head. If I look at my watch I see the watch, watchstrap, face, hands and so on, then I have got to put them together to get it into one piece.

The arms and legs are apart and away from me and they go on their own. That's when I feel I am the other person and copy their movements, or else stop and stand like a statue.

I have to think of what I am going to do all the time and that takes up a lot of energy and when I am doing something I am aware of my every movement.

I can't move if I am distracted by too much noise. I can't help stopping to listen. That's what happens when I am lying in bed. If there's too much noise going on I can't move. Say I am walking across the floor and someone suddenly switches on the wireless, the music seems to stop me in my tracks and sometimes I freeze like that for a minute or two.

If I am doing something then I start thinking of what I am doing, that locks me up in a sense. For example, if I drop something and stoop to pick it up, if I start to think of myself in that position and what I am doing, that locks me up in that position. If you keep thinking of where your body is it gets locked up.

If I am going to sit down, I have got to think of myself and almost see myself sitting down before I do it. All this makes me move much slower now. I prefer to think out movements first before I do anything, then I get up slowly and do it. I have to do everything step by step, nothing is automatic now. Everything has to be considered.

I find it very difficult to do things now, just everyday things like shaving, things that you do immediately you get up. Just things I used to do without thinking, like hanging your coat up or taking your tea. I am very easily put off now—by noises or people speaking to me. It's trying to concentrate on two things. Sometimes I have just to cut everything short and sit down.

Sounds sometimes make me feel dizzy.

It's not that I can't concentrate right, it's just that I can't concentrate on the major issues. I get fogged up with all the different bits and lose the important things in the picture. I find myself paying attention to all sorts of tiny things instead of getting on with the things I should be doing.

If I am talking to someone they only need to cross their legs or scratch their heads and I am distracted and forget what I was saying.

information (Payne 1959). Although there is no evidence that the term describes either a structural or a functional entity, there is some heuristic value in assuming that a central filter is operative in normal mental functioning and defective in schizophrenia, for this assumption helps explain both how the normal individual's consciousness is protected from being flooded by the innumerable stimuli to which he is exposed and why the schizophrenic's consciousness is not (Chapman 1962, Venables 1964). Indeed, almost all the cognitive changes reported by patients in the earliest stages of schizophrenia (see Table 12) (McGhie 1961), as well as the abstract and somewhat overlapping generalizations into which their experiences can be translated (see Table 13), can be described in terms of this unifying concept.

The notion that the schizophrenic suffers from a malfunctioning central filter might account for not only his increased awareness

TABLE 13. *Cognitive Disturbances in Early Schizophrenia*

CHANGES IN ATTENTION AND PERCEPTION

Extreme "openness" to stimuli

Distractibility of attention

Loss of focal direction of attention so that it is directed radially and diffusely

Loss of freedom to direct attention at will

Inability to distinguish relevant from irrelevant stimuli, that is, to distinguish object from field; individual thus pays an unusual amount of attention to the background features of the perceptual matrix

Sensory perception, for example, changes as colors and shapes become more vivid

Speech perception is impaired. Patients are unable to appreciate the content because of their preoccupation with form and have difficulty in following conversations, the more so when more people are taking part

Inability to distinguish stimuli of one sense modality from those of another

A response to one sense modality, for example, may be triggered by stimulation of another; normally discrete sensory channels become diffuse

Inability to distinguish internal from external stimuli

Increasing "self consciousness" in literal sense

Loss of spontaneity of motility caused by heightened awareness of sensations and volitional impulses

Need to plan and execute each action "step by step"

LACK OF ABILITY TO CONTROL, DIRECT, AND INHIBIT THINKING

Overinclusive thinking

Associative sequences are not distinguished from logical sequences and in some areas inappropriately replace them

Abstract and concrete thought levels are not distinguished so that there is a fluidity between them

BLOCKING

Thought processes are easily interrupted by both external and internal stimuli and heightened sensory input but also why realms of thinking usually confined to the dreaming state begin to dominate his waking behavior and why long-forgotten memories may come vividly to the fore and assume major importance. This concept may also explain why the schizophrenic appears more sensitive than the nonschizophrenic to interpersonal events, why he pays as much attention to the paracommunicative as to the communicative aspects of social intercourse (Bateson 1956), and why he may again start to utilize ways of thinking he had discarded many years before. Some aspects of his cognitive mode are sometimes referred to as "primary process" thinking, which in its most typical form uses one object or person to symbolize another, equates wishes with actions, and fails to distinguish between parts of an object and its whole (Freud 1900). In certain respects, such thinking resembles (and has often been compared with) the cognitive mode prominent in childhood, dreaming, artistic creativity, and the working of the unconscious.

SCM IN OTHER SYNDROMES

Since cognitive disturbances of a similar kind may also be seen in a number of other conditions, problematic questions of differential diagnosis can arise (Tucker 1969). Patients in the manic phase of *manic-depressive disease* often resemble schizophrenics in that they, too, report accelerated thinking and a sense of unusual clarity. Schizophrenics, on the other hand, often exhibit a manic-like hyperactivity, euphoria, and grandiosity. The distinction between the manic and the schizophrenic can be particularly difficult when the patient's prior or family history offers no clue, and his cognitive mode is devoid of the other disturbances summarized in Table 13. In some cases, the illness's course suggests differences. The manic patient's symptoms tend to be more constant than those of the schizophrenic: his accelerated thinking and his sense of unusual clarity are generally uninterrupted, while those of the schizophrenic are usually interspersed with blocking and perplexity; similarly, the schizophrenic patient who is elated will feel this way only briefly, while the manic's euphoria is likely to be persistent. Another distinction is that symptoms like hyperactivity, optimism, euphoria, and grandiosity tend in the manic to increase in concert, while in the schizophrenic such symptoms, if seen at all, are more likely to progress individually, each at its own rate. Unlike the manic, then, the schizophrenic may be euphoric without being hyperactive and then reverse the pattern.

The schizophreniform cognitive mode (scm), either alone or in combination with delusions, hallucinations, unusual memories, and bizarre social behavior, may also be seen in *organic brain syndromes* of almost every conceivable cause (see Chap. 11), and the clinical picture, at least initially, may be hard to distinguish from that seen in schizophrenia. When such symptoms arise after a head injury (see p. 423), withdrawal from a cns depressant (see p. 296), or the ingestion of stimulants (see p. 319), hallucinogens (see p. 321), or antidepressants (see p. 604), the correct diagnosis usually can be made if a complete *history* can be obtained. The patient's history is not always reliable, however: he may be confused, not know what agents he took, or be afraid of getting into trouble. When schizophreniform symptoms appear in connection with encephalitides, seizure disorders, brain tumors, cerebrovascular accidents, or degenerative diseases, the history may be of less relevance, and the diagnosis of organic disease will depend on the identification of characteristic *neurologic symptoms* or *findings*. In some cases, neither organic findings nor cause can be demonstrated, and the patient is misdiagnosed as schizophrenic for some time before the organic basis of the symptoms becomes evident. The nature of a patient's hallucinations offers an additional clue: auditory hallucinations are more suggestive of schizophrenic, and visual hallucinations of organic disorders. A *mental status examination* may also be useful, for the organic patient is more likely to be dysmnesic and disoriented than the schizophrenic. This distinction is not always feasible: some schizophrenics are so delusional or uncommunicative that it is impossible to determine what they remember or understand of where or who they are. The problem is compounded by the fact that disordered sleep is as typical a symptom of organic delirium (see p. 413) as it is of acute schizophrenia and can further aggravate preexisting disturbances in thinking, memory, and orientation. As a result, the distinction between organic and schizophrenic disorders can sometimes be made only after the patient's sleep has returned to normal. Organic patients who are sleeping well rarely exhibit scm, while schizophrenic patients continue to do so. If, however, a patient remains or becomes disoriented and dysmnesic after his sleep disturbance subsides, organic disorder may well be suspected. Finally, when a patient is believed to be schizophrenic but responds to ect or drug treatment in an uncharacteristic manner, such as by becoming excessively drowsy or confused or failing to improve, it is necessary to reconsider the diagnosis and undertake an even more vigorous search for organic factors (see also p. 642).

Patients with acute and chronic *anxiety neurosis* may also have some features of scm: accelerated thinking, increased sensitivity to insignificant stimuli, easy distractibility, depersonalization, and heightened self-consciousness. While such symptoms resemble those seen in schizophrenia, they differ in that they generally last only as long as the anxiety attack itself and are not associated with a feeling on the part of the patient that the objects he perceives seem more vivid than they did in the past. A patient with an anxiety neurosis may also have some sleep difficulty and, especially in the midst of an episode, some impairment in his social behavior, but these problems are neither so great nor so likely to progress as they are in the patient with a schizophrenic episode. The distinction between an anxious patient who shows scm and a schizophrenic is not always easy, however, for anxiety, like all other neurotic symptoms, can be a precursor of schizophrenic illness (Chapman 1966, Slater 1965). Whether or not an apparently neurotic symptom is in truth the forerunner of a schizophrenic episode will be clarified only by the passage of time. Nevertheless, such a progression should be suspected when the patient in question 1/ has a previous or family history of schizophrenic disorder, 2/ experiences incessant or crippling anxiety, or 3/ suffers from profuse or persistent cognitive disturbances.

THE RELATIONSHIP OF SCM TO OTHER SYMPTOMS IN THE COURSE OF SCHIZOPHRENIC ILLNESSES

Scm is so common in patients who are diagnosed as acutely schizophrenic that, for purposes of defining the syndrome, it could almost be viewed as the feature without which the diagnosis cannot be made. The fact that schizophrenic patients often report having had scm for months or years before developing other symptoms, and that some describe their entire clinical picture as if it were solely a reaction to scm has led to the speculation that scm is not merely a cognitive style but the basic disorder that, by its severity, determines many of the patient's other symptoms.

Patients with acute schizophrenic episodes, for instance, often ascribe their anxiety, depression, elation, sense of depersonalization, and perplexity to their cognitive disorder; those developing the catatonic and paranoid types often report that their motility changes or delusional ideas are efforts to cope with, adapt to, or diminish the cognitive disorder and thus to fend off the discomfort it evokes (Chapman 1966). This speculation must be viewed with some caution, though, for scm is also seen in patients with other psychiatric disorders and in individuals without any overt psychiatric illness at all and could in any case scarcely be seen as the cause of a patient's sleep disorder or hallucinations.

Whether SCM is viewed as a basic symptom of the disorder, a predisposing cognitive style, or an epiphenomenon of the underlying disease, it is so commonly present by the time a patient's symptoms are sufficiently well defined that almost any clinician would consider him acutely schizophrenic, that it might almost be considered a *necessary* criterion for the diagnosis. Its occurrence in other disorders precludes its being a *sufficient* criterion to establish the diagnosis, however, and we shall therefore describe a number of other symptoms that, in association with SCM, lend further support to the diagnosis of schizophrenia.

ACUTE SCHIZOPHRENIC EPISODES

The extent to which the patient's cognitive disorder impairs his ability to cope with or understand his everyday world and the consequences to which this will lead depend on the severity and duration of the illness and on the individual's premorbid personality structure. The patient whose cognitive disorder is brief in duration or mild in degree may experience no more than a few days of confusion or a minor rotation in the way he views his world. One whose disorder is severe and persistent, however, will almost of necessity experience a profound alteration in his sense of subjective reality and, in addition, may develop a wide range of apparently related symptoms.

Initially, the patient may take pleasure in his new sense of awareness and his newfound ability to sense special significance in what he sees; he may even believe that his understanding of the world has increased. He may feel somewhat elated or start to ruminate about religion, art, psychology, or the meaning of life. As his disorder progresses, however, and he begins to realize that his ability to function and his comprehension of the world around him have become impaired rather than enhanced, his pleasure is likely to fade; he may then become increasingly anxious, perplexed, and depressed and, in an attempt to diminish his confusion, start to develop obsessional thinking. As his ability to focus his attention or otherwise direct his thought processes dwindles, he becomes increasingly fearful of being swamped by a tide of impressions he cannot control (McGhie 1965). He starts to view his relationship to his environment as one in which he is no longer able to exert initiative, reconcile current with previous experiences, or distinguish between his own thoughts and feelings and his reactions to external stimuli. Gradually, he loses his sense of identity and feels increasingly alienated, even from himself.

When the clinical picture is confined to these symptoms, it may be labeled as an acute schizophrenic episode. At the beginning of the illness, however, the patient's symptoms tend to fluctuate or even disappear entirely for brief periods. While such vagaries can make it hard to assess the patient's disorder, a patient whose symptoms were severe enough to cause him to be referred for treatment is likely to have experienced a change in his sleep patterns as well.

In most cases, the patient's *sleep disorder* starts as difficulty in falling asleep (DFA). Whether and how quickly total insomnia ensues varies. Around the time the patient begins to lose sleep, he is likely to report that his dreams have become longer, more frequent, and more vivid. Thereafter, nightmares occur in which everyday fears are expressed in a symbolic fashion, and familiar faces and voices appear distorted or possessed of a special, usually fearful significance. Next, just before he falls asleep or just after he awakens, he may have dreamlike experiences that seem so real that, even after he gets up, he may behave as if they were (hypnagogic or hypnopompic hallucinations (Feinberg 1967). This can of course be embarrassing and may be dangerous as when he was defending himself against an aggressor in his dream and assaults the first person he encounters upon rising. With the progression of his illness, dreamlike experiences and hallucinations may occur even while he appears fully awake and increase to the point where they dominate his entire subjective experience and govern all his waking behavior. When he reaches this state, he may indeed fulfill what Jung (1909) described in saying: "Let the dreamer awake and walk about as one awakened and we have the clinical picture of dementia praecox."

Once the clinical picture of an acute schizophrenic episode has developed, the illness may take one of several courses. In most cases, the symptoms recede within a few weeks. When they do not, they are usually joined or replaced by others. The appearance of motility changes, hallucinations, a primitive revivification of old memories and conflicts, delusional interpretations of experience, and social withdrawal mark the emergence of more complex clinical syndromes such as *acute catatonic, paranoid,* and *schizoaffective* types of schizophrenia. These additional symptoms develop less frequently in the first or second schizophrenic episode than they do in the later ones, perhaps because the first episodes tend to be brief.

Why these new symptoms develop is not known. Some patients

offer explanations, but who can say whether these explanations are accurate? For example, the patient may say that he is moving more slowly or more deliberately in order to reduce his perceptual bombardment and thus diminish his discomfort. He may describe his delusions as if they were efforts to understand the unusual sensations he is experiencing. Such explanations have given rise to the view that "the end clinical picture is determined, in part, by how the individual patient reacts to his deficiencies in perception and cognition and what methods of self-help he employs, some electing to maintain a restriction of all motor activity including speech, others deciding to relinquish such strategies at the price of performing in a disorganized fashion" (Chapman 1966).

The patient's age and the speed with which his illness progresses also appear to have some bearing on the kind of symptoms he will develop and thus on the subtype of schizophrenia to which his disorder will be assigned. Rapidly progressing illnesses, such as *acute catatonic schizophrenia,* are most common in middle or late adolescence; marked by motor symptoms, affective lability, and unsystematized delusions; and likely to remit fairly quickly. Those that progress more slowly, like *paranoid schizophrenia,* are more common in the late twenties and early thirties; marked by neurotic symptoms, more stable affective disturbances, and systematized delusions; and less likely and slower to remit. That mixture of schizophrenic and affective symptoms labeled *schizoaffective schizophrenia* is considered to fall between these extremes, in that the symptoms tend to occur in the early and mid-twenties and to develop and recede more slowly than catatonic and more rapidly than paranoid symptoms.

In *acute catatonic* episodes, the patient's cognitive functioning deteriorates within a very few days; his sleep disturbance, which almost invariably begins with difficulty in falling asleep (DFA), usually develops into total insomnia within days or at most a few weeks; and his anorexia develops with equal rapidity. Whether or not the motility changes, as suggested above, are volitional efforts to cope with alterations in sensory input, they are in any case the most typical symptoms of catatonic illnesses and indeed the criteria for making the diagnosis. The patient may either be hyperactive and excited (in which case he is usually overtalkative and elated as well) or inhibited and withdrawn (in which case he is usually mute, depressed, negativistic and, in particularly severe cases, stuporous).

Fluctuations between hyperactive and inhibited states are common, as is stereotyped and manneristic motor behavior. The catatonic patient's explanations for his unusual feelings or sensations are often grotesque. He may believe that the world is about to be destroyed or that his heart or brain has been replaced with a mechanical substitute. In many cases, the hallucinations and delusions involve destroying or controlling others or being destroyed or controlled by them; in some, they mirror the patient's affective lability: accusing or insulting voices alternate with others that confer great powers on him. These symptoms are overwhelming and in such constant flux that the delusions developed to explain them must be mended and amended so rapidly and so often that they are devoid of any well-integrated systematization. Bizarre, violent, assaultive, automutilatory, and even suicidal behavior may occur either as a result of the delusional ideas or as a response to hallucinated commands. Even when the patient seems immobile and stuporous, he looks so tense and explosive that those around him feel apprehensive and uncomfortable—and not without reason, for he may well become excited and assaultive without obvious provocation. The observer's sense of impending danger is indeed so typical a reaction to the inhibited catatonic that it might well be considered a valid diagnostic criterion.

In *paranoid schizophrenia,* the characteristic cognitive disorder usually develops over a period of several months. Compared to the catatonic patient, the paranoid patient's cognitive impairment progresses slowly; it permits him to come upon delusional ideas in a far more leisurely manner and requires him to formulate only a few "insights" a week in order to encapsulate his bewilderment or explain his symptoms. His delusions are thus more systematized, more plausible, and easier to integrate into his personality structure. As a result, his views may seem quite reasonable for some time, so that he is unlikely to be seen by a psychiatrist until his illness has been in progress for months or years (see also Chap. 5).

SCHIZOAFFECTIVE DISORDERS

The term *schizoaffective schizophrenia* (Cobb 1943), sometimes used to refer to patients showing both schizophrenic and affective features, has been criticized on the grounds *1/* that it elevates to the status of a separate clinical entity what is either but one phase in the course of a schizophrenic illness or a mixture of two distinct disorders, and *2/* that the psychopathology, premorbid personality, prognosis, and treatment response of these patients are by no means distinctive enough to warrant adding a subtype to the group of schizophrenias (Fish 1962, Mayer-Gross 1960). There is much merit in these objections, for affective symptoms are not the exception but almost the rule in schizophrenia (Kraepelin 1896). States of euphoria and depression are the first and for some time the only manifestations of some incipient schizophrenic episodes. Such symptoms can also occur in the midst of an episode, though in such cases they are usually overshadowed by the patient's other symptoms. Affective symptoms are, moreover, particularly common in the recovery phase (Bowers 1967), either as a part of the illness' course or as a result of the tranquilizers or the ECT the patient has received. The converse —that schizophrenia-like symptoms occur in the course of an affective disorder—is also no rarity. Both manic and depressed patients often show paranoid or otherwise delusional features and may even hallucinate.

Despite these objections, we find the concept of some operational value. In the first place, its use makes it possible to avoid a more specific diagnosis at the outset of the illness when there is no way of knowing its outcome. Moreover, the notion that there is a clinical category between schizophrenia and manic-depressive disease helps explain why patients labeled as manic-depressive at the time of their first hospitalization often appear increasingly schizophrenic with each confinement. Finally, it is our experience that patients who show both kinds of symptoms in fairly equal admixture and, in addition, show them throughout the course of a given episode require a different form of treatment from those who are manic, depressed, or schizophrenic only.

CHRONIC SCHIZOPHRENIA

Patients whose thinking or behavior has appeared schizophrenic for a number of years eventually develop a clinical picture that, for want of a better generic term, may be called *chronic desocialization:* they become apathetic, callous, socially awkward, or inappropriate; in some cases, they may even appear demented. Symptoms of this kind are prominent in the disorders customarily classified as *hebephrenic, simple,* or *chronic undifferentiated* schizophrenia, and may also be seen in adults who were autistic or schizophrenic during their childhood and did not recover completely (see p. 369); they seem to result from both the protracted cognitive disorder and its social consequences.

When left to his own devices, the schizophrenic patient tends to have little conventional contact with others. He refrains from meeting people or making acquaintances, he avoids social situations, and he may even rebuff those who approach him. In many cases, his social behavior is so incomprehensible and bizarre that it causes him to be ostracized and avoided. If his behavior gets bad enough, he will be hospitalized and thus further deprived of conventional social intercourse. Unlike the normal person, who learns to assess his own impact in terms of the reactions of those around him and is thus enabled to modify his behavior to conform to the expectations of others, the schizophrenic tends to derive little benefit from the social feedback to which he is exposed. His behavior may be so odd that those around him will treat him in an unconventional, unhelpful, or even hostile way. Even when others try to ignore his odd ways and respond to him just as they would to anyone else, as may occur in a therapeutic community (see p. 508), he may mistake their intentions or interpret their behavior in an idiosyncratic or even delusional manner.

Since the chronic schizophrenic's symptoms are caused, at least in part, by the impoverishment and distortion of his social feedback, it follows that the environment to which he is exposed during the acute phase of the illness has a significant bearing on whether and when he will develop symptoms of desocialization. It can determine how quickly he is referred for treatment: if his family is socioeconomically deprived or culturally estranged, if it permits or encourages irrational and disordered thinking, or for some other reason ignores his bizarre behavior and does nothing to stop it, he may not see a doctor until his illness has been in progress for so long that his social deterioration is well advanced (Gillis 1965). The patient's environment during the time of an acute illness also affects the extent of his withdrawal and isolation. Whether the patient is hospitalized or remains at home, the more he is permitted to withdraw, the more desocialized, the harder to treat, and the less likely to recover he becomes.

Symptoms of chronic desocialization are not limited to schizophrenic patients. Indeed, if a patient's only symptoms are social incompetence, retardation, apathy, or an oddly motivated callousness, and his examination and history reveal no scm in either the present or the past, his symptoms are less likely to represent a chronic schizophrenia than

1/ the long-term consequences of an inadequate social environment on a person with perceptual handicaps, learning disabilities, or a mild mental deficiency,

2/ an unusual form of an inadequate or histrionic personality disorder,

3/ the late sequelae of organic brain damage, or

4/ a protracted depression in a person with a schizoid personality.

The term used most commonly to describe chronically desocialized schizophrenic patients (perhaps because it is the broadest) is *chronic undifferentiated schizophrenia*. In general, this label intends to convey the idea that the patient has been schizophrenic for some time, exhibits delusions, hallucinations, motor symptoms, or unusual mannerisms, and has developed the symptoms of chronic desocialization. Neither this term nor the others describe discrete syndromes, however. Innumerable combinations of symptoms exist, and there is little agreement on the criteria for assigning a particular disorder to one or another of the diagnostic categories. What, for example, is the difference between a *simple* and a *hebephrenic* schizophrenia? Some clinicians distinguish between them on the basis that the simple form does not show hallucinations, delusions, or motor symptoms, while the hebephrenic may, but as these symptoms are not obligatory in the hebephrenic either, the distinction has obvious flaws. Others consider the age at which the patient becomes ill as the distinguishing feature and label as hebephrenic all schizophrenic illnesses that first appear during adolescence and, continue on a chronic course. Still others use the term hebephrenic to refer to all patients whose most striking features include silliness, clowning, prankish behavior, and labile and inappropriate affect. Perhaps the distinction rests only on the amount of drive or volition the patient exhibits: the hebephrenic's peculiar behavior, philosophical concerns, fluctuating moods, and inability to hold a job despite great ambitions and efforts seem based on *wanting something,* while the simple schizophrenic's blandness, vagueness, drifting, and menial employment seem based on *wanting little or nothing.* Seen thus, a hebephrenic girl's promiscuity might derive from a search for pleasure or a sense of importance, while the promiscuity of a simple schizophrenic girl would stem from her indifference to the situation and her consequent disinclination to resist sexual advances.

With the passage of time, distinctions blur, particularly if the patient has caused enough social embarrassment to be hospitalized.

The institutionalized patient rapidly fades into the gray anonymity of the chronic ward, and for him such issues as promiscuity, unemployment, and social embarrassment are over. Even if he were eventually to recover from the cognitive disorder, the paucity of medical care extended to the back-ward schizophrenic might well permit the event to pass unnoticed. Even the patient himself may consider his hospitalization justified or prefer the hospital setting to any other. Indeed, such patients often provide the loudest protests against rehabilitation programs that threaten to propel them into a world of which they had never felt a part and to which they do not wish to return (Braginsky 1966).

LATENT SCHIZOPHRENIA

The final, perhaps somewhat questionable, category of schizophrenic illness is that in which the affected individual does not show (or shows only rarely) such symptoms as delusions, hallucinations, or bizarre social behavior, but, over an extended period, does display other symptoms or personality traits so similar to those seen both in the families of schizophrenics and in individuals who are or subsequently become schizophrenic that it is assumed that his disorder is in fact a *forme fruste* (Mayer-Gross 1960) of the same disease. The concept that a disorder could be considered schizophrenic even if it did not show the classical symptoms was first introduced by Bleuler (1911), who used the term *latent schizophrenia* to refer to certain irritable, odd, moody, or withdrawn individuals whom he considered to be suffering from a mild form of the illness. This term has been criticized on the grounds that it unnecessarily broadens the concept of schizophrenia and that it is illogical to speak of an illness as latent except in retrospect. The underlying notion has, however, been perpetuated to some extent by the construction of a number of related diagnostic labels: *pseudoneurotic schizophrenia* (Hoch 1949), *borderline state* (Knight 1953), *pseudopyschopathic schizophrenia* (Dunaif 1955), *schizoid personality* (Bleuler 1941, Kretschmer 1926), and a host of others. Whatever the term, the implication is the same: the individual's symptoms or behavior do not at first glance appear schizophrenic but derive from the same factors that in another patient would cause the more typical form of the disease.

The kinds of behavior and symptoms shown by such individuals range from obsessional thinking, hypochondriasis, panphobia and pananxiety to drug addiction, litigiousness, argumentativeness, shyness and delicacy, eccentricity, bigoted piety, fanaticism, suspiciousness, and hypersensitivity (Bleuler 1941). While individuals with such traits are not always "really" schizophrenic, they are more likely than normals to develop an overt psychosis (Ugelstad 1968), and they may, moreover, when given phenothiazines, abandon some of their unusual behavior patterns and become less likely to decompensate. Even in these patients, the manifest symptoms may seem connected with an underlying cognitive disturbance. The latent schizophrenic might appear obsessional because he has learned to cope with his confused thinking by becoming pedantic and unusually precise, writing meticulously detailed notes to himself, and planning future events in minute detail. Another might appear hypochondriacal because his unusual somatic experiences lead him to consult one physician after the next, though in such cases the bizarreness of the symptoms he describes and the suspiciousness or reproachfulness with which he complains about the physician's inaction or ineffectiveness might betray the underlying disorder. In some cases, a latent schizophrenia masquerades as drug addiction: the patient finds a drug that keeps his discomfort in check and exhibits no obviously schizophrenic symptoms until he stops taking it (see p. 312). Even a paranoid patient may not be immediately identifiable as schizophrenic: if his delusional ideas are not too far removed from reality, and especially when he makes a conscious effort to mislead those around him, his explanations for being argumentative, litigious, suspicious, or in pursuit of some girl who exhibits no apparent interest in him may for some time appear reasonable and hard to dispute.

The disorder labeled *pseudoneurotic schizophrenia* also falls into this category. In the typical case, the patient falls ill during his late 20s or early 30s (Hoch 1962), and, despite being lucid and devoid of delusional ideas, shows numerous neurotic symptoms, the most characteristic of which are pananxiety and panphobia. These patients may decompensate intermittently into a frank psychosis, but even in the interim period their symptoms tend to fluctuate. That the patient can develop a number of characterologic and neurotic ways of coping with his disorder seems to be caused in part by the alternating periods of cognitive dysfunction and reintegration he experiences that permit him to use many of his premorbid coping mechanisms and to establish a wide variety of new ones as well.

TREATMENT OF SCHIZOPHRENIC ILLNESSES WITH ACUTE FEATURES

The treatment of schizophrenic illnesses can be arbitrarily divided into three periods of varying goals and lengths. The goal of the *first phase* is to enable the patient to engage in meaningful discussions with his physician and transact with those around him with some measure of comfort and effectiveness; this can usually be achieved within a few weeks. The length of the *second phase* is less predictable; it lasts until the patient has established a durable relationship with his physician, no longer needs close supervision, and, if hospitalized, is well enough to be discharged. The *third phase* of treatment aims toward the patient's readjustment to the community; how long it should last—or whether indeed it should ever end—must be decided from case to case.

The First Phase of Treatment

The Treatment Setting

Some general comments regarding the choice of treatment setting and its effect on the patient's treatment and the course of his illness have been made in Chapter 2. While most of these statements are applicable to the acutely ill schizophrenic, special problems arise in trying to provide him with protection and structure without making him excessively dependent.

Patients with acute schizophrenic illnesses are more likely to need *hospitalization* than those who are neurotic or depressed. When the illness is florid, the patient is unable to engage in a meaningful discussion or collaborate with his doctor, which makes it harder to understand or protect him. Since he may be dangerous to both himself and the community and, if untreated, is likely to get worse, hospitalization, which makes the patient easier to protect and to treat, is often the wisest first step. A comprehensive treatment program may be initiated more rapidly in the hospital setting than would be feasible or safe in outpatient treatment. Despite these advantages, hospitalization may undermine the long-term goals of treatment (see also p. 135) by showing the acutely ill schizophrenic how quickly it relieves his distress and thus teaching him how to escape from stress by becoming ill and dependent. It is preferable, therefore, to avoid hospitalization whenever possible.

The best yardsticks for measuring the patient's need for hospitalization are his sleep pattern, the rate at which his illness has progressed, and the extent of demonstrable danger. Outpatient care may be attempted when 1/ the sleep loss does not exceed two hours nightly, 2/ the illness has progressed relatively slowly, and 3/ the patient has made no overt threats to himself or the community. Inpatient care will be mandatory, however, when the patient is delusional or subject to imperative auditory hallucinations, for his behavior is then likely to be unpredictable. Patients whose illnesses are this severe usually have such other symptoms as severe sleep loss, confusion, or bizarre behavior that make the need for hospitalization obvious. The following comments on the treatment of acute schizophrenic illnesses assume that the patient is hospitalized, but are, with minor modifications, equally applicable to outpatient treatment.

The optimal treatment setting for the acutely ill schizophrenic may be defined as that which is most conducive to his comfort and collaboration (Storms 1969). Experiments with subjects whose ability to assess the relevance of stimuli is impaired by being given hallucinogenics, or deprived of sleep or sensory stimulation, suggest that the discomfort, sense of portentousness, and perceptual disturbance that these individuals experience can be mitigated by an ordered sequence of meaningful stimuli (Bliss 1959, Davis 1960, Freedman 1961, Heron 1961, Rosenzweig 1966, West 1962, Williams 1959). Experience confirms what these investigations suggest: that the acutely ill schizophrenic responds best to a consistent, simple, and well-structured environment that repeatedly presents him with meaningful information concerning his situation and the behavior to which he is expected to conform (Spadoni 1969). The more confused and disoriented the patient is, the simpler his environment should be. If hospitalization and medications do not diminish his confusion and agitation and his behavior is intolerably disruptive, it may be necessary to isolate him from other patients until his condition improves.

Isolation rooms should not be used, however, if any other solution is possible; they certainly should not become a routine way of maintaining a ward's serenity. All too often, they are more of a therapeutic hindrance than a help, for a patient can become just as uncomfortable from being understimulated as from being overstimulated: autistic fantasies, paranoid ideas, and agitation may increase. The effect on other patients must also be considered:

some suffer vicariously or become fearful that they too will be isolated; others regard the event as an instructive example of how to "get away from it all" by being "locked up."

Unfortunately, the alternatives to isolation rooms require elements that are hard to come by, such as a high staff-patient ratio or a well-organized social structure that encourages patients to take responsibility for each other (Almond 1968). The use of isolation can be avoided or shortened by providing the patient with a nonintrusive companion—a special nurse, another patient in partial remission, or even a family member—who can help him test reality and become familiar with his environment. When the patient's unruly behavior is being either ignored or encouraged by his fellow patients or is causing them to ostracize him, the situation must be discussed in patient-staff meetings, and every effort must be made to involve other patients in staying with him, watching him, and encouraging his resocialization (Detre 1970, Fleck 1969, Rubenstein 1966).

Somatic Aspects of Treatment

Phenothiazines have today largely replaced the classical sedatives in the treatment of the agitated schizophrenic, for they not only have a more protracted tranquilizing effect but also are less likely to augment his confusion. Even more important than the phenothiazines' immediate calming effect, however, is their efficacy in relieving such symptoms as anxiety, perplexity, insomnia, withdrawal, hallucinations, delusions, and affective disturbances (Casey 1960, Kurland 1962, May 1964, NIMH 1964). They can also prevent the development of new symptoms, and protracted use often prevents chronic desocialization (Goldberg 1965). Indeed, it is of such vital importance that the patient receive phenothiazines quickly that it is warranted to give them in liquid or parenteral form if he is initially too fearful, delusional, or insightless to collaborate.

The choice of phenothiazines proceeds in accordance with the guidelines presented in Chapter 14, which may be summarized as follows:

1/ Patients whose most prominent symptom is marked agitation are given "sedating" phenothiazines such as chlorpromazine (Thorazine).

2/ Those whose agitation is less marked are given "intermediate" phenothiazines such as perphenazine (Trilafon).

3/ Those who show little or no agitation at all are given either one of the intermediate or one of the more alerting phenothiazines, such as fluphenazine (Prolixin).

4/ Patients whose illnesses appear refractory to phenothiazines or who tolerate phenothiazines poorly may be given reserpine, butyrophenones, or thioxanthenes.

In *acute schizophrenic illnesses,* treatment should begin with a moderate dose of a phenothiazine, which should be repeated at fairly frequent intervals and, if necessary, increased. Fifty mg of chlorpromazine, 4 mg of perphenazine, or 1 mg of fluphenazine should be given at hourly intervals until the patient either reports that he is feeling better or falls asleep. Thereafter, the dosage is titrated according to his symptoms, ability to sleep, and social behavior. The total daily dosage required at this stage is usually six to 12 times as large as the individual doses listed above and is given in three to five divided doses throughout the day. Typical dosage schedules would thus be chlorpromazine 100-200 mg, 4-5 times daily, perphenazine 8-16 mg, 4-5 times daily, or fluphenazine 2-5 mg, 3-4 times daily.

In *acute catatonic episodes,* the patient's behavior can become so dangerous that the rapid institution of therapeutic measures of heroic proportions becomes necessary. Phenothiazines like chlorpromazine (Thorazine), usually in doses of 800-1,200 mg, but as much as 2,000 mg daily, or perphenazine (Trilafon), usually in doses of 48-64 mg, but up to 96 mg daily, should be given on the first day. Since these dose levels often lead to hypotension or extrapyramidal side effects, the patient's physical condition must be carefully monitored. Most catatonic patients given doses of this magnitude behave more reasonably and sleep better within a short time. An early sign of improvement is that the patient's systolic blood pressure—which, at this stage of illness, is usually 30 mm to 40 mm above normal—returns to its premorbid level. If the patient's sleep and social behavior do not improve within 48 hours or improve only after he is given the highest dosage levels, intramuscular injections of reserpine, 2 to 5 mg, 3 times daily, should be given in addition to the phenothiazines. If these measures are effective, the dosage should not be changed for a minimum of 10 days. If, however, the patient does not respond to phenothiazines or reserpine within 48 to 72 hours, his blood pressure remains high, his sleep loss severe, or his behavior impulsive and disruptive, he should be given one or two electroshock treatments daily until his sleep improves. Thereafter, ECT may be discontinued since drug treatment alone usually suffices to maintain and further the improvement.

The somatic treatment of *paranoid schizophrenic* illnesses follows the same general principles, with the exception that antidepressants may be needed after the patient's agitation diminishes. A more detailed discussion of their management may be found in Chapter 5 where, in order to highlight their contrasts and similarities, schizophrenic and nonschizophrenic paranoid syndromes are discussed together.

In the *schizoaffective schizophrenias* of the *manic* or *excited type,* intermediate or sedative phenothiazines alone, such as perphenazine (Trilafon), 32 to 64 mg daily, or chlorpromazine (Thorazine), 600 to 1,000 mg daily, should be used initially, but if this is not effective, it may be necessary to turn to a brief course of ECT (see p. 648). *Schizoaffective disorders* of the *depressed type* sometimes respond to phenothiazines alone, but usually respond better when the patient is also given an antidepressant. Treatment with an antidepressant-phenothiazine combination is, in any case, superior to the use of antidepressants alone, and is started by giving the patient an intermediate phenothiazine, such as perphenazine in doses of 32 mg to 48 mg daily for a week or ten days. At this time, an antidepressant, such as imipramine (Tofranil), 75 to 150 mg daily, is added. After the patient's sleep has been restored (or if it has been good from the outset), an alerting phenothiazine like fluphenazine (Prolixin), 10 to 15 mg daily, may be substituted for the perphenazine. Once the patient's mood has lifted, the antidepressant dosage should be gradually reduced. While antidepressants can usually be discontinued entirely after 12 to 18 months, some patients fare best by taking these agents indefinitely. The use of lithium carbonate has also been recommended in the treatment of acute schizoaffective disorders (Rice 1956), regardless of the type. This drug, though, can aggravate excitement and heighten paranoid ideation, and should therefore be given in conjunction with a phenothiazine or other major tranquilizer (see p. 192).

Psychotherapeutic Aspects

Until the patient's sleep has improved and his psychotic symptoms have stopped disrupting his social relationships, it is important that all aspects of his treatment and environment remain uncomplicated. Psychotherapy, for example, should be limited to frequent, brief, supportive contacts in which patient and doctor discuss only the most immediate problems in the patient's everyday life. Long or complex discussions should be postponed until the patient is sleeping better, his psychotic symptoms have receded, and his social functioning has improved. Even at this time, however, the discussions should be approached gingerly and if, in their course, it is noticed that the patient's delusions have not fully receded, and especially if these delusions include the therapist, the transactions should be simplified once more in the sense that the therapist limits them to a brief explanation of the real situation.

Although much has been learned about the way schizophrenic patients and their families interact (Lidz 1966), too little is known to permit unequivocal or uniform recommendations concerning the family's involvement in the patient's treatment. In some circumstances, family members must be involved, in others excluded; usually they need support, sometimes they may also need treatment; sometimes treatment or counseling for them is indicated for the patient's sake, more often for their own. In some cases, the patient and family should be seen together, either at intervals or at all times; in others, treatment proceeds best when they are seen separately. A more comprehensive discussion of these questions and of the indications for family treatment may be found in Chapter 13.

When the patient is so ill that the question of hospitalization arises, it is likely that his family will become involved. By meeting with them, the clinician can obtain additional information regarding the patient's condition and determine whether they are able to offer the patient enough support and supervision to stay out of the hospital. If his condition is grave or his family too confused, rejecting, hostile, or intellectually limited to help him, hospitalization is usually the best course, because it ensures that his treatment will proceed without undue complications and permits him to be separated from a family that is, at least at that time, noxious for him. The decision to hospitalize the patient because of his family's inability to care for him properly, however, should not be regarded as a decision to separate him from his family permanently. There are situations, to be sure, in which a protracted or even a permanent separation of patient and family seems desirable, but a decision of this kind can be made only after the family's transactional style has been observed for some time.

The relatives of schizophrenic patients frequently seem somewhat strange—stranger perhaps than the families of patients with other illnesses (Alanen 1966)—but this does not by any means demonstrate that this strangeness is causally related to the patient's difficulties (Schopler 1969) or that he would fare better if he were living alone. The family's peculiarity or psychopathology may make it harder to work with them, but it can also make it easier: their own struggles with psychological problems may lead them to be especially supportive toward their afflicted relative and particularly tolerant of his difficulties. Moreover, even though some schizophrenic patients' families obstruct the therapist's intentions and plans, this is neither so frequent as commonly believed nor by any means unique to the families of schizophrenics. Indeed, there seems to be little correlation between obstructionism and those factors usually considered pathogenic. On innumerable occasions, we have seen classically overprotective, confusingly ambiguous, domineering, and ambivalence-promoting parents who, perhaps because they recognized and felt guilty about their own failings, have encouraged the patient to cooperate with the physician and have tried their best to do so themselves. If a parent seems irrationally insistent that his child can and *must* get well, we should not deride this as denial or overprotectiveness, as is commonly done, for it is at times the only force that keeps the patient out of the hospital, socially active, and involved in treatment, and thereby prevents the development of chronic desocialization. No matter how limited the family's support may be, it is usually a far better defense against the patient's social isolation than halfway houses, patient social clubs, or any of the other artificially erected facilities that we can provide.

These are not the only reasons for maintaining a patient's family ties and seeking to involve his family in his treatment. An additional motive is that we want to develop the kind of relationship with them that will enable them to pay heed to our recommendations and, if necessary, can be used to help them modify their behavior. When the patient is hospitalized, his family should be encouraged to visit him. This gives us an opportunity to observe and influence the patient-family transactions, and may help the acutely ill patient accept and feel less threatened by his new surroundings. Just after admission, he may be so disturbed that visitors can stay for only a few minutes at a time, but longer visits are usually feasible within a few days. If the patient does not wish to see his family, we will initially respect his wishes and explain the situation to them, but as he starts to get better, we must try to make sense of his reluctance, if necessary by insisting on a few joint meetings.

THE SECOND PHASE OF TREATMENT

The second phase of treatment begins when the patient's sleep has improved and his psychotic symptoms no longer interfere with his ability to communicate with those around him and take care of his most immediate personal needs. Its goal, which is to restore to the patient primary control over his activities, is attained when he is well enough to function outside a hospital and continue treatment on his own.

Psychotherapeutic and Environmental Aspects

After the patient's sleep has improved and he is in reasonably good contact with his environment, he should be helped to examine the conflicts and stresses operative both in his current situation and in the time just before his more serious symptoms began. If these discussions seem unproductive, it is sometimes useful to invite the patient's family to participate in them. The initial *meetings with a patient's family* usually take place in the shadow of the distressing events that preceded referral and can be a fertile field for increasing dissension. They should therefore be limited to gathering information about the patient's and family's background and answering their questions regarding treatment. Later meetings will offer the physician a greater opportunity to understand the familial relationships, and these may well become the focus of the discussions. Even at this time, however, the physician should urge the participants to avoid discussing excessively painful issues until the patient's thinking has become lucid enough to permit his full-fledged participation. Such meetings may well be disturbing to the participants, but it is far better that their difficulites with each other be aired while the patient is hospitalized than that they be left to erupt after he leaves. Nevertheless, when such meetings affect the patient adversely, the advisability of continuing them must be reassessed. A few hours of agitation or one sleepless night would not be sufficient cause to discontinue them, but a more prolonged upset indicates that the patient is not yet ready to take part.

Once family meetings have become tolerable for the participants, the therapist may use them as a laboratory in which to 1/ observe the way the patient and family behave toward each other, 2/ comment on their behavior and its consequences, 3/ suggest new ways of communicating and interacting, and 4/ offer the participants a setting in which to practice these new ways while learning them. Clear intrafamilial communication is important for psychiatric patients just as it is for other people; it is of even greater benefit to the schizophrenic, for he is especially prone to confusions or delusions when presented with messages that must be understood on several levels. In some cases, the therapist may need to act as the family's interpreter until, under his guidance, all concerned learn to communicate with candor and understanding. When the patient's illness is particularly embarrassing or trying for his family or their behavior toward him is unusually unconventional, it may be useful to treat both patient and family in a group composed of other patients and families. (Further comments on these and other techniques of family therapy will be found in Chapter 13.)

Attempts to improve the patient's interaction with his family should be combined with efforts to *educate* him (and them) about the illness. They should not be spared the discouraging news that some schizophrenic illnesses relapse, but rather should be taught to recognize the prodromal signs, such as disturbances in sleep or cognitive functioning. They should be impressed with the importance of promptly reporting any symptoms that should arise. When maintenance drug treatment is indicated, they must understand why this recommendation is made and why it is unwise to reduce or discontinue the drugs without the physician's agreement (see p. 97).

The best way to tell whether the patient is ready for increased freedom or for hospital discharge is to observe his transactions with those around him. At the beginning, while he is still restricted to the hospital, the major criterion of social improvement is his behavior toward other patients, visitors, and staff during ward activities and therapy meetings. Once his biologic and social functioning approximates the premorbid level, he may leave the hospital for limited periods, first in the company of relatives or other patients, and finally alone. If he tolerates this well, brief home visits may be permitted, and then a trial return to work. If an even more gradual transition from hospital to everyday life is desired, it can be stretched out over a period of several weeks, in which the patient leaves the hospital to pursue his regular activities during the day but returns to the hospital each night; or spends his nights at home and his days in the hospital. This gradual succession of steps enables the psychiatrist to examine the patient's response to the increasing stress of everyday situations. If all goes well and the patient's sleep or behavior do not suffer from his increased social involvement, it is time to make plans for his discharge.

Somatic Aspects

Throughout the second phase of treatment, decisions about the patient's drug requirements are based on his ability to take part in the psychotherapeutic transactions and to tolerate the gradual steps toward discharge described above. Since the purpose of this phase is to prepare the patient for discharge, and since the drug dosage required in the first phase may diminish the alertness required for functioning in the outside world, the patient's drugs are usually lowered toward the end of the second phase. The diminution should be gradual, and a minimum of 10 days should elapse between one reduction and the next. After each step, the patient's condition should be reassessed to determine whether the lower dose level suffices to prevent the recurrence of symptoms. At the time of his discharge, he should be taking enough medication to ensure sound sleep and to enable him to relate to his environment with some comfort and effectiveness. Typically, doses of 24 to 32 mg of perphenazine (Trilafon) or 8 to 12 mg of fluphenazine (Prolixin) provide ample protection when the patient is beginning the extramural or third phase of treatment. For the next three to six weeks, drug dosage should not be reduced further, but can be raised if his symptoms recur.

Once the acute phase of illness is over and the hallucinations, delusions, agitation, and difficulty in falling asleep have disappeared, many patients show *depressive symptoms,* such as anergia, apathy, lassitude, early morning awakening, withdrawal, and even suicidal ideation (Bowers 1967, Cohen 1964, Ploticher 1962, Steinberg 1967). This change in symptoms is a source of discomfort and danger. The physician is often so engrossed with the patient's thought disorder per se that he fails to view the depression and suicidal potential with the seriousness they deserve (Achté 1966). In some cases, the depressive symptoms are caused by the major tranquilizers the patient is taking (Simonson 1964); in others, such symptoms have been present from the onset, but remain unnoticed until after delusions, hallucinations, and bizarre thinking are no longer prominent (Shanfield 1970). But there is no way of knowing in the individual case, and even if it were known that they were drug-induced, it might be unwise to lower the patient's dosage, as this might cause his thought disorder to recur. Whatever their cause, they often remit within a few weeks; when they do not, an antidepressant like imipramine (Tofranil), 75 to 150 mg daily, should be added. If the upper dose range is needed, it should be approached gradually, for antidepressants can reactivate sleep disturbances, cognitive disorders, delusions, and hallucinations. If this should occur, the dosage of antidepressant should be reduced for one to two weeks and then raised again. In many cases, antidepressants are ineffective and a course of ECT becomes necessary, but even this may not relieve the patient's depressive symptoms, which in some instances continue for many months.

To what extent the patient's new and troubling image of himself contributes to the depressions following acute schizophrenic episodes is hard to say. It is our impression, in any case, that suicidal ideation often develops after the patient discovers that he is too anergic to function as he did before he first fell ill and therefore assumes that he is permanently impaired. Often, he will experience much relief from being assured that his anergia is transient; and, since his depression and self-denigration are likely to increase each time he cannot perform as he expects to, he should be urged to assume only those responsibilities that he can shoulder with comfort. Part-time employment may be better at first; a woman may need extra help with her household; a student may be well advised to limit his course load or to drop out of school for a time. This kind of protection and cushioning should not go on indefinitely, however; after the patient has been out of the hospital for a number of months, he may need to be urged to get back into harness, lest his dependent adjustment become permanent.

The Endpoint of Hospitalization

The patient's release from the hospital marks only the border between the second and third phase of treatment and does not by any means signify that we consider him fully recovered. It is not only unnecessary but untherapeutic and unrealistic as well to insist that his health be restored before he is discharged. Some patients take months or years to become as well as they once were, and many never return to their premorbid level. Nonetheless, after some time in the hospital, most patients can safely return to the outside even if some of their symptoms persist. In many cases, the extent of the patient's improvement can be gauged only after he is discharged, for his performance in the stable, all-too-comfortable, and dependency-inducing confines of the hospital does not necessarily correspond to the way he will cope with the harsher demands of the world outside. Even more important, his further improvement may hinge on his discharge, for any difficulties he may have in participating in community and family activities are best overcome if they are discussed while he is experiencing them. Indeed, if we are to consider skillful and comfortable handling of extramural activities an important criterion of remission, it is a veritable contradiction in terms to speak of a hospitalized patient as "cured" (Bachman 1970).

The length of the second phase will depend in some measure on how long the patient was ill before his treatment began. Patients with *acute catatonic* and *acute undifferentiated* illnesses usually consult physicians a few days or weeks after the onset of their most acute symptoms and often feel and look so much better after 10 to 14 days of vigorous treatment that they seem ready to leave the hospital. Patients with *paranoid* schizophrenia, on the other hand, tend to come to medical attention only after their symptoms have been in progress for some months or years and usually take a correspondingly longer time to achieve the same level of improvement. Rapid improvement may well be gratifying to both patient and doctor, but can compromise the patient's further course if too quickly followed by discharge. Some patients, to be sure, are so frightened by the dramatic sequence of events and so impressed with the rapidity of their improvement that they voluntarily continue in treatment after discharge. More commonly, however, rapid recovery and discharge permit the patient to deny the severity of his illness, cause him to ignore the physician's further recommendations, and thus pave the way for a relapse. This kind of self-defeating sequence is less likely to occur in a patient who has been hospitalized for some months: having had time to contemplate the consequences of his illness and to develop a meaningful relationship with his physician, he will be more disposed to remain in treatment even after his discharge.

The desire to have the patient enter outpatient treatment as early as possible must, then, be tempered by our awareness of the adverse effects of premature discharge. The diminution of symptoms is thus a far less realistic endpoint of hospitalization than the assurance that the patient will continue his treatment as long as he needs to (Zolik 1968). Considerations of this kind can occasionally justify prolonging the patient's hospital stay by a few weeks.

THE THIRD PHASE OF TREATMENT

Once the patient leaves the hospital, three goals measure the success of his treatment. The most immediate and most important is that he continue his treatment. The second is that his transition to the world outside, his resocialization, and his return to premorbid social functioning proceed smoothly. The third goal is that he become well enough to function without any treatment, but this ought not to be overemphasized, for the propensity to schizophrenic decompensation is often lifelong. The achievement of these goals rests on both the efficacy of the earlier phases and the psychotherapeutic and pharmacologic measures taken during the final phase.

Since psychiatrists who treat hospitalized patients often maintain no outpatient practice, many patients must transfer from one doctor to another at the time of discharge. In such situations, a smooth transition and the continuation of treatment can be best assured if the patient starts seeing his outpatient therapist during his final weeks of hospitalization and continues his meetings with his hospital doctor for several weeks after his discharge. The two therapists should, of course, be in touch with each other during the weeks both are treating the patient.

During the earlier phases of treatment, the complexities of the doctor-patient relationship should be discussed only to the extent required to prevent the patient from doing anything that would interfere with his treatment (such as prematurely leaving the hospital, returning to work, discontinuing his medications, or interrupting his psychotherapy); but after discharge the focus of discussion may become a good deal broader. It may be of some value to explore the way the patient and doctor affect each other and the rules, both stated and unstated, that govern their relationship. Such discussions may eventually be expanded to a search for *patterns in the patient's behavior* as exemplified in this relationship. An understanding of these patterns may help the patient achieve a better understanding of his social impact, for his way of relating to the therapist is likely to reflect the way he relates to others, and the doctor's reactions to him are likely to resemble the reactions of others. When such patterns interfere with the patient's pursuit of his life goals, their consequences should be examined, and their background may need to be explored.

Group therapy meetings, patient clubs, hospital activities, and community social functions are helpful adjuncts to the patient's resocialization. Patients who have not previously worked or whose occupational skills have suffered from disuse should be offered vocational counseling and training, encouraged to find a job, and advised on how to keep it. These activities are social in the sense that they involve other people, but require only superficial social competence. Comfort and skill in handling intimate relationships, on the other hand, may be far harder to achieve. Indeed, when a patient has a long history of difficulty in getting close to others, he should be cautioned against becoming involved in an intimate friendship or romance until he has made some progress in acquiring at least the most superficial social skills, has been working for some time, and has thus shown that he can transact comfortably in less demanding situations. Each of these steps can be difficult; one function of the patient-doctor transactions is to explore the difficulties and their causes and, so far as possible, prepare the patient to overcome them.

THE TERMINATION OF TREATMENT

After the patient has been free of acute or disabling symptoms for a period of six to 12 months, decisions are required concerning his further treatment. In making these decisions, the following questions are of particular relevance:

1/ Has the patient had previous episodes of schizophrenic illness? If so, how many has he had and how far apart were they?

2/ How long was he ill before receiving treatment?

3/ How well is he functioning at present, and how does this compare with the years before his acute symptoms developed (or, if he has had previous episodes, with the periods between them)?

4/ How disabling or dangerous were his symptoms at the height of the current or previous episodes?

5/ Was the current episode preceded by any stress that might have contributed to his falling ill?

The answers to these questions will help the clinician decide whether and for how long the patient should continue to take drugs, and whether he needs to continue in intensive psychotherapy or might do just as well if his visits were briefer, less frequent, or discontinued entirely.

Since many patients remain well only if they are given *maintenance medications* (Engelhardt 1967, Gantz 1965, Gross 1961, Morton 1968, Wessler 1963, Winkelman 1964), and since recurrences can have tragic consequences, the decision to discontinue drugs cannot be made lightly. Using the listed questions as guidelines, then, a patient is a candidate for maintenance drug treatment if

1/ he has had several episodes of illness within the space of a few years, or

2/ he has been continuously psychotic for two or more years, and

3/ no obvious precipitants can be found that help explain either the current or any earlier episode;

4/ the symptoms of this or previous episodes endangered his life or his chance of returning to his prior social situation,

5/ his (or his family's) prior behavior or current attitudes suggest that he would not immediately consult a physician should his symptoms recur;

6/ despite having been on drugs for some years, his remission is incomplete in the sense that he continues to show residual symptoms that exacerbate whenever his drugs are decreased, or

7/ he had been socially impaired for an extended period before his acute symptoms arose but now functions fairly well.

On the other hand, a patient who has had but a single brief episode, and that precipitated by a severe or unusual stress of some kind, and who had always functioned well before his symptoms began would not meet our criteria for maintenance medication. The individual patient's situation is rarely as clear-cut as these examples, however, and the physician must decide which of the two it approximates more closely.

As a general rule, we try to discontinue a patient's drugs after a first episode of schizophrenic illness. We wait until his symptoms have been quiescent and his social functioning restored for a period of six to 12 months; then, over a six-month period, we gradually reduce his drug dosage until he is taking no drugs at all. During this time, and for at least 12 months thereafter, the patient must be closely observed. If he develops a sleep disorder or any of the other symptoms that characterized his original illness, or if his social functioning declines, the drug dosage is increased to the point where these difficulties once more subside, are held at this level for three or four months, and then lowered again. We continue our effort to discontinue the patient's drugs for a period of one to two years. If, even after so long a period, each attempt is followed by a resurgence of symptoms or a deterioration of social functioning, we assume that the patient will remain ill for some time, stop exposing him to the fluctuations inherent in the withdrawal attempts, and arrange to continue his medications indefinitely. In some cases, we try to lower the patient's drugs again three to five years later, but this rarely succeeds.

Reports concerning the patient's past and present social functioning may prompt a decision to use maintenance medications even after a single episode of acute illness. We are therefore likely to give a patient drugs for at least two years if, even before his acute symptoms began, his personality and performance had been severely disturbed and his achievements had compared poorly with those of his peers—especially if the administration of phenothiazines had not only diminished recent psychotic symptoms, but also improved the individual's social functioning beyond its premorbid level. If, even after he has been on drugs for two years, withdrawal causes the previous difficulties to return, we continue the drugs indefinitely.

In any case, maintenance medication is indicated when a patient has had several episodes of illness, each of which occurred while he was not taking drugs and remitted after he resumed taking them. This decision usually follows the second episode of illness, but may be delayed until after the third if the first two episodes 1/ so rapidly followed each other that what appeared as a second might have been no more than a relapse of the first, 2/ were so mild and so far apart that it seems unnecessary to subject the individual to the hazards and inconveniences of long-term drug administration in order to avoid some distant and easily manageable recurrence, or 3/ were each preceded by some event that seems to have so reasonable a relationship to the development of the illness that the double occurrence might be viewed as a coincidence and not as evidence of a chronically relapsing course. This last criterion, of course, is the weakest: a temporal correlation between a stress and a subsequent illness can readily imply causation where, in reality, the two events are only accidentally linked in time. The patient who develops the symptoms of an acute schizophrenic episode immediately after some kind of stress—cortisone administration, the prolonged use of hallucinogens, going away to college, or encephalitis—is, to be sure, less likely to develop such symptoms again than one whose symptoms appeared without provocation, but he is also less likely to be free of such symptoms permanently than the person who has never had such symptoms at all. In the presence of an antecedent stress, we might thus be more willing to lower a patient's drugs and more reluctant to start him on maintenance medication, but would not shorten the length of time after recovery that we continue to see him. The meetings need not even be long or frequent, especially if the patient's relationship to the doctor seems stable enough to ensure that he will call if difficulties arise, but it is essential that these meetings continue for a year or two after the patient's symptoms recede.

The criteria used in deciding how frequently the patient and doctor should meet and how long their meetings should be are similar to those used in deciding how long the patient should be given drugs. In general, the patient should remain involved in a psychotherapeutic relationship as long as his social functioning continues to improve. Once his performance has reached a plateau that equals or exceeds his premorbid level or, despite changes in therapist and type of therapy, he continues to function poorly, it is reasonable to try to determine whether his functioning would decline if his contact with the therapist were reduced. To this end, we gradually shorten the duration of the meetings and lengthen the intervals between them until the patient is seen for 10 to 15 minutes every six to eight weeks. If the patient's social functioning has been and remains good, the further course depends on whether he is still taking drugs. If he is not taking drugs, the meetings are gradually spaced further and further apart until he shows he can tolerate even a six-month interval between meetings without running into difficulties. At this time his treatment can be discontinued entirely. Naturally, if the patient's social performance remains poor or he is still taking drugs, he must continue to be seen, but the intervals between visits can be as long as three months and the meetings themselves quite brief. Even a patient who does not need or benefit from psychotherapy and who does not take medication should be seen in a brief followup visit every three to six months if his previous illness was so severe that it is imperative to guard him against the danger of an undetected relapse.

In some cases, the patient's social functioning declines as the length or frequency of his therapy meetings is reduced. If the decline is mild, we may do nothing in the hope that he will soon find adequate substitutes for the therapeutic relationship; if it is marked or continues for more than six months, further psychotherapy is indicated and may remain so indefinitely. In some cases, the patient must receive both drugs and psychotherapy for an extended period. This is especially true of those patients whose premorbid adjustment was poor or whose illness was prolonged, for such individuals tend not only to have a poorer prognosis but also—as evidenced by the length of time they functioned poorly before being referred— to stem from a family that is uninformed, noncorrective, excessively tolerant of psychopathology, or reluctant to permit treatment. Prolonged treatment can make the entire difference between a downhill course and rehabilitation for a patient of this kind (Lee 1965), and it is essential that vigorous followup efforts be made. If the patient misses an appointment, he should immediately be called or even visited, and this should be followed by a letter reminding him of his next appointment time. In some cases, it is helpful to enlist the collaboration of a visiting nurse or even the patient's employer; in others, to hold regular meetings with the patient's family, in which to explore and, if necessary, correct their attitudes toward his illness and treatment.

The divergence of opinions regarding the indications for maintenance medication rests in part on the fact that most studies aimed at assessing its effects vary widely in the *type* and *dosage* of drug used and in the *time span* during which its effectiveness was judged. Indeed, until these factors are standardized (Katz 1962), our conviction that patients who are given "enough" of the "right" drug tend not to relapse will be no more than a feeble generalization.

While there is no solid evidence to show that any particular *type* of phenothiazine protects the patient against future relapse better than others, we tend to avoid using sedating phenothiazines like chlorpromazine (Thorazine) or thioridazine (Mellaril) as maintenance medications. In the first place, when these drugs are given in doses high enough to prevent relapse, they have been reported to have deleterious long-term effects (see p. 589). This is less true of the more alerting phenothiazines, which, being effective at far lower dose levels, are also less likely to make the patient drowsy, impair his reaction time, or otherwise interfere with his normal daytime functioning. The patient's subjective reaction to the drug helps to determine its long-term effect. In our experience, patients taking sedating phenothiazines are more likely to complain about the way the drug makes them feel and more likely to stop taking it than those taking alerting ones.

In most instances, a *maintenance dosage* of 12 to 16 mg of perphenazine (Trilafon), 8 to 12 mg of trifluoperazine (Stelazine), or 6 to 8 mg of fluphenazine (Prolixin) daily affords sufficient protection against relapse. In some cases, however, somewhat higher maintenance doses (Rosati 1964), such as 16-24 mg of perphenazine, 15-20 mg of trifluoperazine, or 10-15 mg of fluphenazine daily, are preferable. The higher doses are in any case more efficient in preventing what has been aptly labeled as the "drug dosage merry-go-round"—that common situation in which the therapeutic relationship and the patient's life adjustment are continually disrupted by the unending cycle of illness → medication → remission → medication reduction → exacerbation → medication increase → remission → medication reduction → and so forth (Forrest 1964). Higher maintenance dose levels are also indicated in patients whose premorbid functioning has not been restored or had always been poor. If, after being given the maintenance dose levels suggested above, a patient remains free of acute symptoms but continues to show some impairment in his social functioning, it may be useful to increase the medication, and if this helps, to continue increasing it every two to three months until the patient either stops improving or develops unmanageable side effects.

As with dosage, there is no definitive answer to the question of *how long* maintenance drug treatment should continue or whether it should ever be discontinued at all. It is known, however, that there is even more difference between the social adjustment of the medicated and the nonmedicated schizophrenic at the end of 12 to 24 months than there is after a briefer time (Engelhardt 1963, Gross 1961). Indeed, from the little that is currently known, it appears that the value of maintenance medication derives less from preserving the patient's comfort between episodes of mental illness than from preventing decompensation when the next bout of illness is "due." Maintenance medication, of course, does not protect the patient against every manifestation of his illness. Even if his initial symptoms have improved and he continues to take phenothiazines as prescribed, he may remain socially awkward or somewhat uncomfortable and, at intervals, have a mild exacerbation of the cognitive disorder (which he will probably experience as an episode of obsessional thinking or anxiety). These episodes do not usually progress further and can be regarded as subclinical relapses, in the sense that the patient would exhibit psychotic symptoms at this time were he not taking medications. With these reservations, however, it is our experience that patients who continue to take the prescribed dose of a major tranquilizer following remission of their first or second episode of schizophrenic illness rarely relapse severely enough to require hospitalization.

That many untreated patients experience but a single episode of schizophrenic illness during their lifetime casts some doubt on the favorable results reported of maintenance treatment. Nevertheless, we have seen many patients whose illnesses had recurred repeatedly for many years and who recover once they are given phenothiazines, remain well as long as they take them, relapse each time they stop taking them, and remit again as soon as phenothiazine treatment is reinstituted. Some of these patients have few or no symptoms when on medicines, while others function only marginally. Yet, however they function, the important thing is that they do not relapse again.

Initially, we thought that the favorable results with patients who took the drugs faithfully were achieved solely because healthier patients are more likely to follow medical recommendations than those with more serious illnesses; that acquiescence to the prescribed medications might thus be a characteristic of patients who, in any case, would have had a better prognosis; and that, conversely, reluctance to take drugs might characterize patients whose prognosis was graver from the beginning. In recent years, as our recommendations to patients and their families have become increasingly firm, we have found that the results are equally satisfactory when the patient is reluctant or unwilling to take the drugs and does so only as a result of family pressure or even frank coercion. The patient's attitude toward taking his drugs or his reasons for doing so are, then, of far less importance to his prognosis than his adherence to the physician's recommendations. Our experiences in this regard should not lead to premature generalizations regarding the long-term effectiveness of maintenance medication, however, for these drugs have been in use only since the mid-1950s, and thus the longest continuous drug-induced and drug-maintained remission has not yet completed its second decade.

TREATMENT OF SCHIZOPHRENIC ILLNESSES WITH CHRONIC FEATURES

The foregoing comments refer chiefly to the treatment of the acute schizophrenic illness or the chronic schizophrenic illness with an acute exacerbation. The chronic undifferentiated, simple, and hebephrenic schizophrenias, however, require a different and usually a far more time-consuming treatment approach. Such patients may show improvement, but they rarely recover completely; in many cases, even the most vigorous treatment efforts achieve nothing or result in only a slight amelioration of the patient's behavior. Indeed, once a patient has been continuously hospitalized for two or more years, his chance of ever returning to the community is less than 10% (Brown 1960). Nevertheless, that even this small percentage of chronically ill patients recover sufficiently to leave the hospital and even to work and that many of these remain well (Linn 1962) justify the time, personnel, and facilities expended in striving for this goal.

The difficulties encountered in rehabilitating the chronically ill schizophrenic patient result from not only his illness but also its social consequences. His thinking is disordered and has been so for a long time, and his behavior has led to a long period of hospitalization, social withdrawal, or ostracism (Tourney 1960) and thus to an impoverishment of his store of information, vocabulary, and transactional skills (Wing 1961, Wynne 1963). In addition, he is likely to have developed compensatory mechanisms, such as systematized delusions or obsessional rituals, which are extremely hard to dislodge. All these factors further impair his thinking, behavior, and social functioning. The net result, after some years, is that the patient is so inadequate that social retraining is well-nigh impossible, and he has been abandoned as hopeless by those most likely to tolerate him if he could improve even slightly—his family and friends.

While a protracted course of alerting phenothiazines often improves the patient's cognitive functions (Clark 1961), his social competence is unlikely to improve unless he is also offered some kind of *long-term social retraining* (Wing 1961). Indeed, one might contrast the treatment of the acutely ill schizophrenic patient with that of the chronically ill patient by saying that the acute requires somatic therapies administered against a background of social retraining and in the context of a psychotherapeutic relationship, while the chronic requires social retraining and a supportive relationship against a background of somatic therapy.

The psychiatrist's persuasion and his offer of emotional and professional support can sometimes convince a reluctant family to take the patient back home or encourage a skeptical community agency to offer him treatment, a job, or a place to live, but the ultimate success of these efforts depends less on the doctor's talents than on the patient's. All such persuasion will come to naught if the doctor cannot restore the patient's social acceptability by helping him to become relatively lucid, able to work, or in some way appealing. At the very least, he must learn to bathe regularly, dress with some decorum, eat inoffensively, and respond appropriately to simple requests. That even these apparently minor goals are achieved so rarely points up the immensity of the rehabilitative task. Intensive efforts to improve the patient's cognitive functioning, stabilize his mood, and broaden his social and vocational skills must therefore precede any attempt at extramural placement, and support in these areas must continue to be offered long after the patient's discharge (Achté 1967, Becker 1967, Esser 1967).

Some hospitals have worked out imaginative programs of social retraining and remotivation (Ludwig 1969, McGee 1968). It might appear to the uninitiated that bibliotherapy, social clubs, patient government, and sheltered workshops serve only to keep patients amused. Properly used, however, such programs can help the patient maintain his ability to transact with others, remain interested in the world around him, and retain his ties with the larger community. Music and dance therapies can also achieve such goals and, in addition, help patients remold the odd and awkward motor patterns that are often fostered by illness and isolation (Shatin 1961). Community volunteers are valuable participants in such programs: their interest in the patient as a person may rekindle his hopes for a different life, even if he has long been resigned to an institutional existence; and their social behavior offers him a model to imitate, as he tries to adapt his own behavior to the demands of the world outside the hospital.

If a patient's work tolerance, social attitudes, and social and occupational skills can be sufficiently improved, gradual exposure to a less sheltered environment may be attempted. Day hospital care (Zwerling 1966), night hospitals (Wulff 1966), halfway houses (Rothwell 1966), or placement with families (Pasamanick 1967) may help ease the transition to life outside the hospital. Thereafter, new problems arise, such as finding a working environment neither too monotonous nor too stimulating and preventing the patient from reverting to his accustomed withdrawal and isolation after working hours. These goals may be fostered and the patient's life enriched by encouraging him to become involved with community agencies; join patient clubs of the kind exemplified by Recovery, Inc. (Wechsler 1960) or Fountain House (Beard 1964); become a hospital volunteer; join a social club or therapy group; go to night school; or take courses in languages or music. Instruction in dancing or public speaking can also be of value in restoring the patient's self-confidence and improving his social skills.

It is essential that the patient's medications, work performance, and living arrangements be reassessed from time to time and that his continuing contact with the aftercare agencies be assured. Premature discontinuation of treatment is dangerous for the chronically ill patient. Any unexplained absence from his home or his job and any failure to show up at a follow-up visit should be viewed as an ominous sign: unless he is promptly reintegrated into the aftercare program, it is extremely likely that his symptoms will worsen and that he will eventually have to return to the hospital. Obviously, all aspects of aftercare—medical, social, and vocational—must be centrally coordinated either by a community agency or by the patient's doctor (Coleman 1967, Hall 1966, Havens 1967). The release of chronic patients after five to 10 years of hospitalization, however, is so recent a development that there are at present few facilities available that can ensure a program of this kind (Hogarty 1968, Lamb 1968, McGowan 1966).

The chronic patient's response to *somatic treatment* is far harder to gauge than that of the acutely ill patient. The criteria used in the treatment of the acutely ill patient—namely, the extent to which his sleep is restored and his excitement abates—are of little value, for the chronic patient often seems to sleep soundly and may well be apathetic, anergic, and inactive to start with. We usually start treatment by giving the chronically ill schizophrenic an alerting phenothiazine like fluphenazine (Prolixin) or trifluoperazine (Stelazine) in doses of 20 to 40 mg daily, but it is hard to decide when or how to modify his regimen. We generally make no changes in the patient's drug dosage for the first three to six months. Then we raise the dosage by 5 mg increments every month or two until the patient either improves or develops unmanageable side effects. As long as he continues to improve, the drug dosage is left unchanged, but whenever his improvement reaches a plateau, we increase the dosage again until no further improvements result from additional increases. It is rarely of benefit to exceed doses of 50 to 60 mg of an alerting phenothiazine daily. If this treatment program is successful, the patient's behavior will become somewhat less bizarre, he will appear less uncomfortable in the course of interpersonal transactions, and the outward manifestations of his discomfort, such as withdrawal and isolation, will diminish. His ability to follow instructions designed to improve his social behavior and to diminish his unattractiveness may be used as a further criterion: the more pressure of this kind he can accept and the better he follows and improves on such instructions without becoming upset, rebellious, increasingly bizarre, sleepless, anorexic, or otherwise symptomatic, the more likely it is that he is receiving the proper treatment.

When phenothiazines alone show little or no effect, other treatment measures may be tried: *the addition of an antidepressant to the phenothiazines* is occasionally helpful (Bennett 1963, Hordern 1963). A protracted course of *reserpine* (see p. 538) may be beneficial, and here, too, the addition of an antidepressant can consolidate whatever gains have been achieved. When pharmacologic treatment measures fail to provide an adequate foundation for the patient's social rehabilitation, his prognosis is grave, and it is justified to use even more vigorous treatment measures. Maintenance ECT (see p. 650) given at weekly, monthly, or even two to three month intervals can sometimes hold the most disruptive symptoms in check for a long time. In some cases, it can restore a patient to a fairly dignified form of extramural functioning for as long as it is administered. *Regressive and "depatterning"* ECT (see p. 650), in which the patient is given a large number of shock treatments at frequent intervals (up to four or six a day for a number of weeks) is also said to relieve some of the more protracted illnesses. Its apparent purpose is to confuse a patient so greatly that whatever rehabilitation efforts are made affect one who is not only completely dependent and infantile, but also as free of delusional ideas as he is of all others. Unfortunately, however, a patient's first coherent words after a series of 40 shock treatments may well be delusional in nature. *Psychosurgery* (see p. 663) has also been used in the treatment of chronic schizophrenics. While it rarely helps them return to the community, it may benefit those who have functioned at minimal work assignments for some time, as in the hospital shop, and could make better use of their opportunities were it not for occasional outbursts of violence that interfere with their activities even within the hospital community (Sargant 1962).

Clearly, the therapeutic optimism expressed in the section on acute schizophrenic illness is not equally applicable to chronic illness. After a patient's thinking has been disordered and he has been locked in his family's attic or on a hospital's chronic ward for many years, he is usually so desocialized that even the most exhaustive psychotherapeutic and somatic treatment efforts are of little or no avail. Full recovery is a rarity; in most cases, little is achieved beyond offering the patient a less chaotic and more dignified adjustment to his illness and environment (Ekblom 1964, Ekdawi 1966, Marjerrison 1964).

PROGNOSIS OF SCHIZOPHRENIC ILLNESSES

That contemporary treatment methods lead to apparent recovery in the majority of acute patients whose illnesses appear just as schizophrenic as those that in the past were considered prognostically grave makes it necessary to redefine the diagnostic significance of the patient's prognosis. The old dictum might be reversed to say that "real" schizophrenics recover and that those whose symptoms look similar but who do not recover are suffering from some other disease. Perhaps, some years hence we will even be able to identify what it is that distinguishes those patients who look schizophrenic and go on to recover from those who look equally schizophrenic but remain ill.

While the improved outcome can be attributed in part to such factors as early referral and diagnosis, modern hospitals, increasing emphasis on psychological and social therapies, greater availability of low-cost outpatient and aftercare clinics, and increased precision in diagnosing illnesses of demonstrably organic origin, the most remarkable decline in the deteriorating courses has occurred since 1954, when chlorpromazine (Thorazine) was introduced. Since that year, the total number of psychiatric patients residing in hospitals has gone steadily downward, even though the national population as a whole has increased and more and more patients with senile psychoses and other organic brain syndromes are admitted to hospitals and remain there permanently (Brill 1959, 1962).

Some investigators have tried to relate the patient's prognosis to the *subtype* of schizophrenia from which he is suffering. Acute schizophrenic episodes with mixed or catatonic symptoms, for example, have long been considered relatively *benign,* while simple and hebephrenic schizophrenias are believed to be more *malignant* Brill 1965). These views have some validity even today, for the symptoms, and thus the subtype, of the illness determine the speed with which the patient is offered treatment, and this in turn influences his outcome (Fossum 1961). As we have noted, acute schizophrenias are rapidly noticeable and show symptoms that prompt immediate referral and treatment. Simple and hebephrenic schizophrenias, on the other hand, are more insidious and less noticeable: the patient's symptoms may not be severe enough to prompt referral until his illness has been in progress for some time. Naturally, this relationship between subtype and referral for treatment is shaped also by factors inherent in the patient's environment. Thus, a patient is likely to remain ill for some time before being treated when

1 / his illness does not disrupt the life adjustment he needs in his particular sociocultural setting;

2 / his illness progresses so slowly that he can mask it by assembling paranoid, somatized, or obsessive-compulsive defenses against it;

3 / his family, classmates, co-workers, and friends find his initial symptoms tolerable;

4 / he comes from an emotionally disturbed family that has trained him to think irrationally or has made him afraid of treatment; or

5 / treatment has not been considered, is ideologically unacceptable, or for economic, geographic, or other reasons is simply unavailable.

These factors may explain both the late referral and the poor prognosis of patients who stem from socioeconomically deprived families (Hollingshead 1958) or whose illnesses have caused them to drift downward socially (Morrison 1959).

The patient's age at the time he falls ill, as we have previously suggested, is related to not only his symptoms, but also the further course of schizophrenic illness. All other things being equal, the younger the patient is at the time he falls ill, the poorer his prognosis is likely to be (Pollack 1968). One way of explaining this observation is that the more "malignant" illnesses become noticeable at a younger age (Harrow 1969); another, that a schizophrenic illness delays or interrupts the development of the patient's personality to such an extent that he remains at whatever level of social and occupational achievement he had reached at the time he became ill (Bashina 1965, Rassidakis 1963). When a young person's behavior is so odd that it causes him to be excluded from those groups in which his peers are developing their social skills, his impaired social functioning may be self-perpetuating (Offord 1969). Even patients who were socially competent before becoming ill may lose some of the skills they had previously acquired if their thinking remains disturbed or they are in a deprived social setting (such as a hospital) for a long enough period (Wynne 1963). There is then some correlation between the subtype to which the patient's disorder is assigned and his prognosis, but it is by no means sufficient to permit accurate predictions in the individual case. This observation is hardly surprising in view of the arbitrary and variable character of the criteria by which most disorders are classified, and a number of attempts have been made to relate the patient's prognosis to factors other than the subtype of his illness (Vaillant 1964a, b).

Stephens' and Astrup's (1963) efforts to identify factors that correlate with a schizophrenic patient's prognosis began with a modernization of Langfeldt's (1937) distinction between the "process" or more malignant schizophrenias and the "nonprocess" or "schizophreniform" types. Later, approaching the problem from a different standpoint, they determined an alternate and equally useful set of prognostic indexes (Stephens 1965): when a patient on admission has five or more of nine easily assessable characteristics, he has a 94% chance of recovering and maintaining his recovery for a five-year period; with four or fewer of these traits he has an 89% chance of *not* recovering. The characteristics that indicate a good prognosis are:

1/ the patient's condition has progressed in no more than six months from onset to full-blown psychosis;
2/ clear precipitating factors can be determined;
3/ depressive features are seen;
4/ the patient is married; and
5/ there is a good premorbid social adjustment and work history.

The prognosis is also better when the patient

    6/ shows no marked emotional blunting,

    7/ expresses feelings of guilt,

    8/ is neither passive nor experiences feelings of influence, and

    9/ is confused or disoriented at the time of the initial examination.

Other valid but less discriminating factors are that the patient

    10/ is considered to have a cyclothymic personality,

    11/ is 20 years or older at the time his psychosis starts,

    12/ has an IQ that is not below average,

    13/ shows no peculiar or bizarre mannerisms,

    14/ has a personality that is not considered schizoid by the physician, and

    15/ has a family history of affective disorder rather than schizophrenia (Astrup 1966, Erlenmeyer-Kimling 1969, Robins 1970).

These correlations are extremely interesting but somewhat outdated, for the sample on which they are based was composed only of hospitalized patients, most of whom were treated in the prephenothiazine era. Since many of the schizophrenics seen today are not hospitalized at all, since most receive phenothiazines early and many continue to take them for an extended period, Stephens' (1968) criteria may be of greater importance as baseline values against which to gauge the results of current treatment methods than as tools with which to predict a given patient's course. Today, for example, a patient's emotional blunting is less relevant than it was in the past, for even the emotionally blunted patient has a good chance of improving if he remains in a hospital and is given phenothiazines for a long enough time (Janacek 1965).

A NOTE ON PERIODIC PSYCHOSES

A number of syndromes that have in common a relatively rapid and regular alternation in mood, activity, and cognitive functioning may be given the generic label of *periodic psychoses*. These illnesses are quite rare, but are of special theoretical interest, not only because they mark the boundary between manic-depressive and schizophrenic reactions, but also because it has long been believed that an understanding of the biologic events that coincide with psychological changes will advance our knowledge of the pathogenesis, and perhaps even of the etiology, of other mental disorders (Stokes 1939).

The extended, lifelong alternation of mood states called *manic-depressive illness* is occasionally, but not usually, of sufficient regularity to warrant inclusion in this group. More typical are those cases reviewed by Bunney (1965), in which a specific duration of manic behavior—24 hours in his cases—alternates with episodes of depressed behavior at regular intervals. The best-described, rapidly alternating cognitive disorder is the one known as *periodic catatonia* (Hardwick 1941), in which brief periods of excitement or stupor (almost indistinguishable from catatonic states) alternate with longer periods of normal behavior or apathy. Ever since these disorders were first described (Kraepelin 1913, Näcke 1893, Pilcz 1901), they have been the subject of intensive investigation. The most notable of the earlier studies were performed by Gjessing (1932a, 1932b, 1935), who not only described and classified these disorders, but also determined that an alternation of nitrogen retention and excretion correlated with the mental state. According to Gjessing, close observation of the temporal relationship between the patient's nitrogen balance and the onset of symptoms throughout several episodes makes it possible to predict when the patient will become ill.

Gjessing sought to mitigate the patient's psychological symptoms by lowering his nitrogen stores with a low-protein diet and the administration of thyroid preparations. Labeling as *Type A* those cases in which stupor or excitement sets in at the beginning of the phase of negative nitrogen balance, and as *Type B* those in which they set in at the end of this phase, he recommended that increasing doses of thyroxin be given intramuscularly, starting eight to 10 days before stupor or excitement begin in Type A, and shortly before they are due to end in Type B. Starting with 2 mg of thyroxin intramuscularly on the first day, he increased the dosage by 1 to 2 mg daily for eight to 10 days and, continuing until the symptoms subsided, reached total doses as high as 40 to 50 mg of thyroxin. When the pulse rate exceeded 140 or became irregular, he discontinued the thyroxin and, once the pulse rate returned to 90, gave the patient dessicated thyroid in doses sufficient to maintain his pulse rate at this level and to keep his basal metabolism rate at +10% to +15%. He kept some patients on this regimen for a number of years and reported that it prevents both nitrogen retention and further episodes of psychosis (Gjessing 1939).

The therapeutic effectiveness of thyroid in disorders of this kind has been confirmed by some authors (Hardwick 1941, Mall 1952) and is made even more plausible by the finding that experimental thyroidectomy in rats can cause periodic phenomena that can be ɪeversed by thyroid administration (Richter 1959). Nevertheless, many patients do not improve on thyroid, and even those who do may, after some time, become and remain refractory, even when the dose is further increased (Hardwick 1941). Such cases may still respond to reserpine or haloperidol (Haldol), but these drugs sometimes achieve their effect only at the price of making the patient apathetic for a prolonged period (Gjessing 1964, 1967).

REFERENCES

Achté, K. A.: On prognosis and rehabilitation in schizophrenic and paranoid psychoses, Acta Psychiat Scand *43* (Suppl 196): 5-217, 1967.

Achté, K. A., Stenbäck, A., and Terä-väinen, H.: On suicides committed during treatment in psychiatric hospitals, Acta Psychiat Scand *42*:272-284, 1966.

Alanen, Y. O.: The family in the pathogenesis of schizophrenic and neurotic disorders, Acta Psychiat Scand *42* (Suppl 189): 1-654, 1966.

Almond, R., Keniston, K., and Boltax, S.: Value system of a milieu therapy unit, Arch Gen Psychiat (Chicago) *19*:545-561, 1968.

Astrup, C.: Prognostic importance of genetic factors in functional psychoses, Brit J Psychiat *112*:1293-1297, 1966.

Bachman, B. J., Anderson, C. M., and Houpt, J. L.: From the therapeutic community to the community, Hosp Community Psychiat, to be published.

Bashina, V. M.: Work capacity and social adaptation of schizophrenic patients who become ill in childhood and adolescence, Int J Psychiat *1*:248-252, 1965.

Bateson, G. J., Haley, D. D., and Weakland, J. H.: Toward a theory of schizophrenia, Behav Sci *1*:256-264, 1956.

Beard, J. H., *et al.*: Three aspects of psychiatric rehabilitation at Fountain House, Ment Hyg *48*:11-21, 1964.

Becker, R. E.: Evaluation of a rehabilitation program for chronically hospitalized psychiatric patients, Soc Psychiat *2*:32-38, 1967.

Bennett, J. L., and Hamilton, L. D.: Sequential use of antidepressant drugs with chlorpromazine in chronic schizophrenia, Psychiat Quart *37*:53-65, 1963.

Bleuler, E.: Dementia Praecox oder Gruppe der Schizophrenien, Leipzig: Deuticke, 1911.

Bleuler, M.: Remission of schizophrenia after shock therapy, Z Ges Neurol Psychiat *173*:553-597, 1941.

Bliss, E. L., and Clark, L. D.: Studies of sleep deprivation: relationship to schizophrenia, Arch Neurol Psychiat *81*:348-359, 1959.

Bowers, M. B., Jr., and Astrachan, B. M.: Depression in acute schizophrenic patients, Amer J Psychiat *123*:976-979, 1967.

Braginsky, B. M., Grosse, M., and Ring, K.: Controlling outcomes through impression-management: An experimental study of the manipulative tactics of mental patients, J Consult Psychol *30*:295-300, 1966.

Brill, H., and Patton, R. E.: Analysis of population reduction in New York State mental hospitals during the first four years of large-scale therapy with psychotropic drugs, Amer J Psychiat *116*: 495-509, 1959.

———: Clinical-statistical analysis of population changes in New York State mental hospitals since introduction of psychotropic drugs, Amer J Psychiat *119*:20-35, 1962.

Brill, N. Q., and Glass, J. F.: Hebephrenic schizophrenic reactions, Arch Gen Psychiat (Chicago) *12*:545-551, 1965.

Brown, G. W.: Length of hospital stay and schizophrenia: A review of statistical studies, Acta Psychiat Scand *35*:414-430, 1960.

Bunney, W. E., and Hartmann, E. L.: Study of a patient with 48-hour manic-depressive cycles: I. An Analysis, Arch Gen Psychiat (Chicago) *12*:611-618, 1965.

Cameron, N.: Reasoning, regression and communication in schizophrenics, Psychol Monogr *50*:1-33, 1938.

Casey, J. F., *et al.*: Treatment of schizophrenic reactions with phenothiazine derivatives: Comparative study of chlorpromazine, triflupromazine, mepazine, prochlorperazine, perphenazine, and phenobarbital, Amer J Psychiat *117*:97-105, 1960.

Chapman, J.: Early symptoms of schizophrenia, Brit J Psychiat *112*:225-251, 1966.

Chapman, J., and McGhie, A.: Comparative study of disordered attention in schizophrenia, Brit J Psychiat *108*:487-500, 1962.

Clark, M. L., et al.: Chlorpromazine in chronic schizophrenic women: 1. Experimental design and effects at maximum point of treatment, Psychopharmacologia (Berlin) *2*:107-136, 1961.

Cobb, S.: Borderline of Psychiatry, Cambridge: Harvard, 1943.

Cohen, S. et al.: Tranquilizers and suicide in the schizophrenic patient, Arch Gen Psychiat (Chicago) *11*:312-322, 1964.

Coleman, J. V.: Community project in behalf of the hospitalized mentally ill patient: The cooperative care project, Amer J Psychiat *124*:76-79, 1967.

Davis, J. M., McCourt, W. F., and Solomon, P.: Effect of visual stimulation on hallucinations and other mental experiences during sensory deprivation, Amer J Psychiat *116*:889-892, 1960.

Davison, K.: Schizophrenia-like psychoses associated with organic brain diseases: Preliminary observations on 50 patients, Newcastle Med J *67*:258-301, 1966.

Detre, T., and Tucker, G.: Psychotherapy for the mentally ill: A redefinition of goals, *in* Abrons, G., and Greenfield, N. S., eds.: The New Hospital Psychiatry, New York: Acad Press, 1970.

Dunaif, S. L., and Hoch, P. H.: Pseudopsychopathic schizophrenia, *in* Hoch, P. H., and Zubin, J., eds.: Psychiatry and the Law, New York: Grune, 1955.

Ekblom, B., and Lassenius, B.: Followup examination of patients with chronic schizophrenia who were treated during a long period with psychopharmacological drugs, Acta Psychiat Scand *40*:249-279, 1964.

Ekdawi, M. Y.: Changes in ward behavior of severely disabled schizophrenic patients: Four years' study, Brit J Psychiat *112*:265-267, 1966.

Engelhardt, D. M., et al.: Long-term drug-induced symptom modification in schizophrenic outpatients, J Nerv Ment Dis *137*:231-241, 1963.

Engelhardt, D. M., et al.: Phenothiazines in prevention of psychiatric hospitalization. IV. Delay or prevention of hospitalization: A reevaluation, Arch Gen Psychiat (Chicago) *16*:98-101, 1967.

Erlenmeyer-Kimling, L., and Nicol, S.: Comparison of hospitalization measures in schizophrenic patients with and without a family history of schizophrenia, Brit J Psychiat *115*:321-324, 1969.

Esser, A. S.: Behavioral changes in working chronic schizophrenic patients, Dis Nerv Syst *28*:141-147, 1967.

Feinberg, I.: Sleep electroencephalographic and eye-movement patterns in patients with schizophrenia and with chronic brain syndrome, Res Publ Ass Res Nerv Ment Dis *45*:211-240, 1967.

Fischer, M., Harvald, B., and Hauge, M.: Danish twin study of schizophrenia, Brit J Psychiat *115*:981-990, 1969.

Fish, F. J.: Schizophrenia, Baltimore: Williams & Wilkins, 1962.

Fleck, S.: Vigilance (orienting behavior), conditional reactions, and adjustment patterns in schizophrenic and compulsive patients, Ann NY Acad Sci, *56*:342-379, 1953.

———: Schizophrenia, *in* Conn, H. F., ed.: Current Therapy, Philadelphia, Saunders, 1969, pp. 736-739.

Forrest, F. M., et al.: Drug maintenance problems of rehabilitated mental patients: Current drug dosage "merry-go-round", Amer J Psychiat *121*:33-40, 1964.

Fossum, A., Astrup, C., and Holmboe, R.: Follow-up study of 1,102 patients with functional psychoses, Proc III World Psychiat *1*:102-107, 1961.

Freedman, S. J., Grunebaum, H. U., and Greenblatt, M.: Perceptual and cognitive changes in sensory deprivation, *in* Solomon, P., et al., eds.: Sensory Deprivation, Cambridge: Harvard, 1961, pp. 58-71.

Freud, S.: Die Traumdeutung, Wien: Deuticke, 1900.

Gantz, R. S., and Birkett, D. P.: Phenothiazine reduction as a cause of rehospitalization, Arch Gen Psychiat (Chicago) *12*:586-588, 1965.

Gillis, L. S., and Keet, M.: Factors underlying the retention in the community of chronic unhospitalized schizophrenics, Brit J Psychiat *111*:1057-1067, 1965.

Gjessing, L. R.: Effect of thyroxine, pyridoxine, orphenadrine-HCl, reserpine and disulfiram in periodic catatonia, Acta Psychiat Scand *43*:376-384, 1967.

———: Studies of periodic catatonia: II. The urinary excretion of phenolic amines and acids with and without loads of different drugs, J Psychiat Res *2*: 149-162, 1964.

Gjessing, R.: Beiträge zur Kenntnis der Pathophysiologie des katatonen Stupors I. Mitteilung: Über periodisch rezidivierenden katatonen Stupor, mit kritischem

Beginn und Abschluss, Arch Psychiat Nervenkr *96*:319-389, 1932a.

——: Beiträge zur Kenntnis der Pathophysiologie des katatonen Stupors II. Mitteilung: Über aperiodisch rezidivierend verlaufenden katatonen Stupor mit lytischem Beginn und Abschluss, Arch Psychiat Nervenkr *96*:393-473, 1932b.

——: Beiträge zur Kenntnis der Pathophysiologie der katatonen Erregung III. Mitteilung: Über periodisch rezidivierende katatone Erregung, mit kritischem Beginn und Abschluss, Arch Psychiat Nervenkr *104*:355-416, 1935.

——: Beiträge zur Kenntnis der Pathophysiologie periodisch katatoner Zustände. IV. Mitteilung: Versuch einer Ausgleichung der Funktionsstörungen, Arch Psychiat Nervenkr *109*:525-595, 1939.

Goldberg, S. C., Klerman, G. L., and Cole, J. O.: Changes in schizophrenic psychopathology and ward behavior as a function of phenothiazine treatment, Brit J Psychiat *111*:120-133, 1965.

Gross, M., *et al.*: Discontinuation of treatment with ataractic drugs, Recent Advances Biol Psychiat *3*:44-63, 1961.

Hall, J. C., Smith, K., and Shimkunas, A.: Employment problems of schizophrenic patients, Amer J Psychiat *123*:536-540, 1966.

Hardwick, S. W., and Stokes, A. B.: Metabolic investigations in periodic catatonia, Proc Roy Soc Med *34*:733-756, 1941.

Harrow, M., Tucker, G. J., and Bromet, E.: Short-term prognosis of schizophrenic patients, Arch Gen Psychiat (Chicago) *21*: 195-202, 1969.

Havens, L. L., and Cubelli, G. E.: Psychiatrist and the state vocational rehabilitation agency, Amer J Psychiat *123*:1094-1099 (Mar), 1967.

Heron, W.: Cognitive and physiological effects of perceptual isolation, *in* Solomon, P., *et al.*, eds.: Sensory Deprivation, Cambridge: Harvard, 1961, pp. 6-33.

Heston, L. L.: Psychiatric disorders in foster home reared children of schizophrenic mothers, Brit J Psychiat *112*:819-825, 1966.

Hoch, P. H., and Polatin, P.: Pseudoneurotic forms of schizophrenia, Psychiat Quart *23*:248-276, 1949.

Hoch, P. H., *et al.*: Course and outcome of pseudoneurotic schizophrenia, Amer J Psychiat *119*:106-115, 1962.

Hogarty, G. E.: Hospital differences in the release of discharge ready chronic schizophrenics, Arch Gen Psychiat (Chicago) *18*:367-372, 1968.

Hollingshead, A. B., and Redlich, F. C.: Social Class and Mental Illness: A Community Study, New York: Wiley, 1958.

Hordern, A., and Somerville, D. M.: Clinical trials in chronic schizophrenia, Med J Aust *1*:40-43, 1963.

Janecek, J., Vestre, N. D., and Zimmerman, R.: Prognostic evaluation of recently admitted psychiatric patients: Basic prognostic data for hospitalized patients, presented at the Annual Meeting of the American Psychiatric Association, New York, 1965.

Jung, C. G.: Psychology of dementia praecox, New York: J Nerv Ment Dis Pub Co., 1909.

Kallmann, F. J., *et al.*: Developmental aspects of children with two schizophrenic parents, Psychiat Res Rep Amer Psychiat Ass, #19 (Dec), 1964, pp. 136-145.

Katz, M. M., and Cole, J. O.: Research on drugs and community care: A review and analysis of recent results and methodological progress, Arch Gen Psychiat (Chicago) *7*:345-359, 1962.

Klaf, F. S., and Hamilton, J. G.: Schizophrenia—A hundred years ago and today, Brit J Psychiat *107*:819-827, 1961.

Knight, R. E.: Borderline states, Bull Menninger Clin *17*:1-12, 1953.

Kraepelin, E.: Lehrbuch der Psychiatrie, Leipzig: Johann Ambrosius Barth, 1913.

——: Psychiatrie, Leipzig: Johann Ambrosius Barth, 1896.

——: Zur Diagnose und Prognose der Dementia Praecox, Allg Z Psychiat *56*:254-264, 1899.

Kretschmer, E.: Physique and character, New York: Harcourt, 1926.

Kringlen, E.: Heredity and environment in the functional psychoses: An epidemiological-clinical twin study, Oslo: Universitetsforlaget, 1967.

Kurland, A. A., *et al.*: Comparative effectiveness of six phenothiazine compounds, phenobarbital and inert placebo in the treatment of acutely ill patients: Personality dimensions, J Nerv Ment Dis *134*:48-61, 1962.

Lamb, H. R.: Release of chronic psychiatric patients into the community, Arch Gen Psychiat (Chicago) *19*:38-44, 1968.

Langfeldt, G.: Prognosis in schizophrenia and the factors influencing the course of the disease: A Katamnestic study, including individual re-examination in

1936, London: Oxford, 1937.

Lee, M. E.: Follow-up study of the post hospital adjustment of mental patients treated in a family oriented psychiatric center, thesis, Smith College School of Social Work, Northampton, 1965.

Lidz, T., Fleck, S., and Cornelison, A.: Schizophrenia and the Family, New York: Internat Univ Press, 1966.

Linn, E. L.: Relation of chronicity in the functional psychoses to prognosis, J Nerv Ment Dis 135:460-467, 1962.

Ludwig, A. M., and Marx, A. J.: Buddy treatment model for chronic schizophrenics, J Nerv Ment Dis 148:528-541, 1969.

MacDonald, N.: The other side: Living with schizophrenia, Canad Med Ass J 82: 218-221, 1960.

Mall, G.: Beitrag zur Gjessingschen Thyroxinbehandlung der periodischen Katatonien, Arch Psychiat Nervenkr 187:381-403, 1952.

Marjerrison, G., et al.: Withdrawal of long-term phenothiazines from chronically hospitalized psychiatric patients, Canad Psychiat Ass J 9:290-298, 1964.

Matussek, P.: Untersuchungen Uber die Wahnwahrnehmung 1. Mitteilung: Veranderungen der Wahrenhmungswelt bei beginnenden, primären Wahn, Arch Psychiat Nervenkr 189:279-319, 1952.

May, P. R., and Tuma, A. H.: Effect of psychotherapy and Stelazine on length of hospital stay, release rate, and supplemental treatment of schizophrenic patients, J Nerv Ment Dis 139:362-369, 1964.

Mayer-Gross, W., Slater, E., and Roth, M.: Clinical psychiatry, Baltimore: Williams & Wilkins, 1960.

McGee, T. F., et al.: Further evaluation of small group living program with schizophrenics, Arch Gen Psychiat (Chicago) 19: 717-726, 1968.

McGhie, A., and Chapman, J.: Disorders of attention and perception in early schizophrenia, Brit J Med Psychol 34:103-116, 1961.

McGhie, A., Chapman, J., and Lawson, J. S.: Effect of distraction on schizophrenic performance: 1. Perception and immediate memory, Brit J Psychiat 111:383-390, 1965a.

———: Effect of distraction on schizophrenic performance: 2. Psychomotor Ability, Brit J Psychiat 111:391-398, 1965b.

McGowan, L., Harrison, R., and Coleman, J. V.: Can mental patients use traditional vocational services, Hosp Community Psychiat, Dec, 1966, pp. 370-372.

Morrison, S. L.: Principles and methods of epidemological research and their application to psychiatric illness, Brit J Psychiat 105:999-1016, 1959.

Morton, M. R.: Study of the withdrawal of chlorpromazine or trifluoperazine in chronic schizophrenia, Amer J Psychiat 124:1585-1588, 1968.

Näcke, P.: Raritäten aus der Irrenanstalt, Zeitschr f Psychiat, April, 1893, pp. 631-672.

National Institute of Mental Health (Collaborative Study Group): Phenothiazine treatment in acute schizophrenia: Effectiveness, Arch Gen Psychiat (Chicago) 10:246-261, 1964.

Offord, D. R., and Cross, L. A.: Behavioral antecedents of adult schizophrenia: A review, Arch Gen Psychiat (Chicago) 21: 267-283, 1969.

Pasamanick, B., Scarpitti, F. R., and Dinitz, S.: Schizophrenics in the Community, New York: Appleton, 1967.

Payne, R. W., and Friedlander, D.: Short battery of simple tests for measuring over-inclusive thinking, J Ment Sci 108:362-367, 1962.

Payne, R. W., Matussek, P., and George, E. I.: Experimental study of schizophrenic thought disorder, Brit J Psychiat 105:627-652, 1959.

Pilcz, A.: Die periodischen Geistesstörungen, Stuttgart: Gustav Fischer Verlag, 1901.

Ploticher, A. I.: Certain problems of the pathophysiology of schizophrenia in the light of data on the development of remissions and recurrences, Soviet Psychol Psychiat 1:58-63, 1962.

Pokorny, A. D.: Problems in psychiatric classification, Int J Neuropsychiat 1:161-167, 1965.

Pollack, M., Levenstein, S., and Klein, D. F.: Three-year posthospital follow-up of adolescent and adult schizophrenics, Amer J Orthopsychiat 38:94-109, 1968.

Pollin, W., et al.: Psychopathology in 15,909 pairs of veteran twins: Evidence for a genetic factor in the pathogenesis of schizophrenia and its relative absence in psychoneurosis, Amer J Psychiat 126:597-610, 1969.

Rassidakis, N. C., et al.: Follow-up study of schizophrenic patients: Relapse and readmission, Bull Menninger Clin 27:33-40, 1963.

Reisby, N.: Psychoses in children of schizophrenic mothers, Acta Psychiat Scand *43*:8-20, 1967.

Rice, D.: Use of lithium salts in the treatment of manic states, J Ment Sci *102*: 604, 1956.

Richter, C. P., Jones, G. S., and Biswanger, L.: Periodic phenomena and the thyroid: 1. Abnormal but regular cycles in behavior and metabolism produced in rats by radiothyroidectomy, Arch Neurol Psychiat *81*:233-255, 1959.

Robins, E., and Guze, S. B.: Establishment of diagnostic validity in psychiatric illness: Its application to schizophrenia, Amer J Psychiat *126*:983-987, 1970.

Rosati, D.: Prolonged high dosage ataractic medication in chronic schizophrenia, Brit J Psychiat *110*:61-63, 1964.

Rosenzweig, N., and Gardner, L.: Role of input relevance in sensory isolation, Amer J Psychiat *122*:920-928, 1966.

Rothwell, N. D., and Doniger, J. M.: Psychiatric Halfway House: A Case Study, Springfield (Ill): Thomas, 1966.

Rubenstein, R., and Lasswell, H. D.: Sharing of Power in A Psychiatric Hospital, New Haven and London: Yale Univ Press, 1966.

Sargant, W.: Present indications for leucotomy, Lancet *1*:1197-1200, 1962.

Schopler, E., and Loftin, J.: Thought disorders in parents of psychotic children, Arch Gen Psychiat (Chicago) *20*:174-181, 1969.

Shanfield, S., et al.: Schizophrenic patient and depressive symptomatology, J Nerv Ment Dis, *151*:203-210, 1970.

Shatin, L., Kotter, W. L., and Dougmore, G.: Music therapy for schizophrenics, J Rehab *27*:30-31, 1961.

Shields, J., Gottesman, I. I., and Slater, E.: Kallmann's 1946 schizophrenic twin study in the light of new information, Acta Psychiat Scand *43*:385-396, 1967.

Simonson, M.: Phenothiazine depressive reaction, J Neuropsychiat *5*:259-265, 1964.

Slater, E. T., and Glithero, E.: Follow-up of patients diagnosed as suffering from "hysteria," J Psychosom Res *9*:9-13, 1965.

Spadoni, A. J., and Smith, J. A.: Milieu therapy in schizophrenia: Negative result, Arch Gen Psychiat (Chicago) *20*:547-551, 1969.

Stafford-Clark, D.: Discussion of: Biochemistry and schizophrenia, Fabing, H. D., Brit J Psychiat *104*:584-588, 1958.

Steinberg, H. R., Green, R., and Durell, J.: Depression occurring during the course of recovery from schizophrenic symptoms, Amer J Psychiat *124*:699-702, 1967.

Stephens, J. H., and Astrup, C.: Prognosis in "process" and "nonprocess" schizophrenia, Amer J Psychiat *119*:945-953, 1963.

Stephens, J. H., Astrup, C., and Weitz, J. W.: Prognostic factors in recovered and deteriorated schizophrenics, presented at the 121st Annual Meeting of the American Psychiatric Association, New York, 1965.

Stephens, J. H., and O'Connor, G.: Long-term prognosis in schizophrenia using the Becker-Wittman Scale and the Phillips Scale, read before the 124th Annual Meeting of the American Psychiatric Association, Boston, Massachusetts, 1968.

Stokes, A. B.: Critical review: Somatic research in periodic catatonia, J Neurol Psychiat *2*:243-259, 1939.

Storms, L. H., and Broen, W. E.: Theory of schizophrenic behavioral disorganization, Arch Gen Psychiat (Chicago) *20*:129-144, 1969.

Tourney, G., et al.: Effect of resocialization techniques on chronic schizophrenic patients, Amer J Psychiat *116*:993-1000, 1960.

Tucker, G., et al.: Perceptual experiences in schizophrenic and non-schizophrenic patients, Arch Gen Psychiat (Chicago) *20*:159-166, 1969.

Ugelstad, E., and Astrup, C.: Study of psychotic patients treated with individual psychotherapy prior to admission in a mental hospital, Brit J Med Psychol *41*: 117-124, 1968.

Vaillant, G. E.: Historical review of the remitting schizophrenias, J Nerv Ment Dis *138*:48-56, 1964a.

———: Prospective prediction of schizophrenic remission, Arch Gen Psychiat (Chicago) *11*:509-518, 1964b.

Venables, P. H.: Input dysfunction in schizophrenia, *in* Maher, B. A., ed.: Progress in Experimental Personality Research, New York: Acad Press, 1964, pp. 1-47.

Wechsler, H.: Self-help organization in the mental health field: Recovery, Inc., a case study, J Nerv Ment Dis *130*:297-314, 1960.

Wender, P. H.: Role of genetics in the etiology of the schizophrenias, Amer J Orthopsychiat *39*:447-458, 1969.

Wessler, M. M., and Kahn, V. L.: Can the chronic schizophrenic patient remain in the community? A follow-up study of 24 long-term hospitalized patients returned to the community, J Nerv Ment Dis *136*:455-463, 1963.

West, L. J.: Hallucinations, New York: Grune, 1962.

Williams, H. L., Lubin, A., and Goodnow, J. J.: Impaired performance with acute sleep loss, Psychol Monogr 73:1-26, 1959.

Wing, J. K., and Freudeberg, R. K.: Response of severely ill chronic schizophrenic patients to social stimulation, Amer J Psychiat 118:311-322, 1961.

Winkelman, N. W., Jr.: Clinical and socio-cultural study of 200 psychiatric patients started on chlorpromazine 10½ years ago, Amer J Psychiat 120:861-869, 1964.

Wulff, M. H.: The evening-patient: Experiences from a rehabilitation hostel for psychiatric patients, Acta Psychiat Scand 42 (Suppl 191):250-259, 1966.

Wynne, R. D.: Influence of hospitalization on the verbal behavior of chronic schizophrenics, Brit J Psychiat 109:380-389, 1963.

Zolik, E. S., Lantz, E. M., and Sommers, R.: Hospital return rates and prerelease referrals, Arch Gen Psychiat (Chicago) 18: 712-717, 1968.

Zwerling, I.: The psychiatric day hospital, in Arieti, S., ed.: American Handbook of Psychiatry, vol. 3, New York: Basic, 1966.

CHAPTER

FOUR

Affective Disorders

DEPRESSION

THE TERM "DEPRESSION" is used in a variety of ways: to describe an individual's lifelong *outlook* or current *mood* without implying that he is ill; to refer to the sadness or tearfulness that arises as a *symptom* of a wide range of psychiatric and nonpsychiatric illnesses; and to describe certain *syndromes* of which sadness and tearfulness are usually the most prominent symptoms, but which generally include certain other symptoms as well: psychomotor retardation, self-derogation, apathy, and somatic complaints ("typical" depressions) (Lehmann 1959). The term is even used to refer to syndromes in which sadness and tearfulness are either not noticeable at all or are overshadowed by such symptoms as headaches, phobias, or obsessional ideas ("atypical" depressions). Finally, it can describe one phase of an illness that, at other times in the individual's life, is manifested by pathologic euphoria (manic-depressive disease).

This confusing multiple usage is partly an outgrowth of the difficulties inherent in distinguishing the person who is disturbed by some event in his life from the one who is mentally ill (Hudgens 1967). Deaths, separations, and occupational setbacks are so often followed by a depressed mood that it is natural to look for such stresses whenever a person seems sad. That the average person feels dejected, becomes tearful, and functions poorly after the death of someone he loves does not explain, however, why one individual remains distraught or gets steadily worse for months thereafter, while another, even if he had been just as close to the person who has died and at first seemed equally moved, is back on his feet within days or, at most, weeks. More significantly, it does not explain why some people become depressed without any apparent reason at all or after an event that seems disastrous to them but innocuous or insignificant to everyone else. The cause of the depression that comes in the wake of a medical illness is equally hard to pin down. That some individuals with fatiguing or debilitating diseases become depressed does not explain why many do not, or why those who do sometimes remain depressed even after their physical condition has much improved (Oswald 1963). The only reasonable way of explaining these events is to postulate a constitutionally (and perhaps even genetically) determined proclivity to depressive symptoms (manifested by a greater frequency of depression and the development of depressions in response to mildly upsetting events and relatively mild physical illnesses), to take note of the increased frequency of depression with advancing age, and to point out that some illnesses produce depressions more readily than others. But we recognize that this merely sweeps the relevant questions under the rug.

DEPRESSIONS FOLLOWING PSYCHOLOGICALLY DISTRESSING EVENTS ("DEPRESSIVE NEUROSES")

Prior to the introduction of antidepressants, the distinction between "reactive" (or "neurotic") and "endogenous" (or "psychotic") depressions was considered of vital importance, but this distinction now seems less sharp and less useful (Kay 1969a, 1969b, Kendell 1970). Current research has cast doubt on the once widely held belief that patients who become depressed immediately after some tragic event (or are for some other reason diagnosed as having a "reactive" depression) make better use of psychotherapy or respond less readily to ECT and antidepressants than those who, because their depressions arise without apparent precipitant, are diagnosed as having an "endogenous" depression (May 1969, Pollitt 1965). In any case, it is now generally agreed that episodes of sadness or depressed mood that seem to arise in response to an upsetting life experience but continue for more than two or three weeks are clinically, therapeutically, and prognostically indistinguishable from those that arise without any precipitant at all and that they may even recur and appear "endogenous" at a later time in the individual's life.

By the time the individual who has suffered a distressing experience asks to see a psychiatrist (if he asks to see one at all), he will usually have weathered the worst. For a few days or weeks, he may have been unable to erase the event or its consequences from his mind and had difficulty in falling asleep or pursuing his regular tasks, but he is usually able to work and take part in most interpersonal transactions within a week and regains his customary level of competence within a month at most (Clayton 1968).

An overhasty decision to offer such an individual treatment can rob him of an important experience in coping with difficulty, deny him the catharsis of mourning, and even lead him to view himself as dependent, fragile, or "sick." The person seen by a physician immediately after he suffers a personal loss should therefore be encouraged to turn to his friends, family, or clergyman for consolation and told to return for reevaluation a week or two later. If his discomfort is severe, he may be offered a mildly euphorizing antianxiety agent such as chlordiazepoxide (Librium), 10 to 20 mg, 3 to 4 times daily, for a week or two. If he is so far from home or so isolated that he has no one to talk to, is in such obvious discomfort that his safety seems in doubt, or is not functioning as well as expected within a reasonable time, more vigorous treatment may be indicated.

The individual who responds catastrophically to an event that seems trivial will sometimes be found to have reacted the same way before to the same kind of event. The person who becomes depressed whenever he has to adapt to a new situation—a new job, the conclusion of a romance, a new school, or a new place to live (Pittman 1968)—may benefit from psychiatric treatment not only because it may help him to cope with his current discomfort but because it may help him improve his adaptive skills or, at the very least, recognize his limitations and learn to identify the kinds of situations he should avoid. If, however, such advice falls on deaf ears and the patient repeatedly makes the same turmoil-producing mistakes, he is probably suffering from a personality disorder (see Chap. 7) and is unlikely to change without long-term treatment.

Depressive Symptoms Associated with Somatic Illness

While the individual whose *mood* is depressed after a difficult life situation can usually be distinguished from the one with an incipient depressive *syndrome* by the brevity and relative mildness of his discomfort, this does not distinguish him from the patient whose depression is a *symptom* of some underlying disease (Altschule 1965). The distinction cannot even be made by establishing the presence of an organic disease, for the medical illness may be as unrelated to the ensuing depression as an upsetting event is to a depressed mood. The problem is usually the other way round, however: the individual's depression is attributed to a life event but in reality is caused by an organic disease. The depression that appears immediately after an apparently depressing event and is therefore thought to be causally related may in fact reflect not sadness but an incipient, as yet unidentified, organic disorder that so impairs the individual's effectiveness that he cannot cope with a problem he might otherwise have been able to shrug off. The difficulty in establishing causal relationships of any kind becomes even more evident on consideration that sadness, intellectual and motor retardation, insomnia, social withdrawal, agitation, vague somatic complaints, weight loss, fatigue, and irritability are precursors and symptoms not only of depressive syndromes but of many other psychiatric and nonpsychiatric disorders as well (Silverman 1968).

Even when the organic illness is manifest, it may be impossible to determine whether a concomitant depression is attributable to the illness, the treatment, the individual's attitude toward either or both, or some totally unrelated occurrence (Kerr 1969, Schwab 1967). For example, when a patient with cancer becomes depressed, anorectic, anhedonic, and sleepless, it is impossible to know whether these symptoms are caused by his pain, his fear of further discomfort and death, a cerebral metastasis, the oddly furtive and incongruously patronizing way in which his family is treating him, or the hormones, chemotherapy, radiation, or surgery being used in his treatment. The difficulty in distinguishing depressive illness and organic syndrome is further exemplified by the patient with cerebral arteriosclerosis whose sadness and retardation make his clinical picture identical to that seen in depressive syndromes (see also p. 404).

Depressive symptoms secondary to organic disease tend to lift if and when the patient's physical condition improves. Thus, if there is any concern that antidepressant therapy will complicate the assessment of the underlying disorder or be incompatible with its treatment, it is preferable to postpone treating the depression until the associated disease is relieved. If, however, the patient's depression seems to be a threat to his life, aggravating his illness, or interfering with his ability to collaborate in his treatment, there may be no choice but to start using antidepressants immediately. Under these circumstances, or if the depression persists even after the underlying disease remits, the treatment follows the same principles as outlined below for other depressive syndromes.

Depressive Syndromes

From the standpoint of symptoms, age, history, and treatment response, depressive syndromes may be classified as typical, atypical, or manic-depressive in character. The *typical depression* is marked by symptoms of sadness, tearfulness, psychomotor retardation or agitation, anorexia, weight loss, diminished ability to concentrate, self-reproach, pessimism, diminished energy, libido, and interest, thoughts of death, suicidal ideas or attempts, insomnia, and early morning awakening (EMA). Neurotic symptoms and cryptogenic somatic complaints may occur but are not the most prominent symptoms (Grinker 1961). The syndrome is more common in women than in men and is most commonly seen in the age group between 45 and 60. Similar episodes are often found in the patient's previous and family history, and recurrences are not unusual. The patient's symptoms tend to be diurnal in character, in the sense that they are worse in the morning than they are at night. The individual episodes may last for six to 18 months, then generally subside, and are more common in individuals with an obsessional or perfectionistic life style and those who are mildly anxious throughout their lives than they are in the general population. The disorders tend to respond fairly rapidly to antidepressants, particularly those of the dibenzazepine group.

The term *atypical depressions* is used to refer to a group of disorders that, despite having a slightly different concatenation of symptoms, have so many similarities with the typical depressions that they are considered related. The most characteristic feature is the presence of cryptogenic somatic complaints (such as headaches or abdominal pain) or neurotic symptoms (such as obsessions, phobias, or anxiety), which replace or overshadow many of the symptoms described above and thus cause the disorder to look markedly different. While the patient may not exhibit, or exhibit only in attenuated form, such symptoms as sadness, fearfulness, and retardation, he usually suffers from insomnia, EMA, and anorexia, and his neurotic or somatic complaints tend to be diurnal in character. The patient tends to be younger than the one with the typical depression and is less likely to have had a previous episode of typical depression. He is also unlikely (but not quite so unlikely as the patient with the typical depression) to have had an episode of mania. These disorders have a relatively good response to antidepressants (perhaps equally good to dibenzazepines and MAOI), with the exception that the patient may complain bitterly of side effects. That these disorders are in fact related to typical depressions and not some unrelated disease that, perhaps by coincidence, also responds to antidepressants is not clearly established but is suggested by the similarity in symptoms (especially the sleep, appetite, and diurnality) and by the observation that such patients often have a family history of depression, develop a typical depression some weeks or months later (Clouston 1903, Hays 1964), or recover from their atypical symptoms and then, perhaps years later, after a new round of "neurotic" or "somatic" complaints, go on to develop symptoms that no longer leave the diagnosis of typical depression in doubt (Bratfos 1968, Brodwall 1947, Post 1968).

The *manic-depressive depression* also has a number of symptoms in common with the typical depressive syndrome, but differs in that the patient exhibits hypersomnia rather than insomnia, shows a striking degree of anergia and no agitation, and exhibits little or no anorexia. His family history, past history, or subsequent course generally include episodes of pathologic euphoria, insomnia, and hyperactivity. While not restricted to younger persons, the average age is younger than that at which typical depressions occur. Such episodes generally last no more than four to six months, are shorter in older than in younger patients, and may eventuate in mania. The individual's personality during his well periods tends to be intact, though he may be subject to subclinical mood fluctuations. Depressions of this kind are generally unresponsive or poorly responsive to antidepressants, somewhat responsive to lithium carbonate, and most responsive to a combination of antidepressants and lithium carbonate or to ECT.

CLASSIFICATION OF AFFECTIVE DISORDERS

The foregoing distinctions among the various kinds of depressions are relevant for classifying affective disorders. A classification of this type must therefore specify

    1/ whether the patient's current symptoms are characteristic of
        a/ a typical depression,
        b/ an atypical depression,
        c/ a manic-depressive depression,
        d/ a manic episode, or
        e/ a mixed syndrome;
    2/ whether he has had previous episodes of mood disorder and, if so, what symptoms he exhibited at that time;
    3/ whether he loses his sleep and appetite in the midst of his depression(s);
    4/ what kind of treatment, if any, has been effective in the past;
    5/ whether his symptoms ever become severe enough to necessitate hospitalization or merely affect his day to day functioning;

6/ whether, after the most acute symptoms subside,

   a/ he becomes entirely free of affective disorder for a protracted period of time,

   b/ he continues to have mild or subclinical symptoms, or

   c/ severe symptoms recur so rapidly that he is continually moving from one round of incapacitating illness to the next.

Although these criteria are by no means exhaustive, they do make it possible to classify most of the affective disorders seen in clinical practice. All kinds of variations exist: the individual who is usually free of symptoms but repeatedly has episodes of mild depression; the one who has always been mildly depressed but suddenly becomes so much more depressed that he requires hospitalization; the one who, over the course of his life, has had several episodes of severe depression and several of severe mania and functions in a mildly hypomanic manner in between; the one who so continually oscillates between severe depression and severe mania that normality becomes but a brief interlude on the road between the extremes; the patient who has one episode of severe depression but thereafter remains completely symptom-free; the individual who usually feels quite well but on a number of occasions develops a mild depression during which he sleeps too much. While this list could be extended to include all the possible permutations, the above criteria tend to cluster into a few fairly common types. The two that can most usefully be distinguished are composed of

1/ individuals who, while slightly obsessional and anxious throughout their lives, episodically become severely depressed but do not ever become manic; tend while depressed to have insomnia and anorexia; and are likely to respond to antidepressants; and

2/ individuals who, though usually well, periodically become severely manic or depressed; show hypersomnia and severe anergia during their depressions (Detre 1970); and tend to respond to lithium carbonate.

This dichotomization is in large measure supported by the work of Angst (1966) and Perris (1966), who found striking clinical differences between individuals who had had numerous episodes of depression but had never been manic (*unipolar*) and those who had had at least one severe episode of each (*bipolar*). Among the observations made is that the average age at the time of the first episode of unipolar disease severe enough to require hospitalization is 45; bipolar episodes first occur around 30. The individual unipolar episode lasts longer and, if ECT is used, requires more treatments before remitting than the bipolar; once recovered, however, the patient with the unipolar disease is less likely to relapse. In both types of disorder, the patient's age has an influence on the duration of the individual episode, but this influence manifests itself differently in each: young manic-depressives remain ill *longer* than older ones while young unipolar depressives remain ill for a *shorter* period than older ones. Genetic differences are also found: some families show a tendency to unipolar disease, others to bipolar disease; and those with a high proclivity for one type rarely show the other, with the exception that unipolar manic diseases (which are in any case very rare) are from this standpoint more like the bipolar than like the unipolar depressive disease. The individual patient with a unipolar disorder tends, when he is not acutely ill, to be insecure, sensitive, or obsessional, while the one with a bipolar disorder tends to be active and sociable. Finally, while both types have a suicide rate 10 to 20 times higher than that of the general population (and the unipolar depressive have, if anything, a higher rate than the bipolars), the life expectancy of the unipolar patient is only 4% lower that that of the general population, whereas bipolar patients have a life expectancy 26% lower that that of the general population, with increased death rate from nearly all causes.

UNIPOLAR DEPRESSIONS

The Typical Depression

In addition to the symptoms described earlier, the patient may complain of indecisiveness, irritability, impaired memory for recent events, incapacity for enjoyment, lack of accustomed feelings of warmth toward and from family members, impotence or frigidity, constipation, and tastelessness of food. The patient may also feel incompetent and inadequate, experience his life as devoid of stimulation or pleasure, consider himself unable to "feel" things or become involved, view his situation as hopeless and unchangeable, and, in severe cases, prefer death to his state of misery and the bleak future he anticipates. While suicidal ideas are common, the patient does not always consider them to be the natural outcome of his gloom and discomfort; in some cases, ruminations about self-destruction arise without any reasoned consideration at all, and the patient describes

them as if they were obsessions he felt forced to think about. Under
these circumstances, the patient may view his suicidal ideas as morbid, alien, and abhorrent and ask to be protected against his impulses.
Some patients report *somatic symptoms;* others experience self-
denigratory, paranoid, or nihilistic distortions of their body image
that cause them to consider themselves ugly, malodorous, or victims
of some unknown and incurable disease (see p. 204). The patient's
thought processes tend to be slowed down or so overwhelmed by
constant rumination that he cannot easily shift his attention elsewhere. The *ruminations* are likely to concern events from the past,
typically those in which he was hurt or mistreated or, conversely, did
something he felt was wrong. His guilt is not limited to his real misdeeds, however, but may encompass imaginary ones as well. Despite
his concern about the pain and trouble he causes or anticipates causing those around him, he often prevails on his family and friends to
listen to long-winded, repetitive, and socially inappropriate confes-
sions of long-past and otherwise long-forgotten "sins."

The depressed patient tends furthermore to *ask for reassurance,*
either directly or by making self-deprecatory or despairing comments. When given such reassurance, however, he mistrusts it or at
best experiences only a brief lifting of spirits. He therefore may demand reassurance again and again to the point that he becomes a
source of annoyance and frustration for those around him. Lassitude
and anhedonia, other characteristic symptoms, may lead the patient
to make a determined *effort to conserve his energy* (which he sees
as vastly depleted). This concern, especially when he is anxious or
phobic about being with other people, may lead him to stop working
and to *withdraw* from all social, athletic, and sexual activities. Not
surprisingly, the patient's actions or, more characteristically, his failure to act, generate and intensify family tensions, cause the traditional
communication channels to break down even further, and thereby
diminish and distort the feedback of regulating cues from the
environment.

The patient who has been depressed for some time may develop
ideas of reference. Initially, these may be limited to a disquieting
feeling that some of the events around him have some special meaning that he does not fully grasp, but this gradually develops into the
conviction that he is, in some way, the central figure of these events.
Unlike the schizophrenic, who ascribes special meaning to every
experience that impinges on his perceptual field, the depressed
patient with paranoid symptoms tends to concentrate on single,
sometimes very minute, events that he considers the clue to his

puzzlement. After three to six months of illness, his entire outlook may be colored by his *paranoid ideas,* and even if he decides to say nothing about his ideas at first, he eventually starts to accuse his relatives or spouse of malevolent plans and infidelities and to misidentify almost everything he hears or sees in a manner consistent with his delusion of being criticized, spied upon, deceived, or persecuted (see Chap. 5).

The most prevalent and often the most overtly disturbing symptom, however, is *impaired sleep.* In many cases, the patient's sleep difficulties begin as mild early morning awakening (EMA). Gradually, this becomes more severe and begins to include sleep continuity difficulty (SCD) and difficulty in falling asleep (DFA) (Zung 1964); finally, he is almost completely unable to fall or to stay asleep. Although the patient's claim that he gets no sleep at all is rarely borne out by his family's observations, the report ought not be discounted, for the feeling of not having slept or of not feeling rested on awakening is, in all probability, caused by disturbances in the depth and continuity of sleep (Mendels 1967).

The patient's report that his sleep is "fine" may be equally misleading. Some patients have sleep difficulty for no more than a week or two and thereafter sleep well. This pattern is particularly common when the patient has suddenly been relieved of external pressures, whether by leaving his job, starting psychotherapy, entering a hospital, or being treated with new indulgence by his family, and is usually associated with other signs of improvement. These changes, however, by their very nature, are temporary; as long as the patient's depression remains active, his sleep will deteriorate again as soon as the pressure mounts.

The Atypical Depression

Since younger patients are less likely to become depressed or, if they do, to develop a typical depression, it is reasonable to assume that, as in other disorders, there is a close relationship between the depressed patient's clinical picture and his age (Sloane 1961). Although it is possible that the younger patient's depression has atypical features because it remits rapidly (Lundquist 1945) and thus exhibits only the prodromal and not the late or typical symptoms of the depression, the relationship between particular symptoms and the age at which the illness occurs is so striking that it is possible to create a general description of the clinical picture for each age group, a *timetable of depressive symptoms,* as it were.

While a continuously sad mood is rare prior to the eighth or ninth year of life, even a child of three can show mood fluctuations marked with tearfulness, temper tantrums, nightmares, anorexia, and transient fears, and one of school age may develop school phobia in addition (see p. 380). At the onset of puberty, the symptoms may include conversion symptoms and, especially in patients later shown to have manic-depressive disease (see p. 381), sullenness, negativism, impulsivity, or histrionic behavior. The depressed adolescent may be irritable and hostile and show a surly rebellious resistance to his parents' orders (Rubins 1968, Toolan 1962). In some instances (again more commonly in those later shown to have manic-depressive disease), this may be accompanied by sexual promiscuity, physical assaultiveness, or other rule-breaking behavior (King 1970). Depressed patients in late adolescence may also have episodes of anxiety and depersonalization, which in the patient in the early 20s are joined by phobic and obsessive symptoms, thus producing the clinical picture that is sometimes referred to as a *phobic anxiety-depersonalization syndrome* (Roth 1960). From the mid-20s through the mid-30s, depressed patients often exhibit anxiety and vague somatic complaints; they may become afraid of fainting, being unable to breathe, or having an uncontrollable anxiety attack if they should leave their homes or go out into a crowd, and as a result become incapacitated. Depressions in this age group are often preceded by a sudden decrease in the patient's sexual activity, to the point of temporary impotence or frigidity. Patients in their late 30s tend to be less anxious than those who are younger, but become increasingly subject to unexplained, persistent, and fairly well-localized somatic complaints (Jacobowsky 1961), such as pains in their head, abdomen, or back (for a discussion of hypochondriasis and conversion neurosis, see pp. 469 and 221). From the early 40s to the late 50s, patients generally show more and more of the typical depressive features and fewer of the earlier symptoms. Systematized delusions of persecution or jealousy may also occur at this age. Patients in their 60s and beyond once again show few features of the "typical" depressions: in these years, organic factors secondary to the aging process give rise to agitated depressions with unsystematized paranoid delusions.

Just as the age-related changes in an individual's psychobiologic makeup permit the construction of the foregoing timetable of depressive symptoms, the age-related changes in an individual's social role and responsibilities permit the construction of a parallel *timetable of depressive life concerns*. That a depressed patient's symptoms develop fairly slowly and his cognitive functioning remains relatively unimpaired explains in part why such patients tend to account for their illness in terms of their current life situations. Unwarranted rumination about the past and unneeded worry about the present, however, are so characteristic of depressive syndromes that it is never certain that the patient's concerns are realistic or that his theories concerning the depression's "cause" are valid. The issues that the depressed patient worries about are indeed similar to those that concern others of his age and circumstance, and it is important not to confuse understanding why he might have become sad with understanding why he has developed a depressive syndrome.

Accordingly, the depressed child tends to be troubled about the way his parents and siblings treat him and about the way he feels about them in return; the depressed adolescent about his value systems, sexual identity, scholastic achievement, and "fitting in" to his group. Young adults generally worry about their choice of career or spouse, or question their preparedness for parenthood, which in women of childbearing age comes to clear-cut expression in postpartum mental illnesses (see p. 194). Later concerns focus on the difficulties they are facing in taking care of their dependent parents. Patients who become depressed in their early 40s are often troubled about having gone as far in their work as they are likely to go; those in the late 40s worry that their performance and advancement is starting to decline. Around this age, they also start to be concerned that their parental role is about to end and that they must now adjust to their lives or marriages without children. In addition, they are likely to be confronted with the problems engendered by the aging, illness, and death of their parents. The concerns of the 40s continue into the 50s, and at this time mesh with worries about declining sexual ability, which in turn give rise to a renewed preoccupation with their adequacy as marital partners and the degree of satisfaction they derive from their spouses. In the 60s, the deaths of spouse, siblings, and friends blend with the fear of being abandoned by one's children and the boredom of retirement. Thereafter, depressed patients focus on their health, their real or potential disabilities, becoming a burden, and, whether stated or not, but always in the background as a major concern, their impending death (Weiss 1961).

The typical depression is thus in some ways merely an artifact (Rosenthal 1968), a description of an advanced stage of depression in the particular age group between 45 and 60 that is most disposed to depressive syndromes: its symptoms and concerns do not represent a separate symptom complex but merely one point on a continuum of depressive symptoms that, in traveling across an age-related scale of biologic reactivity, consecutively reflect the problems associated with each period of life.

Treatment of Unipolar Depressions

INDICATIONS

While it is usually the depressed patient's impaired functioning and social impact that prompt his referral, biologic criteria must also be used to assess the severity of his illness. It is thus necessary to gauge not only his discomfort, immobilization, and despair; his environment's ability to cope with him; and the dangers foreshadowed by suicide threats or attempts; but also the severity, persistence, and progression of his sleep disorder and anorexia. The obvious difficulties in evaluating social and intrapsychic factors make the assessment of the biologic ones doubly important. Sleep loss in excess of three hours a night is, next to attempted suicide, the most frequent concomitant of any depression severe enough to warrant hospitalization, and this means that, whatever the setting, situation, or ostensible reasons for referral, by the time the patient's depression has progressed to the point that it seriously disturbs his sleep, it also prevents him from coping with or being tolerated by his environment. As the sleep deficit mounts, the dangers increase: impaired judgment, impulsive behavior, and delusional thinking may follow (see Table 2).

In most cases, the depressed patient consults the psychiatrist of his own accord or with a minimum of urging by his family or his family doctor and is a willing, even if somewhat skeptical, collaborator in the treatment program. When, however, his sense of despair leads him to view a psychiatric consultation either as futile or as an obstacle to an already formulated plan of committing suicide and he rejects treatment, the family must be informed of the consequences of his not receiving treatment and what, if anything, they should do to see that he does. When they learn that the vast majority of depressed patients, treated or not, will eventually feel better again, they may wonder whether it might not be simplest just to let things take their own course. What speaks against this idea is that the untreated patient may take the one step that can thwart recovery: commit suicide. Only rarely will a sophomoric discussion of the patient's "right" to commit suicide develop, for the patient, at this point, is obviously unable to think rationally or make decisions for himself, and there is as little question of rights as there would be with a child.

The untreated depression generally lasts between six and 18

months and in some cases for several years. Throughout this period, the patient may be severely uncomfortable, socially and occupationally unable to function, and constantly prey to suicidal impulses. By the time his illness remits, his family relationships, his economic position, and his job security may be so gravely compromised that his recovery from the depression may seem inconsequential in the total context of his life. We therefore consider immediate treatment imperative and advise the family to exert whatever influence they can to implement this. When the situation is grave and there is no other way to arrange for his treatment, we urge them to have the patient hospitalized, even without his consent.

TREATMENT SETTING

The choice between hospital and outpatient treatment can be problematic: premature hospitalization is crippling and embarrassing; unduly postponed hospitalization, dangerous. Using the criteria outlined in Chapter 2, we prefer to treat the depressed individual as an outpatient only when this is unlikely to compromise his safety or comfort or to interfere with the efficiency of his treatment. To the assessment of suicidal risk outlined on page 56 may be added the observation that suicidal ideas are so common in depressive syndromes (Guze 1970, Pitts 1964, Silverman 1968) that the patient who denies having any such thoughts at all must be suspected of concealing them and thus considered in even greater danger than the one who discusses them without hesitation (Havens 1967). Even when safety and comfort are not the prime motives, hospitalization may be preferred from the standpoint of relieving the patient of his fear of being alone and protecting him from the pressure of outside obligations and the discomfort he may experience in social transactions with exasperated friends and relatives. Their intolerance of the patient's constant demands and the anguish and apprehensiveness they feel as a result of his condition may indeed become so extreme that it must be taken into account in deciding on hospitalization.

SOMATIC TREATMENT

For reasons that are discussed on page 635, drug treatment has today largely replaced electroshock therapy in the management of depressive syndromes. The most effective drugs in restoring the depressed patient's premorbid mood and activity level are the so-called *antidepressants,* a term used to refer to certain dibenzazepine derivatives like imipramine (Tofranil) and monoamine oxidase inhibitors

(MAOI) like phenelzine (Nardil). The patient's depression and psychomotor retardation (at least by the time he comes for treatment) may be of less immediate importance than his protracted insomnia and agitation, which, in addition to causing severe discomfort, can confuse the diagnostic picture. It is thus advisable to combine the administration of antidepressants with that of *phenothiazines,* which (whether or not they have a beneficial effect on the patient's mood disorder) rapidly relieve insomnia and agitation in most cases and thus provide the patient and family with the first glimmer of hope that something useful can be done. The use of phenothiazines is particularly important when there is any possibility that the patient might in reality be suffering from schizophrenia since, without phenothiazines, antidepressants can cause schizophrenic symptoms to become even more severe. Phenothiazines should thus be used first, when the patient is young or has delusional ideas, when his illness has had a rapid onset, and when there is a previous or a family history of schizophrenic illness.

If the patient has been taking CNS depressants, such as alcohol, sedatives, or "minor" tranquilizers (see Table 35), it is important that he stop. This is by no means an easy task, since depressed patients often come to depend on such agents after discovering that they provide an immediate (even if transient) euphoria and have a rapid effect on their sleep difficulties. The patient who has taken such drugs because of his depression must be warned that CNS depressants are addictive, in the sense that they must be used in ever increasing amounts to achieve the desired effect and produce severe discomfort when withdrawn if previously taken in sufficiently high doses for a long enough time; that their long-term effect is to heighten and not to relieve depression (Stafford-Clark 1957); that they are likely to impair his judgment and, when readily available, may become an all too convenient vehicle for an impulsive suicide attempt. Despite such warnings, the patient may continue to take these agents —either openly or covertly—and in some cases it may be necessary to hospitalize him to ensure that he does as he is told (see Chap. 9).

Unless the patient's prior use of CNS depressants dictates a more gradual procedure, the phenothiazine dosage should be rapidly increased to whatever level is needed to improve his sleep. Intermediate phenothiazines like perphenazine (Trilafon) or prochlorperazine (Compazine) are preferable for this purpose to phenothiazines like chlorpromazine (Thorazine) or thioridazine (Mellaril), which, while more sedating, tend to cause hypotension, a side effect that is especially undesirable in view of the fact that the antidepressant that will subsequently be added is also likely to lower the patient's blood pressure (see Table 33). Although somewhat higher doses can be used in the closely supervised hospital setting, an outpatient is given 4 mg of perphenazine every two to four hours, up to a total of 16 mg, from the time of his initial visit until 8 PM on the same day. The patient should be advised to retire by 10 PM and shortly before may be given 50 to 100 mg of a mild sedative antihistamine like diphenhydramine (Benadryl). At 9 PM and at hourly intervals until 3 AM, he should receive 2 mg of perphenazine. Whenever he falls asleep, the phenothiazine schedule is interrupted, but if he awakens before 3 AM, it may be resumed until that hour. Thereafter, no further medications should be given, although the patient should be encouraged to remain in bed until morning. The patient (or family) is instructed to call the physician the following morning in order to report on his sleep and on the total amount of medication required and to receive instructions for the coming day's medications (see Table 10).

The second day's dosage is computed from that of the first. If, for example, the patient got no sleep at all, he would have received a total dosage of 30 mg of perphenazine (Trilafon). If he did sleep, even if only briefly, this figure might be somewhat lower. The second day's schedule should consist of four individual doses at four-hour intervals (say, at 8 AM, 12 noon, 4 PM, and 8 PM), each equal to about one fourth of the total dose of phenothiazine taken on the first day. From 9 PM that evening until 3 AM, the patient should again be given 2 mg of perphenazine every hour while awake. On the third day, he is again given the previous day's total dosage in four divided doses, and again 2 mg hourly are given at night. This program will often lead to a marked improvement in the patient's sleep within three or four days and at the outset may even have a beneficial effect on his mood. The effect on the patient's mood is inconstant and tends to be transitory, however; thus, as soon as the patient's sleep starts to improve, antidepressants should be added.

Antidepressant Medication.   Antidepressants of the imipramine (Tofranil) group tend to be safer and more effective than MAO-inhibitors and should therefore be used first. In the first two days, the dosage of imipramine is 25 mg, tid; for the next two, 25 mg, qid, after which the dose is increased to 50 mg, tid. Slower increases are indicated for the patient who has a cardiovascular disease or CNS disorder or exhibits a marked drop in blood pressure. When other antidepressants are used, the dose levels will differ (see Table 37), but the rate of increase should be approximately the same. To allay the patient's and family's concern, they should be warned in advance that imipramine is likely to cause blurred vision and dryness of mouth.

The behavioral changes follow a predictable sequence. There is usually little change until the patient has been taking at least 100 or, more commonly, 150 mg of imipramine for five days. Around this time, his relatives may report that he has periods in which he seems somewhat more active and that he can occasionally be seen to smile. The patient will generally deny this, however, and for the next few days report that he feels as bad as ever. Between the tenth and fourteenth day, the patient himself may begin to notice some improvement, though he will probably continue to voice despair and pessimism and deny that the improvement is lasting or meaningful. It is often not until after he has been taking a full therapeutic dose for three to four weeks that he feels—sometimes gradually, sometimes suddenly—that the "lights have gone on" and starts to have hope for the future.

Between the tenth and the fourteenth day of treatment, some patients exhibit agitation and difficulty in falling asleep, some (particularly those over 50) exhibit memory disturbances, and a few even become delirious. Such episodes usually subside within three to four days whether additional treatment is offered or not and are often followed by a marked improvement. If, however, the patient's discomfort is severe, chlordiazepoxide (Librium), 30 mg daily, may be of value.

During these first weeks, the daily imipramine dosage is increased from 150 to 200 or even to 300 mg, if, and only if, the expected sequence of amelioration fails to occur. Once the patient begins to improve, the phenothiazines should be reduced as rapidly as the patient's sleep permits: the daily dose of perphenazine can usually be reduced by 6 to 8 mg weekly unless and until the sleep difficulty recurs, at which point the reduction schedule is halted. If, after a week or so, the patient's sleep is again improving, the schedule may be resumed, though perhaps somewhat more gradually. The antidepressants should not be reduced with equal rapidity, however: for a period of eight to 12 weeks after the patient's symptoms have remitted, the dose of antidepressant should remain unchanged. Thereafter, an attempt should be made to lower it by about one third (as from 150 to 100 mg of imipramine daily). This dose should then be maintained for at least three weeks, after which the daily dosage is lowered by 25 mg every three weeks until a dose level of 50 mg daily is achieved. This level is then maintained for about six weeks and thereafter reduced to 25 mg daily. Naturally, if in the course of these medication changes there is an exacerbation in the patient's symptoms and his sleep difficulties or mood fluctuations recur, the antidepressant reduction schedule must be halted or even reversed. It is, in any case, usually best not to discontinue the medication entirely until the patient has been free of symptoms for a minimum of six months.

A patient who becomes depressed during menopause and exhibits anxiety attacks, cold sweats, and "hot flashes" (Neugarten 1965) may, with the approval of her gynecologist, be given conjugated equine estrogens (such as Premarin) in doses of 1.25 to 5.0 mg daily (Kupperman 1967, Wallach 1959, Wilson 1963), as this often diminishes the frequency and severity of the autonomic symptoms and will in some cases mitigate the depression as well (Greenblatt 1965).

The "atypical" depressions that are most common in younger patients and are characterized both by the symptoms described above and by such other symptoms as anxiety, phobias, depersonalization, and conversion may be treated in much the same manner as the typical ones, but their management is usually more problematic. When given antidepressants of the imipramine type, the patient's discomfort may for a time become more severe, his sleep disturbance get worse, and the side effects—xerostomia, dyspnea, and dizziness—seem unbearable. Such complaints are usually fairly innocuous and, even if nothing is done, tend to subside within the same three to four week period required for the depressive symptoms to lift. If, however, the patient finds the new symptoms so intolerable that he threatens to stop taking the prescribed medication, it may be useful to give a mild sedative such as chlordiazepoxide (Librium), 20 to 30 mg, or diazepam (Valium), 6 to 10 mg, daily for a few weeks. The frequency with which such side effects emerge when drugs of the imipramine group are given to patients with atypical depressions and, even more, the belief that such patients have a better therapeutic response to MAOI (Sargant 1961) has prompted some clinicians to use MAOI from the outset in atypical depressions.

The Exacerbation of Symptoms.   Throughout the course of treatment, the patient's sleep and symptoms may fluctuate. Transitory setbacks are common, particularly around the time of the menstrual period or when a viral or other illness supervenes. Even a mild exacerbation cannot be ignored, however, and it is important to determine whether it signifies drug toxicity, improvement, incipient relapse, or drug withdrawal, or is caused by some completely unrelated event. An increase in agitation in the first two weeks of taking an antidepressant may represent *drug toxicity* and can be relieved by giving a mild sedative. It can also mean that the patient is *schizophrenic,* especially if he becomes increasingly delusional, in which event an increase in the phenothiazine dosage or a decrease in the antidepressant dosage is indicated. If, after his most acute symptoms diminish, the patient reexperiences symptoms he had at an earlier stage of his illness (such as anxiety, somatic complaints, or obsessional thinking), and there has not been a recent drug reduction, this reexperiencing in all probability represents a transient *rollback phenomenon* of the kind described on page 53 and requires no intervention. If the patient's symptoms first develop soon after the antidepressant dosage is reduced, he is either experiencing withdrawal symptoms or has suffered a relapse. Symptoms that arise within two weeks of reducing or discontinuing one or more of his drugs and are associated with gastrointestinal distress and tremulousness are probably *effects of drug withdrawal* and will subside spontaneously within a week or ten days. Symptoms that develop more than ten days after a drug reduction and are associated with insomnia, sadness, agitation, anergia, or despair or are similar to those that prevailed at the height of the illness in all likelihood represent a *relapse,* especially if they persist for more than two weeks. Under these circumstances, and particularly when the patient's sleep difficulties progress rapidly, the antidepressant dosage should once more be increased, followed by increases in phenothiazines, if needed.

The Treatment of Recurrent Depressions. While the titration of medication against symptoms described above may need to be continued for 12 to 18 months (in older persons even longer), the individual episode of depression generally comes to an end in the sense that the patient can eventually be withdrawn from antidepressants entirely without running the risk of immediate relapse. This does not necessarily mean that there is no further reason for concern, for while it is true that many persons who have had one depressive episode do not ever have another, it is equally true that others experience such episodes repeatedly. The *long-term administration of antidepressants* is admittedly far less effective in preventing new rounds of depression than the long-term administration of phenothiazines is in preventing schizophrenic episodes; nevertheless, patients who have had three or more depressive episodes (especially those with a family history of recurrent depressions) should be continued on antidepressants even when they are symptom-free.

Maintenance treatment with lithium carbonate has also been recommended in recurrent depression whether or not the individual has had an overt manic episode (Baastrup 1967).

Management of Illnesses Refractory to the Initial Course of Medications.   The optimistic statement that most patients with depressive syndromes respond favorably to treatment is valid only statistically. Some patients, especially men, do not improve even after they have been taking 200 to 300 mg of imipramine (Tofranil) for six weeks. Under these circumstances, the imipramine should be discontinued for seven days and an MAO-inhibitor, such as phenelzine (Nardil), substituted. Those who do not respond to the first type of antidepressant, however, are less likely to respond to the second and thus present difficulties in treatment.

If a patient improves after being given an antidepressant and, while still taking it, becomes depressed again, it is possible that he has become tolerant to the drug's antidepressant effect and that his drug dose should be increased (Horwitz 1968). If this is not helpful, it may be worthwhile to try to reactivate his responsiveness by giving him 3 to 5 mg of reserpine intramuscularly twice daily for two days (Kuhn 1961). Still other patients achieve only partial improvement on a particular medication regimen. Certain antidepressant-phenothiazine combinations, for example, seem to cause such severe anergia or somnolence that the patient's daytime functioning suffers until the phenothiazine dosage is reduced. Occasionally, a patient, despite feeling more cheerful and functioning more effectively, remains anhedonic for a year or even longer, says that he is not yet feeling "up to par," expresses constant fear of relapse, and experiences episodes of anxiety, "stomach flutters," and palpitations. If these or other residual symptoms last longer than six months and are unresponsive to medication, four to six electroconvulsive treatments may produce a satisfactory remission.

ECT should also be used when the patient shows little or no improvement after a four to six week trial with one representative of each of the two groups of antidepressants. Our reluctance to administer ECT to the depressed patient until it is demonstrated that he is refractory to drug therapy does not stem from the old shibboleth that its use is immoral or from the conviction that it is more dangerous or less effective, but from concern regarding its effect on the patient's self-image and future collaboration and the social impact of the memory disturbance that often follows ECT. ECT is, however, the treatment of choice when the patient

1/ is in acute danger of committing suicide;

2/ has on previous occasions responded poorly to antidepressants and well to ECT;

3/ refuses to take drugs;

4/ suffers from some disease that precludes the use of antidepressants; or

5/ develops intolerable side effects.

Although no magic number of ECTs can be suggested, we rarely give fewer than three treatments and continue until the patient feels some relief or is becoming mildly confused. Then we give three further treatments, and stop. A sequential combination of antidepressants and ECT is often superior to the use of either alone, and it is believed that pretreatment with antidepressants reduces the number of convulsive treatments required to ensure a stable remission (Oltman 1960). This observation may be an artifact, however: the number of ECTs required may be lower or the response to ECT better following a course of antidepressants only because the use of antidepressants postpones the use of ECT. Thus, by the time the physician decides to use ECT, the illness (which is usually self-limited in any case) might have reached a more benign stage or be about to remit spontaneously. While the value of using an antidepressant before giving ECT may be debatable, it is generally agreed that antidepressants sustain remission after a successful course of ECT. If a patient who has previously responded poorly to antidepressants recovers fully on ECT and then relapses despite taking antidepressants, a new or longer course of ECT may be required. Should this pattern continue, it may be necessary to administer prophylactic or maintenance ECT at two to four week intervals over a period of months or years (see p. 650).

PSYCHOTHERAPY

The principles for using the various kinds of psychotherapeutic encounters that are spelled out in Chapter 13 are with certain modifications applicable to depressive syndromes as well. In the first phase of treatment, the therapist must cope with the patient's despair, suicidal ideation, self-induced social isolation, passivity, irritating manner, and self-deprecatory assessment of his own worth and competence. Once these have subsided, the patient's tendency to regress must be countered and a rapid return to his usual activities encouraged. Finally, the patient must be helped to decide whether a long-term psychotherapeutic involvement is warranted or whether (and how) the treatment relationship should be terminated. Discussions of the patient's premorbid life style or factors in his past that might be causally related to his illness may be required at some time in the course of his treatment, but should be postponed until he is well enough to tolerate them and the patient-doctor relationship is stable enough to permit him to explore such matters without becoming so upset that his symptoms return or he terminates treatment.

The *initial phase of treatment* is difficult for both participants. The patient is unable to talk, and often to listen; what little he says may consist solely of complaints, self-derogatory comments, and doubts concerning the future. While some patients—particularly those who have previously been ill—are not pessimistic about the outcome of their illness (Harrow 1966), many feel hopeless, view any effort to communicate as futile, and consider the therapist foolish for believing it worthwhile. The limited scope of the patient's discussions, his disdain for the psychotherapeutic process, and the repetitive and monotonous manner in which he presents his litany of despair may render him hard to listen to and—whether or not the therapist acknowledges it—annoying to be with (Tabachnick 1961). Despite these difficulties and frustrations, every effort must be made to involve the patient in an intimate and trusting relationship, both as a bulwark against suicide and as an instrument for persuading him to follow the physician's instructions.

The therapist's success in establishing a collaborative relationship with the patient depends on the way their attitudes and personalities mesh, on his ability to tolerate the patient's unusual social behavior, and on the patient's assessment of the therapist's expertise. If the therapist's comments and inquiries reflect familiarity with the illness, the patient may start to appreciate that neither he nor his illness is so unique or unfathomable as he had thought; that the therapist can be viewed as knowledgeable and possibly helpful; and that the therapist's optimism may be based on experience, not just the desire to reassure him as his friends and family do. It will become obvious to him that the doctor has seen similar cases if he "knows" that the patient gets bored with television, is unable to concentrate enough to read or to understand what he reads, finds himself unattractive when he looks in the mirror, feels empty and emotionally blunted, feels worse in the morning than in the evening, wakes up in the middle of the night and, unable to go back to sleep, fretfully lies in bed or gets up to pace. The patient's doubts about the efficacy of treatment may be further allayed when the physician demonstrates his awareness that the patient views the therapist's expression of optimism as fraudulent, believes himself to be the "one in a million" who will prove an exception (Kline 1969), and is convinced that the therapist understands neither the severity of the depression nor the relevance of the things about which he is depressed.

Even if a meaningful relationship can be established in the first meeting or two, the patient's apathy and despair may again supervene and cause the relationship to falter. For this reason, the patient and doctor should meet frequently enough to establish a basic level of rapport until the patient's mood lifts. These meetings should be fairly short. In their course, the therapist will inevitably be exposed to the patient's demands for reassurance. Knowing that these requests are usually insatiable and apt to be traps for the unwary and that responding to them is of transient value at best, he may be tempted to respond impatiently and let the patient know how tedious he finds them. Since the patient generally stops making such demands at the end of the acute phase, which lasts only a few weeks, the reassurance he requests may safely be given again and again.

When the illness has impaired the patient's ability to transact with his friends and family, group therapy may be indicated. Joint meetings with the patient and his family may also be useful, for in the typical case the illness will have caused much unspoken and unresolved friction between them. In the beginning, the main purpose of *group therapy* is to expose the patient to a certain amount of social stimulation and to offer him the encouragement of patients who have recovered from similar illnesses. It is therefore unnecessary (and may even be harmful) to insist that the patient participate actively until he feels comfortable enough to do so. A therapy group should initially be an adjunct to, not a substitute for, individual meetings; follow-up treatment, however, can often take place in the group setting alone.

At the outset, *family meetings* will be used to gather information about the patient's illness and life situation and to ensure the collaboration of his relatives. As treatment progresses, they can be used to help the patient cope with whatever family pathology contributed to his illness, to support his relatives in their often difficult assignment of spending time with him, and to help them cope with the guilt, anger, and confusion that his condition has evoked. Reassurance and information will in most cases be effective: the more they know about depressions, the more helpful they are likely to become. It is thus of value to point out to the family that the patient's ruminations, apathy, and imperviousness to reassurance reflect illness rather than their incompetence or his perversity; that most depressive illnesses respond to treatment fairly rapidly; that the patient will probably withdraw all or most of the accusations he is currently making as soon as his mood lifts; and that it is natural for them to respond to his accusations and apathy with anger until they can redirect their anger toward its logical target, the illness itself, and understand that the patient is in fact as unable as he appears to act differently or "pull himself together."

A psychotherapeutic relationship serves also to protect the patient from the consequences of his indecisiveness and poor judgment. When the patient is so insecure about his own judgment that he is unable to make even minor decisions, the therapist or family should make them for him rather than permit him to torture himself with needless ruminations. Such major decisions as leaving a girlfriend, a wife, or a job should always be postponed until the patient is in better condition. The patient's conviction that he must take a less demanding job if he wishes to recover or that he will never be an adequate spouse and should therefore separate may be based on his distorted view of the situation and, if acted on precipitously, can be a later source of disadvantage and regret. When a decision does not brook delay, the therapist must act as a sounding board for the patient's thinking, offering him (and sometimes insisting that he accept) a more realistic perspective of his situation than his illness allows. The depressed patient may be striving beyond his limits to demonstrate a high level of competence because he erroneously believes that his job situation is tenuous or that pushing himself will hasten his recovery. By demanding too much of himself, however, he will become even more inclined to failure and thus even more discouraged and liable to suicide. Patients should therefore be advised to limit rather than expand their activities until their mood starts to improve.

The foregoing recommendations have focused more on the establishment of an intimate doctor-patient relationship, the providing of advice, support, reassurance, and stimulation, and the protection of the patient from unwise decisions than they have on exploring the patient's psychodynamics or family relationships. This emphasis is intentional, for the acutely depressed patient may be so retarded in his thinking and speech that he is unable to answer complex questions and may erroneously consider this inability to be further evidence of his incompetence and "incurability." Even if he is verbal, his reports about the past and his notions concerning the causes of his depression are so colored by his illness that the possibility must always be entertained that they are retroactive falsifications or attempts at denial. It is in any case unwise to engage the severely depressed patient in a discussion of his own contribution to his illness, as this will almost invariably deteriorate into an inappropriate recital of his real or imagined faults and sins (Taylor 1969). Furthermore, even if it were (as it is not) possible to document the widely held view that internalized anger plays an important role in the mechanism of depression (Friedman 1970, Gershon 1968, Harrow 1970), it is not useful to permit or encourage the patient to vent such feelings. The patient who is able to express such emotions may consider himself disloyal and feel even guiltier; the one who is not may view his inability to do what he thinks the doctor wants as evidence that his illness is incurable and his treatment futile. The therapist, moreover, should spare the family gratuitous interpretations or guilt-provoking questions, for the most immediate consequence of such comments is to cause them to distort what they tell him. The *tour de force* in which the uninformed therapist deals out the roles and components of guilt as though they were cards in a game of bridge is today undertaken only by novices. Even the mildest interpretive comment, when premature, can cause the relatives to feel so guilty or angry that they pull away from the patient and refuse to collaborate with the doctor. These consequences should be avoided at all costs, as they may well increase the inherent danger of suicide and place formidable obstacles in the path of outpatient treatment.

The *second phase of treatment* usually proceeds fairly well by itself; the patient starts to talk about returning to work and gradually picks up the pieces of his former life. In rare cases, he has become so used to pleading inability for disinclination that he continues to use this explanation even after his depression lifts. This kind of regression is particularly common in adolescents and can become a way of life unless it is countered with increased pressure to perform. When the patient's passivity continues for months after his symptoms subside or is based on long-standing feelings of inferiority, he must be involved in intensive psychotherapy as soon as he is able to tolerate some degree of self-examination (Beck 1967).

In the *third phase of treatment,* which begins once the acute symptoms have receded and the patient has resumed his previous activities, he and the therapist must decide together whether and how long treatment should continue. Although the criteria for this decision are by no means simple, we tend to recommend *long-term therapy* for those patients who

1/ show unresolved conflicts even after their mood has improved;

2/ are in a life situation that has been and can again become a source of trouble;

3/ have a long-standing personality disorder that makes them offensive, inadequate, or sensitive, requiring that they be socially retrained, given continuous advice, or taught how to cope with everyday stresses; or

4 / have recurrent episodes of suicidal depression.

Even when there is no indication for long-term therapy, however, we recommend regular visits for a period of three months and follow-up visits at three-to-six-month intervals for 18 to 24 months after the symptoms subside.

After the decision to terminate has been made, the patient may attempt to hold on to the therapist as a source of support. While the therapist's round-the-clock availability throughout the most critical phase of the illness may have taught the patient to reach for the telephone instead of an overdose, it may in time stimulate his dependency needs to such an extent that he finds it hard to stop calling. This does not occur so often as might be expected, however. Even if the patient's regressive tendencies and concern about abandonment are stimulated by a discussion of termination, the end is uneventful far more frequently than the literature on termination would lead one to believe. When the patient does become upset at this juncture, it may be of value for him to recognize that his desire to have someone to lean on conflicts with the existential reality that he is all alone. Such discussions will in any case serve as a vehicle for exploring the indications for continued psychotherapy.

Other issues must also be discussed with the patient in the final stage of treatment, not the least of which are the limitations inherent in treatment: the dependent patient may remain as dependent as he was before getting ill, and the obsessive-compulsive patient may continue to count license plate numbers. Whatever the current disorder's precipitant might have been, and whatever the patient's personality type, level of insight, or life situation is, he should understand that his chance of becoming depressed again is higher than that of someone who has never had an episode of this kind. In the face of these reservations, it is remarkable how often patients who have recovered from a depressive syndrome describe themselves as feeling better than ever and attribute their sense of well-being to the transactions between themselves and their doctors. That a mental illness steers some people into their first encounter with a relatively intelligent and sympathetic human being may explain why they believe that the illness was the "best thing that ever happened" to them, but it is also a pathetic commentary on the quality of many human relationships. Excessive enthusiasm for the results of treatment must be viewed with suspicion, however, for the patient's newfound pleasure in life may be a sign of hypomania (see p. 189).

BIPOLAR AFFECTIVE DISORDERS

The term manic-depressive *disease* is preferable to manic-depressive *psychosis* in referring to bipolar affective disorders, for the latter would seem justified only when the patient's behavior is irrational or leads to social consequences catastrophic enough to warrant hospitalization (Gottlieb 1950). Mild, regularly recurring mood shifts that last for weeks or months at a time are sometimes called *cyclothymic personality disorders,* and are distinguished only in that they have never before led to such disastrous behavior. Until recent years, the natural history of bipolar affective disorders has been tragic. Its course is long, the patient's life expectancy is shortened, his life functioning is intermittently disrupted by episodes of poor judgment and eccentric behavior that lead to catastrophic social consequences, and he may spend as much as a third of his life in a mental hospital (Oltman 1962).

That this illness appears simple and that full recovery is common makes it the more provocative and intriguing. Yet, while improved pharmacologic measures that can prevent or abort new episodes seem to be in the offing, the surest way for a patient to avoid the disastrous social consequences of this illness is to establish an enduring relationship with a physician with whom he and his family can collaborate. Until this occurs and until he learns to recognize his symptoms early enough to report for treatment at the first sign of trouble and then do what he is told, even potentially effective treatment measures will fail. Before this kind of relationship develops, however, patient and physician usually go through two or three episodes together, gradually establishing rapport during the insightful periods of the patient's remission.

Depressive Phase

CLINICAL FEATURES

The major difference between the depressive phase of manic-depressive illness and the typical unipolar depression is that the patient exhibits less psychomotor agitation, insomnia, and anorexia, but more anergia. Although many bipolar depressives complain that their sleep is not restful, most sleep more than they do during their well periods, and some consider this their only source of satisfaction or way of escaping the discomfort of the depressive phase. Since the symptoms are similar in most other respects, they need not be described here.

It might seem that the bipolar depressive's repeated experience with the ebb and flow of the symptoms would permit him to feel more optimistic than the unipolar depressive. This is not the case, however, for the patient usually feels the same sense of despair anew and, even if willing to recall his previous remissions, is unable to rid himself of the feeling that this is the episode from which he will never get better. These fears, while exaggerated, are not completely unjustified. The depressive phase of bipolar disease is appreciably less responsive to antidepressants than the acute phase of unipolar disease, and it is still too early to know whether the promising results that have been reported with lithium carbonate will stand the test of time (see page 610). As in the typical unipolar depressions, a dibenzazepine derivative like *imipramine* (Tofranil) is the first antidepressant used. During the first week, the dosage is rapidly raised to 150 mg daily. Thereafter, the daily dosage is raised by 50 mg increments weekly until the patient is either feeling better or receiving a dosage of 300 or even 400 mg daily. If, even after two to three weeks at this dose level, the patient's mood does not improve or improves only slightly, the imipramine is discontinued over a 10 to 14 day period to avoid withdrawal symptoms (see page 604), and an MAO-inhibitor like *phenelzine* (Nardil), 15 mg, 3-4 times daily, substituted. If this too proves ineffective, the more toxic but sometimes more effective MAOI *tranylcypromine* (Parnate) can be tried. If, during previous bouts of depression, one antidepressant has proved superior to the others, it will of course be the first to be used.

If, on the other hand, during the current episode of illness or during previous ones, the patient has been given both kinds of antidepressant without avail, a course of *lithium carbonate,* increased until the serum lithium level reaches 1.5 mEq/1, should be tried. The use of lithium in the treatment of the depressive phase as well as the maintenance therapy aimed to check recurrences is conducted along the same lines as the treatment and prevention of the manic phase, that is, relatively high doses for the episode itself followed by a lower maintenance dose (see below). Although the extent to which lithium therapy is helpful in depressions is not yet established, it is our impression that depressions associated with manic-depressive disease, particularly those accompanied by hypersomnia, respond favorably to lithium. In some of our cases, the drug had only a moderate effect on the patient's mood, but hypersomnia and anergia diminished, and the *simultaneous administration of antidepressants* (even if they had previously had no effect) produced considerable improvement in mood as well.

Should lithium carbonate alone or in combination with antidepressants also fail, a course of ECT may be indicated. The comments made earlier (see p. 178) regarding the number and frequency of ECTs required for the treatment of unipolar depressions also apply to the treatment of the bipolar types.

Some patients become manic after being given an antidepressant. Although it is rarely possible to determine whether the shift is caused by the drug or by the natural course of the illness, the antidepressant should be reduced or withdrawn and, if the situation warrants, a phenothiazine added. If the manic phase then subsides and the patient again becomes depressed, it seems reasonable to assume that there was some causal relationship and that antidepressants should be given in smaller doses, if at all. If the manic symptoms persist or recur even after the antidepressant has been stopped and phenothiazines have been tried, the patient should receive lithium carbonate or ECT as described below for mania.

A strong, *supportive relationship* with the therapist is of vital importance during the depressed phase of manic-depressive disease to help the patient feel less discouraged about his condition and to mobilize him as soon as possible. When the depressive phase follows a prolonged and chaotic manic episode, his overtaxed physician and family may well greet his despair of ever recovering from his anergia and depression with an untherapeutic "Amen" and do little to encourage his becoming more active. Even the patient may fear the return of the manic state and, despite occasional expressions of nostalgia, withdraw from all activity in the hope of averting a recurrence. The fear of relapse, moreover, can compound the patient's feelings of inadequacy—feelings that derive from his depressive outlook and his awareness that he is periodically unable to function adequately—and thus encourage him to assume a defeatist attitude toward both his illness and his life. Since with the passage of time this will intensify his withdrawal and passivity, it is essential that a psychotherapeutic relationship be established as rapidly as possible.

Manic Phase

Manic episodes may arise both during symptom-free periods and after depressive episodes. Many patients are practically never asymptomatic, some having continual fluctuations in mood at all times, others being slightly depressed or mildly hypomanic. The style and development of the frank manic episode depends on the patient's age, premorbid personality, life situation, and occupation. In younger patients, the individual episode may appear expansive, pseudopsychopathic, and rebelliously antisocial; in older ones, it may appear as a frenzied effort to succeed in business or school, an effort that, at least initially, can be very effective. At what point in the episode the patient will turn to a psychiatrist depends largely on his previous experience. During the first few episodes, he may not appear until his condition is fairly well advanced, particularly if he is naturally eccentric or his environment is able to tolerate his hyperactivity and grandiosity. Even in subsequent episodes, he may at the outset feel so well that he is reluctant to report his symptoms to the physician, pretends he is sleeping well, responds to his environment's objections to his grandiose schemes by laughing and saying he was "just kidding," and in short denies having any symptoms at all. This state of euphoria is not universal, however, and some patients—especially those in the midst of the transition from depression to mania—show such intense sadness and anxiety that, despite voicing much gaiety, they are distinctly uncomfortable and consult a physician rapidly.

That the cardinal features of the manic phase—euphoria, expansive plans and desires, accelerated associations, hyperactivity, and insomnia—are observed in a number of other disorders, the most notable being catatonic excitement and the prodromal phase of a deliriform organic brain syndrome, presents certain problems in *differential diagnosis* (see p. 113). The manic phase of manic-depressive illness can be distinguished from catatonic excitement because the manic patient is usually older, has a history of mood swings, and has taken weeks or months rather than days to develop the behavioral symptoms and sleep disorder. Episodes of manic behavior seen in the course of acute and chronic brain syndromes (such as thyrotoxicosis, frontal lobe damage, tumors, and general paresis) can be distinguished from the manic phase of bipolar disease by the absence of previous manic episodes and the presence of organic findings. Particular attention must be paid to the possibility of an underlying organic disease when a patient remains confused and dysmnesic even after his sleep has improved, especially when his affect appears unusually labile. Whether the schizoaffective schizophrenia with manic features is merely a mixture of schizophrenic and manic disease, as some authors contend, or a distinct disease entity is hard to determine, especially because the patient with a manic episode often exhibits delusional and hebephrenic features (Welner 1964) (see also p. 119).

(see also p. 119).

CLINICAL FEATURES

The transitional phase from normal to hypomanic may be nearly imperceptible. The patient who becomes manic while recovering from a depression may start by telling himself that his previous feelings of tension and pessimism were foolish and that he should be more "realistic." He feels better at long last, and both he and the family are relieved that the period of stagnation has passed. As time passes, however, the patient begins to mention *"plans."* First he speaks of them only as "ideas," and his family encourages him; he shares all his decisions or actions with them, and they do not oppose his ideas so he does not become hostile (Schwartz 1963). From time to time, someone may mildly question some of the plans or ask for more details, but they quickly withdraw their questions and stifle any objection for fear that the patient will become depressed again. The patient's mood may show some fluctuations, but these are usually no greater than those experienced by the clinically well, and the only way to tell whether his mood and behavior are morbid would be to compare them with those seen in previous episodes (Jacobson 1965). Some patients invariably pursue the same grandiose project; others signal the onset of each manic episode with such signs of hyper-alertness as *irritability, acute hearing,* and *speeded thinking.* Not uncommon is a hypersensitivity to light that causes the patient to wear sunglasses, even indoors, while offering the most varied and unlikely explanations for this strange practice: he looks better in sunglasses, has lost his regular prescription glasses, or the like.

When the patient first starts to decompensate, he often functions quite well at work. He may sell far more than anyone in his company or develop plans for the expansion of his business that on the surface seem quite sensible. If the patient has had a previous episode, his psychiatrist and family may have occasional doubts but will then berate themselves for being too conservative and for not encouraging the patient to exploit fully his newfound business acumen and intellectual gifts. As the patient describes his *feeling of well-being* and his successes, and expresses gratitude to his physician for getting him through his depressive illness, the physician may begin to feel pride in the accomplishments of his charge. This false sense of security may continue even after the patient starts to give parties for his employer, take gifts to his co-workers and doctor, and speculate in the stock market, for in this phase he may be successful and well-liked, exude

a general sense of well-being and good fellowship, and provide pleasure for everyone around him. The physician will quite justifiably
become concerned, however, when he hears that the patient has hired
a secretary to go around with him to carry out his "brilliant" ideas
and notices that he has taken to wearing increasingly fashionable
and colorful clothes, grown a moustache, bought a new watch, and
made a down payment on a brand-new car. At this time he may try
to set some limits on the paitent's behavior. Since the manic patient's
response to a request that he moderate his behavior is to become irritable and hostile, asking him to refrain from new purchases and
observing his ability to do as he is told is an excellent way to determine whether his expansiveness is a normal variant of good feeling
or whether it is driven and morbid.

A young girl who considered herself ugly and unable to get a date
in her depressive episode may start her manic phase by having her
hair done more frequently. The physician may beam with satisfaction
when she starts to "go steady," or reports a B, or even an A, for a
school composition on which her teacher has noted "Full of good
ideas." The doctor may not become concerned until the girl brings
her "steady" into her therapy session, describes two or three different
boys as her "steady," and signs up for 22 school credit hours and a
full-time job. Soon she will be dating nightly, perhaps several times
during one night. Her sex life may appear to be promiscuous, even
while little genital sexual activity occurs.

The first signs of the housewife's manic phase may be that she is
cleaning her house more vigorously, buying books on exotic cooking,
or looking for a part-time job. That she is entering box-top contests
may not seem odd until it is learned that she is engaged in many
dozens of them and has recruited her neighbors to provide her with
additional labels. Soon she may try to persuade her husband to buy
a new house, at which time he may learn that she has already been
discussing this prospect for weeks with a real estate agent.

As the patient moves toward a frank manic episode, his productions take on a *mildly psychopathic* tinge. When the physician expresses skepticism about the burst of activity, the patient may start
to tell lies that make it obvious that he considers himself "smarter
than the doctor." Even if he has already been given a sedative, it will
cause only the mildest improvement in his sleep and will not prevent
him from *staying up all night* when he has a date, *overspending* on
various "important" gadgets and appurtenances, taking on new com-
mitments, making long-distance telephone calls, starting *litigation*
with a neighbor regarding a long-disputed property line, or writing

letters to prominent persons regarding his proposals for changing the world. Often the patient shows an increasing degree of *confusion* or becomes *delusional,* the more so if he starts to drink during a manic episode. That alcoholics often come from manic-depressive families and that many manic-depressives are alcoholics even before they become patently manic explains why many manic-depressive patients are hospitalized with the diagnosis of alcoholism and the manic symptoms are not detected until they are withdrawn from alcohol (Mayfield 1968).

TREATMENT

While the physician's clinical judgment during the depressive phase is based largely on the information the patient volunteers about his mood and the degree of anergia and apathy he exhibits, the manic phase—and with it the effectiveness of the somatic treatment being employed—is best gauged by close observation of the patient's sleep patterns. Until the manic episode subsides, the patients will be unable to sleep normally or stay in bed throughout the night. Thus, the ability to maintain regular sleep is an excellent measure of improvement. The patient will offer many explanations, some of which sound quite plausible, for not wanting to "waste time" by sleeping or, while in the hospital, needing to talk with the staff or with other patients about his "problems," and for preferring to do this in the hours between 10 PM and 4 AM, when the particular nurse's aide or attendant who "understands" him best is on duty. For this reason, it is important to give the patient specific instructions about the time he is to go to bed and get up, such as being in bed at 10 PM and rising no earlier than 6 AM.

The *drug of choice* in the acute manic episode is lithium carbonate. Administration of this drug may have to be delayed for one or two days until the required laboratory examinations have been completed. In the interim, the patient can be given a phenothiazine or haloperidol (Haldol) in doses sufficient to keep him manageable. This rarely dampens the symptoms entirely, however, and once the laboratory examinations (see p. 608) are completed, the patient is given 300 mg of lithium carbonate tid for the first day, the dose thereafter being increased by 300 mg daily until the patient's sleep is restored or his serum lithium level (which must be monitored regularly) reaches 1.5 mEq/l. Further details concerning this method may be found on pages 606-611.

As soon as the symptoms are under control and sleep becomes normal, the dose of lithium (or if the patient also receives a major tranquilizer, this drug first) is gradually reduced until the serum level is between 0.8 and 1.2 mEq/l. The drug dosage is kept at this level for an additional eight to 12 weeks, unless symptoms recur, at which time the dose is raised again and the higher dose maintained for an additional four to six weeks before being reduced again.

Since lithium is effective in preventing manic episodes and seems in some cases to mitigate the depressive phase as well, *maintenance therapy* is obviously indicated when the patient has had several manic episodes. Some clinicians are in favor of maintenance therapy even when the patient has had only one manic and one depressive episode, on the consideration that such patients already represent a "high risk" group. As it is impossible to predict the frequency of recurrences, decisions concerning maintenance therapy require careful consideration of such factors as the nature and severity of the previous attacks, the duration of the symptom-free intervals, the patient's age and premorbid personality, and the presence of cyclothymic disorder or frank manic-depressive disease in the patient's family. Thus if the patient's acute episodes (or any one of them) have been severe or socially disruptive or led to a loss of impulse control; if the symptom-free interval was less than two years; if the patient was less than 30 years of age at the time of the first episode; if for some years before the episode that prompted referral he had increasingly severe cyclothymic personality changes; and if he comes from a family in which two or more members have affective disorders or have committed suicide, maintenance therapy seems justified on the basis of one manic and one depressive episode and is definitely indicated if he has had two manic episodes. The more of the features above that are present, the greater the disease-associated risks and the less arbitrary the decision to place the patient on maintenance doses. For maintenance lithium therapy, a dose sufficient to achieve a plasma level of 0.6 to 1.2 mEq/l (usually 600 to 1,200 mg daily) is given. This dose is increased whenever the patient's customary mood becomes somewhat hypomanic, especially if he simultaneously experiences some loss of sleep.

Patients who do not respond to lithium carbonate alone and those who, either because they exhibit mixed symptoms from the outset or because they become more confused, delusional, or bizarre while taking lithium, are labeled atypical manics, manic-depressives with schizophreniform features, or schizoaffective schizophrenics, should be given moderate to high doses of *phenothiazines or haloperidol* (Haldol) *along with the lithium carbonate* during the acute episode and low doses of these agents during the maintenance phase of therapy (Aronoff 1970, Lipkin 1970). If this does not help, they should be tried on *phenothiazines* alone, and if this too is unsuccessful, a course of ECT should be instituted.

ECT will also be necessary if the patient's manic excitement is unmanageable from the outset or becomes refractory to drugs in the course of his treatment. The number of ECTs required for the treatment of the manic episode, like the phenothiazine dosage, may be titrated against improvement of sleep. The patient should be given ECT daily or even twice daily until for two nights in a row, he is sleeping at least an hour more than he had, at which time it may be reduced to every other day. Once he is able to sleep six to eight hours nightly, ECT may be discontinued. It is customary to give a few more treatments in order to stabilize the results, but the necessity for such additional treatments has not been proved (Kalinowsky 1961). Most manic episodes are exceptionally responsive to ECT; some even "break" after the first or second treatment. A total of four to six treatments may thus be sufficient, especially if the patient is then given lithium or a phenothiazine which, even if it does not cause the manic episode to subside, may prevent it from recurring. When, however, discontinuation of ECT leads repeatedly to recurrence—and also in the rare circular type of disease in which mania and depression alternate with only brief or no symptom-free intervals—*maintenance* ECT, at intervals of one, two, or even four weeks, may be necessary, though in such cases another try with lithium carbonate should be made first. Unfortunately, ECT may impair the patient's memory and with it his ability to understand and remember what has happened to him. As a result, he may fail to learn how important it is to communicate early and effectively with his physician in the event of future episodes, and it thus becomes more difficult to protect him from the illness' social consequences. Furthermore, when patients find ECT uncomfortable or experience problems with their work or social affairs as a result of their retrograde amnesia, they are likely to be fearful of receiving ECT again and thus reluctant to report an incipient illness in the future.

Most therapists find *psychotherapeutic encounters* with an acutely ill manic patient a taxing proposition. Initially, the patient's comments and behavior can be entertaining and his style engaging, but within hours or days those around him begin to consider him an obnoxious and overwhelming busybody who attempts to control his doctor and, if hospitalized, the entire life of the institution in which he has been placed. Attempts to set limits on his activity only heighten his irritability, and he soon becomes hostile and may even become paranoid. As further limits are set, he transgresses further, and a frustrating cycle is set in motion. To avoid or at least to diminish the effects of this cycle, it is best to protect the patient from any situation that could provide additional excitement. He should be excluded from group therapy, community meetings, or social programs until he can sit through the entire program without making a fool of himself. It may also be of value to place him in a quiet semidark room with a calm, taciturn companion.

The psychotherapist's first task is to try to limit the content of the discussion to a single topic. This may appear impossible, but when the matter is pursued with some vigor, the patient will sometimes consent to stay on one track. At times, particularly during the transitional period from the manic to the depressive phase, it is possible to get the patient to admit how sad and afraid he feels beneath his confident and euphoric facade. By simply acknowledging his appreciation of the patient's discomfort, the doctor can sometimes "break" the manic mood and cause a considerable (if only temporary) improvement in his social behavior. Once he has started to demonstrate some restraint in the one-to-one setting, his ability to tolerate more stimulating events can be tested by involving him in a therapy group.

Initially, he should be urged to talk little and to try to avoid monopolizing the group's time. As soon as he can perform circumspectly in this setting and can tolerate (and be tolerated by) a therapy group, some of the initial restrictions can be lifted. He may be allowed to take part in the hospital's social and recreational program, to receive longer visits from his family, and, if these go well, to make some visits to his home. His ability to tolerate such experiences without developing new symptoms, especially new difficulties in sleeping, will serve as a valuable index by which to gauge his readiness to be released from the hospital.

POSTPARTUM ILLNESSES

The relative frequency of psychological difficulties following childbirth stands in striking contrast to their relative rarity during pregnancy itself. Hyperemesis gravidarum, to be sure, is often seen in the first trimester, but is no longer considered unequivocally psychogenic (Majerus 1960). And, while previously well-compensated pseudoneurotic or schizophrenic patients sometimes experience an exacerbation of obsessive-compulsive concerns during the period of quickening, patients with preexisting mental illnesses tend to improve or recover during the second and most of the third trimester of pregnancy (Pugh 1963). At the very end of the third trimester and after delivery, however, preexisting mental illnesses often flare up again (Nilsson 1967). The symptoms are usually identical to those the patient had before becoming pregnant, with the exception that they show a more labile affect and that the patient's thoughts and concerns tend to focus on the childbearing experience.

DEPRESSED MOOD IN THE POSTPARTUM PERIOD

Many women experience a transient period of elation after giving birth, and this is in turn often followed by a period of *postpartum "blues."* During this time, the patient may have episodes of tearfulness and anxiety, but usually sleeps and eats relatively well and, given a chance to rest, recovers in a matter of days (Yalom 1968). In rare cases, the patient remains mildly depressed for a few months (Pleshette 1956) and may at times be sufficiently uncomfortable to need a mild sedative, but her social functioning usually remains fairly intact. Such difficulties may be viewed as mildly exaggerated stress responses related to the taxing period of pregnancy and delivery and are similar to those that follow other exhausting medical or surgical conditions.

ACUTE DELIRIOUS STATES IN THE POSTPARTUM PERIOD

An episode of confusion and total insomnia with hallucinations and unsystematized delusions that develops abruptly within five days of delivery and recedes equally rapidly (usually after a terminal sleep; see p. 414) is properly called an *acute postpartum delirium.* That such syndromes are usually toxic or infectious in origin is suggested by their having become less common since the introduction of aseptic obstetric techniques and antibiotics (Boyd 1942, Kenin 1962, Oltman 1965). As in other deliriform brain syndromes, the patient usually recovers spontaneously, but can be made more comfortable with adequate hydration, nutrition, nursing care, and vigorous treatment with phenothiazines (see p. 416).

THE POSTPARTUM MENTAL SYNDROMES

The legitimacy of considering the *postpartum mental syndrome* a discrete nosologic entity has long been considered a fair topic for futile debate; nevertheless, most clinicians will acknowledge that women who become mentally ill some weeks after delivery tend to display a characteristic combination of affective and confusional features. In addition to severe sleep loss and obsessional thinking (Jansson 1963), the patient will exhibit a progressive, long-term, low-grade depression, punctuated by sudden outbursts of sadness or rage; and a progressive, long-term, low-grade, sometimes fluctuating confusion punctuated by episodes of paralyzing perplexity. This syndrome may develop in the wake of an acute postpartum delirium or after an uneventful interval of a week or two following delivery, when the patient gradually starts to lose sleep and thereafter exhibits more and more of the features above. The full clinical picture emerges within three to four weeks of delivery, but on occasion may not be seen for as long as two or three months, in which case the patient's sleep and social functioning decline somewhat more gradually, sometimes so gradually that the prodromata have gone unnoticed and are recalled only in retrospect.

Numerous studies have sought to determine which, if any, of the biologic changes and stresses that occur during and immediately after pregnancy might contribute to the development of these syndromes (Marcé 1858, Robin 1962, Thomas 1959, Tobin 1964, Treadway 1969). Efforts have also been made to determine whether a given premorbid personality pattern (Jansson 1963) or a specific attitude toward pregnancy (Biskind 1958, Saunders 1929) influences the occurrence of these syndromes. It seems probable that the characteristic features are in fact the result not of a discrete clinical entity but of the psychosocial and biologic events that inevitably surround pregnancy and delivery. Whatever her predisposition, the new mother's new tasks give her symptoms a content and her concerns a focus. Whether or not she wants the responsibility for her baby's care or feels able to cope with it, she must accept it; the complexities of infant care force a relentless and stress-provoking confrontation with responsibility that an ill person may be unable to handle (Brew 1950, Madden 1958, Yarden 1966). This can be extremely fatiguing, require a sacrifice of her sleep, and, perhaps because of the endocrine changes that occur at this period, have an even more deleterious effect on her functioning than it would under normal circumstances.

Clinical Features

The confusion and perplexity of the patient with a postpartum mental syndrome are marginal in the sense that organizing events (such as contact with another person or an assigned, specific task) tend to diminish them. When, however, no one is with the patient or she is the only person responsible for planning and executing some job, she may become perplexed and disorganized. This in turn can make her so anxious that she cannot endure being alone and so emotionally incapacitated that she cannot perform even the simplest household chore (Chapman 1959). Such a state of affairs prompts many patients to want to visit or move in with their mothers or mothers-in-law; or to telephone their physician or their friends (regardless of how far away they may live) for advice and support. At the same time, their inability to act independently makes them shy away from more complex social relations. The net result of these difficulties is that patients feel inadequate, and concern about this then becomes a topic to brood about.

When the patient is not exposed to any organizing social stimuli, her ruminations are frequently concerned with psychological issues, such as the source of the conflicts. This tendency seems even more pronounced in patients who have just started psychotherapy and try to use their discussions with their doctors to encapsulate their perplexity. The patient may attribute her difficulties to having married too young and having been denied her chance to develop some independence. These ruminations can be fairly painful, as they are often concerned with a great sense of failure. In many cases, the patient will describe herself as "a girl sent to do a woman's job," and express fear that she will be unable to handle any emergency that may arise, such as her baby's becoming sick. In severe cases, the patient becomes afraid of doing harm to the baby or even to her other children.

During episodes of disorganization, the patient may exhibit histrionic emotional outbursts and become physically abusive. Since such episodes are, in addition, often accompanied by feelings of depersonalization, both the patient and those around her may erroneously conclude that she is "acting." The more often she experiences such outbursts, the more likely she is to fear that she will kill or harm her baby; her tendency to obsess may even lead her to ruminate constantly about this possibility. That the husbands of these patients often appear to be silent, intellectualizing, withdrawn, unavailable for affective exchange, and as a result somewhat impatient with their wives' emotionally charged outbursts has been considered of etiologic significance, but may merely mean that a husband of this kind will have difficulty in providing the patient with the well-structured setting she needs and thus add to the likelihood of her becoming perplexed and disturbed. The communication problem between husband and wife may be intensified by his anger about her seemingly histrionic behavior and vague complaints and by the illness' fluctuations, which alternately kindle and then extinguish the hope that things will go well.

Treatment

It is unsafe to permit a patient with a postpartum mental syndrome to remain home by herself during the acute stage of her illness because being alone will further disorganize her and increase her anxiety and thus endanger the lives of both baby and mother (Harder 1967). In many cases, the patient must be hospitalized until she has learned enough about her illness or established a strong enough relationship with a therapist to call for help when she needs it. Fluctuations in the illness may make additional hospitalizations necessary, but readmissions are usually much shorter than the first stay. In some cases, it may be of value to have the mother bring the baby with her to the hospital; this can provide the therapist with an opportunity to observe the mother-child interaction directly and to supervise the mother's care of the child until it has become sufficiently routinized to be unlikely to disorganize her (Main 1961).

Should it be possible to manage the patient at home, a companion is extremely useful. All too frequently, however, the patient engages in a constant struggle with supervision of any kind, and while this may be psychodynamically understandable, it makes proper care much more difficult. Mothers and mothers-in-law are most often available to help in such cases, but the patient will almost invariably resent their presence and see it as a further demonstration of her own inadequacy. It is thus preferable to obtain help from a friend, paid companion, or baby nurse; although this does not usually prevent similar difficulties, it will at least not cause permanent familial disaffection.

The woman with a postpartum mental syndrome often expresses a desire to go to work. The therapist should support such a notion, for a job can be therapeutic, especially when it provides the patient with the structure and organization she needs and thus offers her an arena in which she does not constantly experience episodes of demoralizing panic. In addition, it will ameliorate her sense of being useless and can obviate the emotional paralysis and immobilization she is likely to experience while attending to her household duties with no one around. Part-time positions are generally to be preferred, for a patient with a full-time job is likely to feel guilty about being away from her home and children. Whatever the work schedule, it is important that both husband and therapist provide moral support and help to assuage any feelings of guilt or inadequacy that the patient may experience.

As in other syndromes, an antidepressant may lift the patient's mood disorder, but it can also increase her preoccupations and difficulties in impulse control. Thus, even though the administration of phenothiazines alone can augment the depressive mood, the first target symptoms must be the impulse disturbance and delusional thinking; only after these are reasonably well suppressed should antidepressant therapy be instituted. In patients unresponsive to phenothiazines, reserpine in doses up to 12 mg daily may be tried, followed by a course of antidepressant therapy. Imipramine (Tofranil) in doses up to 400 mg daily may be necessary to relieve both the depression and the obsessional rumination. Antidepressants and tranquilizers have a far greater effect on the patient's affective response than they do on her confusional symptoms, which tend to be favorably affected only by the passage of time. Patients whose confusion, perplexity, and disorganization increase during the premenstrual and menstrual periods sometimes benefit from continuous administration of an ovulatory suppressant with low progestogen content such as norgestrel (Ovral). In rare instances, ECT may also be helpful and, while not usually tried unless the patient has suicidal or infanticidal preoccupations that do not respond to drugs, may produce rapid clearing of all symptoms.

Prognosis and Preventive Measures

While for some patients the postpartum syndrome represents their only bout of mental illness, for others it is but the first or most recent episode of a manic-depressive or (more rarely) schizophrenic illness, in which case the long-term prognosis is that of the underlying disease (Protheroe 1969). The short-term course may in either case be fairly stormy and, in some instances, the illness can last for a year or more. Even after the patient reaches what appears to be a clinical remission, she may for some time experience periodic episodes of perplexity, confusion, and impulsivity (Tetlow 1955).

That patients who have had a postpartum mental syndrome are more likely to develop another than those without such a history has led some physicians to advise against their having more children. Pregnancy need not have a deleterious effect, however, and can even lead to substantial improvement. Patients who become pregnant in the midst of a postpartum mental syndrome often become more comfortable during the period of gestation, and some, remembering the comfort that preceded delivery, may even become pregnant on purpose. But pregnancy cannot be considered a therapeutic recommendation, for such remissions usually last only as long as the pregnancy does, and a relapse at this juncture can lead to the even more problematic situation in which the psychotic mother has yet another young child to care for. Finally, since it is impossible to predict when or whether the illness will recur, the physician's recommendations concerning future pregnancies must take into account the extent of the patient's recovery, the severity of the illness at its worst, and, most important, the circumstances and desires of the patient and husband (see p. 460).

REFERENCES

Altschule, M. D.: Nonpsychologic causes of depression, Med Sci 16:36-40, 1965.

Angst, J.: Zur Ätiologie und Nosologie endogener depressiver Psychosen, Monograph, Gesamtgeb Neurol Psychiatrie Heft 112, Berlin: 1966.

Aronoff, M. S., and Epstein, R. S.: Factors associated with poor response to lithium carbonate: A clinical study, Amer J Psychiat 127:472-480, 1970.

Baastrup, P. C., and Schou, M.: Lithium as a prophylactic agent: Its effect against recurrent depressions and manic-depressive psychosis, Arch Gen Psychiat (Chicago) 16: 162-172, 1967.

Beck, A. T.: Depression: Clinical, Experimental, and Theoretical Aspects, New York: Hoeber, 1967.

Biskind, L. H.: Emotional aspects of prenatal care, Postgrad Med 24:633-637, 1958.

Boyd, D. A., Jr.: Mental disorders associated with childbearing, Amer J Obstet Gynec 43:146-163, 1942.

Bratfos, O., and Haug, J. O.: The course of manic-depressive psychosis, Acta Psychiat Scand 44:89-112, 1968.

Brew, M. F., and Seidenberg, R.: Psychotic reactions associated with pregnancy and childbirth, J Nerv Ment Dis 3:408-423, 1950.

Brodwall, O.: The course of manic-depressive psychosis, Acta Psychiat Scand 22:195-210, 1947.

Chapman, A. H.: Obsessions of infanticide, Arch Gen Psychiat (Chicago) 1:12-16, 1959.

Clayton, P., Desmarais, L., and Winokur, G.: Study of normal bereavement, Amer J Psychiat 125:168-178, 1968.

Clouston, T. S.: The prodromata of the psychoses, and their meaning, Rev Neurol Psychiat 1:781-791, 1903.

Detre, T., et al.: Hypersomnia and manic-depressive disease, to be published. 1970.

Friedman, A. S.: Hostility factors and clinical improvement in depressed patients, Arch Gen Psychiat (Chicago) 23: 524-537, 1970.

Gershon, E. S., Cromer, M., and Klerman, G. L.: Hostility and depression, Psychiatry 31:224-235, 1968.

Gottlieb, J. S., and Tourney, G.: The depressive illnesses: Their diagnosis and treatment, J Chronic Dis 9:234-248, 1959.

Greenblatt, R. B.: Estrogen therapy for postmenopausal females, New Eng J Med 272:305-308, 1965.

Grinker, R. R., *et al.:* Phenomena of Depressions, New York: Hoeber, 1961.

Guze, S. B., and Robins, E.: Suicide and primary affective disorders, Brit J Psychiat *117:*437-438, 1970.

Harder, T.: Psychopathology of infanticide, Acta Psychiat Scand *43:*196-245, 1967.

Harrow, M., and Amdur, M. J.: Guilt and depressive disorders, to be published.

Havens, L. L.: Recognition of suicidal risks through the psychologic examination, New Eng J Med *276:*210-215, 1967.

Hays, P.: Modes of onset of psychotic depression, Brit Med J *2:*779-784, 1964.

Horwitz, W. A.: Physiologic responses as prognostic guides in the use of antidepressant drugs, Amer J Psychiat *125:*98-106, 1968.

Hudgens, R. W., Morrison, J. R., and Barcha, R. G.: Life events and onset of primary affective disorders: Study of 40 hospitalized patients and 40 controls, Arch Gen Psychiat (Chicago) *16:*134-145, 1967.

Jacobowsky, B.: Psychosomatic equivalents of endogenous depression, Acta Psychiat et Neur *37-39* (Suppl 160-167):253-260, 1961-1963.

Jacobson, J. E.: Hypomanic alert: Program designed for greater therapeutic control, Amer J Psychiat *122:*295-299, 1965.

Jansson, B.: Psychic insufficiencies associated with childbearing, Acta Psychiat Scand *39* (Suppl 172):156-168, 1963.

Kalinowsky, L. B., Hoch, P. H., and Grant, B.: Somatic Treatments in Psychiatry; Pharmacotherapy; Convulsive, Insulin, Surgical, Other Methods, New York: Grune, 1961.

Kay, D. W. K., *et al.:* Endogenous and neurotic syndromes of depression: Factor analytic study of 104 cases. Clinical features, Brit J Psychiat *115:*377-388, 1969a.

———: Endogenous and neurotic syndromes of depression: 5 to 7 year follow-up of 104 cases, Brit J Psychiat *115:*389-399, 1969b.

Kendell, R. E., and Gourlay, J.: Clinical distinction between psychotic and neurotic depressions, Brit J Psychiat *117:*257-266, 1970.

Kenin, L., and Blass, N. H.: Mental illness associated with the postpartum state, Clin Obstet Gynec *5:*716-728, 1962.

Kerr, T. A., Schapira, K., and Roth, M.: Relationship between premature death and affective disorders, Brit J Psychiat *115:* 1277-1282, 1969.

King, L. J., and Pittman, G. D.: Six-year follow-up study of 65 adolescent patients: Natural history of affective disorders in adolescence, Arch Gen Psychiat (Chicago)

22:230-236, 1970.

Kline, N. S.: Depression: Its diagnosis and treatment, *in* Modern Problems of Pharmacopsychiatry, vol. 3, Basel and New York: Karger, 1969, pp. 67-74.

Kuhn, R.: Veränderungen der Symptomatik und des Verlaufs der Psychosen durch Medikamente, Phänomenologie und Psychodynamik des Therapeutischen Vorganges, Proc III World Congr Psychiat *3:* 448-453, 1961.

Kupperman, H. S.: Menopausal woman and sex hormones, Med. Asp Hum Sex *1:* 64-68, 1967.

Lehmann, H. E.: Psychiatric concepts of depression: Nomenclature and classification, Canad Psychiat Ass J *4* (Spec Suppl): S1-S12, 1959.

Lipkin, K. M., Dyrud, J., and Meyer, G. G.: The many faces of mania: Therapeutic trial of lithium carbonate, Arch Gen Psychiat (Chicago) *22:*262-267, 1970.

Lundquist, G.: Prognosis and course in manic-depressive psychoses: Follow-up study of 319 first admissions, Acta Psychiat Neurol (Suppl 35):5-95, 1945.

Madden, J. L., *et al.:* Characteristics of postpartum mental illness, Amer J Psychiat *115:*18-24, 1958.

Main, T. F.: Mothers with children on a psychiatric unit, *in* Linn, L., ed.: Frontiers in General Hospital Psychiatry, New York: Internat Univ Press, 1961, pp. 150-166.

Majerus, P. W., *et al.:* Psychologic factors and psychiatric disease in hyperemesis gravidarum: Follow-up study of 69 vomiters and 66 controls, Amer J Psychiat *117:* 421-428, 1960.

Marcé, L. V.: Traité de la Folie des Femmes Enceintes des Nouvelles Accouchées et des Nouvices, Paris: J. B. Baillière et fils, 1858.

May, A. E., Urquhart, A., and Tarran, J.: Self-evaluation of depression in various diagnostic and therapeutic groups, Arch Gen Psychiat (Chicago) *21:*191-194, 1969.

Mayfield, D. G., and Coleman, L. L.: Alcohol use and affective disorder, Dis Nerv Syst *19:*467-474, 1968.

Mendels, J., and Hawkins, D. R.: Sleep and depression: A follow-up study, Arch Gen Psychiat (Chicago) *16:*536-542, 1967.

Neugarten, B. L., and Kraines, R. J.: "Menopausal symptoms" in women of various ages, Psychosom Med *27:*266-273, 1965.

Nilsson, A., Kaij, L., and Jacobson, L.: Postpartum mental disorder in an unselected sample: Psychiatric history, J Psychosom Res *10:*327-339, 1967.

Oltman, J. E., and Friedman, S.: Treatment of depressive states with Marplan, Amer J Psychiat 116:848-849, 1960.

———: Life cycles in patients with manic-depressive psychosis, Amer J Psychiat 119: 174-176, 1962.

———: Trends in postpartum illnesses, Amer J Psychiat 122:328-329, 1965.

Oswald, I., et al.: Melancholia and barbiturates: Controlled EEG, body and eye movement study of sleep, Brit J Psychiat 109:66-78, 1963.

Perris, C., ed.: A study of bipolar (manic-depressive) and unipolar recurrent depressive psychoses, Acta Psychiat Scand 42 (Suppl 194):1966.

Pittman, F. S., Langsley, D. G., and DeYoung, C. D.: School phobics may grow into work phobics, Amer J Psychiat 124: 1535-1540, 1968.

Pitts, F. N., Jr., and Winokur, G.: Affective disorder III: Diagnostic correlates and incidence of suicide, J Nerv Ment Dis 139:176-181, 1964.

Pleshette, N., Asch, S. S., and Chase, J.: Study of anxieties during pregnancy, labor, the early and late puerperium, Bull NY Acad Med 32:436-455, 1956.

Pollitt, J. D.: Suggestions for a physiological classification of depression, Brit J Psychiat 111:489-495, 1965.

Post, F.: The factor of aging in affective illness, in Coppen, A. and Walk, A., eds.: Recent Developments in Affective Disorders. A Symposium (Brit J Psychiat Special Publication No. 2), Ashford, Kent: Headley, 1968, pp. 105-116.

Protheroe, C.: Puerperal psychoses: Long term study 1927-1961, Brit J Psychiat 115: 9-30, 1969.

Pugh, T. F., et al.: Rates of mental disease related to childbearing, New Eng J Med 268:1224-1228, 1963.

Robin, A. A.: Psychological changes of normal parturition, Psychiat Quart 36:129-150, 1962.

Rosenthal, S. H.: Involutional depressive syndrome, Amer J Psychiat 124 (Suppl):21-35, 1968.

Roth, M.: Phobic anxiety-depersonalization syndrome and some general aetiological problems in psychiatry, J Neuropsychiat 1:293-306, 1960.

Rubins, J. L.: Holistic approach to the psychoses: Part I: Affective psychoses, Amer J Psychoanal 28:139-155, 1968.

Sargant, W.: Drugs in the treatment of depression, Brit Med J 1:225-227, 1961.

Saunders, E. B.: Association of psychoses with the puerperium, Amer J Psychiat 85: 669-680, 1929.

Schwab, J. J., et al.: Diagnosing depression in medical inpatients, Ann Intern Med 67:695-707, 1967.

Schwartz, D. A.: Review of the "paranoid" concept, Arch Gen Psychiat (Chicago) 8:349-361, 1963.

Silverman, C.: Epidemiology of depression—A review, Amer J Psychiat 124:883-891, 1968.

Sloane, R. B.: Depression: Diagnosis and clinical features, J Neuropsychiat 2 (Suppl):S11-S14, 1961.

Stafford-Clark, D.: Discussion in Proc Roy Soc Med 50:615-617, 1957.

Tabachnick, N.: Countertransference crisis in suicidal attempts, Arch Gen Psychiat (Chicago) 4:64-70, 1961.

Taylor, F. K.: Prokaletic measures derived from psychoanalytic technique, Brit J Psychiat 115:407-419, 1969.

Tetlow, C.: Psychoses of childbearing, Brit J Psychiat 101:629-639, 1955.

Thomas, C. L., and Gordon, J. E.: Psychosis after childbirth: Ecological aspects of a single impact stress, Amer J Med Sci 238:363-388, 1959.

Tobin, S. M.: Emotional depression during pregnancy, Science 143:677-681, 1964.

Toolan, J. M.: Suicide and suicidal attempts in children and adolescents, Amer J Psychiat 118:719-724, 1962.

Treadway, C. R., et al.: Psychoendocrine study of pregnancy and puerperium, Amer J Psychiat 125:1380-1386, 1969.

Wallach, S., and Henneman, P. H.: Prolonged estrogen therapy in postmenopausal women, JAMA 171:1637-1642, 1959.

Weiss, J. M. A., Chathan, L. R., and Schaie, K. W.: Symptom formation associated with aging: Dynamic pattern, Arch Gen Psychiat (Chicago) 4:22-29, 1961.

Welner, J., and Marstal, H. B.: Symptoms in mania: Analysis of 279 attacks of manic-depressive elation, Acta Psychiat Scand 40 (Suppl 180):175-176, 1964.

Wilson, R. A., and Wilson, T. A.: Fate of the nontreated postmenopausal woman: Plea for the maintenance of adequate estrogen from puberty to the grave, J Amer Geriat Soc 11:347-362, 1963.

Yalom, I. D., et al.: "Postpartum blues" syndrome, Arch Gen Psychiat (Chicago) 18:16-27, 1968.

Yarden, P. E., Max, D. M., and Eisenbach, Z.: Effect of childbirth on the prognosis of married schizophrenic women, Brit J Psychiat 112:491-499, 1966.

Zung, W. W. K., Wilson, W. P., and Dodson, W. E.: Effect of depressive disorders on sleep EEG responses, Arch Gen Psychiat (Chicago) 10:439-445, 1964.

CHAPTER

FIVE

Delusional and Paranoid Syndromes

Pᴇᴏᴘʟᴇ ᴜɴᴅᴇʀsᴛᴀɴᴅ ᴛʜᴇ ᴡᴏʀʟᴅ ᴀʀᴏᴜɴᴅ ᴛʜᴇᴍ in so wide a variety of ways that it becomes extremely difficult to distinguish between thinking that is delusional and thinking that merely does not conform to the majority view. Indeed, anyone who calls another's views delusional postulates implicitly that his own way of understanding the world represents objective fact. Such a premise begs so many philosophical questions (Matussek 1948, Mayer-Gross 1950), however, that the psychiatrist's only practical recourse is to ignore them entirely and persevere in the generally accepted, though disturbingly dogmatic, definition that a person has a delusion *when he adheres to a wrong or unreasonable idea from which no logic or experience can dissuade him.* As used in psychiatry, the term "delusional" is intended to convey that the patient's views diverge greatly from those generally accepted and to imply that the nature of the views or the tenacity with which they are held is based on a morbid process (Arthur 1964).

That most people consider certain ideas inaccurate does not mean that anyone who steadfastly clings to them is paranoid or deluded; if it did, Communists, Jehovah's Witnesses, or southern Republicans could be considered mentally ill. These labels need not even apply to the person who erroneously believes that he is being taken advantage of or is in some danger, for some people are merely unusually cautious and prefer to expect the worst. A woman who believes her husband's grandiose or persecutory ideas may be a participant in a *folie à deux* (Greenberg 1956, Lasegue 1877), but unless her belief disrupts her own social functioning or she persists in her views even after her husband is hospitalized, it is difficult to know whether she is mentally ill or only excessively loyal. In such a situation, the border between illness and erroneous ideas becomes even fuzzier, for a woman who becomes involved in a *folie à deux* is likely to be so isolated that she is not exposed to the natural corrective forces of consensual validation. How can it be determined whether her isolation is a result of her own or her husband's mental illness or whether her adherence to her husband's ideas is not simply her way of maintaining a precarious marital adjustment?

Delusional thinking occurs in so many illnesses that its presence alone is pathognomonic of none (Cameron 1959a, Katz 1964). It is seen in acute brain syndromes, acute undifferentiated or paranoid schizophrenia, manic episodes (Welner 1964), chronic brain syndromes, chronic alcoholism (Johanson 1964, Langfeldt 1961), and prolonged or severe depression. Yet, in each of these illnesses the delusional ideas have certain assessable *features*—their extent, constancy, content, affective coloration, associated symptoms, and consequences—that follow regular patterns. These patterns allow the clinician to assign to the syndrome a diagnostic label that is operationally valid, in the sense that it enables him to construct a treatment plan and to make some tentative predictions regarding the illness' course. We have chosen to discuss the delusional syndromes together in this section despite their disparate origins, because of *1/* the practical importance of distinguishing between delusional patterns, *2/* the dangers these illnesses have in common when the patient translates an inaccurate thought into action, and *3/* the similarity of the precautions required to avert such dangers.

CLASSIFICATION OF THE DELUSIONAL SYNDROMES

Three questions help to distinguish one delusional illness from another:

1/ Are the delusional ideas systematized?

2/ Does the patient show signs of intellectual impairment at the time of examination?

3/ Do the delusions reflect or imply a depressed mood? That is, are they self-derogatory or concerned with death or disabling illness? Does the patient believe he is being persecuted because of his evil ways?

Table 14 schematizes two extreme prototypes of delusional syndromes, the distinction being the degree to which the patients' delusions are systematized. Most syndromes lie somewhere between the two extremes; and to some extent the location of a particular syndrome on an imaginary continuum between them correlates with both its other symptoms and its clinical course and can suggest a

TABLE 14. *Typical Patterns Seen in Delusional Syndromes*

TYPE OF DELUSION	TYPE A NONSYSTEMATIZED	TYPE B SYSTEMATIZED
Nature of "evidence"	Massive number of clues unified by constantly changing explanations	Isolated and minute clues interpreted within a stable, complete system
Pervasiveness of delusions	Global, concerning all life areas	Restricted to well-delineated areas; usually concern interpersonal relationships
Confusion and disorientation	More frequent	Less frequent
Hallucinations	Frequent	Rare, almost never visual
Affect	Labile	Often depressive in early stages; occasionally remains so
Retardation	Rare	More frequent
Anxiety	Ubiquitous	Variable
Agitation	Frequent	Occasional
Sleep disorder	DFA at beginning; usually develops into total insomnia	Variable; SCD and EMA in early stages; may develop into total insomnia but when illness is prolonged sleep may also become normal again
Age of onset	Younger	Older
Onset and progression of illness	Faster	Slower
Illnesses in which seen	Acute brain syndromes Acute schizophrenic episodes Manic episodes Chronic brain syndromes (when severe)	Chronic paranoid schizophrenia Prolonged depressions Chronic brain syndromes (when intellectual impairment is mild) Paranoid personality disorders
Social functioning	Grossly disturbed	Sometimes relatively intact

treatment program. We have labeled as Type A those delusional ideas that are nonsystematized, in the sense that their character, object, and content are constantly changing; and as Type B those delusional ideas that are parts of a complex, stable system of misunderstanding and misinterpretation.

Type A delusions usually *pervade all areas* of the patient's thinking; they are most frequent in *younger* persons and in those suffering from illnesses of relatively *acute onset* (Nathan 1964). Patients with this kind of delusion tend to be *confused* or disoriented, especially in regard to time sequences; occasionally, the confusion extends to the patient's own identity and to that of those around him; in rare instances, he is not even aware of where he is. Such individuals tend also to be *anxious* and agitated and to have a rapidly progressing sleep disorder, usually difficulty in falling asleep (DFA). Clinical pictures of this kind can be seen in acute brain syndromes, acute schizophrenic and manic episodes, and far-advanced chronic brain syndromes. They are generally responsive to phenothiazines and reserpine.

Type B delusions are often *circumscribed,* in the sense that they relate only to a particular area of the patient's life; they are more frequent in *older* persons and in illnesses of relatively *slow onset.* Patients showing Type B delusions tend to be fairly *lucid* and well-oriented and to have a slowly developing sleep disorder, often early morning awakening (EMA). Although they usually perceive the events around them in a factually correct manner, they nevertheless have erroneous ideas about the meaning of their perceptions and the intentions of those around them. (Cameron 1959b). The clues on which they base their delusional network are generally minute and would appear insignificant to most other people. Characteristically, when these patients see a physician, they spend more time and energy in trying to prove that the evidence they believe they have found is authentic and valid than they do in outlining their delusional system or discussing its probable meaning and consequences. Type B delusions are more commonly seen in mild chronic brain syndromes, chronic paranoid schizophrenias, paranoid personality disorders, and severe or protracted depressive syndromes. Phenothiazines usually diminish the pressure of the delusions without affecting their content and may compound the patient's retardation and depressive ideation. In many cases, the patient's delusional ideas start to recede only after treatment with phenothiazines is supplemented with antidepressants or ECT.

In the paranoid syndromes showing Type A delusions, the patient feels exposed to so many stimuli and is so puzzled by the events of his life that he can understand his experiences only by constantly constructing new delusional ideas or rearranging old ones; as a result, his delusions are *unsystematized.* The patient with Type B delusions finds minute clues—a single dish out of place, a missing car key—and uses them to substantiate an extensive and *systematized* confabulation of intention and meaning.

DETERMINANTS OF THE CONTENT

It is not always clear why a patient has a particular kind of delusion or why, if he falls ill again after many symptom-free years, the delusions tend to be similar or even identical. Social factors seem to play some role: sexual delusions are more common in women than in men, and delusions of grandeur are more common in patients with an upper- rather than lower-class background (Sarvis 1962). A partial explanation for the content of the paranoid patient's delusions may lie in the process of *projection,* the individual's tendency to perceive the moods and motives of others in terms of his own. The wife who is concerned that her husband finds her old and unattractive and that he might thus have good reason to prefer another woman may erroneously start to see his statements and actions as a confirmation of her fears. The extent to which the patient's delusions reflect real life problems or psychological issues of long standing does not appear to be determined only by the nature of such problems and concerns; it is related also to the speed with which the illness develops and the psychobiologic integrity of the affected person. Delusions that develop slowly can use the patient's real life experiences as building blocks, so that the more slowly the illness develops, the easier it is for the patient to fit his experiences into his system, and the harder it is to determine that his ideas are inaccurate. Delusions that arise during an extended course of depression, therefore, tend to maintain a relatively stable theme and to sound plausible to the patient's environment; indeed, they may continue to seem plausible to the patient even after he remits. As a result, even after he abandons the idea that he *is* being followed or that his phone *is* being tapped, he may continue to believe that he *was* being followed or that his phone *was* being tapped; in short, he concludes that his suspicions were accurate in the past, but for the present his persecutors have stopped tormenting him. In the course of an acute schizophrenic episode, on the other hand, the patient's bizarre experiences develop so quickly that his explanations for them are patently absurd to others and, once he remits, even to himself.

SIMILARITY TO SYMPTOMS OF OTHER ILLNESSES

The differential diagnosis of the Type A delusions has been discussed in Chapter 3. In some ways, the Type B delusion is akin to the *confabulation* typically seen in chronic organic brain syndromes in that the delusion represents the individual's effort to make sense out of a perceptually disturbed world and to deny the inexplicability of his experiences, while the confabulation seeks to make sense of a world disturbed by memory loss and to deny this loss. Confabulations, however, are given a special coloration by the dysmnesic elements, so that errors occur, first in the realm of time, and later in terms of place and person. Distortions of meaning and intention, when they occur, are usually fleeting and secondary.

The similarities between the delusional ideas of Type B syndromes and the confabulations of organic illnesses are highlighted by the phenomenon called *anosognosia* (Babinski 1914, Weinstein 1955). That this inability or refusal to acknowledge some obvious sensory or motor impairment (sometimes called the "denial of illness") has an organic and not solely an adaptive basis is suggested by its almost exclusive occurrence in patients with lesions of the CNS. Anyone who has tried to persuade an anosognosic hemiplegic that his arm is paralyzed and has heard the patient tenaciously cling to the explanation that he is merely keeping it still in order not to disturb the bedclothes, or that the limb held limp before him is not his own, is reminded both of the senile patient's confabulations and of the complex rationalizations, explanations, and outright prevarications offered by the paranoid patient defending his view that he is being pursued by criminals disguised in masks and wigs.

The tenacity of the Type B delusion lends it the character of the *obsessional idea*. The close relationship between the two is suggested in clinical experience: during the remission of a paranoid illness or in the initial stage of a relapse, many patients report that they are unable to stop thinking about bizarre topics. For example, a man who reports having been convinced for over a year that his wife is having an affair with their parish priest may relinquish his ideas after being treated, declare them erroneous, and feel embarrassed about having harbored them. If after being free of symptoms for several months, his medications are reduced, but his initial disorder is not yet relieved, he may report that he is once more ruminating about his wife's feelings toward their priest. It is particularly interesting that during the initial stage of the relapse patients often continue to consider ideas of this kind irrelevant and erroneous, yet complain of being unable to stop thinking about them, for it demonstrates how obsessional thoughts can be precursors of delusional ideas.

It is sometimes hard to determine whether a patient has a systematized delusion with depressive content or a *chronically depressed self-image* (Retterstöl 1966). The distinction between the two rests largely on the extent to which the patient's view of himself diverges from the judgment of those around him. Thus, a woman who throughout much of her life has erroneously viewed herself as unintelligent, inadequate, and unattractive, and feels that this accounts for her being snubbed by her acquaintances, differs only quantitatively from a woman who considers herself wicked and feels that this has prompted foreign agents to pursue her. In the first instance, the woman's cognitive functioning remains relatively intact with the result that she can so skillfully and understandably incorporate her view of herself into her interpretation of everything that happens to her that her position becomes unassailable by logic or experience, and even her friends and acquaintances may come to accept her severe judgment of herself. This is less true in the second instance, for the ideas are so full of logical flaws and absurdities that her acquaintances are unable to accept them. Her illness thus becomes obvious more quickly, and she is referred for treatment at an earlier and perhaps more easily reversible stage.

The distinction between the Type B delusional syndrome and the protracted depression is made even more difficult because the two often coexist (Schaeffer 1970). Type B delusions, moreover, occur more frequently in patients whose self-image has long been depressed, particularly when they have been isolated (Kretschmer 1950). The same cause-and-effect questions obtain for the observation that paranoid patients have a higher than average incidence of divorce in their histories. Does the paranoia stem from the isolation induced by divorce, or is their propensity to divorce caused by their suspiciousness or morbid jealousy (Langfeldt 1961, Rimon 1964)? Marriage counselors often see couples of whom one member is, and has long been, so irritable, demanding, and subclinically paranoid that the other wants to separate. In many cases, offering the querulant partner the same treatment (including medications) that he would receive if he had a more florid paranoid syndrome can diminish his irritability and suspiciousness to the extent that the spouse becomes more satisfied and the marriage remains intact. The frequency with which such situations arise underlines the importance of considering this diagnostic possibility in evaluating what seems like a garden-variety marital conflict and of ensuring that marriage counselors have available to them the collaboration of an experienced clinician (Dupont 1968).

TREATMENT

The indications for treatment are fairly clear-cut in illnesses that demonstrate the unsystematized delusions described as *Type A:* the symptoms are so pervasive and bizarre and so rapidly and completely disrupt the person's social and occupational functioning that it is not difficult to determine that he needs treatment and, in most cases, hospitalization. The slow, insidious onset of the *Type B* paranoid disturbances may not, however, permit such easy judgments. When, for example, a mild to moderate depression is in progress, it may be some time before delusional thinking becomes apparent. At the beginning, the patient may seem somewhat snappish, ask himself or others more questions than he usually does, or make a few self-derogatory comments. Gradually, the questions and accusations become more and more systematized, until he exhibits frankly paranoid delusions of persecution or jealousy. By the time the illness is full-blown, the delusions, suspiciousness, agitation, and hostility may be so prominent that they eclipse the patient's disturbed mood. In such situations, the delusional ideas are often limited to certain aspects of the patient's life—his marriage or a neighbor—and leave enough areas of his life intact that his social and occupational functioning diminishes little until later on.

Even the patient who appears relatively lucid may need treatment urgently, as delusions often lead to embarrassing or dangerous behavior. Paranoid patients are arrested by the police ten times as often as other mental patients (Rappeport 1965). They are particularly dangerous to the objects of their delusions (Shepherd 1961) and, since one patient in five attempts suicide (Johanson 1964), to themselves as well. Their lack of insight usually leads them to reject treatment or, having consented to see a doctor, to stop coming after a few meetings. For these reasons, it is important to observe closely any patient whose history or presentation suggests that he has been or may become violent or who has delusional ideas that, if true, would lead even a normal person to behave destructively. If his environment cannot cope with his behavior or there is doubt about his remaining in treatment, the patient should be hospitalized.

SOMATIC TREATMENT

In general, the somatic treatment of Type A delusional illness parallels that outlined for schizophrenic disorders (see p. 127), while that of Type B paranoid syndromes parallels the management recommended for depressive syndromes (see p. 172). Since it is often hard to distinguish between the two types (Shepherd 1961), and since the first order of business is to diminish the pressure of delusional material, patients of either type should initially be given phenothiazines. After 10 to 20 days on a phenothiazine such as perphenazine (Trilafon), 32-64 mg per day, Type A delusions generally recede markedly or disappear, while those of Type B persist without alteration in content but with greatly diminished urgency. The patient with a Type B syndrome may be considered ready for antidepressant medication when he no longer uses every conference to prove to the physician the great significance of the hair he found on an old suit, or when, as a manifestation of the "rollback" phenomenon (see p. 53), there is a reemergence of the sadness that was overshadowed by his hostility or the early morning awakening (EMA) that was overshadowed by total insomnia.

If the patient's delusions do not remit and his behavior remains unchanged despite prolonged pharmacologic and psychotherapeutic attempts, ECT may be helpful. While some patients are freed of their delusional ideas permanently after ECT, others show only temporary or partial improvement. As soon as ECT's amnesic effect (which can initially cause them to become so forgetful that they cannot even recall their delusions) wears off and their memory improves, they may either reexperience the same delusions or (as is equally true of patients given medications) merely stop experiencing their persecution as ongoing but recall and believe in the delusions they experienced in the past. Maintenance electroshock therapy, in which the patient is given one treatment every one to four weeks, may be helpful in chronically relapsing conditions, and regressive electroshock therapy, in which two to four treatments are given daily for a number of weeks (see p. 650), may be warranted in desperate, long-term illnesses. The effectiveness of these measures is, however, quite variable.

When the patient's delusional syndrome takes place in the context of an organic disease, somatic treatment should be postponed, if possible, until the organic condition is investigated and treated. The treatment may also need to be modified, as delusions occurring in a patient with an organic brain syndrome often respond to doses of medications far lower than those recommended above and, whether Type A or Type B, do not usually require the addition of an antidepressant (see Chap. 11).

PSYCHOTHERAPY

The psychotherapeutic and environmental management of the nonsystematized Type A delusional illnesses is described in the section on deliriform syndromes (see p. 416) and schizophrenic disorders (see p. 125). In this section, we will concentrate on the management of the systematized Type B delusional illnesses, like paranoid schizophrenia and paranoid depressions.

Establishing a psychotherapeutic relationship with the "healthy part of the patient" was in the past a tedious, time-consuming, frustrating, and usually unsuccessful endeavor. Today it is greatly facilitated by somatic therapies. What makes this effort so difficult, and so important, is that the patient who develops a paranoid syndrome has become socially isolated because he purposely withdraws from social transactions and behaves so strangely that he is ostracized (Bullard 1960). Furthermore, many patients who develop delusional symptoms are isolated at the time they fall ill, and their isolation may have long antedated their illness (Cameron 1959a, Shepherd 1961). Because this isolation can compound the disorder by making it impossible for the patient to use his friends and family for reality testing in the way that nonparanoid individuals can, resocialization techniques, such as group and family therapies, may be the only avenues to adaptation and reality.

While patients with Type A delusional syndromes should be excluded from group treatment programs until their most acute symptoms subside (see p. 129), those with Type B delusional syndromes may fare best when group therapy is the first psychological treatment offered. Groups often seem to know just when the patient's delusional ideas can be questioned without making him try harder to prove them and can influence him to take some distance from such ideas. If, as commonly happens, the patient's delusional system involves the behavior of his family, or if his family has had difficulty in distinguishing what the patient imagines from what has really occurred (as in the *folie à deux* or *folie à famille*), family treatment should be added. It is also important that difficulties the patient may have had with his family during or as a result of the illness be discussed and resolved before he leaves the hospital, as he will need their help and support in remaining socially active, continuing with his treatment, and thereby avoiding new difficulties (Greenspan 1961). Since family meetings initiated too early in the course of treatment can lead to further disaffection, accusations, and ultimatums, it is best to postpone them until they are likely to proceed more smoothly. In determining the right time for such meetings, it is helpful to observe the patient's behavior in his therapy group: when he can tolerate the comments of those in the group and has become responsive to them, he is probably ready to tolerate family meetings.

Therapists sometimes engage in major contortions to avoid stimulating paranoid feelings toward themselves. In order to foster the patient's confidence and to promote his trust, they may avoid all contact with his relatives, neither gathering data from them nor informing them about the patient's course. The patient may find such behavior unusual, however, and become more rather than less suspicious of the therapist's motives. In the few situations we have seen where coincidences occurred that could have supplied a patient with entirely plausible evidence for his delusional system, we have found that he did not incorporate such data into it. Oddly enough, it is often sufficient simply to tell the patient at the time of the first meeting that he may in the future want to involve the doctor in his delusions, but should resist doing so. Since discussion of any kind instead of lessening tends to strengthen delusional ideas, it is not helpful to humor the patient by pretending to believe them. Indeed, after the initial interview, it is wisest to express no further interest in the delusions and even actively to discourage the patient from discussing them. In some cases, it is possible to increase the patient's distance from his delusions by showing him that he becomes even more delusional when confronted with painful issues or exposed to some other form of stress.

As the patient starts to develop a relationship with the therapist, he may want to discuss the possibility that his delusions are true and may even ask the doctor to join him in "fully investigating" the bizarre ideas. When this occurs, he should be told that his insistence on holding such discussions, despite knowing his doctor's view about them, indicates that his illness is continuing and that he is not yet ready to tolerate any liberalization of his privileges. While discouragement of this kind can be criticized on the grounds that it teaches the patient to conceal, rather than abandon, his ideas and thereby causes him to be released from supervision prematurely, we have found that individuals released from the hospital rarely discuss or act on delusions that they were persuaded to keep to themselves during confinement. Further, we have found no evidence that this form of discouragement promotes evasiveness in patients who would otherwise speak more frankly. Indeed, the opposite seems to be far more common: successful dissimulation is possible only after the pressure of delusional material has diminished and is often the first step toward recovery. At this time, it usually becomes possible to engage the patient in discussions of his life situation that rapidly become far more interesting to him than his futile and constantly discouraged attempts to discuss and document bizarre ideas. Indeed, the patient's interest and participation in realistic discussions strongly suggest that his delusions are in fact diminishing and that his recovery is proceeding.

OUTCOME OF DELUSIONAL SYNDROMES

Unless the patient is suffering from a severe and irreversible organic brain syndrome, Type A delusional syndromes usually subside within a few weeks or, at most, a few months. Those of Type B, on the other hand, may continue for months or years and, in some cases, do not remit at all. There are four possible outcomes:

1/ The patient's delusional thinking persists and continues to determine his social behavior.

2/ The patient remains actively delusional but, having begun to appreciate the social consequences of voicing or acting on his delusions, keeps them to himself. (He may believe that so many people are involved in whatever plot he fears that it is wisest to say nothing and to pretend ignorance.)

3/ The patient stops interpreting his current experiences in a delusional manner, but continues to believe that his previous interpretations were correct. (If he has experienced delusions of persecution, he may come to believe that his former tormentors have desisted and is usually prepared to let "bygones be bygones.")

4/ The patient no longer has any delusions, understands that his former ideas were erroneous, and is aware that he has been ill.

These outcomes, which usually occur in the above sequence and are reflected in increasing social competence, may also be considered stages of recovery. While most patients show at least some degree of improvement, many remain at one of the intermediate stages for some time, sometimes partly believing, partly doubting, and partly ignoring their current and past ideas (Retterstöl 1967). Even those who appear fully recovered from their illness may exhibit brief lapses in reality testing under pressure. Relapses can also occur after decades of freedom from symptoms. It is remarkable how often the symptoms are similar to those of an earlier episode. Patients who previously showed paranoid jealousy may make identical accusations toward their husbands or wives, even when in the interim they have remarried; patients with the genealogic delusion of being highborn may seek to claim identical hereditary rights as before; those who believed certain organizations were pursuing them may name the same organizations, even when they no longer exist.

A knowledge of the usual temporal sequence of remission is helpful in determining the optimal dosage of medication and the duration of treatment. Whenever a patient has remained for an extended period at a given but not final stage of amelioration, his medications should be increased. When, despite increases, the patient's symptoms remain at a plateau for 12 to 24 months, the medication may be gradually lowered until his symptoms once more become worse. A patient who believes that he is no longer being persecuted but that he was being pursued in the past should receive more medication, but if he does not improve further after receiving the increased dosage for 12 months, it should be gradually reduced until he is taking no drugs at all, provided that such withdrawal does not lead to the exacerbation of symptoms. When paranoid symptoms return after the drug dosage is lowered or discontinued, the patient's medicines should once more be increased, and a prolonged or possibly even permanent program of drug administration may be indicated. The extent to which the patient collaborates in such medication adjustments is limited by the nature of his disease, however: paranoid patients are known to discontinue their drugs more readily than other patients, a tendency that considerably limits the frequency of good long-term outcomes, which may well depend on protracted drug treatment (Mooney 1965, Wilson 1967).

REFERENCES

Arthur, A. Z.: Theories and explanations of delusions: A review, Amer J Psychiat *121*:105-115, 1964.

Babinski, J.: Contribution à l'étude des troubles mentaux dans l'hémiplégie organique cérébrale (anosognosie), Rev Neurol *27*:845-847, 1914.

Bullard, D. M.: Psychotherapy of paranoid patients, Arch Gen Psychiat (Chicago) *2*:137-141, 1960.

Cameron, N.: Paranoid conditions and paranoia, in Arieti, S., ed.: American Handbook of Psychiatry, New York: Basic, 1959a, pp. 508-539.

———: The paranoid pseudo-community revisited, Amer J Sociol *65*:52-58, 1959b.

Dupont, R. L., and Grunebaum, H.: Willing victims: Husbands of paranoid women, Amer J Psychiat *125*:151-159, 1968.

Greenberg, H. P.: Crime and folie à deux: Review and case history, J Ment Sci *102*:772-779, '956.

Greenspan, J., and Myers, J. M., Jr.: A review of the theoretical concepts of paranoid delusions with special reference to women, Penn Psychiat Quart *4*:11-28, 1961.

Johanson, E.: Mild paranoia: Description and analysis of fifty-two in-patients from an open department for mental diseases, Acta Psychiat Scand *40* (Suppl 177):5-100, 1964.

Katz, M. M., Cole, J. O., and Lowery, H. A.: Non-specificity of diagnosis of paranoid schizophrenia, Arch Gen Psychiat (Chicago) *11*:197-202, 1964.

Kretschmer, E.: Der sensitive Beziehungswahn, ed 3, Berlin: Springer, 1950.

Langfeldt, G.: Erotic jealousy syndrome, Acta Psychiat Scand *36* (Suppl 151):7-68, 1961.

Lasègue, C., and Falret, J.: La Folie À Deux, Ou Folie Communigueé, Annales Medico-Psychologiques, t.XVIII, 1877 (translated by Michaud, R., in Amer J Psychiat *121* (Suppl):1-23, 1964.

Matussek, P.: Psychotisches und nicht-psychotisches Bedeutungsbewusststein, Nervenarzt *19*:372-380, 1948.

Mayer-Gross, W.: Psychopathology of delusions, Congrès International de Psychiatrie I, Tome I. Paris, 1950, pps. 59-87.

Mooney, H. B.: Pathologic jealousy and psychochemotherapy, Brit J Psychiat *111*:1023-1042, 1965.

Nathan, R. J.: Age of patient and diagnosis of schizophrenia, Arch Gen Psychiat (Chicago) *11*:185-191, 1964.

Rappeport, J. R., and Lassen, G.: Dangerousness—arrest rate comparisons of discharged patients and the general population, Amer J Psychiat *121*:776-783, 1965.

Retterstöl, N.: Paranoid and Paranoiac Psychoses, Springfield (Ill): Thomas, 1966.

———: Jealousy-paranoiac psychoses: Personal follow-up study, Acta Psychiat Scand *43*:75-107, 1967.

———: Paranoid psychoses associated with unpatriotic conduct during World War II, Acta Psychiat Scand *44*:261-279, 1968.

Rimón, R., Stenbäck, A., and Achté, K.: A sociopsychiatric study of paranoid psychoses, Acta Psychiat Scand *40* (Suppl 180): 335-347, 1964.

Sarvis, M. A.: Paranoid reactions: Perceptual distortion as an etiological agent, Arch Gen Psychiat (Chicago) *6*:157-162, 1962.

Schaeffer, D. L.: Patterns of premorbid and symptom behaviors in schizophrenic and depressed women, J Nerv Ment Dis *150*:449-465, 1970.

Shepherd, M.: Morbid jealousy: Some clinical and social aspects of a psychiatric symptom, Brit J Psychiat *107*:687-753, 1961.

Weinstein, E. A., and Kahn, R. L.: Denial of illness: Symbolic and physiological aspects, Springfield (Ill): Thomas, 1955.

Welner, J., and Marstal, H. B.: Symptoms in mania: An analysis of 279 attacks of manic-depressive elation, Acta Psychiat Scand *40* (Suppl 180):175-176, 1964.

Wilson, J. D., and Enoch, M. D.: Estimation of drug rejection by schizophrenic in-patients, with analysis of clinical factors, Brit J Psychiat *113*:209-211, 1967.

CHAPTER

SIX

Neurotic Disorders

TRADITIONAL VIEWS OF THE NEUROTIC DISORDERS

IN EVERYDAY LANGUAGE, the word *neurotic* is used so widely that it has lost all but a pejorative meaning. It is used to refer to people who misbehave, act stupidly, or obtain pleasure in unusual ways; to those who are lazy, unmotivated, or unwilling to acknowledge their inadequacies; and to those who ignore their environment's demands or their own needs. Physicians sometimes use the term "neurotic" interchangeably with the term "functional" to describe somatic complaints for which they can find no organic basis. In strict psychiatric usage, however, the term has a far narrower application and denotes only a particular group of syndromes, which are further categorized according to their most striking symptom as anxiety neuroses, conversion neuroses, dissociative, phobic, obsessive, compulsive, depressive, neurasthenic, depersonalization, or hypochondriacal neuroses. These syndromes are traditionally grouped together because it is believed that

 1/ they can be distinguished from psychotic disorders by virtue of being milder, less disabling, and less likely to be associated with cognitive disturbances;

 2/ they are psychogenic and devoid of organic causation;

 3/ the symptoms derive from the patient's anxiety and the way he handles it, the primary difference between one neurotic illness and another being that the anxiety is handled differently; and

 4/ psychotherapy is the only effective treatment for them.

Unfortunately, none of these views has survived the test of time. The borderline between "neurosis" and "psychosis" is fluid; cognitive disturbances are ubiquitous in psychiatric disorders (Beck 1963, Salzman 1966); and the severity of the incapacitation does not necessarily distinguish the two. Patients with neurotic syndromes can be just as uncomfortable and crippled in their social, familial, and occupational functioning as those called psychotic. That neurotic patients often relate their symptoms to conflicts, events, and attitudes of an earlier time has been taken to mean that these disorders are psychogenic, but patients with clearly defined medical illnesses such as cancer or multiple sclerosis are equally liable to offer psychological interpretations of their symptoms. Nor should the neurotic patient's propensity to concentrate on past events be seen as evidence of psychological causation, for old memories can be stirred up by all kinds of events, ranging from lesions of the temporal lobe to depressions or hearing a familiar tune. For most people, explaining the present in terms of the past is preferable to not being able to explain it at all, and especially likely to occur in the psychiatric setting where for theoretical reasons this kind of thinking is encouraged. Moreover, neurotic symptoms are not restricted to patients with neurotic illnesses and indeed are fairly common in the general population (Agras 1969, Bailey 1928, McCall 1969, Roth 1959, Schilder 1938).

There is equally little evidence for the view that neuroses represent efforts to defend against anxiety (Lader 1968), for they are not only ineffective in this regard but, if the patient's account is to be believed, tend to frighten and upset him. Relieving such symptoms, regardless of means, moreover, usually makes the patient feel better and does not lead to substitute symptoms (Eiduson 1968). Finally, it is impossible to demonstrate that neurotic symptoms result from life conflicts or unusual stresses, or that psychotherapy improves the immediate or the long-term outcome (Giel 1964).

Because neuroses are assumed to be caused, at least in part, by some form of intrapsychic conflict and because individuals who have such disorders are sometimes hard to get along with, the distinction between *neurosis* and *personality disorder* has become so blurred that the first is sometimes called "symptom neurosis" and the second "character neurosis." There are, however, good reasons to uphold a distinction: it is true, to be sure, that individuals with a propensity to acute anxiety attacks are often insecure, even when they are not acutely anxious; that those who develop phobias may always have been inordinately concerned about new experiences; that patients with conversion symptoms are often histrionic in other areas of their lives; and that patients with an obsessive-compulsive neurosis are often exact and meticulous. But it is equally possible that an individual whose personality was previously unremarkable can also—sometimes quite suddenly—develop neurotic symptoms that are completely incongruent with his premorbid personality (Kanner 1957).

CLASSIFICATION OF NEUROTIC DISORDERS

Although classifying neurotic disorders according to their most prominent symptom facilitates statistical manipulation, it does not provide a clear picture of the individual patient, who is usually suffering from a combination of rapidly fluctuating symptoms and is apprehensive and upset about his condition as well. Our discussion of neurotic disorders, nevertheless, will follow the traditional diagnostic system, with the exception that we have included depressive neuroses in Chapter 4, where all disorders marked by depressed or elated mood are discussed together in the hope of clarifying certain differential diagnostic issues. Discussing neurotic and affective disorders separately does not mean to imply that the two are mutually exclusive. On the contrary, many neurotic syndromes have so much in common with depressions that they may be viewed as "depressive equivalents." Like depressions, many neurotic disorders relapse repeatedly and are associated with changes in sleep patterns and appetite, especially early morning awakening (EMA), hypersomnia, and anorexia; diminished sexual interest; a family history of depression, a good response to antidepressants (Cole 1964, Goldman 1962, Haddock 1965, Jakab 1960, Klein 1964, Sargant 1961); and subsequent depressive episodes. Such similarities are most striking in phobic and obsessive neuroses (Kessell 1968, Marks 1970, Noreik 1970, Terhune 1949), but can also be seen in other neurotic syndromes, particularly in patients over 30.

CLINICAL FEATURES AND COURSE OF NEUROTIC DISORDERS

ANXIETY NEUROSES

When people speak of *anxiety*, they refer not only to a normal spring of human motivation, a mental symptom, or a cause of mental symptoms, but also to the discomfort that arises at times of danger, the signal that precedes it, or a morbid discomfort that can occur even when there is no impending danger at all. Difficult as the term may be to define (Cattell 1958, Rioch 1956), the experience is fairly easy to describe. Everyone who has been in a situation of danger and uncertainty will have had the quite normal response of fearfulness, sweating, dry mouth, fast heartbeat, pounding in the chest, diarrhea, restlessness, muscle tension, breathlessness, hyperventilation, trembling, giddiness, tightness in the chest, and butterflies in the stomach. As the experience is universal, it can be considered *morbid* only when the symptoms are excessive, continue long after the danger is past, arise when there is no manifest danger, or interfere with the individual's pursuit of his normal life. Although such episodes may occur in a variety of organic syndromes (see Table 4) and as a precursor of most psychiatric illnesses, we will comment only on those anxiety states in which, even after some time, no other symptoms emerge so that the anxiety may be considered independent of any other condition.

A distinction is often made between *acute* and *chronic* anxiety neuroses. Patients usually describe the former in terms of its somatic signs, their free-floating anxiety, and their puzzling sense of impending doom. These symptoms can last from less than a minute to an hour or more; once they subside, the patient usually feels weak and exhausted. Episodes of acute neurotic anxiety occur rarely in persons who are generally symptom-free and in no way unusually fearful or sensitive to stress, maintain a well-integrated personality, and demonstrate good social functioning. More commonly, the patient has always been fairly anxious, and the acute episodes are merely punctuation marks in a long course of low-level anxiety. Patients with a propensity for acute attacks of anxiety also tend to show a persistent, nonprogressive difficulty in falling and remaining asleep (DFA and SCD) (Winokur 1963); their sleep loss does not generally exceed one or two hours a night, however. Nightmares from which the patient awakens in fright are common, especially around the time of acute attacks.

It is important to ascertain whether the anxiety that a given individual experiences is a normal stress response, symptomatic of an anxiety neurosis, or symptomatic of or prodromal to some other disease. However, this distinction can be as difficult as drawing the line between morbid depression and sadness, for, whatever its cause, the anxiety itself looks and feels much the same (Chapman 1966, Garmany 1955, Hays 1964). One of the few distinguishing features of the anxiety attack that is symptomatic of an anxiety neurosis is that the patient rarely attributes the attack to a precipitating event and almost never tries to explain or interpret his symptoms. Even if he does report some ostensibly significant event, it usually bears no temporal relationship to the onset of symptoms. Another distinguishing feature of neurotic anxiety is that it tends to fluctuate in intensity, while the anxiety that portends schizophrenic decompensation is incessant, and the patient's sleep, cognition, and social functioning become manifestly disturbed within days. The anxiety that precedes a depressive syndrome may fluctuate for a few days or weeks, but is then augmented or replaced by more obvious symptoms of depression like retardation, tearfulness, anorexia, EMA, and despair.

Individuals who are chronically fearful and oversensitive are said to have a *chronic anxiety neurosis*. Dreading acute anxiety attacks, such patients often take exaggerated steps to "protect" themselves, refusing to leave the house or engage in social situations they consider too strenuous. Such measures are almost invariably unsuccessful, and result only in a further disruption of the patient's relationships to his friends and family. Even those who do not have acute anxiety attacks tend to respond to stress in a demonstrably disproportionate way. In most cases, the patient also shows a lack of self-confidence and other features commonly found in depression and has difficulty in concentrating, making decisions, and—at least while he is under stress—maintaining precision in his occupational tasks (Cattell 1958, Winokur 1963).

HYSTERICAL NEUROSES

These neuroses were for a time the last tenacious citizens of that proud, ancient, and once overpopulated diagnostic province known as *hysteria*. In former days, it was a melting pot not only for its current residents but also for such incongruous bedfellows as depersonalization neurotics, individuals with unrecognized atypical seizure disorders, narcoleptics, somnambulists, inadequate psychopaths, malingerers, the emotionally labile and immature, and—last but by no means least—that large group of individuals whose major problem is their flair for the dramatic. Those who loved this colorful land and appreciated the hospitality it extended to any patient unwilling to settle elsewhere were saddened by the gradual emigration of most of its inhabitants and, vowing revenge on the plague of reason that had decimated the land, succeeded (in DSM-II) in forcibly repatriating the *"hysterical personalities,"* offering only the insignificant compromise that they could also be considered *"histrionic."* Such loyalty to this almost deserted province was understandable, for, as Miller (1960) has said, "history records the hysteric as the best friend any theoretician ever had." As evil spirits, wandering organs, split consciousness, repressed conflicts, and transference of feelings were postulated and exorcised by the healers and in turn gratefully confirmed by the sufferers, it became clear how useful it was to place under one diagnostic roof any syndrome in which the patient's suggestibility and gullibility were both high and contagious.

What is most striking about all these syndromes is their effect on the observer, especially one who is called on for help. Confident that he understands, better than any other, what is wrong and will be able to provide the necessary relief, the treatment ceremony traditionally begins with the healer's showing great enthusiasm about both the individual patient and the syndrome at large. More often than not, however, the elation rapidly gives way to disappointment and finally to mutual recrimination. The parallel between this kind of doctor-patient relationship and that of lovers has not been lost on observers, and because such patients are also suggestible and occasionally provocative, they have often been thought to eroticize their life relationships, particularly those with physicians.

The disappointment that follows the initial enthusiasm is caused by numerous factors. That the patient's intellectual functioning is grossly intact makes it increasingly difficult for the doctor to empathize with the patient's bland affect and inattentiveness to certain life events, which, together, are labeled *la belle indifférence* and thought to be pathognomonic of these syndromes. In addition, since these symptoms are often indistinguishable from outright fraudulent manipulations of the environment used to obtain special privileges or "secondary gains," the doctor may gradually come to feel that he is being put on and taken in. In many ways, the doctor's disenchantment with both patient and syndrome is similar to the response of persons who become interested in hypnotic phenomena, which are similar to the hysterical ones, in that they too are characterized by selective inattention, constriction of consciousness, easy suggestibility, and heightened eroticization of the relationship.

To avoid the overinclusiveness of the past, the use of the term *hysterical neurosis* is currently restricted to individuals who show varying degrees of selective inattention to particular elements of their internal or external environment, as manifested by conversion symptoms and such symptoms of dissociation as fugue states, amnesia, and multiple personality. That the term *conversion* was originally meant to imply that the patient had converted an unconscious conflict into a symptom has covered the syndrome with an unassailable etiologic cloak that, far from clothing it, has denuded it of any phenomenologic significance. To understand the way the term conversion is used currently, it must be recognized that symptoms that are

a/ *dissimulable* (in the sense that a patient could pretend to have them even when he does not) and

b/ *cryptogenic* (in the sense that thorough examination of the patient provides no evidence of disease or disorder that would explain their occurrence)

may be viewed as evidence of

1/ some as yet undiagnosed disease,
2/ malingering,
3/ hypochondriasis, or
4/ conversion neurosis.

The last of these diagnoses is particularly likely if

1/ the symptoms entail a *loss or disorder of function;*
2/ the symptoms are *illogical,* by which is meant that

a/ they *make no anatomic, physiologic, or medical sense,* as when the patient describes a hemianesthesia that ends precisely at the midline or cites multiple or migratory complaints that defy a unitary explanation, or

b/ the organ or *organ systems* that would be expected to malfunction if the symptoms were "real" can be shown to be *intact,* as when the EEG of a patient who reports total deafness shows an arousal response whenever there is a loud noise;

3/ the symptoms are *psychologically understandable* in the sense that they

a/ *symbolize* his feelings, as when an individual suddenly becomes blind after seeing a horrifying event, or

b/ are well suited to help him achieve some goal (or *secondary gain*) such as receiving attention or avoiding an unwanted situation without taking responsibility for the decision, as when an abruptly occurring paralysis prevents a man from taking a job in which his inadequacy would become evident, or recently developed nightly headaches prevent a frigid woman from having intercourse with her husband;

4/ the individual has such a propensity to overdramatize every event in his life and to behave in a way always so replete with excitement, interpersonal chaos, and fits of temper that he is considered to have a *histrionic personality;*

5/ he is *easily suggestible* in the sense that he rapidly accedes to any hint as to the possible etiology of the condition, confirms having a large number of other symptoms that he thinks the examiner might expect, or experiences a dramatic relief of symptoms in response to interventions that could have only a placebo effect;

6/ he appears *bland and indifferent* toward his symptoms even when they are the kind that would severely frighten the normal person; or

7/ he has had *cryptogenic, dissimulable, and illogical symptoms* so often that he is considered to have a *propensity* for them.

Defining a syndrome in which diagnosis involves so wide a variety of criteria creates manifold problems. Quite apart from the fact that an underlying organic disease can almost never be ruled out and malingering almost never proved, it seems arbitrary and artificial to distinguish between cryptogenic dysfunction and cryptogenic symptoms of other kinds; to distinguish between hypochondriasis and conversion on the basis of the patient's attitude toward his symptoms, excessive and unreassurable preoccupation with them being labeled as hypochondriasis and indifference to them as conversion; or to distinguish between either of these syndromes and psychophysiologic disorders on the basis that the latter must occur in an organ innervated by the autonomic nervous system (Whitlock 1967).

It is equally problematic to limit the diagnosis of conversion to individuals who are suggestible or have a histrionic personality, as the propensity to cryptogenic symptoms may also be found in persons whose behavior is circumspect, relaxed, and mature (Chodoff 1958, Kretschmer 1926, Stephens 1962, Ziegler 1960, 1962). Finally, it does not appear useful from the standpoint of treatment or prediction to label an unexplained physical symptom as a conversion solely because it appears to be related to the patient's psychological situation or can be made to disappear by psychological means, because incontrovertibly organic symptoms can also be triggered by psychologically important events; used to achieve conscious and unconscious goals; and disappear after a psychological intervention. Two young women, both of whom were thought to have conversion neuroses, have served to impress these principles on us. The first was referred for psychiatric evaluation because she was unable to swallow immediately after she performed fellatio on her brother; the second because of a severe opisthotonos and headache that was relieved immediately after she received a subcutaneous injection of saline into her neck. Further evaluation showed both to have encephalitis, the second with fatal outcome.

If the term *conversion* is used as a synonym for "cryptogenic" or "hard to explain," conversion symptoms can occur not only in conversion neuroses but also in malingering, schizophrenia, alcoholism, compensation neurosis, psychopathy, epilepsy, drug addiction, mental retardation, manic-depressive disease, drug reactions, and in patients who are later found to have brain tumors, leukemia, myasthenia gravis, multiple sclerosis, hyperparathyroidism, etc. (Gatfield 1962). For these reasons, we restrict the term *conversion neurosis* to individuals who repeatedly develop dissimulable symptoms that are cryptogenic or illogical and are not subsequently found to have some other organic or psychiatric cause (Farley 1968, Perley 1962, Woodruff 1967, 1969). While a complete list of such symptoms would undoubtedly comprise a compendium of semiology, the most common types of dysfunction that occur in patients with conversion neuroses are: blindness, deafness, aphonia, globus hystericus, motor paralyses, paresthesias, anesthesias, unsteady gait, blackouts, and fits.

Both the individual conversion symptom or dissociative episode and the propensity to develop such symptoms may have organic determinants. Such symptoms are by no means uncommon in patients with known organic diseases (McKegney 1967), demonstrable seizure disorders, or an atypical EEG (Ackner 1954, Bingley 1958, Williams 1956, Ziegler 1954); at times of endocrine change (premenstrual, postpartum, and menopausal periods); after head injuries (Thompson 1965); and in the early stages of schizophrenia (Slater 1961). Moreover, even though these symptoms are often triggered by upsetting events, most individuals who respond to a crisis in this manner either have been anxious for most of their lives or were irritable and depressed even before the event. Sleep deprivation may also contribute to the development of such symptoms: soldiers who develop fugues, amnesias, or conversion symptoms on the front lines have frequently had no opportunity to sleep for some days before their symptoms began.

All too often, the patient's symptoms seem so unreal and his bland reaction to them so suspicious that the physician performs an inadequate workup, ignores even the most obvious organic symptoms, and uses the label "conversion hysteria" merely as a polite circumlocution for the word "liar." The possibility of an underlying organic or psychiatric (particularly depressive) disease should not be ignored, however, as whenever long-term follow-up studies are done with patients originally labeled *hysteric,* a high percentage is found to have some other disorder that would explain either the symptom or the propensity for such symptoms (Slater 1965). This finding is not even an indictment of the original diagnostic procedures, for a valid diagnosis is often impossible until some months after the initial examination, when the illness begins to display its true character.

Obsessive-Compulsive and Phobic Neuroses

The distinction made in the United States between obsessive-compulsive and phobic neuroses is not observed in Europe, where the term "obsessional symptoms" includes phobias; intrusive ideas, images, ruminations, or impulses; and compulsive acts (Henderson 1962). This lumping together has much to recommend it, as these symptoms are often seen concurrently and are similar in that the patient experiences them as morbid or unreasonable and attempts to resist them. We discuss obsessive-compulsive and phobic symptoms together not only because of their similarities, however, but also because of their differences, which, though often minute, are nonetheless important in predicting the patient's course and planning his treatment.

Some situations, like danger or embarrassment, are so generally disliked that apprehensiveness and attempts at avoidance are considered quite normal. Other situations are generally so well tolerated that one who fears or seeks to avoid them is considered odd. Nevertheless, almost everyone has a few things he prefers to avoid even though he can stand them if he must: heights, bridges, the feel of a particular texture, the rustling of silk, or the like. A phobia thus cannot be viewed as morbid unless the feared situation, object, or idea can be avoided only by a marked rearrangement of the individual's life; causes him such anxiety in merely thinking about it that his social functioning suffers; or is so widespread that it cannot be avoided.

The term *phobia* is somewhat arbitrary, as it refers only to a particular kind of aversion. If the patient's discomfort relates only to a particular person, it is in all likelihood considered no more than an *antipathy,* even if he concedes that his discomfort with the person in question is unreasonable or disadvantageous. If he is uncomfortable not only with particular people but with most people, he may be labeled *schizoid.* In fact, the label *phobic* is usually restricted to the individual who becomes anxious when confronted with a particular object or physical setting, and aversion to people is labeled phobic only when it extends to certain kinds or groups of people, such as crowds, doctors, or policemen. The name assigned to both the discomfort and the way the individual copes with it is derived from the nature of the phobogenic object: agoraphobics fear open places, zoophobics avoid animals, and an alphabet lies between.

Because precision, orderliness, and the careful consideration of alternatives are necessities of everyday life, the distinction between the pathologic and nonpathologic occurrence of obsessional and ruminative thinking is at once delicate and important. A person's desire to have everything around him in order or his habit of starting each day by making a detailed list of what he has to do may be considered either efficient or obsessional, but is unlikely to be viewed as morbid unless it grossly interferes with his day-to-day activities. An automobile driver's need to perform complex mental computations while driving, in order to determine whether the license plate numbers of the cars that pass by are perfect squares, is more obviously obsessional, but even this, in itself, does not stamp him as ill. The label of illness does seem justified, however, when an individual is so constantly preoccupied with certain feared or unwanted thoughts or impulses that he cannot concentrate on anything else, and his social functioning suffers. If he realizes that his thoughts or fears are absurd, struggles against them, and is made even more uncomfortable by the awareness that he is unable to exclude them from his consciousness, his thinking may be called pathologically *obsessive*.

Compulsive behavior may be defined as an obsessional symptom that manifests itself in the repeated performance of one or more specific acts or rituals for no purpose other than to avoid the sense of anxiety experienced while resisting the impulse to do so. In some ways, this compulsion to perform a task in order to avoid a buildup of anxiety has much in common with the subjective experience of the individual given a posthypnotic suggestion. It has been compared with the child's endeavors to ward off fears or undo forbidden impulses by setting himself irrelevant tasks of prevention or atonement ("step on a crack and you break your mother's back") and has also been related to the rituals involved in superstitions or religious observances. But again these comparisons have a number of flaws. Ritualistic, unchosen, useless, and repetitive behavior is also seen in patients with organic brain syndromes and in children who have become autistic at so young an age that one could scarcely credit them with this kind of abstracting ability.

The distinction between phobic and obsessive-compulsive syndromes is not easy, for many patients show mixed or transitional forms. In some cases, the patient's compulsive behavior is related to a *phobia* (as when he must wash all food he eats because he fears it is unclean); in some, it stems from *obsessional ruminations* (as when he keeps thinking he is covered with germs and scrubs his hands till they are raw and bleeding); and in others, the patient confesses that he has no idea why he is engaging in such behavior except that it makes him feel less anxious. The symptoms may even appear sequentially, as when a patient starts by being *obsessionally* concerned about germs; then *phobically* avoids touching certain objects he considers germ-laden; and finally no longer considers avoidance sufficient protection and starts washing his hands *compulsively*. (The transition from phobic avoidance via compulsive behavior to *delusional* thinking takes place when he goes on to consider himself "contaminated," appreciating less and less the absurdity of his fears.)

The degree to which the patient is able to keep the symptoms in check is an important differentiating feature. The *phobic* patient can maintain his comfort by avoiding the phobogenic object, but, try as he may, the *obsessive-ruminative* patient is unlikely to find an effective avoidance maneuver. Patients with *compulsive* symptoms may or may not find ways of controlling their symptoms: those whose urge to blaspheme increases in church can try to think about unrelated matters or, failing in this, stay home. A further distinction between purely phobic neuroses and those with obsessional features is that phobic symptoms emerge and disappear more readily. Phobic symptoms, indeed, can arise so suddenly that the patient knows just when in his life he first had them and can date the onset of the current episode with precision; moreover, if he gets better, all or almost all his symptoms subside so that he can usually report exactly when he is symptom-free. This is less true of scrupulous, ruminative, or compulsive patients. Although their presenting symptoms can occasionally be precisely dated, they are more likely to be an intensification of a preexisting meticulousness or moral rigidity. In addition, obsessive-ruminative and compulsive symptoms remit less frequently, more slowly, and less completely than phobic ones, and some degree of social impairment usually remains (Ingram 1961, Pollitt 1960).

These disorders can also be distinguished in terms of their social consequences. In the *obsessive-compulsive neurosis*, patients are apt to suffer "spontaneity insufficiency" (Skoog 1965). Peer and community relationships are the first to decline, particularly for individuals who had habitually shown a distant and relatively mechanical orientation toward personal ties even before developing a recognizable illness; family relationships generally become disturbed next; and the patient's ability to work declines last. The sequence is different in *phobic neurosis*. Because the phobia may extend to objects encountered in getting to work (like automobiles or elevators), the individual's occupational competence may suffer first; community and peer relationships are affected later; and family relationships last of all. Unlike the obsessive patient, whose behavior promotes distance in interpersonal relationships, the phobic patient's difficulties with his family seem less of his doing than of theirs. The longer his illness lasts, the less likely it is that his family will continue to tolerate his demands for special consideration, and the more irritated they will become with the way he demands objective and extremely time-consuming evidence of their love and their willingness to stand by him.

Biologic symptoms may be seen in both kinds of disorders, but will not serve to differentiate between them. Sleep disturbances are not uncommon, especially DFA in obsessive-compulsive patients (Skoog 1965). Whether the obsessive-compulsive's sleep difficulty is primary or secondary may be impossible to determine: do his bedtime rituals stem from his inability to sleep, or is it the other way around? Neither disorder affects the patient's appetite, though he may develop a secondary eating disturbance when he is overconcerned about cleanliness, when prolonged obsessive-compulsive handwashing precedes each meal, or when particular kinds of food are the phobogenic objects.

While the patient's symptoms may remain stable from the onset to the resolution of the disorder, they are more likely to progress. Except for those instances in which the individual loses his intellectual distance from his symptoms and becomes frankly psychotic, decompensation entails only an extension of the initial symptoms and a further decline in social functioning. The obsessional thoughts, compulsive rituals, or phobogenic objects become more diversified, frequent, crippling, and isolating. The *neutrality and distance* of the patient's concerns also change, the objects of the phobic patient's concerns becoming less distant and less neutral, those of the obsessional patient more distant and more abstract. The phobic's dislike of exotic foods proceeds to a fear of eating in restaurants, then to a concern about canned foods, until finally, even in his own home, he must supervise the preparation of meals from raw to finished product. The obsessional individual's occasional worries about his differences with his wife proceed to daily ruminations about his general life situation, and finally to an internal dialogue about such abstract matters as the meaning of life or the value of searching for a meaning that is so incessant that the constant thinking and the struggle against it preclude all other mental or social activity. Either group of symptoms can be the forerunner of a depressive syndrome; obsessive-compulsive symptoms, of schizophrenia. As the decompensation proceeds toward schizophrenic psychosis, thoughts that were initially alien take on an increasingly imperative quality. Having blasphemous thoughts while in church extends to a fear of expressing them, then to the feeling of being compelled to blaspheme, and finally to the sense of being "commanded" to do so.

Whether the decompensation is merely an extension of the initial symptoms or a forerunner of psychosis, it will, in all likelihood, be preceded or accompanied by anxiety, increasing sleep difficulty, and anorexia. These symptoms offer a basis for predicting the patient's course, for as long as the patient's anxiety or insomnia continues, his other symptoms are likely to get worse; once sleep and tranquility return, they will recede or at least remain stable.

OTHER NEUROSES

The validity of legitimizing chronic fatigue in hypersensitive individuals with a sleep disturbance by calling it *neurasthenic neurosis* is questionable in our opinion. If it is of recent origin, it is almost invariably prodromal to or an accompaniment or sequel of some other physical or mental illness; and if of long standing, it might better be viewed as a manifestation of an asthenic personality.

Episodes during which an individual experiences himself as affectless, feels that the objects he perceives (or he himself) are somehow unreal, observes himself with the detachment of a spectator, or behaves in a robot-like manner are called *depersonalization*. Such episodes can occur in a wide variety of situations that alter or diminish the individual's alertness. They can occur as a result of sleep deprivation, in individuals with a compulsive personality, in the prodromal phase of a schizophrenic illness, and before and during depressions (especially those with obsessional features). While the propensity to develop depersonalization symptoms repeatedly may be considered neurotic, a large percentage of otherwise "normal" individuals may develop mild and transient symptoms of this kind from the age of six on (Sedman 1963).

Hypochondriacal neuroses, in which, either because of certain symptoms or without any symptoms at all, an individual obsesses about having some dangerous physical disease, are in some ways a cross between a conversion hysteria and an obsessional neurosis with a little depression and paranoia thrown in for good measure. Their treatment is basically that of depression and is further discussed in Chapter 12.

THE TREATMENT OF NEUROTIC DISORDERS

INDICATIONS FOR TREATMENT

Hidden in the plethora of studies describing the treatment of psychoneurotic disorders is the paucity of those that are controlled or of practical value. Most reports fail to establish criteria by which the diagnosis is made or the severity measured; few distinguish between improvement in the patient's adaptive skills and improvement in the presenting symptoms; and few acknowledge that neurotic syndromes remit spontaneously so often that it is difficult to assess treatment success. The majority are restricted to the ambiguous results of psychotherapeutic interventions; only recently have any well-designed studies sought to assess the effectiveness of somatic therapies.

For this reason, the physician has little beyond his clinical experience and his individual preferences and prejudices on which to base a decision whether treatment should be offered and what kind it should be. Ideally, he should use the same criteria that are pertinent in other illnesses (see p. 84). To what extent does the treatment protect the patient's life, occupational skills, reputation, and personal relationships? How rapidly is it effective? How long does the effect last? Does it cause the patient's social and biologic functioning to improve? And how does the treated patient's course compare with that of the untreated? This last question is of course the most pertinent in assessing the results of treatment, and any answer to it must take into account what little is known about the natural history of the neurotic disorders.

THE NATURAL HISTORY OF NEUROTIC DISORDERS

Neurotic symptoms that appear immediately after a stressful event are usually benign; they disappear within hours or days, often soon after the stress is relieved. Those that occur without a preceding stress may persist or fluctuate over many months. At times, the patient's symptoms remit and relapse at such regular intervals, looking and developing so similarly each time that the disorder brings to mind recurrent mood disorders.

Acute anxiety attacks usually last no more than one to two hours; even the propensity to react in this way may last no longer than a few weeks or months. Occasionally, the patient will remain symptom-free thereafter; more commonly, episodic relapses occur, particularly when a new stress arises. Indeed, anxiety neuroses usually occur in persons whose entire life style is so pervaded with insecurity, inadequacy, and fearfulness that the periods between acute attacks are marked by long-term, low-level anxiety. In any case, most acute episodes have so brief a natural course that the success of the innumerable interventions proposed in their treatment—psychological, pharmacologic, or both—may derive more from their natural tendency to remit rapidly than from the specific therapeutic measure used.

Dissociative neuroses generally last for a period of a few minutes up to a few days. While amnesic symptoms and fugue states that have persisted for months or even years have been reported, this long duration generally occurs only in persons who might have some special motive for such symptoms, such as having escaped from prison or having deserted their wives. In such cases, there can be genuine doubt about the reported amnesia, particularly because these patients usually seem relatively comfortable until they are "cured" or in some other way reminded of their former existence. *Conversion* symptoms of brief duration often remit as soon as a suggestion intended to induce a remission is made. This is less likely to occur when the patient's symptoms are of long standing, have an organic determinant, entitle him to a pension, or enable him to control his family.

Patients with *obsessive-compulsive neuroses* tend to have a bleaker outlook than those with other neurotic disorders. In some cases, their illness continues uninterruptedly for years; in others, the course fluctuates or the illness gets progressively worse; in still others, the course is phasic, and the illness may partially remit for years before relapsing once more. Although such patients are rarely disabled completely and most improve somewhat, they rarely recover fully (Ingram 1961, Kringlen 1964, Pollitt 1960). *Phobic neuroses* generally have a more benign course, especially for the short-term. Even without treatment, they generally recede gradually but completely in eight to ten months; those offered treatment may improve more rapidly. The outlook is not unclouded, however, for patients who have recovered from one such episode often develop another at a later time. Moreover, phobic neuroses that have lasted for a year or more may bring about a systematic utilization of avoidance maneuvers that becomes a way of life (Errera 1963), and the individual, despite being fairly comfortable and productive, may continue to avoid certain objects or situations indefinitely.

Although it is impossible to predict at the time a neurotic illness begins whether it will eventually become chronic or cause severe incapacitation, the younger the individual is, and the more insidiously his symptoms arise, the poorer his prognosis. The likelihood of a chronic course is also greater when the patient's history is devoid of a precipitating event or prodromal symptoms, such as anxiety or depression (Skoog 1965). The patient has a relatively good chance of recovering quickly and fully if his illness starts with anxiety, sleep difficulty, anorexia, or a depressed mood, but not so good a chance if such symptoms appear fairly late in the illness' course. When, for example, a patient with a long-standing obsessional illness becomes depressed and is given the standard dose of an antidepressant, his depression may lift, but his primary obsessional illness is likely to remain relatively unaffected.

The examination of the patient with a long-standing neurotic disorder often reveals that the symptoms themselves are less striking than the way in which both patient and family have changed their lives in order to adapt to the illness. In extreme cases, their entire lives revolve around the disability. Since most symptomatic neuroses do not grossly impair the patient's ability to think, work, communicate intelligibly, or interact warmly and affectionately with his family, those around him may not even protest the demands made on them. Moreover, the more gradually the patient's illness develops, the harder it may be for them to notice how much is demanded and the easier it is for them to adapt. By the time they become aware of the unusual circumstances in which they have become enmeshed, the situation may be bizarre and the irritation they feel may seem sudden and unfair.

Whether grudging or amicable, however, the family's acquiescence to the patient's demands can lead to new problems. After his symptoms have been in progress long enough to become the nodal points of a new adjustment, they may become the focal points of secondary gain. When they get out of hand or he uses them to justify making his family do things they would otherwise be able to avoid, frustration and anger mount. The housewife's fear of being home alone may induce her husband to give up his "poker night," but when he brings her for treatment, it may be hard to determine whether the impetus is his sense of captivity or hers. It is thus unquestionably valuable to pinpoint the secondary gains that the illness helps the sufferer achieve, but this coincidental result of the disease process must not be confused with its cause (Cameron 1963, Dancey 1957, Katz 1963). Nevertheless, the advantages that have accrued to the patient during his illness and his fear of making any efforts beyond those involved in his flight from the symptoms may perpetuate his social withdrawal and cause him to continue his unusual adaptive maneuvers even after his illness remits.

THE SETTING OF TREATMENT

Most neurotic patients are ambulatory and can be treated while living at home. Despite their innocuous appearance, however, the symptoms can interfere with biologic functions—notably eating and sleeping—exhaust and exasperate the family, and disrupt the patient's functioning to such an extent that extramural treatment becomes impossible. Hospitalization may thus be indicated when a patient's travel phobia prevents him from visiting the doctor's office or his fear of medicines causes him to refuse to take what is prescribed. It may also be useful when the family has converted the home into a pseudohospital in an effort to adapt to the patient's demands or the neurotic disorder itself has subsided but both patient and family have settled into an arrangement that contributes to a continuation of the now outdated immobilization.

PSYCHOTHERAPY

Although there are as many approaches to psychological treatment as there are therapists and patients, it is generally agreed that patients who have an understanding of their discomfort and of their life situation suffer less than those who do not. Since most therapists believe that such understanding is facilitated by exploring past experiences, an attempt to uncover and deal with conflicts that mold the patient's way of dealing with his world is usually a part of any treatment effort. The neurotic patient wants more than understanding, however: he wants most of all to have his symptoms relieved. Being rational and free to choose whether and with whom his treatment will proceed, he is far more able than the psychotic patient to influence the dialogue between himself and the therapist. Inevitably, these discussions focus in large measure on what the patient sees as the problem: his symptoms.

In neurosis, as in other illnesses, the clinician's efforts are directed to the *symptoms themselves,* to their *consequences,* and to their *causes.* Psychotherapists differ in their approach to a given illness most notably in the degree and manner of their concentration on one or another of these three aspects. We shall use the psychotherapeutic treatment of phobias to illustrate some of these methods, but with a few modifications the same techniques may be applied to the treatment of other neurotic disorders as well.

The therapist who focuses on the *manifestations* of the symptoms may repeatedly point out how harmless the phobogenic objects are, advise the patient on how best to avoid them (as by changing jobs), or exhort him to make a greater effort to tolerate them. Some therapists try to diminish the patient's fears by bringing him into contact with the phobogenic object—either gradually or suddenly (Wolpe 1961). Therapists who use *desensitization* techniques urge the patient to visualize successive situations that are increasingly like those he fears (see p. 490). Some therapists seek to minimize the patient's concern about his symptoms by making light of them or by friendly *bantering* (Coleman 1963); others urge the patient to *exaggerate his fearfulness* to such an extent that it eventually seems ridiculous to him (Frankl 1960). All these efforts suggest behavioral or attitudinal change to the patient, and their effect is enhanced by the patient's trust in the therapist and his confidence in the therapist's knowledge or professional reputation. This effect is most pointedly illustrated in hypnotic techniques, when the *posthypnotic suggestion* is made that the feared object or situation can be faced with less dread, or the fear is displaced to a different and less commonly encountered object (Gill 1959).

Other therapists concentrate on the *consequences* of the phobia. They believe that an exploration of the patient's attitude toward the affected life areas will clarify what purposes—conscious and unconscious—his symptoms enable him to achieve. If the phobia's most obvious effect is that it disturbs the patient's family, the therapist may explore the patient's feelings toward them or may even invite them to take part in the discussions with the patient, in the hope that this will help to unravel the transactional aspects of the patient's symptoms (Berne 1961, 1964). One useful measure in studying such parameters is to ask the patient directly just how his life would be different if he were not afraid to do the things that he fears.

Another therapist may try to discover the *causes* for the patient's choice of a particular phobogenic object. He may try to determine what previous experiences the patient has had with the objects he fears or ones that are similar. If he believes that the feared objects symbolize earlier fears or conflicts and that the patient's fears will diminish when he understands what they mean, he may attempt to decode these symbols and uncover the psychological roots of the disorder. Free associative techniques in which the patient says everything that comes to his mind occasionally make this easier. Some therapists use narcosynthetic techniques (see p. 661), hypnosis, or a combination of these, in order to facilitate such explorations; but others feel that the patient's resistances should be studied, not bypassed, so that both patient and doctor can better understand his personality structure (Reich 1949). They will try to determine which topics the patient has the most difficulty talking about and how his resistance to doing so shows itself.

That the range of psychological efforts is so wide leads to two conclusions: each physician finds ways that he considers most comfortable and suitable to the therapeutic situation, and not one of these ways is of such obvious or universal advantage that it overrides the physician's individual preferences. Our own approach, which is as much a reflection of our personal point of view as those listed above, is discussed at greater length in the chapter on psychotherapy (13). It is not demonstrable that any of the psychotherapeutic techniques necessarily alleviates symptoms, or if it does (as in the desensitization treatment of monosymptomatic phobias uncomplicated by anxiety, depression, or social problems), that the beneficial effects can be sustained even if treatment is continued. Nevertheless, it appears likely that the opportunity to discuss and explore one's general life situation with an interested, intelligent human being enhances life adaptation in both the ill and the well. This can be a special dividend, giving the patient, after the symptoms subside, a somewhat broader understanding of what motivates him and others and increasing his ability to think and communicate with others about himself and his world.

SOMATIC TREATMENT

While the final word on the relative merits of somatic and psychological therapies in neurotic disorders has by no means been spoken, the value of somatic therapy in the individual case at least can be assessed fairly quickly (Kellner 1970). We have found the following criteria helpful in determining whether a neurotic illness is likely to **respond** to somatic therapy and to which of the available treatment measures it is likely to respond best. In general, patients with neurotic disorders who have difficulty in falling asleep (DFA), show overt anxiety with neurovegetative symptoms, or are between 12 and 40, respond best to sedatives, minor tranquilizers, and in some cases phenothiazines; while those who have early morning awakening (EMA), anorexia, or a cyclic course, or are between 40 and 65, respond best to antidepressants. This dichotomization should not be overvalued, however, for there are so many transitional forms and admixtures of anxious and depressive components that it is often best to give a combination of medications (Winkelmann 1965).

The temporal sequence of sleep disorder and neurotic symptoms may help predict how the patient will respond to drug treatment. When the neurotic disorder is associated with a sleep disturbance from the outset, both the neurotic symptoms and the sleep disorder may be expected to respond to somatic therapies directed to the sleep disorder. When the sleep disorder develops during the course of the illness, it will usually respond to somatic therapies, but the neurotic symptoms themselves are less likely to do so. When the patient sleeps fairly well throughout the course of the illness, somatic therapies are usually of little benefit, and in any case unnecessary, because the patient is likely to recover fairly quickly even without treatment. Nevertheless, if his symptoms persist for six months or more, and particularly if they start to invade areas of social, familial, or occupational functioning that were previously intact, medication should be tried.

While most physicians would agree that the effectiveness of drug treatment can be assessed only if the patient is given a high enough dose for a sufficient period of time, the neurotic patient's drug regimen tends to be discontinued more rapidly than the psychotic's. That there is less evidence for the value of drugs in neurotic than in psychotic disorders, and that the neurotic patient who experiences side effects is more rational and thus better equipped to plead a convincing case against continuing a given drug, tends to make the physician take such complaints more seriously than he would if the patient were psychotic. As a result, he is less likely to override the patient's objections, more likely to give him permission to discontinue the drug, and thus less likely to find out how he would fare if he were to continue for the full course.

While "drug-induced" discomfort can usually be mitigated by reassurance or minor adjustments in dosage, drugs can, in some cases, aggravate the patient's original symptoms or provoke side effects that he builds into his illness. Phenothiazines can aggravate symptoms of depersonalization and conversion, and drug-induced extrapyramidal symptoms are so common in neurotic patients that it is almost as though they had some particular sensitivity of the basal ganglia. Even using a drug can become a focus for a patient's neurotic complaints, as when he becomes phobic about taking pills or obsesses about the precision with which they must be taken or about what taking them means. If such problems outweigh the therapeutic advantages of the drug's use, there may be no choice but to change or discontinue them.

Side effects are less common with the minor tranquilizers, such as meprobamates, benzodiazepines, and barbiturates (see Table 35). These agents will relieve the patient's anxiety, at least initially, and are indicated when the patient's discomfort is of mild or intermittent character. Barbiturates, 15-30 mg, 3-4 times daily; meprobamate (Miltown or Equanil), 200 mg, 3-4 times daily; or benzodiazepines like chlordiazepoxide (Librium), 10-20 mg, 3-4 times daily, often provide prompt relief from discomfort and enable the patient to sleep. In acute anxiety attacks, chlordiazepoxide, 25-50 mg p.o. or i.m., usually aborts the attack within 20 to 30 minutes. Higher doses should not be given for more than four or five days, lest tolerance and dependence develop, with the consequence that the drug not only loses its effectiveness but causes withdrawal symptoms that compound the patient's anxiety; with prolonged use, such agents may also intensify the depressive components of the illness (see p. 173). Since most patients tolerate minimal doses of minor tranquilizers quite well for an extended period of time, their prolonged use may be indicated in chronic anxiety, obsessive-compulsive, and occasionally even in phobic neuroses.

When antidepressants are used, they should be given in approximately the same doses as used in the more typical depressive syndromes (see p. 174): imipramine (Tofranil), 75-100 mg daily, or phenelzine (Nardil), 45-60 mg daily (Kelly 1970). In some cases, the patient may become more anxious than before, but the exacerbation of symptoms is usually temporary. If the discomfort does not subside within a few days, chlordiazepoxide (Librium), 20-30 mg daily, may be added for a week or ten days and then gradually reduced.

When phenothiazines are used in neurotic disorders, the dosage should be much lower than that in schizophrenic or depressive syndromes. *Sedating phenothiazines* like chlorpromazine (Thorazine) should be avoided, for they tend to make the patient feel even worse and can aggravate conversion symptoms and depersonalization. *Alerting phenothiazines* such as trifluoperazine (Stelazine) or fluphenazine (Prolixin, Permitil), 1-2 mg, up to three times daily, are somewhat better tolerated and often helpful; *reserpine* in doses no higher than 0.25-1.0 mg, 3-4 times daily, may also be used, particularly in the treatment of chronic anxiety neuroses.

Since the foregoing measures are only moderately effective, many other more vigorous procedures have been tried. In obsessional illnesses and in some persistent phobic reactions, *high doses of imipramine,* up to 400 mg daily (Geissman 1964, Tellenbach 1963), have been found surprisingly successful. Moreover, patients with obsessional and conversion neuroses that have been refractory to all other efforts may improve on a regimen that starts with *reserpine* (3 to 6 mg daily), adds *imipramine* (75-100 mg, daily) ten days later, and maintains this *combination* for a three-month period. If the patient improves, the reserpine may be gradually discontinued over a two-to-three month period, and if the patient thereafter continues to do well, the imipramine may be discontinued. In some obsessional neuroses, after years of suffering, and especially when anxiety or depression dominate the clinical picture, *psychosurgery* (see p. 663) may be a last resort. *Hallucinogens* have also been reported of value in some cases (see p. 662), and *lithium carbonate* when the disorder has a cyclical course (see p. 606).

When a phobic neurosis neither remits spontaneously nor responds to psychotherapy or pharmacotherapy, and particularly when it is accompanied with EMA or a depressed mood, ECT may be indicated. ECT can also be tried in intractable obsessive-compulsive disorders, but usually benefits only those patients whose disorder shows a distinct affective component. This component may be masked, so that a diagnostic interview, following an intravenous injection of methamphetamine (Methedrine), 15-30 mg in 10 cc of saline over a 5-15 minute period, may be of value (see p. 659). If, in the course of an interview of this kind, the patient becomes markedly depressed, there is a fair chance that ECT will be helpful, but if obsessional ideation increases or delusional thinking appears, ECT may cause the individual's symptoms to exacerbate and should therefore be avoided.

REFERENCES

Ackner, B.: Depersonalization. II. Clinical Syndromes, J Ment Sci *100*:854-872, 1954.

Agras, S., Sylvester, D., and Oliveau, D.: Epidemiology of common fears and phobia, Compr Psychiat *10*:151-156, 1969.

Bailey, P., and Murray, H. A.: Case of pinealoma with symptoms suggestive of compulsion neurosis, Arch Neurol (Chicago) *19*:932-945, 1928.

Beck, A. T.: Thinking and depression: I. Idiosyncratic content and cognitive distortions, Arch Gen Psychiat (Chicago) *9*: 324-333, 1963.

Berne, E.: Transactional Analysis in Psychotherapy, New York: Grove, 1961.

———:Games People Play: The Psychology of Human Relationships, New York: Grove, 1964.

Bingley, T.: Mental symptoms in temporal lobe epilepsy and temporal lobe gliomas, Acta Psychiat Neurol *33* (Suppl 120):1-151, 1958.

Cameron, N.: Personality Development and Psychopathology: A Dynamic Approach, Boston: Houghton Mifflin, 1963.

Cattell, R. B., and Scheier, I. H.: Nature of anxiety: Review of thirteen multivariate analyses comprising 814 variables: Present confusion in conceptualization; necessary methodological conditions for solving the problem, Psychol Rep *4* (Suppl 5):351-388, 1958.

Chapman, J.: Early symptoms of schizophrenia, Brit J Psychiat *112*:225-251, 1966.

Chodoff, P., and Lyons, H.: Hysteria, the hysterical personality and "hysterical" conversion, Amer J Psychiat *114*:734-740, 1958.

Cole, J. O.: Therapeutic efficacy of antidepressant drugs: Review, JAMA *190*:448-455, 1964.

Coleman, J. V.: Banter as a psychotherapeutic intervention, Amer J Psychoanal *22*: 1-6, 1963.

Dancey, T. E., and Sarwer-Foner, G. J.: Problem of the secondary gain patient in medical practice, Canad Med Ass J *77*: 1108-1111, 1957.

DSM-II: Diagnostic and Statistical Manual of Mental Disorders, ed 2, prepared by The Committee on Nomenclature and Statistics of the Amer Psychiat Ass, Washington, DC: Amer Psychiat Ass, 1968.

Eiduson, B. T.: Two classes of information in psychiatry, Arch Gen Psychiat (Chicago) *18*:405-419, 1968.

Errera, P., and Coleman, J. V.: Long-term follow-up study of neurotic phobic patients in a psychiatric clinic, J Nerv Ment Dis *136*:267-271, 1963.

Farley, J., Woodruff, R. A., Jr., and Guze, S. B.: Prevalence of hysteria and conversion symptoms, Brit J Psychiat *114*: 1121-1125, 1968.

Frankl, V. E.: Paradoxical intention: Logotherapeutic technique, Amer J Psychother *14*:520-535, 1960.

Garmany, G.: Emergencies in general practice: Acute anxiety and hysteria, Brit Med J *2*:115-117, 1955.

Gatfield, P. D., and Guze, S. B.: Prognosis and differential diagnosis of conversion reactions (a follow-up study), Dis Nerv Syst *23*:623-631, 1962.

Geissmann, P., and Kammerer, Th.: L'imipramine dans la nevrose obsessionnelle: Étude de 30 cas (Imipramine in obsessional neurosis: Study of 30 cases), Encéphale *53*:369-382, 1964.

Giel, R., Knox, R. S., and Carstairs, G. M.: Five year follow-up of 100 neurotic out-patients, Brit Med J *2*:160-163, 1964.

Gill, M. M., and Brenman, M.: Hypnosis and the Related States, New York: Internat Univ Press, 1959.

Goldman, D.: Effect of 'energizers' on neurotic patients, Dis Nerv Syst *23*:632-639, 1962.

Haddock, J. N.: Place of obsessions, compulsions and phobias in psychiatric diagnosis and treatment, J South Med Ass *58*:1115-1121, 1965.

Hays, P.: Modes of onset of psychotic depression, Brit Med J *2*:779-784, 1964.

Henderson, D., and Batchelor, I. R. C.: Henderson & Gillespie's Textbook of Psychiatry, London: Oxford, 1962.

Ingram, I. M.: Obsessional illness in mental hospital patients, Brit J Psychiat *107*:382-402, 1961.

Jakab, I.: Erfahrungen mit Tofranil bei endogenen und reaktiven Depressionen, Wien Med Wschr *110*:259-260, 1960.

Kanner, L.: Child Psychiatry, ed 3, Springfield (Ill): Thomas, 1957.

Katz, J.: On primary gain and secondary gain, Psychoanal Stud Child *28*:9-50, 1963.

Kellner, R.: Drugs, diagnoses, and outcome of drug trials with neurotic patients. A survey, J Nerv Ment Dis *151*:85-96, 1970.

Kelly, D., et al.: Treatment of phobic states with antidepressants. A retrospective study of 246 patients, Brit J Psychiat *116*: 387-398, 1970.

Kessell, A.: Borderlands of the depressive states, Brit J Psychiat *114*:1135-1140, 1968.

Klein, D. F.: Delineation of two drug-responsive anxiety syndromes, Psychopharmacologia (Berlin) 5:397-408, 1964.

Kretschmer, E.: Hysteria, New York: Nerv & Ment Dis Pub, 1926.

Kringlen, E.: Prognosis in obsessional illness, Acta Psychiat Scand 40 (Suppl 180):155-158, 1964.

Lader, M., and Sartorius, N.: Anxiety in patients with hysterical conversion symptoms, J Neurol Neurosurg Psychiat 31: 490-495, 1968.

Marks, I. M.: Classification of phobic disorders, Brit J Psychiat 116:377-386, 1970.

McCall, R. J.: Dispensable and the indispensable in psychopathological classification: Neurosis and character disorder in the 1952 and 1968 DSM's, Int J Psychiat 7:399-403, 1969.

McKegney, F. P.: Incidence and characteristics of patients with conversion reactions: I. General hospital consultation service sample, Amer J Psychiat 124:542-545, 1967.

Miller, M. H., and Chotlos, J. W.: Obsessive and hysterical syndromes in the light of existential consideration, J Exist 1:315-329, 1960.

Noreik, K.: A follow-up examination of neuroses, Acta Psychiat Scand 46:81-95, 1970.

Perley, M. J., and Guze, S. B.: Hysteria—Stability and usefulness of clinical criteria, New Eng J Med 266:421-426, 1962.

Pollitt, J. D.: Natural history studies in mental illness: Discussion based on a pilot study of obsessional states, Brit J Psychiat 106:93-113, 1960.

Reich, W.: Character Analysis, New York: Noonday, 1949.

Rioch, D. McK.: Experimental aspects of anxiety, Amer J Psychiat 113:435-442, 1956.

Roth, M.: Phobic anxiety-depersonalization syndrome, Proc Roy Soc Med 52: 587-595, 1959.

Salzman, L. F., et al.: Conceptual thinking in psychiatric patients, Arch Gen Psychiat (Chicago) 14:55-59, 1966.

Sargant, W.: Physical treatments of depression: Their indications and proper use, J Neuropsychiat 1 (Suppl):s1-s10, 1961.

Schilder, P.: Organic background of obsessions and compulsions, Amer J Psychiat 94:1397-1416, 1938.

Sedman, G., and Reed, G. F.: Depersonalization phenomena in obsessional personalities and in depression, Brit J Psychiat 109:376-379, 1963.

Skoog, G.: Onset of anancastic conditions: Clinical study, Acta Psychiat Scand 41 (Suppl 184):1-82, 1965.

Slater, E.: The thirty-fifth Maudsley lecture: "Hysteria 311," Brit J Psychiat 107:359-381, 1961.

Slater, E., and Glithero, E.: Follow-up of patients diagnosed as suffering from "hysteria," J Psychosom Res 9:9-13, 1965.

Stephens, J. H., and Kamp, M.: On some aspects of hysteria: Clinical study, J Nerv Ment Dis 134:305-314, 1962.

Tellenbach, H.: Über die Behandlung phobischer und anankastischer Zustände mit imipramin, Nervenarzt 34:133-138, 1963.

Terhune, W. B.: The phobic syndrome: Study of eighty-six patients with phobic reactions, Arch Neurol (Chicago) 62:162-172, 1949.

Thompson, G. N.: Post-traumatic psychoneurosis—Statistical survey, Amer J Psychiat 121:1043-1048, 1965.

Whitlock, F. A.: Aetiology of hysteria, Acta Psychiat Scand 43:144-162, 1967.

Williams, D.: Structure of emotions reflected in epileptic experiences, Brain 79: 29-67, 1956.

Winkelman, N. W., Jr.: Three evaluations of a monoamine oxidase inhibitor and phenothiazine combination, Dis Nerv Syst 26:160-164, 1965.

Winokur, G., and Holemon, E.: Chronic anxiety neurosis: Clinical and sexual aspects, Acta Psychiat Scand 39:384-412, 1963.

Wolpe, J.: Systematic desensitization treatment of neuroses, J Nerv Ment Dis 132:189-203, 1961.

Woodruff, R. A., Jr.: Hysteria: Evaluation of objective diagnostic criteria by the study of women with chronic medical illnesses, Brit J Psychiat 114:1115-1119, 1967.

Woodruff, R. A., Jr., Clayton, P. J., and Guze, S. B.: Hysteria: Evaluation of specific diagnostic criteria by the study of randomly selected psychiatric clinic patients, Brit J Psychiat 115:1243-1248, 1969.

Ziegler, D. K., and Paul, N.: On the natural history of hysteria in women: Follow-up study of twenty years after hospitalization, Dis Nerv Syst 15:301-306, 1954.

Ziegler, F. J., and Imboden, J. B.: Contemporary conversion reactions II. Conceptual model, Arch Gen Psychiat (Chicago) 66:279-287, 1962.

Ziegler, F. J., Imboden, J. B., and Meyer, E.: Contemporary conversion reactions: Clinical study, Amer J Psychiat 116:901-909, 1960.

CHAPTER
SEVEN

Personality Disorders

CLASSIFICATION

THE TERM "PERSONALITY DISORDER" refers to certain characteristic behavioral patterns that develop early in the individual's life and produce a persistent, usually lifelong constriction in his gamut of responsiveness. There is to be sure some dispute over which of these patterns are legitimate objects of medical concern and at what level of disability they become so; whether some of them represent mild or prodromal forms or variants of other more clearly defined mental disorders; and whether they are all discrete enough entities to warrant different labels or are separated by artificial boundaries (Small 1970). Nevertheless, they are generally categorized into the following subtypes:

1/ the *paranoid personality* (see also Chap. 5), characterized by hypersensitivity and rigidity in interpersonal relations, a conspicuous tendency to blame and ascribe evil motives to others, jealousy, envy, unwarranted suspiciousness, extreme stubbornness, and excessive self-importance;

2/ the *cyclothymic* (or *affective*) *personality* (see also Chap. 4), characterized by recurrent periods of unwarranted elation (marked by warmth, friendliness, high energy, and enthusiasm for competition) alternating with periods of unwarranted sadness (marked by worry, pessimism, low energy, and a sense of futility);

3/ the *schizoid personality* (see also Chap. 3), characterized by shyness, aloofness, introversion, avoidance of close or competitive relationships, inability to express hostility directly, and autistic thinking;

4/ the *explosive* (or *epileptoid*) *personality* (see also Chaps. 10 and 11), characterized by low frustration tolerance manifested by feelings of rage, usually coupled with outbursts of verbal abusiveness or physical violence, which are not only disproportionate to the stimulus (if there was indeed any provocation at all) but also strikingly different from the individual's usual behavior. While some individuals of this kind take pride in their "short fuse" and the fact that they let no real or imagined slur pass without putting the offender in his place, the majority regret and are puzzled by their behavior during such episodes. The alternate label, epileptoid personality, has been chosen to suggest the phenomenologic link to psychomotor seizures, the primary behavioral differences being that the individual with an explosive personality is not amnesic for the episodes in question and shows no other evidence of a seizure disorder.

5/ the *obsessive-compulsive personality* (see also Chap. 6), characterized by an inability to relax and excessive concern with adherence to standards of conscience, conformity, hygiene, or orderliness;

6/ the *histrionic personality,* characterized by excitability, emotional immaturity and instability, vanity, self-centeredness, and attention-seeking self-dramatization (see also Chap. 6);

7/ the *asthenic personality,* characterized by easy fatigability, low-energy level, lack of enthusiasm, marked incapacity for enjoyment, and oversensitivity to physical and emotional stress;

8/ the *passive-aggressive personality* of the *passive-dependent type,* characterized by helplessness, indecisiveness, and a tendency to cling to others; or the *passive-aggressive type,* characterized by pouting, stubbornness, procrastination, inefficiency, and passive obstructionism;

9/ the *inadequate personality,* characterized by ineffectual responses to intellectual, social, emotional, and physical demands, inadaptability, ineptness, lack of physical and emotional stamina, poor judgment, and social incompatibility; and

10/ the *antisocial personality,* characterized by a propensity for being in trouble; failure to profit from either experience or punishment; inability to maintain loyalty to any person, group, or code; callousness, hedonism, and irresponsibility; marked emotional immaturity and lack of judgment; a tendency to avoid taking the blame for misdeeds by blaming them on others or explaining them so that they seem warranted, reasonable, and justified.

DISTINCTION BETWEEN SITUATIONAL, SYMPTOMATIC, AND "TRUE" PERSONALITY DISORDERS

In evaluating behavior of the kind described above, it is important to establish whether it represents

1/ a "situational personality disturbance," by which we mean the response of a normal person attempting to cope with or derive gain from an unusual situation,

2/ the symptoms of an intercurrent medical or psychiatric illness, or

3/ the lifelong maladaptive style that may legitimately be called "personality disorder."

Behavior consistent with the clinical picture of a personality disorder may thus have quite disparate causes. Attention-seeking self-dramatization, the typical sign of the histrionic personality disorder, for example, looks the same whether it appears in a normal individual who considers it the best way to hold onto the person he loves; as the first manifestation of a schizophrenic episode; or in an individual whose formative years were spent in a provocative family setting that abounded in histrionic role models and who has used such behavior throughout his life.

The *situational personality disturbance* may be to some extent a function of predominant learned response patterns, but its characteristic feature is that it is limited in time and place to the circumstances in which it is required (Block 1968, Endler 1966) and, at least quantitatively, is at variance with both the individual's previous life style and his image of himself. Typical examples may be found in the seemingly paranoid, but nonetheless quite appropriate, hypersensitivity and suspiciousness characteristically seen in fugitives and conspirators; and in the seemingly passive-aggressive prisoner of war who, finding that his captors become frustrated when he refuses to speak, becomes increasingly stubborn and taciturn.

When behavior identical with that seen in the "true" personality disorder occurs as a *symptom* of a medical or psychiatric illness, the diagnosis of the basic illness can be quite difficult, for the behavioral symptoms can be so prominent that they overshadow the individual's other symptoms. In some cases, the behavioral idiosyncrasies represent only an intensification of the individual's ordinary response patterns. Traits that were previously barely perceptible come to dominate his entire personality and are thus, at least from a quantitative point of view, inconsistent with his former lifestyle and self-image. In other cases, entirely new behavioral manifestations occur, their nature depending to some extent on the type of illness. If, for example, the patient's illness is one that episodically or consistently impairs his energy level (such as narcolepsy, diabetes, or chronic depression), he is likely to develop *passive-aggressive* behavior patterns. If his illness is associated with cognitive dysfunctioning and confusion, making it necessary for him to organize elaborately his behavior and thinking (as in the early phases of a schizophrenic episode or in a senile dementia), his behavior may well become *compulsive*. Protracted mental illnesses, in particular, may result in constricted adjustment patterns that leave a residual *inadequate* personality disorder even after the original illness remits.

Antisocial behavior is an especially common symptom of other mental illnesses. It may be seen in *schizophrenia* (page 123), *paranoid syndromes* (p. 210), *mental retardation* (p. 356) and, not infrequently, as the first sign of an *organic brain syndrome* (p. 443). *Manic-depressive disease,* too, may lead to bouts of anti-social behavior (Schipkowensky 1968). In the typical case, the antisocial act is committed in the midst of a manic phase, but this is often not realized, especially when the ensuing depression coincides with the individual's arrest or hospitalization and is considered a consequence of his having been caught. If the depressive phase does not occur until after the legal threat has diminished, the charges have been dismissed, or the sentence suspended, the events may be interpreted psychodynamically, the patient's depression being viewed as a result of his desire to be punished.

The characteristic features of *true personality disorders* are that they develop at an early age, persist throughout the individual's life, are consistent with his self-image, and represent his life-style. Since most persons tend to use one particular set of coping mechanisms more than others, we consider the predominance of a single mode of response to life events a disorder only when there is evidence that it affects a person's flexibility sufficiently to hinder him in attaining his immediate or long-term goals.

This constriction in adaptive skills is rarely the individual's sole reason for seeking treatment, however, for the average person with a personality disorder views his reliance on a limited number of responses not as illness but as "the way he is." Only those who are psychologically very sophisticated, or who have encountered a situation that they want to, but cannot, master behaving as they do, will go to a therapist complaining of their own social style. Such requests for treatment are indeed so rare that other possibilities must be considered, as that the individual is in fact suffering from some intercurrent physical or mental illness and that this or some unaccustomed stress is overtaxing his already limited adaptive resources, producing impaired functioning or unusual discomfort (Coleman 1967).

A study of the individual's reactions to the examiner during the first meeting may reveal the nature of the personality disorder, but the range of information required for a judgment concerning its treatment requires supplementary data. The patient's relatives and associates, by describing his past and present behavior, can help the physician distinguish between the acute reaction that is, likely to be situational or symptomatic in nature and the protracted pattern of the "true" personality disorder. *Family meetings* will also help the clinician determine the patient's family role and assess the stresses to which he is likely to be exposed. Such meetings are of particular value for individuals with an antisocial personality, for the family's encouragement of the patient's corruption may be unidentifiable without first-hand observation of their interaction with him.

It is also of value to examine the patient's functioning in other social settings. A *therapy group* is particularly suitable for this purpose because it offers the examiner an opportunity to observe the patient's role-taking abilities and social competence (Eliasoph 1963). In this setting, the person with a neurotic illness will usually show a good capacity for understanding and responding to the needs of those around him; the one with a dyssocial personality may understand their needs and motives but, having rejected the traditional modes of social behavior, respond to them in an unconventional manner; the person with an antisocial personality can respond to their needs only in a limited way: he tends to form temporary alliances with certain group members, not in order to offer them friendship or understanding, but to exclude other members of the group or to attack and undermine the therapist. Finally, the person whose behavior disorder is symptomatic of some other mental illness tends to distort the motives of others, is unable to differentiate clearly between their motives and his own, expresses his feelings poorly or inappropriately, or demonstrates other symptoms that clarify the diagnosis.

TREATMENT

For centuries, the behavioral styles seen in personality disorders have been attributed to immutable individual differences. Any attempt to change such traits was considered not only futile but perhaps even immoral. As a result, almost no data are available about the efficacy of the various treatment possibilities, and no clear-cut guidelines can be offered.

One path to obtaining such data as far as *drug treatment* is concerned consists of treating the patient's personality disorder as if it were an abortive form of the treatable syndrome it most closely resembles (Heston 1970) and giving him whichever drug would be effective for that illness. Phenothiazines, for example, have been found useful for patients with schizoid personality disorders; and antidepressants or lithium carbonate for patients with cyclothymic and obsessive-compulsive personalities (see p. 239). Less clearly documented but worth trying are phenothiazines alone or in combination with antidepressants for patients with paranoid personality disorders; and diphenylhydantoin (Dilantin), a major tranquilizer, or a combination of the two for patients with explosive personalities. Minor tranquilizers, antidepressants, or a combination of the two have been tried for patients with histrionic, asthenic, and passive-aggressive personalities on the (admittedly undocumented) assumption that chronic anxiety or depression might play a prominent role in this type of maladaptive behavior.

Our conviction that a person who is troubled about the way others respond to him will benefit from exposure to the views of others and from developing some understanding of himself moves us to advise some kind of *psychotherapy* in most cases, in the hope that this will provide the individual with a setting in which he can identify his current style, learn new ways of coping with stress, and practice the new techniques he learns. While the kinds of psychotherapeutic techniques that may be used are outlined in greater detail in Chapter 13, it should be noted that most self-referred patients seek treatment because their adaptive style has created difficulties with their families at a particular juncture in their life and that they are rarely interested in long-term therapy. We try, therefore, to see the patient together with his parents or wife (and often his children as well) and generally stop seeing them soon after the crisis has passed. If the first set of meetings has been of benefit, we find it useful now and then to offer a kind of refresher course: when a crisis arises or the effect of the last meetings has dissipated and they all revert to their old ways, the therapeutic contact is renewed just long enough to help alleviate the difficulties. In this way, each crisis provides an opportunity to focus on the family's communication problem and to teach them to accept each other's limitations and avoid isolating the patient.

ANTISOCIAL BEHAVIOR

DIFFERENTIAL DIAGNOSIS

The frequency with which individuals who have engaged in antisocial activities are called to the psychiatrist's attention and the strength of the community's insistence that he deal with them make it advisable to discuss antisocial behavior at some length. In most cases, the individual's past history will give the clinician some clues to the proper diagnosis. Single antisocial acts, like single aberrant acts of any kind, obviously do not suffice for a diagnostic label. However, when the individual repeatedly behaves in an antisocial manner, shows no symptoms or signs of another illness, and has engaged in antisocial acts for so long that other symptoms would have emerged if his antisocial behavior were symptomatic of some disorder, the clinician must try to determine whether his behavior represents

1/ an *antisocial personality disorder,* once called "psychopathic personality" or, some years earlier, "moral insanity";

2/ a *dyssocial personality disorder,* by which is meant either

a/ *social maladjustment without manifest psychiatric disorder,* as exemplified by the professional criminal or the marginal businessman who believes that his prime obligation is to look out for himself, or

b/ a *group delinquent reaction,* as exemplified by the member of the adolescent gang; or

3/ an *explosive personality disorder.*

Whether and to what extent these represent distinct clinical entities is hard to say, for there is undoubtedly much overlap between them. Nevertheless, despite the diversity of traits seen in individuals who repeatedly engage in antisocial behavior, Cleckley (1955), by calling attention to a number of features that many of these individuals have in common, has identified what amounts to a discrete, distinguishable, and, in any case, fairly familiar syndrome (see Table 15). He explains why many, and at times all, of these apparently unrelated characteristics are observed in psychopaths in terms of an underlying cognitive disorder that he calls "semantic aphasia." This notion is shared to some extent by Miller (1964), who believes that the psychopath is *impaired in his ability to appreciate the passage of time.* Experiencing his world as existing only in the present, realizing that he, like everyone around him, has a wide range of choices what he shall become, recognizing that the selection of one life-goal means the abandonment of others, and unwilling to abandon any of his potentialities, he may be unable throughout his life to choose any single commitment or goal, and, choosing none, surrender them all. Coupled with this disturbance is a *concretistic approach to human communication* that, especially

TABLE 15. *Clinical Features of the Antisocial Personality*

1. Superficial charm and intelligence	8. Shallowness of affective reactions
2. Absence of delusional thinking	9. Specific loss of insight, with an ability to rationalize behavior so that it appears warranted, reasonable, and justified
3. Unreliability, untruthfulness, insincerity, and irresponsibility	
4. Lack of remorse or shame	
5. Inadequately motivated antisocial behavior	10. Unresponsiveness in general interpersonal relations
6. Propensity for trouble, poor judgment, and failure to learn from punishment or experience	11. Fantastic and uninviting behavior (especially after drinking)
	12. Rarity of successful suicide
7. Pathologic egocentricity and incapacity for love, expressed by callousness, hedonism, and the absence of real loyalties to any person, group, or code	13. Impersonal, trivial, and poorly integrated sex life
	14. Failure to follow any life plan

(Modified with permission from Cleckley, H.: *The Mask of Sanity: An attempt to Clarify Some Issues About the So-Called Psychopathic Personality*, ed 3, St. Louis: Mosby, 1955.

when it redounds to the individual's advantage, is seen as manipulative or opportunistic. When the average person promises to repay a personal loan "very soon," he means in a matter of days or weeks, but the psychopath, reproached two years later, seems genuinely indignant as he explains that there was no precise time limit set.

Along with the disregard for social rules, many psychopaths show a remarkable *propensity for being caught.* Whether this represents some Dostoevskian need to be punished or results from the individual's failure to appreciate the nuances of social conventions and expectations is not known (Halleck 1966). It takes a relatively high level of abstract thinking to break the law successfully, however, and—despite their opinions to the contrary—psychopaths as a group have *no higher intelligence than the general population.* Nonetheless, the psychopath's *view that he is smarter than most people* cannot be completely disregarded. Undoubtedly, his freedom from the usual social inhibitions enables him to take and shift roles and positions with a rapidity that the average person would find impossible. The speed with which the confidence man finds just the right explanation for his victim's objections is indeed remarkable to observe, and it is an ability that can no longer be exercised by individuals who, in the process of aging, become less psychopathic. Nevertheless, the fairly frequent observation of such incidents as an individual's breaking into a liquor store at night, passing by the store the next morning to discuss the mysterious theft with the owner, and then "accidentally" dropping one of the stolen bottles from his coat pocket gives support to the theory that there may indeed be some "need to be caught" (Alexander 1930). The notion that many psychopaths hide an extreme degree of moral rigidity beneath their manifest amorality is made even more plausible by the observation that such individuals often become strong adherents of some puritanical cult when they experience a long-term remission.

Individuals manifesting *dyssocial behavior without manifest psychiatric disorder* as a consequence of a predatory occupation or adherence to the values of a deviant social group are believed to differ from those with an antisocial personality in their ability both to develop genuine interpersonal ties and to avoid conflict with the law. That an individual has a criminal occupation or belongs to a morally deviant group does not prove that he is dyssocial rather than antisocial, of course, for psychopaths as a rule are greatly attracted to criminal occupations and may go far out of their way to find or join morally deviant groups. The distinction lies rather in the success with which the individual pursues his endeavors, whatever they may be. The psychopath is generally so unstable and undependable that even the criminal or morally deviant group relegates him to a position of little importance or rejects him outright. The distinction between dyssocial and antisocial personalities is further underscored by the observation that individuals showing antisocial behavior before adolescence generally continue to do so thereafter, and almost never achieve the level of stability that would permit their behavior to be called merely dyssocial.

The individual engaged in a *group delinquent reaction* (which is, strictly speaking, a sociologic and not a psychiatric statement), on the other hand, is likely to have exhibited few antisocial symptoms until, during adolescence or young adulthood, he joins a subculture (like the "hippies" or a street gang) that openly disregards conventional social codes. Such individuals tend to engage in antisocial activities in response to the peer group's social pressure and its objections to the traditional social rules. That their activities are morally repugnant to the community at large does not deter the disaffected participants from viewing their way of life as satisfactory, particularly since their definition of success is likely to be as unconventional as their behavior (Haley 1969, Stojanovich 1969). In some cases, however, even when the individual seems totally committed to his new, untraditional way of life, he may abandon it as suddenly as he joined it and, perhaps wiser for the experience, return to his previous path.

The individual who habitually engages in *antisocial behavior involving physical violence* is not usually Cleckley's type of psychopath (unless drunk). He may be a dyssocial hoodlum functioning as his gang's paid "enforcer" or an individual with an explosive personality. That individuals engaging in episodically explosive and antisocial behavior can be further categorized is suggested by Gibbens' (1961) description of certain delinquent adolescents whom he calls *hysterical psychopaths,* whose antisocial behavior is periodic, who move from one dramatic crisis to another, are intelligent, cooperative, and almost too ready to admit that they are grossly unstable, commit pointless crimes bound to be detected, and punctuate their behavior with suicide attempts when things go wrong; and by Tong's (1960) description of individuals who exhibit abnormally high reactivity to stress, short-lived but profound disturbances in sleep and appetite, and agitated, panicky, or chronically anxious behavior, which may include suicidal gestures, physical violence, and sexual assaultiveness. Recent studies suggesting that aggressiveness, tall stature, and XYY chromosomes are often associated (Jacobs 1965, 1968, Price 1967) raise interesting questions concerning the role of genetic factors in the development of explosive and antisocial personalities. Chromosomal aberrations seem to be associated with so wide a variety of mental disorders, however, that the specificity of this constellation may be more apparent than real (Daly 1969, Hook 1970, Sundequist 1969).

That antisocial behavior has not been satisfactorily categorized and that different authors may thus use different terms (like antisocial, psychopathic, dyssocial, or explosive) to describe the same phenomena or, conversely, the same term (like antisocial) to describe different phenomena may account for the wide divergence of opinion concerning the cause, characteristics, and course of the "typical" disorder. Thus, while there may be some individuals who pursue a trouble-studded, antisocial existence without manifest anxiety or other signs of neurosis, the majority show a wide variety of neurotic symptoms and personality problems. In a retrospective study of children seen in a child guidance clinic 20 years before, Robins (1966) has documented that the more antisocial traits an individual displays, the more likely he is to have neurotic or somatic symptoms, and that these symptoms, like the antisocial traits, are likely to have been present ever since childhood. The individual who, as an adult, behaves antisocially may thus during his childhood have exhibited irritability, aggressiveness, difficulty in relating to his peers, lying, stealing, truancy, fire-setting, cruelty to animals, and teasing behavior toward younger children and, in addition, may have exhibited hyperkinesis, tics, nail-biting, thumbsucking, stuttering, sleep disturbances, enuresis (or encopresis), and specific learning deficits, particularly dyslexia (Jonsson 1967) (see also Chap. 10).

Even if a satisfactory phenomenologic categorization of antisocial behavior were achieved, it would not resolve the etiologic questions that, in this field as elsewhere in psychiatry, involve the relative significance of organic or environmental factors. Adverse environmental conditions (such as a broken home and particularly the absence of the father; being reared in an antisocial environment, in poverty, or by an alcoholic) are so often associated with antisocial behavior (Gregory 1965, Jonsson 1967) that they have been thought etiologically relevant. This may be too simple an explanation, however, for the parent who is antisocial or alcoholic or abandons his children may well have transmitted his unusual traits to the child as part of the latter's genetic endowment (Christiansen 1968, Heaton-Ward 1963). The role of organic factors is further supported by the observation that the antisocial individual (especially the violent one) is more likely than the general population to show neurologic dyfunctioning, to be illegitimate, to have been subjected to intrauterine trauma in the course of an unsuccessful abortion, to have received inferior pre- and postnatal care, and to exhibit signs of other mental disorders, especially paranoid ideation, mental retardation, and sexual psychopathology (Hertzig 1968, Miller 1969, Rochford 1970, Skelton 1969, Stott 1962). It is also known that individuals who exhibit antisocial behavior have a high incidence of first degree relatives who are alcoholics, drug addicts, or hysterics (Guze 1969); and that antisocial behavior occurs in individuals whose families and rearing environments are free of adversity (Oleinick 1966, Stevens 1969).

However the causal relationship is assessed, the individual's family situation is so unquestionably related to his subsequent behavior that it has become possible to identify with some accuracy the child who is likely to become delinquent (Tait 1969). Predictions based on Glueck's Prediction Table (see Table 16), which encompasses five interpersonal family factors, can, if applied at school entrance (five and a half to six years), discriminate with a high degree of accuracy between those children who will and those who will not subsequently become delinquent. That relatively accurate predictions can also be made for the child of two and a half to three years is particularly interesting because the factors on which the predictions at this age are based are partially biologic but may influence subsequent family relationships. As Glueck himself has put it (1966):

> the influences of the home environment, even when they are criminogenic, operate *selectively* to propel towards maladjustment and delinquency certain children who are characterised by specific traits

which enhance their vulnerability. Individuals differ in the degree of permeability or affinity to the elements in the social and cultural milieu in which they find themselves and to which they are subjected. It is the *concatenation* in the particular individual of factor-trait interpenetrations of these influences from divergent sources that determines whether, at a certain point of pressure, resistance to antisocial self-expression will break down.

TREATMENT OF ANTISOCIAL BEHAVIOR

The effort to provide psychotherapy for the individual with an antisocial personality disorder and thereby to modify his pathologic way of perceiving and responding to social order is usually doomed before it begins. In most cases, he attends only because of the pressure exerted by his family, employer, or probation officer. Such outside pressures may sometimes provide the extra impetus toward treatment that the individual himself has long thought necessary, but more often than not the help he requests is in truth the last thing he wants. Although psychopaths do seem to experience anxiety, neither the discomfort nor the negative social feedback to which they are exposed seems to promote the internalization of social rules and conventions that would be required to modify their behavior (Lykken 1957). Even when, as may occur after a crisis, the individual's anxiety about his behavior or its consequences is great enough to lead him to ask for help on his own, this desire usually dissipates as soon as his initial discomfort declines, and he soon falls back into the pattern of giving no thought to his past or future (Schmideberg 1961).

The psychopath's treatment course is as repeatedly punctuated by failure as his life is: he may fail to appear at the therapist's office because he becomes involved in some other activity while on the way or because he considers the therapist just another of the authority figures he has come to dislike. The psychopath rarely allows those around him to remain neutral toward him, and the physician almost invariably finds himself setting rigid limits on the patient's behavior, acting punitively, and thus propelling the patient out of treatment; or identifying with the patient to such an extent that he appears to condone, and thus to encourage, his antisocial behavior (Rosen 1965). Even when the therapist is flexible enough to adapt to the patient's changing needs, most psychopaths remain unable to view their lives as a meaningful sequence, to tolerate the frustration that therapy entails, or to meet such simple

TABLE 16. *The Glueck Prediction Tables for Identifying Potential Delinquents* *

FIVE-FACTOR TABLE TO IDENTIFY POTENTIAL DELINQUENTS AT 5½-6 YEARS

SCORE CLASS	DELINQUENCY RATE %	NONDELINQUENCY RATE %
Under 250	16.0	84.0
Over 250	79.1	20.9

Predictive Factors	Delinquency Scores
Discipline of boy by father	
Firm but friendly	9.3
Lax	59.8
Overstrict or erratic	71.0
Supervision of boy by mother	
Suitable	9.9
Fair	57.5
Unsuitable	83.2
Affection of father for boy	
Warm (including overprotective)	33.8
Indifferent or hostile	75.9
Affection of mother for boy	
Warm (including overprotective)	43.1
Indifferent or hostile	86.2
Cohesiveness of family	
Marked	20.6
Some	61.3
None	96.9

THREE-FACTOR TABLE TO IDENTIFY POTENTIAL DELINQUENTS AT 5½-6 YEARS

SCORE CLASS	DELINQUENCY RATE %	NONDELINQUENCY RATE %
Less than 140	8.6	91.4
140-200	58.2	41.8
200 or over	89.0	11.0

Predictive Factors	Delinquency Scores
Supervision of boy by mother	
Suitable	9.9
Fair	57.5
Unsuitable	83.2
Discipline of boy by mother	
Firm but kindly	6.1
Erratic	62.3
Overstrict	73.3
Lax	82.9
Cohesiveness of family	
Marked	20.6
Some	61.3
None	96.9

* (Modified with permission from Glueck, E. T., and Glueck, S.: Identification of potential delinquents at 2-3 years of age, Int J Soc Psychiat *12*:5-16, 1966).

TABLE 16. *The Glueck Prediction Tables for*
Identifying Potential Delinquents * (continued)

FIVE-FACTOR TABLE TO IDENTIFY POTENTIAL DELINQUENTS AT 2-3 YEARS

SCORE CLASS	DELINQUENCY RATE %	NONDELINQUENCY RATE %
Less than 225	11.1	88.9
225-275	48.8	51.2
275 or over	89.7	10.3

Predictive Factors	*Delinquency Scores*
Pathology of parents †	
Absent	17.7
Present	59.1
Attachment of parents to child	
Both attached	30.8
One or both indifferent or hostile	75.8
Extreme physiologic restlessness in childhood	
Absent	36.5
Present	66.5
Nonsubmissiveness of child to parental authority	
Absent	24.8
Present	78.0
Destructiveness of child	
No evidence	35.7
Evidence present	74.2

† Defined as evidence of alcoholism, delinquency, emotional disturbance, or mental retardation in one or both parents.

These tables are utilized by rating the patient on each factor, adding the delinquency scores next to each factor, determining the score class of the individual's total delinquency score, and determining the likelihood of delinquency in that score class.

requirements of the psychotherapeutic contract as promptness, regular attendance, and the payment of even a symbolic fee. Outpatient treatment is therefore usually not feasible, and the individual is eventually sent to a hospital, residential center, or jail by a frustrated psychiatrist or judge, at which time treatment proceeds under even franker duress.

Although some therapists object when the court or a law enforcement agency insists that the patient be treated in a residential setting, it has been shown both with criminals (Craft 1969, Stürup 1948) and with addicts that coercive measures enhance the success of treatment (see p. 317). Since the crucial ingredient of successful therapy is in all likelihood long-term exposure to adequate role models, treatment in a *residential setting* may indeed be the only way to ensure that the continuity of this exposure not be imperiled by the patient's being jailed or dropping out.

Individual psychotherapy may play some part in the patient's treatment, but most residential centers are more geared to work programs and discussion groups that focus on the patient's difficulties with peer relationships and authority figures. The individual's difficulties in day-to-day living with others suggest that the treatment setting should initially foster dependency and encourage autonomy only after his customary ways of coping with stress have been discouraged and new methods successfully introduced. Group work is usually combined with a flexible but directive educational approach, best described as a protracted exercise in acceptable social behavior. Insisting that the patient go through the motions of behaving like a "decent" and "civilized" person, even though he does not at first feel like or understand why he should be one, may, if repeated often enough, provide him with sufficient positive feedback to understand and appreciate that such behavior entails rewards. And this may in turn motivate further changes. These goals are by no means easy to achieve, for the only lesson the psychopath with his disordered time sense and lack of appreciation of consequences is capable of learning from his environment's disapproval is that antisocial behavior has deleterious *short-term consequences*. Since what he needs most to learn is that it also has deleterious *long-term consequences*, it is sometimes useful not to punish him immediately when he misbehaves but to postpone punishment until some arbitrarily selected time, days or perhaps even weeks later.

Despite its stresses, the residential treatment center, if properly organized, can provide the patient with an existential experience, a sense of belonging, and a feeling of competence much like that induced by hallucinogens or religious conversion, and thus so restructure his perception of the world around him as to change his behavior. To lead a group of this kind requires experience, flexibility, a capacity for rapport, and charisma far more than it requires medical training. Not surprisingly, the most successful residential centers are run by youth workers, social workers, or rehabilitated delinquents, who are not viewed as authority figures and are well-suited to promote self-criticism and reflection.

Keeping the patient in a residential setting is as difficult as keeping him in outpatient treatment, for psychopaths have an uncanny ability to form corrupt alliances in which they persuade their relatives, or even their therapists, to give them a "vote of confidence" by dismissing them from treatment. When the patient is a minor or has strong family ties, his family must be involved if untimely discharge is to be prevented. They should be instructed neither to take the patient back home nor to support him financially if he drops out, escapes, or otherwise sabotages his treatment. This instruction often falls on deaf ears, however, and the patient may soon be back home without having changed at all.

While the psychopath's short-term prognosis is fairly poor, his behavior often "matures out" by the time he is 40 (Glueck 1943, Robins 1966). If his psychopathic behavior is still prevalent at this time, it is likely to continue for the rest of his life. The outlook is somewhat brighter for the dyssocial individual who, despite having learned aberrant social rules, is capable of forming strong personal ties. Such individuals can change rapidly, if they find someone whom they like and with whom they can identify. Even in well-organized residential treatment centers, however, three quarters of the residents go on to have two or more reconvictions (Gibbens 1959, Hartelius 1965). The high relapse rate is an index of not only our ignorance concerning effective treatment but also our inability to predict outcome with enough precision to know just who should not be released (Stang 1967, Whittet 1968, Williams 1969). Because the individual with a history of assaultive behavior, alcoholism, seizures, or other evidence of neurologic disorders is known to be more likely to engage in future violence than the one whose crimes have been against property alone (Guze 1965, Skelton 1969), decisions concerning the release from confinement of the aggressive psychopath must take these elements of his history into account.

Pharmacotherapy and other biologic treatments are also of little help here. The possibility that some psychopaths suffer from altered brain functioning has been considered, following the observation that a significant number of subjects who behave in an antisocial manner have EEGs with 14 and 6 cycles per second positive spike patterns and other maturational defects (Gibbs 1951, Hill 1952). While there is general agreement that seizure disorders and other evidence of neurologic dysfunctioning are present in a significant percentage of individuals with antisocial personalities (McKerracher 1966, Sayed 1969), there is much doubt that the 14 and 6 patterns are uniquely diagnostic (Lombroso 1966, Wiener 1966) or that they represent an indication for anticonvulsant therapy (Klein 1967, Lefkowitz 1969). Nevertheless, patients with episodically occurring impulse control disturbances may occasionally benefit from 200 to 400 mg daily of diphenylhydantoin (Dilantin) (Boelhouwer 1968), even when they show no other evidence of seizure disorder. That psychopaths over 25 who have immature EEG patterns have a more favorable prognosis than those with a normal EEG (Gibbens

1959) seems paradoxical, but suggests that EEG immaturity signals a delayed maturational process that may still "catch up," a speculation that finds further support in the previously mentioned observation of a decline in antisocial behavior after the age of 40 (Cason 1946).

Recently, it has been suggested that the psychopath's constant, apparently senseless search for stimulation serves to counter a profound inner experience of sameness and emptiness and that his response to social order is akin to the normal person's response to a sensory deprivation experience (Quay 1965). Interestingly, this striving for excitement and affectively charged experience bears certain similarities to the behavior of some depressed adolescents and young adults who seek stimulation by cutting themselves with razors, engaging in drag racing, or playing "chicken," with the explanation that this makes them feel "alive" and "real." The boredom and dysphoria experienced by these patients is sometimes associated with obsessive personality features (McKerracher 1968, Rinzler 1968), in which case a three- to six-week course of high doses of antidepressants may be worth trying—since nothing else seems to help. The one notable exception in which drugs are useful in combating antisocial behavior is the patient with an explosive personality whose response to stress takes the form of bursts of aggressive or self-destructive behavior accompanied by anxiety and insomnia. These patients often improve markedly after a number of months on phenothiazines or reserpine. The possibility cannot be excluded that psychopharmacology, at some future date, may contribute to the treatment of personality disorders or that some biologic treatment measure will be found that will help restore adequate social functioning, either by altering stress reactivity or accelerating brain maturation. Far-fetched as this interesting speculation has sounded since it was first proposed (Ayd 1964), it must be remembered that our concept of schizophrenia has sustained no less profound a revision since the advent of psychopharmacology.

REFERENCES

Alexander, F.: Neurotic character, Int J Psychoanal 11:292-311, 1930.

Ayd, F. J.: Need for additional psychopharmaceutical drugs, J Neuropsychiat 5: 462-463, 1964.

Block, J.: Some reasons for the apparent inconsistency of personality, Psychol Bull 70:210-212, 1968.

Boelhouwer, C., Henry, C. E., and Glueck, B. C., Jr.: Positive spiking: Double blind control study on its significance in behavior disorders, both diagnostically and therapeutically, Amer J Psychiat *125:* 473-481, 1968.

Cason, H., and Pescor, M. J.: Statistical study of 500 psychopathic prisoners, Public Health Rep *61:*557-575, 1946.

Christiansen, K. O.: Threshold of tolerance in various population groups illustrated by results from Danish criminological twin study, *in* deReuck, A. V. S., and Porter, R., eds.: The Mentally Abnormal Offender, Boston: Little, 1968, pp. 107-120.

Cleckley, H.: The Mask of Sanity: An Attempt to Clarify Some Issues About the So-Called Psychopathic Personality, ed. 3, St. Louis: Mosby, 1955.

Coleman, J. V.: Social factors influencing the development and containment of psychiatric symptoms, *in* Scheff, T. J., ed.: Mental Illness and Social Processes, New York: Harper, 1967, pp. 158-168.

Craft, M.: Natural history of psychopathic disorder, Brit J Psychiat *115:*39-44, 1969.

Daly, R. F.: Mental illness and patterns of behavior in 10 XYY males, J Nerv Ment Dis, *149:*318-327, 1969.

Eliasoph, E.: Paradigm for differential groupings of male adolescent offenders, Berkshire Farm Monogr *1:*5-21, 1963.

Endler, N. S., and Hunt, J. McV.: Sources of behavioral variance as measured by the s-r inventory of anxiousness, Psychol Bull *65:*336-346, 1966.

Gibbens, T. C. N.: Treatment of psychopaths, J Ment Sci *107:*181-186, 1961.

Gibbens, T. C. N., Pond, D. A., and Stafford-Clark, D.: Follow-up study of criminal psychopaths, J Ment Sci *105:*108-115, 1959.

Gibbs, E. L., and Gibbs, F. A.: Electroencephalographic evidence of thalamic and hypothalamic epilepsy, Neurology (Minneap) *1:*136-144, 1951.

Glueck, E. T., and Glueck, S.: Identification of potential delinquents at 2-3 years of age, Int J Soc Psychiat *12:*5-16, 1966.

Glueck, S., and Glueck, E.: Criminal Careers in Retrospect, New York: Commonwealth Fund, 1943.

Gregory, I.: Anterospective data following childhood loss of a parent: I. Delinquency and high school dropout, Arch Gen Psychiat (Chicago) *13:*99-109, 1965.

Guze, S. B., and Cantwell, D. P.: Alcoholism, parole observations and criminal recidivism: Study of 116 parolees, Amer J Psychiat *122:*436-439, 1965.

Guze, S. B., Goodwin, D. W., and Crane, J. B.: Criminality and psychiatric disorders, Arch Gen Psychiat (Chicago) *20:*583-591, 1969.

Haley, J.: Amiable hippie: New form of dissent, Reflections (Merck Sharp and Dohme Publication) *4:*1-11, 1969.

Halleck, S.: Psychopathy, freedom and criminal behavior, Bull Menninger Clin *30:*127-140, 1966.

Hartelius, H.: Study of male juvenile delinquency, Acta Psychiat Scand *40* (Suppl 182):7-138, 1965.

Heaton-Ward, W. A.: Psychopathic disorder, Lancet *1:*121-123, 1963.

Hertzig, M. E., and Birch, H. G.: Neurologic organization in psychiatrically disturbed adolescents: Comparative consideration of sex differences, Arch Gen Psychiat (Chicago) *19:*528-537, 1968.

Heston, L. L.: Genetics of schizophrenic and schizoid disease, Science *167:*249-256, 1970.

Hill, D.: EEG in episodic psychotic and psychopathic behaviour: Classification of data, Electroenceph Clin Neurophysiol *4:* 419-442, 1952.

Hook, E. B., and Kim, D-S.: Prevalence of XYY and XXY karyotypes in 337 nonretarded young offenders, New Eng J Med *283:*410-411, 1970.

Jacobs, P. A., *et al.:* Agressive behaviour, mental subnormality and the XYY male, Nature *208:*1351-1352, 1965.

——: Chromosome studies on men in a maximum security hospital, Ann Hum Genet *31:*339-347, 1968.

Jonsson, G.: Delinquent boys, their parents and grandparents, Acta Psychiat Scand *43* (Suppl 195):1-264, 1967.

Klein, D. F., and Greenberg, I. M.: Behavioral effects of diphenylhydantoin in severe psychiatric disorders, Amer J Psychiat *124:*847-849, 1967.

Lefkowitz, M. M.: Effects of diphenylhydantoin on disruptive behavior, Arch Gen Psychiat (Chicago) *20:*643-651, 1969.

Lombroso, C. T., *et al.:* Ctenoids in healthy youths: Controlled study of 14- and 6-per-second positive spiking, Neurology (Minneap) *16:*1152-1158, 1966.

Lykken, D. T.: Study of anxiety in the sociopathic personality, J Abnorm Psychol *55:*6-10, 1957.

McKerracher, D. W., Loughnane, T., and Watson, R. A.: Self-mutilation in female psychopaths, Brit J Psychiat *114:*829-832, 1968.

McKerracher, D. W., Street, D. R. K., and Segal, L. J.: Comparison of the behaviour problems presented by male and female subnormal offenders, Brit J Psychiat *112:*891-897, 1966.

Miller, M. H.: Time and the character disorder, J Nerv Ment Dis *138:*535-540, 1964.

Miller, P. R.: Outcasts and conformers in a girls' prison, Arch Gen Psychiat (Chicago) *20:*700-708, 1969.

Oleinick, M. S., *et al.:* Early socialization experiences and intrafamilial environment, Arch Gen Psychiat (Chicago) *15:* 344-353, 1966.

Price, W. H., and Whatmore, P. B.: Behaviour disorders and pattern of crime among XYY males identified at a maximum security hospital, Brit Med J *1:*533-536, 1967.

Quay, H. C.: Psychopathic personality as pathological stimulation-seeking, Amer J Psychiat *122:*180-183, 1965.

Rinzler, C., and Shapiro, D. A.: Wrist-cutting and suicide, J Mount Sinai Hosp NY *35:*485-488, 1968.

Robins, L. N.: Deviant Children Grown Up: Sociological and Psychiatric Study of Sociopathic Personality, Baltimore: Williams & Wilkins, 1966.

Rochford, J. M., *et al.:* Neuropsychological impairments in functional psychiatric diseases, Arch Gen Psychiat (Chicago) *22:* 114-119, 1970.

Rosen, I. M.: Treatment of character disorders, Dis Nerv Syst *26:*221-224, 1965.

Sayed, Z. A., Lewis, S. A., and Brittain, R. P.: Electroencephalographic and psychiatric study of thirty-two insane murderers, Brit J Psychiat *115:*1115-1124, 1969.

Schipkowensky, N.: Affective disorders: Cyclophrenia and murder, *in* deReuck, A. V. S., and Porter, R. eds.: The Mentally Abnormal Offender, Boston: Little, 1968, pp. 59-75.

Schmideberg, M.: Psychotherapy of the criminal psychopath, Arch Crimin Psychodyn *4:*724-735, 1961.

Skelton, W. D.: Prison riot: Assaulters vs defenders, Arch Gen Psychiat (Chicago) *21:*359-362, 1969.

Small, I. F., *et al.:* Passive-aggressive personality disorder: Search for a syndrome, Amer J Psychiat *126:*973-983, 1970.

Stang, H. J.: Diagnostic and prognostic study of a material comprising abnormal Norwegian delinquents, Acta Psychiat Scand *43:*111-120, 1967.

Stevens, A., and Wehrheim, H. K.: Psychiatry and juvenile delinquency: Causative factors and treatment, Behav Neuropsychiat *1:*14-20, 1969.

Stojanovich, K.: Antisocial and dyssocial: Entities or shibboleths?, Arch Gen Psychiat (Chicago) *21:*561-567, 1969.

Stott, D. H.: Evidence for a congenital factor in maladjustment and delinquency, Amer J Psychiat *118:*781-794, 1962.

Stürup, G. K.: Management and treatment of psychopaths in a special institution in Denmark, Proc Roy Soc Med *41:* 765, 1948.

Sundequist, U., and Hellström, E.: Transmission of 47, XYY Karyotype?, Lancet *2:*1367, 1969.

Tait, C. D., and Hodges, E. F.: Potential delinquents followed all juvenile years, read at American Psychiatric Association Convention, Miami, Florida, May, 1969, Crime and Delinquency, to be published.

Tong J. E., and Murphy, I. C.: Review of stress reactivity research in relation to' psychopathology and psychopathic behavior disorders, J Ment Sci *106:*1273-1295, 1960.

Whittet, M. M.: Medico-legal considerations of the A9 murder, Brit J Med Psychol *41:*125-138, 1968.

Wiener, J. M., Delano, J. G., and Klass, D. W.: EEG study of delinquent and non-delinquent adolescents, Arch Gen Psychiat (Chicago) *15:*144-150, 1966.

Williams, D.: Neural factors related to habitual aggression: Consideration of differences between those habitual aggressives and others who have committed crimes of violence, Brain *92:*503-520, 1969.

CHAPTER
EIGHT

Sexual Disorders and Deviations

TRADITIONALLY, disturbances in the completion and enjoyment of the sexual act are classified with psychophysiologic disorders, while sexual deviations, perhaps because they have long been considered a manifestation of otherwise aberrant behavior, are classified with personality disorders. For the sake of convenience, however, we will discuss all types of sexual disturbance together in this chapter.

Until very recently, the community considered itself entitled to dictate its members' sexual behavior and was prepared to enforce its mores by prohibitions and punishments. More and more of the legal restrictions against untraditional sexual practices have been lifted in the past few years, but the attitude persists that certain practices, even if they are no longer a crime, are sick and that the individual and the behavior concerned are legitimate objects of medical concern. Many sexual deviations undoubtedly stem from, are associated with, or lead to social and psychological difficulties, but the fact that an individual engages in sexual behavior that deviates from the patterns the community overtly approves does not, in itself, suffice to label him mentally ill. The question is fortunately more theoretical than practical, for the individual with a sexual problem is usually seen by a psychiatrist only when he feels troubled about it, was troubled to start with, or when his behavior has disturbed his social adaptation and caused difficulties with his partner or with the law.

The interest in human sexuality that the psychiatric profession has expressed for decades has led it to welcome patients with sexual problems and given it a unique opportunity to study these problems and propose methods for their relief. It is thus with some sense of embarrassment that we acknowledge that the causes are understood no better today than they were a century ago. Moreover, even though the recommendation that the sexually troubled individual consult a psychiatrist is quickly at hand, the only thing known about the results of intervention is that most of the reports are at variance with each other.

THE NORMATIVE CONTINUUM

The intensity and direction of a person's sexual desires and the way in which they are expressed cannot be labeled simply normal or abnormal, but must be placed on a continuum. Very few people are always potent, invariably homosexual, or exclusively masochistic. There is probably no one who can have a satisfactory sexual relationship with *any* partner, in *any* manner, at *any* time. Some people are unwilling or unable to have a sexual relationship with anyone at any time, regardless of the manner. Others restrict their behavior —and sometimes their fantasies as well—to one sex or style, and many, of course, to a single partner. Given a particular partner or situation, one person is usually able to perform satisfactorily and with enjoyment, another may do so only rarely, and another not at all. The individual's sexual behavior is also influenced by his mood, his feelings toward and the willingness of the partner at hand, the availability of the partner he desires most, and his physical and psychological health. Ability is often—but not always—determined by desire, and both are further affected not only by external circumstances, light or darkness, nudity or clothing, danger of discovery or its absence, but also by the individual's sex, age, and culture (Parsons 1942, Whyte 1943), and the biological cycles that govern his or her moods.

Almost everyone has sexual interests that go beyond the ventro-ventral heterosexual coitus within marriage that society overtly considers acceptable. Moral training, fear of consequences, availability of willing partners, and information regarding techniques affect whether and to what extent these desires are fulfilled. The customs and tolerance of the environment, as well as the individual's attitude toward himself, will affect whether he or his environment see his behavior as a deviation or an offense. Kinsey, for example, has shown how imprecise the label *homosexual* is. Between adolescence and the age of 45, 50% of the men and 28% of the women he interviewed had been homoerotically aroused; 37% of the men and 13% of the women had had at least one orgastic homosexual experience; and 18% of the men and 8% of the women had had as much homosexual as heterosexual experience for a period of several years. However, only 4% of the men and 3% of the women had been exclusively homosexual throughout their lives (Kinsey 1948, 1953).

Much the same can be said for *fetishism,* which—especially in men—is a common component of sexual arousal. The mildest form entails only a heightened degree of attraction to a particular part

of the female body—eyes, breasts, or hair. In the individual designated a fetishist, this may be exaggerated to the extent that he can
be aroused by only a certain item of clothing, such as an article of
lingerie. In some cases, the individual attains maximal pleasure by
stealing the item from a shop or a clothesline, and his referral for
treatment results from his having been arrested.

The notion that all sexual behavior lies on a continuum is not
intended to suggest that there is no such thing as pathologic sexuality, but to emphasize that an individual's deviation from conventional sexual interests or practices can be defined as pathologic only
when he or his environment are dissatisfied with his situation or
his sexual behavior is clearly related to an underlying disease. In
some cases, the individual's dissatisfaction results solely from his
appreciation that his behavior is aberrant and his concern that this
proves he is sick; this can often be dispelled by providing him with
adequate information. In others, he is concerned with the impact his
behavior has or, if it were known, could have on those around him.

EXAMINATION

While the importance of the *medical history* and *physical examination* should not be overrated in cases of sexual dysfunctioning,
the psychiatrist must do what is necessary to identify those patients
whose further evaluation should be undertaken by the endocrinolo-
gist or urologist. Although the evidence presented for the hereditary
character of such sexual deviations as homosexuality (Heston 1968,
Kallman 1952) is equivocal, a *family history* should be obtained, as
the occurrence of similar deviations in other family members will
affect the way the patient is seen both by himself and by those
around him. It is even more important, however, to gather data
regarding the stability and harmony of the rearing environment, and
especially the presence or absence of an adequate, like-sexed person
with whom the patient was able to identify. Information concerning
the patient's *sexual development* is also of value: the age at which
heterosexual activity was initiated (if ever); the nature and extent
of the individual's dating habits, sexual behavior, and fantasies at
different ages during his life; the age at which the current problem
(or even a different one) first arose; whether his sexual desires or
behavior were ever different and, if so, what his life circumstances
were at such times. The patient's sexual history cannot be assessed
in a vacuum, however, but must be viewed in the context of his
general social functioning. When the individual's sexual difficulties

are linked (as often they are) with other behavioral aberrations, an attempt must be made to determine which is the chicken and which the egg or whether both are merely different aspects of an identical core disturbance. Since changes in an individual's sexual drive and an intensification of deviant patterns can result either from changes in his interpersonal relations or from functional and organic mental syndromes, a *social history* should be obtained and a thorough *mental status examination* performed on any patient whose sexual difficulties are of relatively recent origin.

IMPOTENCE, FRIGIDITY, AND INCREASED SEXUAL DESIRE

When a man is unable to engage in the sexual act to his own satisfaction, the cause may be a specific or general lack of interest or inability to tumesce, maintain an erection, ejaculate when he wants to, or experience an orgasm (Cooper 1969a). The inability to have or maintain an erection, which is the most narrow definition of the term impotence, may be attributable to *mechanical causes, the use of drugs* (such as alcohol, opioids, and other CNS depressants; ganglion blockers and other antihypertensive agents; antidepressants, phenothiazines, or estrogens) or a host of *endocrine, metabolic and CNS disorders,* such as hypogonadism, hypothyroidism, diabetes, chronic infection, hepatic disease, nutritional deficiencies, depressions, lesions of the brainstem or spinal cord, and peripheral neuropathies (Dingman 1969, Federman 1967, Jacobs 1948, McDowell 1968, Rubin 1967, Scheig 1969), but these account for less than 10% of the cases (Kaufman 1967). Aging is of course a prime cause of declining sexual interest and impotence (see Table 17). Because impotence occurs in many mental illnesses; because psychological inhibitions, consciously suppressed homoerotic desires (Cooper 1969b), and marital disharmony can lead to disinclination or impotence; and because many impotent men are episodically anxious as well (though not necessarily concomitantly), it is often assumed that most impotence is *psychogenic.* This assumption has so little foundation, however, that it would be more accurate to call impotence *cryptogenic* except in those cases where the effect of the individual's psychological state has been clearly established.

To some extent, the *treatment* of impotence depends on what is known of its etiology. A mechanical cause like phimosis can sometimes be treated specifically, as with circumcision, and a systemic one like testicular failure with replacement therapy. When the

TABLE 17. *Impotence and Aging*

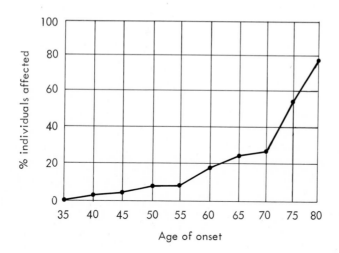

Kinsey, A. C., *et al.: Sexual Behavior in the Human Male,* Philadelphia: Saunders, 1948.

impotence is due to the individual's psychological inhibitions, the patient and sometimes his partner as well may benefit from sex education or psychotherapy. Marital disharmony can be either the precursor or the consequence of sexual problems. The episodically anxious man with episodic impotence sometimes needs only to be reassured that his disability is temporary, while his sexual partner is counseled to be patient and active in rearousing him, lest his fear of impotence diminish his sexual ability and set into motion a vicious cycle (Masters 1970). If such simple measures are not effective and the therapist suspects that the transactional pattern between the partners is disturbed, a detailed inquiry into the events that precede the unsuccessful attempts at sexual union may help the couple to understand the subtle ways in which they bring each other to mutual failure or contribute to the undermining of spontaneity. If even these measures fail, more intensive marital counseling or psychotherapy may be indicated.

The pharmacotherapy of impotence has so venerable a tradition that the concocters of aphrodisiacs may be considered the most ancient forebears of today's pharmaceutical chemists. The older aphrodisiacs—strychnine, yohimbine, and especially cantharides— were dangerous to use but often gave good results, for impotence tends to be transient, and almost any intervention can succeed for the first two or three nights when both physician and patient are confident that it will. While the same might be said for the treatment of premature ejaculation, there may be some truth in recent reports citing a higher success rate with thioridazine (Mellaril), 200 mg one hour before bedtime, than with placeboes (Doepfmer 1964, Singh 1963), particularly since such patients show marked autonomic lability and anxiety. Antidepressants may also be helpful, as decreased sexual interest, frigidity, and impotence occur in a high percentage of depressed subjects (Kral 1958). Testosterone has also been used in the treatment of impotence, but seems useful only when the disorder is secondary to androgen deficiency (Grumbach 1967).

What has been said of male impotence is with appropriate modifications generally applicable to the woman who complains of an inability to be sexually stimulated, except that birth control pills, structural or inflammatory diseases of the pelvis, and prolonged or painful delivery must be added to the list of causes (Brady 1967, Huffer 1970, Kane 1969). Furthermore, while most women consider orgasm an important criterion of satisfaction in the coital act, some place excessive importance on achieving it in each coital experience. Similar overemphasis may be given to the desire to reach climax simultaneously with the partner or without additional clitoral stimulation. Fortunately, many misconceptions, like the argument that a female requiring clitoral stimulation to achieve orgasm is "phallic" and suffers from a disturbance of feminine identity, have been disposed of by systematic investigation (Masters 1966). As in the treatment of impotence, meetings including both husband and wife may be indicated. An explanation of the anatomy and physiology of sexual behavior and of the numerous sexual techniques that can be used to enhance enjoyment may provide the couple an education they sorely need and help them to overcome certain inhibitions about discussing their sexual desires, expectations, and dissatisfactions. In some cases, the achievement of sexual satisfaction can be facilitated by relatively simple suggestions: more extended foreplay without pressure on either partner to proceed to coitus; mutual mapping out of each partner's erogenous zones during protracted caressing sessions; a more rostral male or a superior female position; oral and manual stimulation of the penis or of the clitoris and mons veneris as an integral part of coitus; or, when too rapid ejaculation by the male is part of the problem, firm pressure on the dorsal and ventral aspects of the coronal sulcus just before ejaculation. Unresponsive cases of impotence, especially if the partner's dissatisfaction has resulted in marital disharmony, may be helped by the use of splinted condoms (known as mechanotherapy) (Russell 1959). In other cases, the physician may suggest that the couple broaden their knowledge of sexual matters by reading about them. We have found *ABZ of Love* (Hegeler 1963) a helpful book for many patients who have been inhibited by misinformation.

While treatment and reeducation programs in which the measures listed above are reinforced by two weeks of daily discussions between both partners and a male-female therapist team have been reported to relieve impotence or frigidity in 80% of cases (Masters 1970), it is too early to know whether such results can be replicated in other centers, and optimism regarding the treatment of sexual inadequacy must be restricted to individuals whose difficulties are of less than two years' duration (Cooper 1970, Johnson 1968).

Whether the complaint of sexual dissatisfaction stems from the husband or the wife, it often conceals far more basic dissatisfactions and rivalries. Outright denial of sexual relations as a "punishment" for the partner's real or alleged misdeeds and the refusal to acknowledge pleasure from the sexual act are among the most common ways in which such rivalries are expressed. Not infrequently, a serious effort to explore marital difficulties is prefaced by talk of sexual incompatibility, which, after the second meeting, is never mentioned again. In such instances, neither explanation nor reassurance can help, and prolonged marital counseling is required.

A sudden *increase in sexual desire* without environmental events that might explain it is rarer than a sudden decline, but may occur in temporal lobe disorders (Falconer 1955, Poeck 1965) and mania, and after the use of such stimulants as amphetamines or cocaine (see p. 319). The paranoid patient with morbid jealousy may also increase his sexual activity, often with the rationalization of trying to cause his or her spouse to be so satiated that the imagined extramarital excursions cease. While the average frequency of sexual outlet for the married person in his mid-twenties seems to be approximately three to four times weekly, this figure is subject to so many influences and to such wide variations in the normal person that only recent increases can be taken into account in assessing what may be pathologic. Such concepts as satyriasis or nymphomania, describing above-average sexual desire and frequency in a man or woman, are usually moral rather than diagnostic; they are most often held by a spouse with a lower level of sexual desire, or, especially regarding women, reflect a puritanical environment.

DEVIATIONS IN THE CHOICE OF
SEXUAL ACTIVITY OR OBJECT

The circumstances under which the sexual deviate sees the psychiatrist, his motives for doing so, and his own view of his aberration all have an important effect on the course of treatment. In most cases, the patient is referred by a court for assessment or treatment after he has been apprehended for his conduct; in others, he will be referred by his attorney, in which case the intent is as frequently to impress the court with the seriousness of the individual's determination to change as it is to obtain treatment. Factors of this kind determine who the psychiatrist sees and thus the reported incidence of certain practices. The fact that the laws do not generally forbid female homosexual practices and are seldom enforced even when they do may have as much to do with the observation that psychiatrists see three times as many male as female homosexuals as the fact that the incidence of homosexual behavior is lower in women than in men (Kinsey 1953). Similarly, social mores being what they are, a woman who wants a diversity of sexual experiences and partners (even if temporarily, as may occur during a manic episode) is far more likely to encounter social difficulties and be referred to a psychiatrist than is a man of similar propensities.

Some individuals complain of deviant inclinations that they do not in fact consummate. An individual may be concerned that he will expose himself in public or that he is "really" a homosexual without ever having engaged in such practices and be so overwhelmed by these concerns that he is not only sexually but socially disabled. When such preoccupations persist, even after thorough discussion with a psychiatrist, they may well be symptomatic of an obsessive-compulsive neurosis or the first sign of a schizophrenic decompensation.

The sexual deviate may consult a psychiatrist because of *internal discomfort* about his condition but more commonly out of concern about its *social consequences*. The homosexual may fear being arrested or being found out by nonhomosexual colleagues and friends. Some sexual deviates confine their abnormal behavior to the performance of the sexual act, while others permit their sexual interests to dominate their entire lives. This latter pattern is best illustrated by the homosexual who devotes a major portion of his time and energy to frequenting homosexual bars, reading books concerning the topic, or using it as a conversational theme, whether with self-justification, self-pity, or such claims as that seven out of ten named historical figures were in truth subject to the same aberrant behavior. Some homosexuals, but perhaps no more than heterosexuals, distinguish themselves by the frequency with which they change partners: some apparently have sexual congress with dozens or even hundreds of new partners within the space of a year.

While there is a slightly higher prevalence of suicide attempts and excessive drinking among female homosexuals (Saghir 1970a), most homosexuals and many other sexual deviates show no disorder in their thinking, demonstrate insight into the unusual character of their life style, are occupationally productive and socially inconspicuous, consider themselves emotionally and sexually satisfied (De Luca 1966, Hopkins 1969, Saghir 1969a, 1969b, 1970b), and can scarcely be considered in need of treatment. Others are troubled by their situation and wish they could change, but no matter how clear their insights or how strong their therapist's urging or their own resolutions may be, continue (like the repentant drug addict—and sometimes with the same nonsensical rationalizations) to frequent the typical hangouts and to engage in flirtations and other activities that can only end with a repetition of the behavior they allegedly want to avoid. The *voyeur,* or "peeping Tom," who complains that his urge simply "drove the car to the left when my home is to the right," and is advised to have his wife pick him up at work each afternoon so that he will not succumb to the urge, will usually present a host of objections to this plan: he is afraid his co-workers will ridicule him; he does not want to tell his wife; he doesn't trust his wife's driving; the whole plan is too inconvenient. And, failing to heed the recommendation, he is soon again caught in a stranger's backyard and imprisoned.

The *results of treatment* are as varied as the goals that are set: avoidance of imprisonment or public scandal; overcoming social isolation; improved self-esteem despite continuation of the aberrant behavior; pursuit of the aberration within a monogamous or emotionally meaningful relationship; improved social comfort and skill; diminution or avoidance of aberrant behavior; partial, equal, or primary use of more traditional sexual patterns; or heterosexual marriage and the establishment of a family. Since the extent of change required to call treatment a success varies from one therapist to the next, and because individuals may for years pursue one type of sexual practice and then, with or without understandable reason, pursue another, statistics on "success" are difficult to assess. The cure rates reported for male homosexuality, for example, range from the 27% reported by Bieber (1962), who considers it possible to alter completely the sexual orientation of some homosexuals in long-term therapy, downward to results ,that do not exceed random changes (Freund 1960). Similar results have been reported in the treatment of female homosexuals (Kaye 1967).

Certain *factors* have been identified *that predispose the patient to change* toward more traditional patterns and. from the beginning alert the therapist to this prospect. The prospects for change increase to the degree that

1/ the individual is young,
2/ he remains in continuous treatment,
3/ his aberration has been of brief duration,
4/ he wants to change,
5/ he has previously engaged in traditional sexual behavior,
6/ his aberration is not obvious,
7/ he seeks to keep it hidden, and
8/ his aberration corresponds to the traditional patterns of his sex (as when the individual is the active male homosexual partner or the passive lesbian).

These differences may, of course, signify only that the aberration is relatively mild, and the better response to treatment should therefore occasion no surprise.

Whether and to what extent even the "successes" succeed is, however, an open question, for the patient may well be dissatisfied with his new life style. Particularly when the apparent success or, worse yet, the therapist's advice has led the patient to marry and even to have children, he may find himself in a union that his scruples prevent him from dissolving, but in which he is unable to achieve emotional or sexual gratification. The traditional marital role he is expected to fulfill may disgust him; even if his spouse makes no sexual demands, he may come to feel inadequate; and eventually he may consider his situation so catastrophic that the only "honorable" solution he sees is suicide.

Since many sexually deviant individuals are not only socially isolated but fear intimacy as well, a combination of *group and individual therapy* can be helpful. The composition of such groups has been widely discussed, but without conclusion. There is dispute, for example, over whether it is preferable to place the homosexual in a group that also has heterosexual members and thus permits a discussion of his total life style rather than just his aberrant sexual behavior (Mintz 1966) or whether he should be placed in an exclusively homosexual group (Hadden 1966). Other treatment attempts include direct suggestion and the so-called "behavior therapies" like *conditioning,* in which the difficulties encountered in each step toward normal sexual behavior are discussed and mastered in tiny increments; and *aversion techniques,* in which the patient is exposed to a painful or unpleasant stimulus together with a stimulus he would otherwise have enjoyed (Feldman 1964, Rachman 1961). These measures have also had little lasting success (Bancroft 1969). *Prison sentences* may protect the community from the deviate's socially repugnant behavior, but do little to change his proclivities. Prisons rarely provide adequate psychotherapeutic care except on paper, and the proximity of many individuals of the same sex in the absence of the other makes them an ideal training ground for homosexuality rather than a dissuading force (Banay 1968).

Pharmacologic treatment, as with phenothiazines (Bartholomew 1968) or estrogens (Whitaker 1959), may diminish sexual desire and thus facilitate a protracted discussion of the problem, but will not by itself alter the direction of sexual interest. Chemical castration can also produce a diminution of sexual interest of inconstant effectiveness. Surgical castration has also been used (Bremer 1959), but is irreversible and mutilating and may cause severe psychological complications, including brief episodes of psychotic decompensation (Wolf 1934). Procedures of this kind must therefore be limited to patients whose aberration is so injurious to the community (intractable sadists, rapists, or pedophiles) that they ask to have their behavior changed at any cost (Stürup 1968). Since treatment is of little benefit, the psychiatrist's most important way of helping such individuals is to *educate the community at large* about deviant behavior, thus helping to vitiate the public opprobrium it arouses. The community's attitude stems not only from its moral repugnance but also from its belief that the sexual deviate is dangerous and possibly assaultive, particularly toward children. These beliefs initiate and maintain a cycle in which the deviate feels isolated, inadequate, and in danger of incarceration and even blackmail, except when associating with the deviant subculture that defensively supports and reinforces his deviation.

One stereotype that arouses the community's concern and imagination with particular vigor is that of the *pedophile,* generally pictured as a demented, middle-aged or elderly stranger, who repeatedly entices helpless children into his car, where he forcibly assaults and penetrates them, thereafter mutilating or even murdering them. Mohr and his associates (1964) have shown, however, that this stereotype is inaccurate in every detail. The intelligence and education of the "typical" offender are in the normal range, and he is more likely to be in his mid-thirties or adolescence than in his late fifties or early sixties. (The adolescent pedophile is labeled more by statute than by good sense, for the typical case entails the 18-year-old boy who is apprehended for having relations with a willing 15-year-old girl.) Most decidedly, the average pedophile is no stranger: 60% to 80% of the offenders are known to the child as a neighbor, family friend, relative, or storekeeper (CSDR 1953). Recidivism studies do not support the idea that the offender's behavior is necessarily repetitive: only 10% to 25% of the pedophiles (homosexuals twice as often as heterosexuals) are reconvicted for the same behavior (Frisbie 1965), and 80% to 90% of the offenses are the first such episodes. Compared to the first offender, however, the individual with a previous record of arrest or conviction (whether for a different sexual offense or some other illegal activity) is far more likely to repeat his sexual offense. The public stereotype also fails to recognize that the average exhibitionist, voyeur, or pedophile is steadily employed, married, and has children of his own. The child, moreover, is rarely as totally ingenuous or helpless as in the stereotype; the older the child, the more likely he is to have consented or even participated actively (CSDR 1954). The majority of acts take place in the home of the victim or the offender and less than a fifth in the offender's car. The nature of the sexual acts depends more on the age and physical maturity of the child than on the pedophile's desire: few offenders (but again more of the homosexual ones) try to penetrate the child; most limit themselves to manual or oral fondling, exposure, and masturbation, especially when the child is prepubertal. How damaging such episodes are is unknown; some authorities believe that the resultant court procedures and police interrogation are a good deal more traumatic for the child than the act itself, which is otherwise quickly forgotten (Mohr 1968).

We do not mean by these comments to recommend the sexual offender as a social companion or babysitter nor to deny that there are individuals who commit sexual offenses repeatedly and represent a danger to the community, but we do want to emphasize that sexual crimes involving violence are extremely rare and committed almost exclusively by individuals suffering from other (usually easily recognizable) mental illnesses (Kivisto 1958). The evaluation of the psychotic sexual offender must obviously proceed with great caution, for even if he recovers from the current episode, he may repeat such behavior should he fall ill again. The danger

of violence is particularly grave when the individual's illness progresses so rapidly that it cannot be checked promptly; when he is
under the influence of delusions or hallucinations and thus unable
to take preventive action; or when his preferred victims are so young
that they are defenseless (Kozol 1966).

Since many pedophiles are socially isolated, group therapy may
be of some value, but what sparse evidence exists suggests that
treatment makes no overall difference in their course: more precisely, heterosexual pedophiles repeat their behavior more frequently and homosexual pedophiles less frequently after treatment.

The highest incidence of recidivism among sexual offenders occurs
in the *exhibitionist,* the individual who repeatedly exposes his
genitalia or starts to masturbate before strangers. While the fright
and potential psychological effect on the victim (almost invariably
a female) should not be minimized, the exhibitionist's behavior
is more a nuisance than a source of physical danger, for he almost
never makes any further advance. His purpose is not (as he may
claim) to excite and thus seduce his victim or (as she may fear)
to proceed to a sexual assault, but merely to see her look of shock
before he or she flees. Since the majority of offenses are not
reported and the majority of offenders neither apprehended nor
convicted, the frequency of reconviction reflects an even higher
prevalence of this behavior. Indeed, the frequency with which small
girls and young women are exposed to such behavior depends only
on the amount of time they spend in parks, public conveyances,
or other semideserted places typically frequented by exhibitionists.
Treatment by psychoanalysis (Karpman 1948), group therapy
(Turner 1961), and deconditioning (Bond 1960) have been
recommended, but the only large-scale study (Mohr 1964) showed
little difference in outcome between treated and untreated offenders. This study's finding that exhibitionists who exposed to adult
females stayed in treatment twice as long and relapsed half as often
as those who exposed to children is consonant with the general
principle that the more nearly the deviant behavior approaches the
norm, the more likely it is to recede.

Transvestism is a form of sexual deviation in which an individual
derives gratification from dressing in the clothes of the opposite
sex. This deviation is often so mild that it comes to the physician's
attention only as an incidental finding, as in the case of the man
who occasionally asks his wife to let him wear her clothes during
the sexual act. In extreme cases, the individual may be unable to
achieve sexual gratification in any other way.

It is not known whether and to what extent transvestism is

related to *transsexualism,* in which an individual feels, despite all physical or genetic evidence to the contrary, that he is inherently of the opposite sex. He may consult a physician to determine what sex he "really" is, but the answer may not be as easy to come by as one might think, for it involves distinguishing between chromosomal, gonadal, hormonal, and morphologic sexuality and must also take into account the sex role assigned to the individual by his rearing environment, the one he currently plays, and the one he feels (Money 1955, 1964, Newman 1970).

In mild cases, behavior therapy may be of some help (Lavin 1961, Thorpe 1964), but in severe ones, the individual's entire functioning is colored by his concern about this topic. Individuals of this kind may change their names, occupations, and clothes to conform to the sex they wish, or believe themselves to be, without in any way considering this a masquerade; and some even go so far as to mutilate themselves to effect their transformation. Not surprisingly, they are almost invariably "homosexual" in their desires, though obviously unable to perform as they would wish. In some cases, the individual feels he will find no peace until he can physically change his sex and comes to the physician for advice on how to accomplish this. Surgical techniques that can fulfill such wishes have become sophisticated in recent years, and it is now possible not only to castrate and penectomize the male transvestite but to construct an artificial vagina (Jones 1968) with which he can achieve orgasm in his new sexual role (Masters 1966) and, via mammoplasty and estrogen administration, provide certain of the secondary sex characteristics, though not fully without hazard as shown by two recently reported cases of breast cancer (Symmers 1968). Similarly, an artificial penis can be constructed for the female with the preservation of orgastic capacity (Benjamin 1967a). The psychological effects of such operations are often quite salutary. If the patient is otherwise reasonably well-adjusted, a sex-change operation, together with appropriate endocrine management, may indeed help him to achieve the satisfaction he expects and alleviate his disconcerting and paralyzing ruminations about sexual identity (Benjamin 1967b, Edgerton 1970, Green 1966, Pauly 1968).

REFERENCES

Banay, R. S.: Sex in prison, Med Asp Hum Sex 2:30-36, 1968.

Bancroft, J.: Aversion therapy of homo-sexuality, Brit J Psychiat *115*:1417-1431, 1969.

Bartholomew, A. A.: Long-acting phenothiazine as a possible agent to control deviant sexual behavior, Amer J Psychiat *124*:917-923, 1968.

Benjamin, H.: Transvestism and transsexualism in male and female, J Sex Res *3*:107-127, 1967a.

———: Transexual phenomenon, Trans NY Acad Sci *29*:428-430, 1967b.

Bieber, I., *et al.:* Homosexuality: Psychoanalytic Study, New York: Basic, 1962.

Bond, I. K., and Hutchison, H. C.: Application of reciprocal inhibition therapy to exhibitionism, Canad Med Ass J *83*:23-25, 1960.

Brady, J. P.: Frigidity, Med Asp Hum Sex *1*:42-48, 1967.

Bremer, J.: Asexualization: Follow-up Study of 244 Cases, New York: Macmillan, 1959.

Cooper, A. J.: Factors in male sexual inadequacy: Review, J Nerv Ment Dis *149*:337-359, 1969a.

———: Sex drive and male potency disorders, Psychosomatics *10*:230-235, 1969b.

———: Frigidity, treatment and short-term prognosis, J Psychosom Res *14*:133-147, 1970.

CSDR (California Sexual Deviation Research): Preliminary Report, January 1953, State of California, Department of Mental Hygiene, the Langley-Porter Clinic, Sacramento.

———: Final Report, March 1954, *Ibid.*

DeLuca, J. N.: Structure of homosexuality, J Project Techn *30*:187-191, 1966.

Dingman, J. F.: Endocrine aspects of impotence, Med Asp Hum Sex *3*:57-66, 1969.

Doepfmer, R.: Über eine neuartige Behandlung der Ejaculatio praecox, München Med Wschr *106*:1103-1107, 1964.

Edgerton, M. T., Knorr, N. J., and Callison, J. R.: Surgical treatment of transsexual patients: Limitations and indications, Plast Reconstr Surg *45*:38-46, 1970.

Falconer, M. A., *et al.:* Treatment of temporal lobe epilepsy by temporal lobectomy: Survey of findings and results, Lancet *1*:827-835, 1955.

Federman, D. D.: Disorders of sexual development, New Eng J Med *277*:351-360, 1967.

Feldman, M. P., and MacCulloch, M. J.: Systematic approach to the treatment of homosexuality by conditioned aversion: Preliminary report, Amer J Psychiat *121*:167-171, 1964.

Freund, K.: Some problems in the treatment of homosexuality, *in* Eysenck, H. J., ed.: Behavior Therapy and the Neuroses: Readings in Modern Methods of Treatment Derived from Learning Theory, Oxford: Pergamon, 1960, pp. 312-326.

Frisbie, L. V., and Dondis, E. H.: Recidivism among treated sex offenders, California Mental Health Research Monograph No. 5, State of California, Department of Mental Hygiene, 1965.

Green, R., Stoller, R. J., and MacAndrew, C.: Attitudes toward sex transformation procedures, Arch Gen Psychiat (Chicago) *15*:178-182, 1966.

Grumbach, M. M.: Gonads: Sex determination and sex differentiation, *in* Beeson, P. B., and McDermott, W., eds.: Cecil-Loeb Textbook of Medicine, Philadelphia: Saunders, 1967, pp. 1320-1336.

Hadden, S. B.: Treatment of male homosexuals in groups, Int J Group Psychother *16*:13-22, 1966.

Hegeler, I., and Hegeler, S.: ABZ of Love, D. Hohnen (trans.), New York: Medical Press of New York, 1963.

Heston, L. L., and Shields, J.: Homosexuality in twins, Arch Gen Psychiat (Chicago) *18*:149-160, 1968.

Hopkins, J. H.: Lesbian personality, Brit J Psychiat *115*:1433-1436, 1969.

Huffer, V., Levin, L., and Aronson, H.: Oral contraceptives: Depression and frigidity, J Nerv Ment Dis *151*:35-41, 1970.

Jacobs, E. C.: Effects of starvation on sex hormones in males, J Clin Endocr *8*:227-232, 1948.

Johnson, J.: Disorders of Sexual Potency in the Male, New York: Pergamon, 1968.

Jones, H. W., Jr., Schirmer, H. K. A., and Hoopes, J. E.: Sex conversion operation for males with transsexualism, Amer J Obstet Gynec *100*:101, 1968.

Kallman, F. J.: Comparative twin study on the genetic aspects of male homosexuality, J Nerv Ment Dis *115*:283-298, 1952.

Kane, F. J., Jr., Lipton, M. A., and Ewing, J. A.: Hormonal influences in female sexual response, Arch Gen Psychiat (Chicago) *20*:202-209, 1969.

Karpman, B.: Psychopathology of exhibitionism: Review of the literature, J Clin Psychopath *9*:179-225, 1948.

Kaufman, J. J.: Urologic factors in impotence and premature ejaculation, Med Asp Hum Sex *1*:43-48, 1967.

Kaye, H. E.: Homosexuality in women, Arch Gen Psychiat (Chicago) *17*:626-634, 1967.

Kinsey, A. C., Pomeroy, W. B., and

Martin, C. E.: Sexual Behavior in the Human Male, Philadelphia: Saunders, 1948.

Kinsey, A. C., et al.: Sexual Behavior in the Human Female, Philadelphia: Saunders, 1953.

Kivisto, P.: Treatment of sex offenders in California, Ment Hyg 42:78-80, 1958.

Kozol, H. L., Cohen, M. I., and Garofalo, R. F.: The criminally dangerous sex offender, New Eng J Med 275:79-84, 1966.

Kral, V. A.: Masked depression in middle aged men, Canad Med Ass J 79:1-5, 1958.

Lavin, N. I., et al.: Behavior therapy in a case of transvestism, J Nerv Ment Dis 133:346-353, 1961.

Masters, W. H., and Johnson, V. E.: Human Sexual Response, Boston: Little, 1966.

——: Human Sexual Inadequacy, Boston: Little, 1970.

McDowell, F. H.: Sexual manifestations of neurologic disease, Med Asp Hum Sex 2:13-21, 1968.

Mintz, E. E.: Overt male homosexuals in combined group and individual treatment, J Consult Psychol 30:193-198, 1966.

Mohr, J. W.: A child has been molested, Med Asp Hum Sex 2:43-50, 1968.

Mohr, J. W., Turner, R. E., and Jerry, M. B.: Pedophilia and Exhibitionism, Toronto: Univ of Toronto Press, 1964.

Money, J., Hampson, J. G., and Hampson, J. L.: Examination of some basic sexual concepts: Evidence of human hermaphroditism, Bull Hopkins Hosp 97:301-319, 1955.

Money, J., and Pollitt, E.: Cytogenetic and psychosexual ambiguity: Klinefelter's syndrome and transvestism compared, Arch Gen Psychiat (Chicago) 11:589-595, 1964.

Newman, L. E.: Transsexualism in adolescence. Problems in evaluation and treatment, Arch Gen Psychiat (Chicago) 23: 112-121, 1970.

Parsons, T.: Age and sex in the social structure of the United States (1942), reprinted in Stein, H. D., and Cloward, R. A., eds.: Social Perspectives on Behavior, Glencoe (Ill): Free Press, 1958, pp. 191-200.

Pauly, I. B.: Current status of the change of sex operation, J Nerv Ment Dis 147: 460-471, 1968.

Poeck, K., and Pilleri, G.: Release of hypersexual behaviour due to lesion in the limbic system, Acta Neurol Scand 41: 233, 1965.

Rachman, S.: Sexual disorders and behavior therapy, Amer J Psychiat 118:235-240, 1961.

Rubin, A.: Sexual behavior in diabetes mellitus, Med Asp Hum Sex 1:23-25, 1967.

Russell, G. L.: Impotence treated by mechanotherapy, Proc Roy Soc Med 52: 872-874, 1959.

Saghir, M. T., and Robins, E.: Homosexuality: I. Sexual behavior of the female homosexual, Arch Gen Psychiat (Chicago) 20:192-201, 1969a.

Saghir, M. T., Robins, E., and Walbran, B.: Homosexuality: II. Sexual behavior of the male homosexual, Arch Gen Psychiat (Chicago) 21:219-229, 1969b.

Saghir, M. T., et al.: Homosexuality: III. Psychiatric disorders and disability in the male homosexual, Amer J Psychiat 126:1079-1086, 1970a.

——: Homosexuality. IV. Psychiatric disorders and disability in the female homosexual, Amer J Psychiat 127:147-154, 1970b.

Scheig, R.: Sexual sequelae of liver disease, Med Asp Hum Sex 3:137-145, 1969.

Singh, H.: Therapeutic use of thioridazine in premature ejaculation, Amer J Psychiat 119:891, 1963.

Stürup, G. K.: Treatment of sexual offenders in Herstedvester, Denmark, Acta Psychiat Scand 44 (Suppl 204):5-62, 1968.

Symmers, W. St. C.: Carcinoma of breast in transsexual individuals after surgical and hormonal interference with the primary and secondary sex characteristics, Brit Med J 2:83-85, 1968.

Thorpe, J., Schmidt, E., and Castell, D.: Comparison of positive and negative (aversive) conditioning in the treatment of homosexuality, Behav Res Ther 1:357-362, 1964.

Turner, R. E.: Group treatment of sexual deviation, Canad J Correct 4:485-491, 1961.

Whitaker, L. H.: Oestrogen and psychosexual disorders, Med J Aust 2:547-549, 1959.

Whyte, W. F.: Slum code (1943), reprinted in Stein, H. D., and Cloward, R. A., eds.: Social Perspectives on Behavior, Glencoe (Ill): Free Press, 1958, pp. 441-448.

Wolf, C.: Die Kastration bei sexuellen Perversionen und Sittlichkeitsverbrechen des Mannes, Basel: Benno Schwabe and Co., 1934.

CHAPTER

NINE

Drug Dependence,
Addiction, and Abuse

THE COMMON DENOMINATOR of a wide range of apparently unrelated behavior patterns is the illegal, socially disruptive, or
medically harmful use of drugs that are pleasurable, relieve anxiety, or, in some other way, affect the individual's perception or
attitude toward life. Efforts to distinguish between different types
of drug users or different patterns of drug use by labeling some
drug dependence, some *drug addiction,* and others *drug abuse* are
of so little clinical value that the terms have come to be used interchangeably. Users come from all economic strata and from all segments of the psychiatric spectrum; the drugs they use, the way
they use them, and the way they get them vary so widely that the
only thing such uses have in common is their lack of medical or
social sanction. As examples in point:

—the young dweller of the Negro ghetto who has taken heroin
regularly since early adolescence and devotes the bulk of his time to
various types of larceny in order to obtain the wherewithal for his
daily dose;
—the alcoholic executive who functions well between bouts with
the bottle, but whose habit constantly raises the specter of lost employment and a broken family;
—the middle-class housewife who, after being given amphetamines
by her family doctor for obesity, discovers she enjoys the effects and
continues to take them;
—the high school or college student who has experimented with
marijuana or LSD, but has no compelling urge to continue.

While there are, strictly speaking, almost as many patterns of
drug use as there are users, a list of the primary factors determining
the nature of drug abuse in the individual case would be relatively
short and include:

1/ The propensity of the agent or agents used to give rise to tolerance and physical dependence.

2/ The individual's willingness, or even eagerness, to experiment with a drug and to continue using it, either immediately or at some later time.

3/ The frequency with which the drug is used.

4/ The drug's effects on the individual's mood, cognitive functioning, occupational competence, and relationships with his family and peers.

5/ The medical hazards to which the individual is exposed each time he uses the drug (acute intoxication) or, after protracted use, withdraws from it (abstinence syndrome).

6/ The psychosocial or medical consequences to which the individual is subject following long-term drug use.

7/ The means, expense, and legality of procuring the drug.

8/ The attitudes, held by both society at large and the individual's own subculture, toward the use of the drug.

1. Tolerance may be said to exist when repeated administration of a given dose of a drug produces a decreasing effect or, stated conversely, when increasingly larger doses must be administered to produce the effects experienced with the original dose. The term *physical dependence* refers to a drug-induced alteration in the individual's physiologic state that manifests itself, when the drug is reduced or withdrawn, in a stereotyped set of physical or psychological changes (usually of discomfort) that can—at least initially—, be reversed by administering more of the original drug.

That tolerance and physical dependence are at least partly caused by the development of biologic mechanisms antagonistic to the drug's original effects is suggested by several observations:

a) The withdrawal symptoms that are indicative of physical dependence on a given drug are generally the opposite of its usual effects. Withdrawal of sedatives is thus followed by excitement, and withdrawal of stimulants by drowsiness and fatigue.

b) Drugs with similar effects (even if of dissimilar composition) tend to give rise to similar abstinence syndromes.

c) Individuals who have become tolerant to one drug are usually tolerant to other drugs that have the same effects, even if the composition of the two drugs is dissimilar (cross-tolerance).

d) Most of the symptoms that result from abruptly withdrawing a given agent can be relieved by giving another drug of the same group (cross-dependence).

A drug's ability to induce tolerance and physical dependence is by no means a *necessary* condition for abuse, since agents lacking these properties are also abused. Nor is it a *sufficient* condition: despite all the uproar about iatrogenic addiction, most people who take a potentially addicting drug over an extended period of time for some specific medical reason stop taking it as soon as the physician stops prescribing it. Nevertheless, after a drug that produces tolerance is used for some time, it is probably being taken in such high doses that, if it also causes physical dependence, the user will have a physiologically reinforced reminder of his need for the drug whenever he starts to withdraw and become increasingly afraid of doing so. This reason for continuing a drug is especially common in the individual who started to take drugs because of his sensitivity to discomfort and his experience that the drug in question relieves it.

2. The individual's *willingness* to experiment with a particular type of drug when given the opportunity, and his *proclivity* to continue its use thereafter or to resume using it after a prolonged period of abstinence, depend in part on the myriad factors subsumed under the vague term *personality*. The notion that drug abusers share certain personality traits that, taken together, could be designated an *add ctive personality* has foundered on the difficulties involved in singling out such traits. To be sure, evidence exists that individuals who use drugs that interfere with their life plans and eventually get them into trouble were often unable to plan ahead and in trouble before resorting to drugs; and that many individuals who are chronically anxious, shy, or depressed enjoy and eventually abuse drugs that relieve these traits. However, there is, at present, no way to predict who, if given the opportunity, will start to abuse drugs or what kind of drug a given individual is most likely to abuse. The individual's socioeconomic situation, rearing, and the resultant social attitudes will all contribute to his decision to take a particular drug or to take drugs at all, but so will a number of other factors, such as his physical condition or state of mind when he first encounters a given drug, the social pressure exerted by drug-using peers, and the local availability of the drug in question. That heroin use is more prevalent among the poor than it is among the middle class cannot be fully explained, then, by the theory that the disadvantaged individual is so lacking in opportunities that he feels he has nothing to lose by taking drugs, while the middle-class individual can usually look forward with some hope, for this theory fails to take into account that even among the poor the proportion of drug users is minute.

It is not surprising that the depressed individual who feels better on amphetamines or the chronically anxious one who feels better on alcohol will continue taking whatever makes him comfortable or return to its use whenever certain symptoms flare up. Nor is it surprising when an individual experiencing withdrawal symptoms tries to stop them by taking more drugs. What is puzzling is why individuals without such symptoms return to drug use, even after they have abstained for months or years. This kind of desire is often called *psychic dependence* and attributed to the effect of the agent abused. In fact, however, the term describes a propensity of the user, not an inherent property of the drug. Indeed, unless it is true that even a single dose of a drug can have such an effect on the individual that he desires it ever after, it must be assumed that psychic dependence is an attribute of the individual's personality and his attitudes toward drug use.

3. It is the *frequency* with which an individual uses a pleasurable and dependence-producing drug that determines whether he eventually uses it continuously, not the mere fact that he takes it. While occasional use is in many cases merely a way station to continuous use, there are without question many individuals who indulge only now and then. Sporadic use of amphetamines, barbiturates, and even heroin is fairly common; and "binge" drinkers (who go for months between bouts) represent a sizable proportion of the problem drinkers. Even agents that produce no withdrawal symptoms (such as hallucinogens) are sometimes taken with increasing frequency, to the point that they become an alternative to coping with life's problems and pursuing real goals, and thus gravely affect the individual's long-term social adjustment. Continuous use is not always associated with physical dependence, however.

4. The drug's *immediate effects* on the individual's perception of the world determine not only who is most likely to enjoy and thus to abuse it but also what the consequences are likely to be. These effects often have a greater influence than the frequency of usage on the individual's social competence and on his peer and family relationships. The continuous user of barbiturates may have far less difficulty with his environment than the binge drinker who stays away from work without notice for a week or ten days every three months, and is thus unable to hold a responsible job, or is so abusive to his family during his drinking bouts that the relationship remains strained even when he is sober. Agents that impair the user's coordination, judgment, or impulse control or cause him to become

somnolent, hallucinated, or excited expose him to such hazards as accidents, social embarrassment, and trouble with the police. They are, therefore, even if taken less frequently, more dangerous for his safety, reputation, and long-term social adjustment than drugs without such effects.

5. The *medical hazards* to which the individual is exposed each time he uses the drug or, after some time of use, withdraws from it, include the hazards mentioned above and such others as overdosage, psychotic decompensation, infections, and withdrawal reactions. The occurrence and severity of these hazards are related to

the nature, amount, and legality of the drug;
the route of administration;
the user's physical and psychological health;
the length of time he has been taking the drug; and
the setting in which it is used or withdrawn.

Accidental overdosage is, for example, most common with drugs procured through illegal channels, for the user can never be sure just how much of the drug or even which drug he is really getting. Heroin is so routinely diluted by the "pushers" that the user who receives an undiluted quantity may experience an overdosage, become comatose, or even die (see p. 308). Hallucinogen overdosage or the substitution of a hallucinogen the user did not expect to receive may give rise to prolonged confusional states. Psychotic decompensation with hallucinations and paranoid ideation can occur, however, after single, ordinary doses of hallucinogens or after protracted use of high doses of stimulants. The user's sophistication has some bearing on the drug's dangers as well: failure to disinfect the injection site or to sterilize the equipment and drugs may cause such medical complications as skin abscesses, hepatitis, tetanus, or septicemia (Louria 1967).

An additional hazard of drug use is that concomitant medical conditions may be neglected. The boisterous and complaining drunk's behavioral symptoms may be so conspicuous that far more dangerous ones like head injuries (see p. 423) and acute pancreatitis (Jones 1965) are overlooked. The drug user, moreover, can blunt such physical symptoms as nausea or pain by increasing his drug use rather than seeing a doctor. Even if he does consult a physician, his complaints may erroneously be interpreted as a maneuver to obtain drugs. This last circumstance is not so common as generally supposed, however, for the typical drug user is afraid of having his habits discovered and, if indigent, so reluctant to use his money for anything other than drugs that he is likely to go out of his way to *avoid* seeing a doctor, even in a medical emergency. The drug user's medical care is, therefore, likely to be spotty at best, and he is in constant danger of misdiagnosis and mistreatment.

6. The *long-term hazards* of drug abuse may be classified somewhat arbitrarily as psychosocial and biologic, but the boundary lines blur in the individual case. It may be hard to determine, for example, whether the decline of the chronic alcoholic's reputation, occupational competence, and social skills are caused by his use of alcohol, by the factors that led him to drink, or by the nutritional deficits, repeated head traumas, and poor sanitary habits to which he is exposed.

7. The *legal regulations* attached to the use and procurement of a given drug have a profound impact on the pattern of abuse. The difference is best illustrated by comparing the use of alcohol with that of heroin. Alcohol is available from reputable companies that are subject to quality control and Federal inspection and do not need to charge for the risks incurred in distribution. It is, therefore, far purer and less expensive than the heroin generally sold on the street. As a consequence, the alcoholic, unlike the heroin addict, need not steal in order to have enough money to buy what he wants; is unlikely to be given a diluted or adulterated product; and need not reject society's rules in toto in order to use the agent he enjoys. Today's heroin user, and increasingly today's marijuana user, can be compared with the drinker of the Prohibition era, who had to consort with gangsters, was exposed to the dangers of homebrew or other adulterated alcohol, and gradually developed a contempt for the law itself.

8. Because the patterns of drug abuse that prevail in a given *community* are a reflection of its *attitudes,* particularly those embodied in its laws, and because not all cultures, not even all those within a single community, have the same attitudes, the patterns of drug abuse vary greatly from one locality and subculture to the next. The community's attitudes, in turn, reflect its economic needs: industrialized societies are usually far harder on the withdrawn, fairly peaceful, but unproductive opiate user than on the noisy, belligerent, but usually still productive alcoholic, while the opposite holds true in those Oriental countries not yet caught up in the drive toward industrialization (Chafetz 1964, Fort 1961, Fraser 1963). Amphetamines and barbiturates occupy a middle position in this

spectrum: when used under medical auspices, there is little community objection; used under other auspices, they are frowned on, but the user is rarely prosecuted.

The attitudes toward drugs that prevail in the prospective user's immediate group also affect his use of such agents. College and even high school students are pressured so vigorously by their peers and by their own curiosity to try LSD and marijuana that the college student of today who has never indulged is considered something of an oddity by his peers. The ghetto dweller's use of heroin, the professional musician's use of marijuana, and the truckdriver's use of amphetamines are other examples of drug abuse patterns that are frowned on by the community at large but tolerated by the subculture in which the individual functions.

GENERAL PRINCIPLES OF TREATMENT AND MANAGEMENT

In few areas of medical practice is the physician confronted with the kind of medicolegal dilemmas that surround the management of drug abuse. When the demands and laws of society are not in harmony with sound medical judgment, the doctor is placed in a delicate and precarious role. Not infrequently, he is forced to engage in complex, inconsistent behavior in order to reconcile professional and social imperatives. Such considerations make it necessary to distinguish between

   —drug users whose treatment raises no question of conflict with community prohibitions and
   —those whose indicated treatment program must be weighed against existing social and legal constraints.

The first category includes the patient who is acutely intoxicated, in the throes of withdrawal, or suffering from one of the medical or psychological disorders that follow drug abuse. Here the physician is free to do whatever he feels is necessary to relieve the patient's distress. He is on similarly safe ground in treating the addict whose habit stems from some treatable disorder, or who has voluntarily sought out the physician for help and will accept the traditional measures for curbing abuse.

The broader problem for the physician arises with the second category, where community precepts are involved. The patient whose drug use presents no hazard to his life or health may seem a questionable candidate for medical treatment, particularly if he has not come of his own volition but has been coerced into doing so by his relatives or a community agency. That drug abuse *per se* is dangerous is debatable and, to a degree, academic, for smoking and overeating are also dangerous, as are mountain climbing, sky diving, and a thousand other activities not prohibited by law. Furthermore, the physician is aware that many of the problems associated with drug abuse are extended or compounded by the very laws intended to relieve them. As a citizen, the doctor may be as concerned as anyone else about the high rate of crime associated with drug addiction, the enormous costs, direct and indirect, that must be borne by the community as a result of the drug user's inability to support himself or his family, and the investigative and correctional personnel required to enforce the laws. But as a medical practitioner whose professional judgment is circumscribed by law and ingrained public attitudes, the doctor must ask himself when and under what circumstances he is willing to assist the community in dealing with individual drug abusers.

Requests for treatment without outside pressure or disingenuous motives are so uncommon that the physician must always try to ascertain the patient's real motives. In some cases, he has come only because his regular source of drugs has been cut off and he hopes to secure enough drugs to tide him over by feigning a desire to withdraw. In others, the visit's prime purpose is to pacify relatives, employers, or the court by exhibiting a desire to reform or, better yet, getting the doctor to agree that he is not really addicted. In yet others, the patient really wants to withdraw, but only in order to enhance the drug's effects. This may occur when the individual finds that his tolerance has reached a level where the discomfort of side effects or the disruption of his day-to-day activities exceeds the pleasure of drug use. Or he may find that he can no longer meet the mounting expense. Such patients may indeed seek help in "drying out" or lowering their intake, but they rapidly become readdicted and repeat this cycle every six to twelve months. Finally, self-referral may stem from a drug-induced depression manifested by symptoms of self-derogation and a desire to reform.

The prevailing attitude on the part of many physicians is to dismiss the patient's reasons for seeking medical consultation as invalid and to impose the community's goal of total abstinence. This difference in goals can create so great a barrier between patient and doctor that it seems important to emphasize here that the situation should be governed by neither the patient's nor the community's attitudes but by the traditional goals of medicine. For the drug user, these goals have the following priority:

1/ improved health and prevention of illness,

2/ increased participation in conventional activities,

3/ decreased participation in criminal activities, and

4/ total abstinence and maximal social functioning (Brotman 1965).

One formidable obstacle to the achievement of these goals is the built-in credibility gap. Not only is the drug user likely to have a diminished regard for the truth; even if he did not, he might feel compelled to distort what he says in the face of arrest or hospitalization. He may understate his drug use, if hospitalized, in order to be placed on a more rapid withdrawal schedule and thus accelerate his release, even if this means drawing on a smuggled-in supply of drugs in the meantime. On the other hand, he may overstate the amount he takes because he *1/* fears the discomforts of withdrawal, *2/* hopes for one final "lift" at the doctor's expense, or *3/* considers a "big habit" a status symbol. The medical dangers of such distortions are obvious: the patient who alleges to take more than he does may be placed on a withdrawal schedule that is, in reality, an overdose; the one who reports less may be placed on a schedule that is too rapid and, in the case of sedatives, can result in convulsions. The patient who understates the amount of drugs he takes can confuse the physician about his general condition, especially if the drug is masking such other symptoms as organic pain or depression or causing symptoms that suggest other disorders. Lethargy, dysarthria, ataxia, abdominal pain, or vomiting can cause a futile search for organic pathology, while hyperalertness, labile affect, paranoid ideation, or blandness in the face of apparent disaster give rise to such diagnoses as schizophrenia, depression, or hysteria. In order to avoid such diagnostic chaos, it is usually wisest to hospitalize the drug abuser for as long as it takes to reexamine and evaluate him in a drug-free state. This will by no means guarantee a correct diagnosis, but it will certainly lower the odds against it.

The priority with which the goals listed above are pursued depends in large measure on prevailing legal restrictions. In opiate abuse, for example, the law has until recently been rigid in its demand that the physician place the goal of abstinence above that of employment. Even if the physician considers the patient one of the small number of users able to keep a job and attend to their other obligations only when taking opiates, he may be prohibited from giving the patient the drugs he needs. Barbiturates and amphetamines, though not as forcefully proscribed, can be procured legally only on prescription, so that the physician must take a stand regarding their use. Alcohol, on the other hand, is available anywhere, so the physician need take no stand at all on the patient's consumption of it.

We mention the effect of the laws in this context only to illustrate the role they play in the treatment process, not to propose their revision or to suggest that it is more therapeutic for the physician to refrain from taking a stand. We do not find the latter position a helpful one, as a matter of fact, and agree with Tiebout (1958) that the attempt to avoid the depriving role is "silly because it denies the obvious, misleading because it is attempting to sugarcoat an unpalatable truth, and a poor example because the therapist is denying reality—behavior at which the patient is already expert." While, the doctor may wish eventually to encourage the patient to abstain, his constraints are usually no stronger than the relationship he has established with the patient. Considerations other than the law may also affect the abstinence timetable: even when the physician considers it preferable for the patient to start treatment without totally abstaining, hoping in time to demonstrate the futility of such efforts, the employer's threat to discharge the patient if he makes a single "slip" may make it necessary to accelerate the program.

The patient's physical condition can also have a marked influence on his treatment. If he is so ill that continued drug use would endanger his life, more radical measures, such as a longer period of hospitalization or an extended stay in a halfway house, may be indicated. The patient's physical condition, too, can limit possible countermeasures, as in the case of the patient with an advanced case of postalcoholic cirrhosis who may be unable to tolerate disulfiram (Antabuse) treatment.

MEASURES USED IN COUNTERING THE DESIRE TO ABUSE DRUGS

As the care, management, and disposition of the problems of drug abuse have been delegated to the agencies of health on the one hand and of law enforcement on the other, both *biologic* and *psychosocial* techniques have been developed. And because the individuals involved are often unwilling to collaborate in the efforts made to help them, these techniques include both *coercive* and *noncoercive* measures. Among the *noncoercive biologic measures* are:

1/ Treatment of whatever medical or psychiatric disorder may underlie the individual's drug use. The most common example is *drug substitution,* in which an individual whose propensity to take drugs is based on a treatable psychological disorder is given a drug that not only controls the symptoms of that disorder as well as or better than the drug he has previously used, but is also less likely to cause physical dependence and tolerance, easier to supervise, and more acceptable socially. Typical examples of drug substitution include the use of diphenhydramine (Benadryl) for the individual who takes drugs to relieve his insomnia; phenothiazines or antidepressants for the one who takes drugs to relieve depression, schizophrenia, or chronic anxiety; hydroxyzine (Vistaril) or chlordiazepoxide (Librium) for the alcoholic with chronic anxiety (see p. 302); or methadone (Dolophine) for the narcotic user (see p. 312).

2/ The administration of an agent that "inactivates" the drug the individual abuses by preventing its usual or desired effects. The most typical examples of this technique are the administration of cyclazocine (and to some extent even methadone) to opiate users (see page 313) and the long-term administration of phenothiazines or reserpine to hallucinogen abusers (see p. 325).

Noncoercive psychosocial techniques include the whole gamut of individual or group psychotherapies: occupational rehabilitation; involvement in groups comprised of individuals who at one time abused similar agents (such as Alcoholics Anonymous or Synanon); and residential treatment of the kind subsumed under the label "therapeutic community." In addition to helping the individual learn new social skills and reinforcing his plan to abstain, these measures may provide him with an alternative source of social stimulation and support, and encourage him, at least for a time, to withdraw from the dyssocial setting in which he has been functioning. Conditioned avoidance techniques, such as the concomitant admistration of apomorphine and alcohol (see p. 304), may also be helpful.

The *coercive biologic techniques* include:

1/ The continuous administration of agents that lead to discomfort when combined with the drug abused. The only agents currently in use for this purpose are disulfiram (Antabuse) or calcium carbimide (Temposil); taken daily, these make the individual sick when he uses alcohol (see p. 304).

2/ A combination of drug detection methods, such as periodic urine testing or the administration of drug antagonists (Cochin 1966, Dole 1966a, Jaffe 1966, Poze 1962), and threats concerning the consequences of being found out.

Coercive psychosocial techniques may be either

preventive, in that the drug abuser is warned that renewed drug use will result in his losing his job, being evicted from his home, or being imprisoned; or

corrective, in that he is removed from his circle of friends by being placed in a work camp or prison, forced to report to a proba-tion officer, or, in the case of the addicted physician, barred from practice or at least from prescribing narcotics by revocation of the appropriate license.

The observation that some alcoholics stop drinking only after they have "hit bottom" has led to a concept of combined preventive and corrective techniques, called "bringing the bottom up," in the sense that the physician urges the family or employer to abandon the patient and let him experience the consequences of his behavior immediately rather than wait until he is so debilitated, confused, and desocialized that he cannot recognize his disaster or take steps to reverse it.

THE PROGNOSIS OF DRUG ABUSE

Our earlier comments about the difficulties inherent in comparing treatment methods or making prognostic statements (see p. 106) are of special relevance in drug abuse. The incidence of improve-ment depends on what definition and criteria are applied. Not surprisingly, most studies concerning prognosis use abstinence as the primary criterion of improvement, but fail to agree on the amount or quality of abstinence that would indicate improvement in the individual case. One study may view as inadequate any result but complete and permanent abstinence from the use of all pleasure-producing agents. Another may measure improvement in terms of the length of continuous abstinence achieved or the amount of time (even if discontinuous) that the individual is free of drug influence after receiving treatment. Many studies concern themselves only with abstinence from the agent first abused and ignore the question of what other drugs the individual may have used thereafter.

Quite apart from the difficulties inherent in defining the degree of abstinence required to demonstrate improvement, or in constructing a follow-up study of long enough duration to give a truly representative sample of the identified drug user's subsequent drug career, there are several objections to the criterion of abstinence itself: an alcoholic could, in theory, be viewed as cured only if he could use alcohol with as much impunity as the nonalcoholic. And what of the former heroin user who, when maintained on methadone, is able to work and assume his social obligations: does the mere fact that he still takes an opioid mean he is not cured?

The criterion of abstinence must for these reasons be replaced (or at least supplemented) by such other criteria of improvement as the restoration of occupational competence and the ability to maintain a stable family relationship. No definitive and replicable studies concerning the drug user's course have been published up to the present, and the only statements on which most observers seem to agree are that:

1/ A sizable number of narcotics users stop taking drugs in their late 20s or early 30s, a process that for want of a better label has been described as "maturing out" (Diskind 1964, Duvall 1963, Hunt 1962, Retterstöl 1964, Winick 1964) (see p. 257). As heroin users who continue to take drugs and engage in criminal activities beyond their fortieth year are unlikely to change thereafter, it follows that the heroin user under 30 has a better prognosis than the one over 40.

2/ The more intact the individual was before he started to use drugs, the higher his previous level of occupational competence and social functioning, the more stable his environment during his formative years, and the more stable his current family relationships, the better his prognosis will be (Davies 1956, Gerard 1962, Miller 1968, Perkins 1970, Smith 1969).

3/ Individuals who abuse opiates, alcohol, or barbiturates have a markedly higher mortality rate and a life expectancy as much as fifteen years below that of the general population. The causes include such hazards as

overdosage, malnutrition, and poor hygiene;

a far higher suicide and accident rate;

a higher propensity to disease of all kinds; and

a marked failure to obtain adequate medical care (Kendell 1966, Retterstöl 1964, Vaillant 1966a).

TYPES OF DRUGS MOST COMMONLY ABUSED

GENERAL DEPRESSANTS OF THE
CENTRAL NERVOUS SYSTEM

The prime characteristic of the drugs in this group is their ability to decrease CNS excitability from the normal level through sedation, hypnosis, and general anesthesia to coma without having a prominent analgesic effect. Included are the anesthetic gases and vapors, alcohol, barbiturates, bromides, chloral hydrate, paraldehyde, non-barbiturate hypnotics like glutethimide (Doriden), methyprylon (Noludar), ethchlorvynol (Placidyl), and ethinamate (Valmid), and such minor tranquilizers as meprobamate (Miltown) and benzo-diazepines like chlordiazepoxide (Librium) (see also Table 35). We discuss these drugs and their abuse together because of the similarities in the symptoms that occur after acute intoxication, chronic abuse, and abrupt withdrawal following protracted use; and because there is some degree of cross-tolerance and cross-dependence among them (see p. 596). In addition, none of these drugs is difficult to obtain: with the exception of alcohol, they require a prescription for legal purchase, but this presents little difficulty, as physicians often feel compelled to give "something" for tension, anxiety, insomnia, or other vague complaints, and these drugs are often the "something" they give; they are also accessible and inexpensive through illegal channels.

Acute Intoxication

The symptoms of *mild to moderate intoxications* are similar for all the drugs in this group. Variances are caused mainly by the quantity taken and the rate at which the particular agent is absorbed, metabolized, and excreted. These differences, in turn, govern the rapidity with which the individual passes through several possibly overlapping stages of behavioral effects: mild excitation, euphoria, and garrulousness (all apparently resulting from a depression of inhibitory centers); relaxation; and, if enough has been taken, dysphoria, ataxia, disorientation, drowsiness, and sleep.

The dose level required to produce such changes varies with the drug and the individual. With alcohol, blood levels beneath 50 mg% generally give rise to little beyond mild euphoria and subsequent relaxation; levels above 100 mg% cause garrulousness, euphoria, labile mood, moderate pupillary dilatation, inconstant nystagmus or lateral gaze, dysarthria, and ataxia; levels above 200 mg%, stupor and coma; and, as the level approaches or exceeds 500 mg%, death. Similar ratios obtain for most of the other drugs in this group, with 10 times the usual hypnotic dose generally being lethal, except in the case of benzodiazepines like chlordiazepoxide (Librium), where amounts 20-30 times the hypnotic dose have been taken without fatal outcome.

The only treatment the patient suffering from *simple intoxication* requires is protection against the consequences of his impaired coordination, judgment, and impulse control. Restoration of alertness can be accelerated by giving the patient a few cups of coffee (each of which contains about 100 to 150 mg of caffeine). The patient who is too nauseated to drink coffee may be given caffeine with sodium benzoate, 250-500 mg, i.m. or i.v., or meth-amphetamine hydrochloride (Methedrine), 5 to 10 mg, in 10 cc of saline, i.v. Some individuals react to depressants (even in small doses) with protracted irritability, excitement, and, in some cases, violence. This condition, known as *paradoxical excitement* after bar-biturate use and as *pathologic intoxication* after alcohol use, usually responds well to a sedating phenothiazine like chlorpromazine (Thorazine), 50 mg, i.m.; if the patient remains excited, this dose may be repeated in 30 to 45 minutes.

As the symptoms of acute intoxication blend into those of *over-dosage*, confusion increases, sleep deepens, deep tendon reflexes diminish, respiration becomes shallow, corneal, gag, and pupillary reflexes are abolished, the typical shock syndrome develops, and, if adequate measures cannot be instituted in time, death super-venes. The dangers of overdosage are particularly great if the patient has taken both alcohol and sedatives, not only because these agents have an additive effect, but also because the odor of alcohol all too frequently leads the physician to believe that the patient is "only drunk" and should be allowed to "sleep it off." It must be remembered, however, that an unusually high proportion of suicide attempts with barbiturates or other CNS depressants are made by individuals intoxicated with alcohol (Achté 1966, James 1963, 1966). Thus, whenever there is any suspicion that the intoxicated person has also taken sedatives, as when his level of drowsiness seems dis-proportionate to the amount of alcohol he is known to have con-sumed, when he is stuporous despite a blood alcohol level below 250 mg%, or when he cannot be awakened after three to four hours of sleep—the physician must immediately investigate the possibility that his drowsiness results from the ingestion of sedatives or that he is unconscious for some completely different reason.

As no specific antidotes are available, treatment consists of keeping the patient alive and preventing potential complications until the drug is metabolized or excreted. Maintaining a patent airway, combating hypoventilation and shock, preventing infection, and hastening excretion with such measures as forced diuresis, alkalinization of the urine, and peritoneal or hemodialysis are the most important ingredients of an effective treatment program (Henderson 1966, Shapiro 1969). Since intensive care can reduce the fatality rate to below 2% (Clemmesen 1961), it is important that the patient be taken to a unit geared to the management of acute poisonings and not treated at home or on an inadequately equipped psychiatric ward.

Chronic Intoxication

The symptoms of *chronic intoxication* with CNS depressants are much like those of acute intoxication, with the exception that the patient's memory, ability to concentrate, and regard for social proprieties deteriorate at the same time that his tolerance to the drug's immediate effects increases. Ataxia, dysarthria, and drowsiness tend to diminish or even disappear after prolonged use; this tolerance has a limit, however, and once the patient's dosage exceeds this limit, such symptoms may reappear. Psychological changes occurring in the wake of chronic intoxication include chronic hyperirritability, blackouts (partial or complete amnesia for the events of several hours, days, and in some cases whole weeks), and deterioration of the individual's personality as manifested by untrustworthiness, impaired judgment, and declining social and occupational competence. Depressions are also extremely common. Although it is hard to say whether the depressions are a cause or an effect of the drinking, alcoholics are known to commit suicide at five times the rate of the general population (Kendall 1966, Kessel 1967, Ritson 1968, Stenback 1965). Paranoid thinking and especially morbid jealousy are also quite common. While the foregoing symptoms may result from the chronic abuse of any CNS depressant, others are related to the particular drug used (such as the dermatoses associated with bromism) or to the associated nutritional and hygienic habits. Jellinek's description of the alcoholic's deterioration (see Table 18), while not fully consonant with our own views, summarizes the salient features of the typical alcoholic's course and is, with some modifications, applicable also to other CNS depressants.

TABLE 18. *The Phases of Alcohol Addiction in Males*

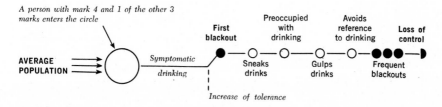

MARKED POPULATION

1. Neurosis or neurotic response pattern
2. Personality inadequacy
3. Psychotic/psychopathologic personalities
4. Hypothetical constitutional liability

PRODROMAL PHASE

Drinking is not conspicuous, and intoxications—limited to evenings except perhaps for weekends—are not severe.

A person with mark 4 and 1 of the other 3 marks enters the circle

AVERAGE POPULATION

Symptomatic drinking

First blackout — Sneaks drinks — Preoccupied with drinking — Avoids reference to drinking — Gulps drinks — Loss of control — Frequent blackouts

Increase of tolerance

CRUCIAL OR BASIC PHASE

Intoxications are the rule, but are still limited to evenings, with hangover the following mornings; onset of solitary drinking varies greatly from one drinker to another, usually occurs in basic phase.

ALCOHOL ADDICTION _____

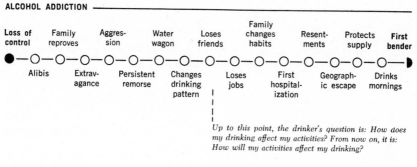

Loss of control — Alibis — Family reproves — Extravagance — Aggression — Persistent remorse — Water wagon — Changes drinking pattern — Loses friends — Loses jobs — Family changes habits — First hospitalization — Resentments — Geographic escape — Protects supply — Drinks mornings — First bender

Up to this point, the drinker's question is: How does my drinking affect my activities? From now on, it is: How will my activities affect my drinking?

ALCOHOL ADDICTION _____

CHRONIC PHASE

With tolerance decreased, drinking becomes nearly constant and the drinker moves on to defeat.

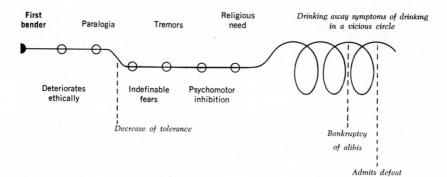

First bender — Paralogia — Tremors — Religious need — *Drinking away symptoms of drinking in a vicious circle*

Deteriorates ethically — Indefinable fears — Psychomotor inhibition

Decrease of tolerance

Bankruptcy of alibis

Admits defeat

TABLE 18. *The Phases of Alcohol Addiction in Males* (continued)

THIS CHART depicts the course of alcohol addiction, which is only the most extreme form of alcoholism. The criterion of alcohol addiction is the loss of control over alcohol intake. It is hypothesized that loss of control will appear in drinkers who have a constitutional liability factor of a physical nature that may be either hereditary or congenital. The hypothesis is based on the observation that many drinkers who drink as much as the addict, over periods of 25 years and more, never come to the stage of loss of control. While no satisfactory laboratory experiments exist on this matter, there are general indications that the constitutional liability factor may be some initial, slight deficiency of carbohydrate metabolism, or of the enzyme system or of certain endocrine relations or a constellation of these factors. The presence of such a physical liability factor may produce alcohol addiction only if psychological tensions should lead to a prolonged heavy use of alcoholic beverages as a sedative. Such heavy use will come about only in the presence of certain social and economic factors. Thus alcohol addiction may be defined as an individual reaction to heavy prolonged alcohol consumption determined by psychological and physical characteristics of the individual under certain social and cultural conditions in his environment. In the absence of the physical constitutional liability factor, but presence of psychological tensions and certain social and cultural factors, other nonaddictive forms of excessive drinking or alcoholism may occur. These latter forms may be regarded as symptoms of underlying psychological or social pathology while alcohol addiction may be viewed as a disease *per se*, which under the conditions described herein is subsequent to symptomatic drinking.

This chart is based on a rigorous statistical analysis of the drinking histories of over 2,000 male alcohol addicts. Every symptom does not appear in every alcoholic, nor do the symptoms occur in every instance exactly in the same sequence. The chart depicts the sequence as it occurs in the majority of alcohol addicts and, in this sense, represents an average. According to various individual and environmental factors, the entire process may take seven to 25 years. The average is 15 years. The different lengths of the lines showing the different phases do not indicate different lengths of duration, but are arbitrarily determined by the number of symptoms which fall into any given phase. While the phases and symptoms depicted here correspond to factual material, the interpretation reflects hypothesis and personal opinion.

THE DOTS represent men and women and the circular arrangement denotes that these persons are acquainted with each other. The serving of alcoholic beverages in this circle may be called a folkway. These people are small users of alcoholic beverages. Compliance with the custom carries a small social reward; it is a minor technique for social acceptance. These small users come into the circle from what may be called the average population and they constitute perhaps 95% of all consumers of alcoholic beverages.

In the left upper corner of the chart is a box designated as "marked population." The meaning of this designation is explained in the text at the right of the box. When such a "marked" person enters the circle and complies with the drinking custom, he may experience considerable relief from the pains which the marks denote. In participating in the "custom" he receives a reward which the others do not receive. Because of that, this person will look for those occasions where his pains will be mitigated or even suspended. He makes the rounds. He does not get actually drunk, but every evening he reaches a stage that may be called "happy glow," which involves fairly heavy drinking.

This form of drinking is a symptom of some underlying psychological or social anomaly. Such drinking lasts until a symptom arises which cannot be explained through the underlying painful condition. This new symptom is the first "blackout" and is explained next.

A BLACKOUT is a partial amnesia without loss of consciousness; intoxication may not be apparent. If it happens frequently after medium amounts of alcohol, the blackout foreshadows alcohol addiction.

When the drinker begins to have drinks of which others do not know (sneaking drinks) and when he is preoccupied with whether there will be enough liquor at some occasion, he gives evidence that drinking means something else to him than to the average drinker. For others it is a custom or part of their diet, but for him it has become a necessity. It has passed from beverage to drug. The avoid-

TABLE 18. *The Phases of Alcohol Addiction in Males* (continued)

ance of speaking about drinking means that he is afraid that people might suspect him of drinking differently from them. These symptoms may occur in any excessive drinker, but when they are coupled with frequent blackouts (3 to 4 times in 10 drinking occasions) after medium amounts, this constellation of symptoms is prodromal to alcohol addiction.

LOSS OF CONTROL means that *after* the ingestion of any small quantity of alcohol a physical demand for that substance is set up which ceases only when advanced intoxication makes further intake impossible. The physiological process underlying this phenomenon is still a matter of surmise (see legend at top of graph). The underlying physiological process becomes active only *after* the ingestion of alcohol and is not responsible for the resumption of drinking several days or weeks later. The drinker resumes drinking because of psychological tensions for which he knows no other remedy or because of a social situation. He is, of course, not aware that he has developed a disorder that makes controlled alcohol intake impossible for the remainder of his life. Loss of control which is the criterion of alcohol addiction develops in the *predisposed* drinker, on the average after eight years of fairly heavy drinking. Psychologically or socially motivated excessive drinkers who lack the constitutional liability factor may show many of the above symptoms, but they do not develop "loss of control." Their drinking behavior may, however, become a grave problem to themselves and society.

Two main systems develop in the crucial or basic phase—a) the system of rationalization, b) the system of isolation. The rationalization first explains to the drinker why he got drunk and why he will not get drunk on other occasions. Later the alibis spread to his family and employment relations and social attitude in general. In this system belongs his attempt to control his drinking by various rules, which never work out (change in drinking patterns), and his belief that living somewhere else would solve the problem (geographic escape). The system of isolation is characterized by aggressions, withdrawal from friends, quitting jobs and protecting his supply of liquor. In consequence of his behavior, his whole family changes its habits. At the beginning of this period he feels persistent remorse, which later is

turned outward into unreasonable resentment. The beginning of morning drinks is a sign that the chronic phase is not far off.

During the preceding phases the drinker, in spite of gross drinking behavior, has limited his intoxication to the evening hours, although he may have commenced drinking some time in the afternoon. He has struggled greatly against neglecting his family and other duties through drinking. Soon after the first morning drinks he finds himself continuing his drinking during the day and may remain intoxicated for two or three days in succession or even longer. This is a behavior that no cultural group condones and that exposes the drinker to grave social punishment. Taking this social risk, which the drinker has avoided probably for 12 or 15 years, is in itself evidence that a grave psychopathological process must have been going on. This behavior is coupled with ethical deterioration and frequently a great deal of paralogic is displayed at this stage. Decrease in alcohol tolerance is often noted at this time. The drinker is beset by nameless fears, tremors and the inability to perform a simple mechanical task (e.g., tying shoe laces) if there is no alcohol in his system. When he takes a drink the symptoms vanish for a while until the effects of alcohol wear off and the symptoms return. A drink is taken again and the symptoms vanish and so on, and now the addict is drinking away the symptoms of drinking. He is drinking in a vicious circle and the drinking becomes obsessive.

At this stage, the alibis of the drinker become so often and severely tested against reality that he cannot keep them up any more and at last admits defeat. At this point he becomes accessible to treatment. The challenging therapeutic problem is to bring about the bankruptcy of the alibis long before it would occur in the normal course of events and thus evoke in the drinker the sincere desire for treatment at a much earlier state.

A summary of lectures delivered by Prof. E. M. Jellinek at the European Seminar on Alcoholism, Copenhagen, October 1951 (copyright by the World Health Organization, Geneva).

Distributed by THE NATIONAL COUNCIL ON ALCOHOLISM, INC., 2 Park Avenue, New York 10016.

Although *chronic alcohol abuse* can have an adverse effect on almost every organ and system in the body, the cause is not always the alcohol itself but the nutritional deficiencies with which the abuse is associated (Brayton 1970, Hines 1969, Isselbacher 1964, Klatskin 1961, Lieber 1969, Lindenbaum 1969, Mendelson 1970a, 1970b). The so-called *Wernicke syndrome*—marked by ophthalmoplegias, nystagmus, ataxia, and peripheral polyneuritis arising either before or together with global disorientation and apathy—is apparently secondary to thiamine deficiency (Victor 1961) and largely reversible. Intravenous administration of 100 mg of thiamine is often followed by dramatic improvement. In the *Korsakoff psychosis,* the patient is relatively lucid and alert and able to perform simple tasks, but displays defects in the acquisition and retention of new impressions and a tendency to confabulate; old memories, habits, and skills are impaired little, if at all (Talland 1965). This disorder is by no means as responsive to treatment as the Wernicke syndrome. Abstinence and adequate nutrition, for a period of six to eight months, may cause a progressive diminution of the symptoms, but recovery is rarely complete, and some learning and memory deficits are likely to persist indefinitely. Should the two syndromes appear simultaneously, the global confusion of the Wernicke overshadows the dysmnesia of the Korsakoff to such an extent that the Korsakoff cannot be identified until the Wernicke recedes. Cirrhosis, hepatic insufficiency, and hepatotoxic effects on the CNS are also extremely common sequelae of chronic alcohol abuse and the associated nutritional deficiencies.

In *chronic bromide intoxication,* the patient complains of headache, anorexia, dryness of the mouth, weakness, and abdominal pain. In severe cases, elevation of CSF pressure, papilledema, confusion, tremor, dysarthria, toxic deliria, and hallucinoses without gross disorientation may occur, the latter especially at night (Levin 1948, 1960). Determination of blood bromide level is important: serum levels over 9 mEq per liter should be considered evidence of bromide intoxication. Treatment consists of the administration of sodium chloride and a diuretic.

The Abstinence Syndrome

For each drug in this group, there is a *daily dose level* that can be considered *safe,* in the sense that most people can, after taking it for some time, abruptly stop doing so without clinically significant consequences. With secobarbital or pentobarbital, for example, this dose is approximately 400 mg daily: anyone who takes less is unlikely to develop a significant degree of physical dependence (Fraser 1958). A person who abruptly withdraws or lowers his intake after regularly exceeding this dose level, or who requires more drugs than he usually takes because an intercurrent medical illness increases his tolerance, will develop abstinence phenomena.

Since the symptoms and signs of the CNS *depressant abstinence syndrome* are similar regardless of which agent is taken (Essig 1964, Haizlip 1958, Hollister 1961a, Selig 1966), Fraser's (1954) description of secobarbital withdrawal is illustrative of the entire group. In the typical case, the patient's drug-induced drowsiness, clouded sensorium, and ataxia diminish four to six hours after his last dose, so that the withdrawal appears to cause a dramatic improvement in his condition. This "improvement" vanishes within a few hours, however, and fresh symptoms start to appear in approximately the following order: anxiety, involuntary twitching, coarse intention tremor of hands and fingers, progressive weakness, dizziness, distortions in visual perception, nausea, vomiting, insomnia, orthostatic hypotension, and hyperreflexia. These symptoms usually reach their maximum intensity on the second day of abstinence, and gradually decline over the next two to fifteen days. In Fraser's study, 79% of the patients had convulsions on the first to fifth day of abstinence, some as often as four times, each convulsion being followed by a temporary improvement in the patient's other symptoms. Within three to six days after withdrawal, 63% had episodes of confusion and delirious psychoses, characterized by disorientation to time and place but not to person, and by visual, haptic, motility, micro-, and auditory hallucinations.

The foregoing symptoms of withdrawal rarely last more than three to five days, at which time the individual usually falls into a terminal sleep of 12 to 16 hours' duration, from which he awakens feeling refreshed and relatively lucid. He may suffer for several weeks thereafter from insomnia and irritability, and some evidence suggests that patients who take sedatives regularly (even if only at bedtime) will show measurable REM and EEG effects for as long as five weeks after they stop (Oswald 1965). Withdrawal of other CNS depressants gives rise to a very similar set of events. The sequence in which the symptoms appear is largely identical, but their duration and severity is determined by

—the agent's rate of metabolism, redistribution, and excretion;
—the user's age, physical condition, and nutritional status; and
—the duration and severity of abuse.

Withdrawal from alcohol, meprobamate, and short-acting barbiturates like secobarbital, all of which are metabolized and excreted fairly rapidly, gives rise to more severe symptoms than withdrawal from chlordiazepoxide or phenobarbital, which are metabolized and excreted more slowly. The abstinence syndrome reaches its peak within two to four days after the withdrawal of short-acting drugs, but not for five to seven days after withdrawal from long-acting drugs. Bromide withdrawal produces few or no symptoms, for the drug is excreted so slowly that abrupt withdrawal automatically leads to a gradual reduction of drug effect.

In its mildest form, the abstinence syndrome is limited to such symptoms as hyperalertness, tremulousness, minor difficulty in falling asleep, and nightmares. Patients who have been using high doses of drugs for an extended period of time, however, may develop convulsions, hallucinoses, and delirium. As a general rule, the greater the drug's anticonvulsant effect and the shorter its action, the greater the likelihood and the earlier the onset of *withdrawal convulsions*. Convulsions are thus more likely to occur and to occur early after withdrawal of short-acting barbiturates and meprobamate, less likely to occur and likely to occur later after withdrawal of long-acting agents like phenobarbital and chlordiazepoxide, and least likely to occur after withdrawal of an agent with little anticonvulsant activity, like alcohol. Patients with a history of seizures are, of course, more susceptible to convulsions.

A postwithdrawal *hallucinosis* (hallucinations in a patient who is otherwise lucid and well-oriented) may begin with a vague and formless hissing or crackling noise (Saravay 1967), but can develop into voices that frighten, accuse, or belittle him or order him to escape, commit suicide, or take some other bizarre or impulsive action. In contrast to the schizophrenic's voices, often experienced as coming from within, the patient experiences the voices as external (Bilz 1959) and feels able to point to their exact location. Visual hallucinations, which the patient explains that he sees but does not believe, may occur in rare instances. This syndrome usually responds well to phenothiazines and readministration of a CNS depressant and generally subsides within three to four days, but the symptoms can reappear every few days for weeks on end. It is important, therefore, to keep the patient under observation in a setting where he can be protected against his own impulsivity for a number of days after his hallucinations seem to have disappeared.

Delirium tremens—a syndrome often seen in, but by no means limited to, alcoholics—is marked by confusion, agitation, insomnia, coarse and persistent tremor (especially of the hands), visual and (in some cases) auditory hallucinations, fever, diaphoresis, and tachycardia, all of which tend to worsen at night. In many cases, the first symptoms are increased irritability and difficulty in falling asleep. The patient may try to relieve these symptoms by drinking more heavily or taking more drugs. This practice may help for a time, but he then starts to have nightmares, to awaken during the night, and soon thereafter to experience visual and tactile hallucinations, often of small, rapidly moving animals or insects crawling on the walls or in his bed. Social contact and sensory stimulation (such as leaving the lights turned on) may interrupt the hallucinations at the outset, but after a few days nothing helps (Gross 1966). About 4% of the patients also have convulsions (Nielsen 1965). While the patient developing delirium tremens has usually been a heavy drinker for at least five years (Nielsen 1965), the length and severity of the delirium are usually determined by the length and severity of the drinking bout that immediately precedes the episode, rather than by the total years of drinking. Almost 40% of the cases are precipitated by trauma or infection (Lundqvist 1961). The delirious state usually subsides within 72 hours; if it lasts longer, the patient must be reevaluated to rule out other causes. The mortality rate for patients with delirium tremens is reported to lie between 3% and 6%; the prognosis is particularly poor for patients with persistent fever, leukocytosis, high blood urea nitrogen levels, and hyperbilirubinemia that does not fall below 5 mg% by the sixth day after admission (Cutshall 1965, Hardison 1966, Victor 1966).

The unreliability of the typical patient's history has important consequences for *the management of withdrawal*. Ideally, the patient would simply report what he has been taking, how much, and for how long, and the physician would prescribe the drugs needed for an optimal reduction schedule and set up a follow-up appointment. This management is likely to be successful, however, only for the patient who, after taking a moderate dose of a minor tranquilizer or sedative for tension or insomnia for a few weeks or months, becomes excessively uncomfortable when he tries to stop and, afraid that he is becoming "addicted," asks for help in withdrawing. In such situations, the patient should be told to continue his highest daily dosage for a two-day period and thereafter to reduce this by about 10% daily over a period of 10 to 14 days. He should be informed what withdrawal symptoms to expect, told that they will subside within a few weeks, and carefully monitored (even if only by telephone) until they do. This ideal situation is rare, however, as the drug user usually exaggerates or understates the amount he takes and, if treated at home, either stops more abruptly than advised or uses his own sources to supplement drugs received from the doctor.

For these reasons, the hospital is usually the safest and most efficient place to achieve withdrawal. The drug user is no more truthful in the hospital, however, than he is at home. Not infrequently, he brings along a supply of drugs or gets his friends to smuggle them into the hospital. Thus, wherever withdrawal takes place, the situation may well remain out of control, and the drug user continue to be exposed to the dangers of delirium and convulsions. It is important, therefore, that any patient who is known or suspected to be taking large doses of CNS depressants be *reintoxicated* before he is withdrawn. This technique has the double advantage of enabling the physician to obtain an independent estimate of the patient's prior drug use and permitting him to start the withdrawal schedule from a known baseline. Reintoxication is especially important for the person who

1/ has been taking CNS depressants with marked anticonvulsant activity (like barbiturates);
2/ has been taking so many different drugs that their total effect is hard to estimate;
3/ shows signs of increasing irritability and tremulousness; or
4/ has a prior history of seizures.

Although reintoxication and withdrawal can be accomplished with the agent the individual has previously used or, indeed, with any CNS depressant, we prefer to use repeated small doses of a short-acting barbiturate like secobarbital, an agent that reaches its peak effect so rapidly and exerts this effect so briefly that the desired dose level is achieved without incurring the dangers of accumulation and overdosage. How soon after admission a reintoxication schedule should begin will depend on the patient's condition and on the amount of time that has elapsed since his last dose. Unless he is drowsy or has just taken his drugs, reintoxication should begin as soon as he enters the hospital and, in any case, as soon as he starts to sober up. One hundred mg of secobarbital is administered orally every hour, until the patient is mildly drowsy and ataxic and his speech is slightly slurred; if he has had a seizure or appears so tremulous that one must be feared, the first doses should be given intramuscularly. Once he is mildly intoxicated, he is given at two-hour intervals as much barbiturate as he needs to maintain this state. The amount of drug required for this purpose over a period of six hours is assumed to be one quarter of his daily barbiturate requirement, the amount he would have to take in order to maintain this state for a 24-hour period. Of this dosage, 90% (divided in four to six doses) is given daily for a two-day period. Thereafter, the amount given is reduced by 10% daily until the patient is receiving less than 300 mg a day, at which point reductions of 75 mg daily may be undertaken (Blachly 1964, Fraser 1953, Isbell 1950). Patients who are debilitated, have a history of seizures, or suffer from other complications should be withdrawn more slowly (Wikler 1968). Librium (chlordiazepoxide), which depresses the patient's respiration less than other CNS depressants and in addition stimulates his appetite, has been found useful in alcohol withdrawal (Kaim 1969): the patient is initially given 50 mg every hour until he is drowsy (up to a total dose of 400 mg) and then withdrawn in a fashion analogous to that outlined above.

Throughout the period of withdrawal, the frequency of administration is gradually reduced until the barbiturate is taken only in the morning and evening. If at any time during this process, the patient shows such signs of impending seizures as tremor and irritability, he must be given additional barbiturates; if he becomes excessively drowsy, a somewhat more rapid reduction is in order. Since the patient can become dehydrated as a consequence of his motor restlessness, sweating, anorexia, and vomiting, his fluid intake and electrolyte balance must be closely observed and, if necessary, adjusted. Parenteral vitamins may be required if the patient is malnourished (Leevy 1965).

While these measures usually prevent the more serious complications of withdrawal, they will not always reverse symptoms that have already developed. The patient who is delirious at the time he is first seen, for example, may not become lucid when reintoxicated. In these cases, excitement can usually be reduced by giving him 25 to 50 mg of a sedating phenothiazine like chlorpromazine (Thorazine) or thioridazine (Mellaril) every three to four hours, as needed. As phenothiazines can facilitate seizure activity, they should be given only if the patient is so agitated that he is in physical danger or cannot be properly cared for, and, in any event, combined with additional doses of barbiturates (see also p. 422.

Measures Used to Counter the Abuse of CNS Depressants

Patients who report that they have taken to the excessive use of barbiturates or alcohol because they are unable to sleep without them will often benefit from *drug substitution,* using diphenhydramine (Benadryl) or hydrozyzine (Vistaril), sedatives that cause no physical dependence and little, if any, tolerance. Mood disorders often underlie the use of CNS depressants since many patients who abuse them are found to have a prior or family history of affective disorder (Pitts 1966, Schukit 1969, Winokur 1968, 1970). Treatment with an antidepressant or lithium carbonate may thus be of value.

Drug substitution is not so successful for patients whose drug abuse rests on a chronic anxiety reaction. In some cases, antidepressants, phenothiazines, reserpine, hydrozyzine (Vistaril), or some combination of these may be helpful; but all too often they offer little relief and other measures must be tried. The safest measure, of course, is psychotherapy directed to providing the patient with the fortitude to bear his discomfort and the strength to resist taking drugs to relieve it. This course has the disadvantage, however, that the patient may return to the use of drugs surreptitiously. An alternative and somewhat paradoxical approach might be to prescribe another agent that, though just as apt to cause physical dependence, can be better controlled. The alcoholic who, when not drinking, is continually anxious might be given a moderate dose of a minor tranquilizer like chlordiazepoxide (Librium) on the rationale that he is likely to find it easier to abstain from drinking entirely than to become a moderate drinker; that 30 to 40 mg of chlordiazepoxide is unlikely to cause physical dependence but may well relieve the symptoms for which he had previously taken alcohol; and that chlordiazepoxide is obtainable only on prescription, while alcohol is freely available so that he is less likely to "pop" an extra pill than he might be to have "just one more drink" if he were trying to become a moderate or social drinker. Substituting a minor tranquilizer for alcohol has the disadvantage, on the other hand, of supporting the patient's pathological view that he needs "something for his nerves" and cannot be expected to control his drinking behavior by himself. He is thus given a ready excuse (if indeed he needs one) to start drinking again.

Psychosocial interventions proceed in three overlapping phases. The first is the establishment of a supportive, perhaps even a dependent, *relationship* with a relatively stable, yet flexible, individual such as a professional therapist or an AA sponsor. The second involves repeated experiences with a *group comprised of individuals with similar problems,* either a formal therapy group or one like Neurotics Anonymous (in the case of the sedative abuser) or Alcoholics Anonymous (in the case of the alcoholic). The *involvement of the patient's family* is often of value in this phase of treatment. The spouse who needs advice about living and coping with the drug user may be advised to join a therapy group along with him or referred to Al-Anon, an AA affiliate that offers its members both practical advice and emotional support. By seeing both husband and wife together, the therapist can explore each partner's complaints about the other and avoid being exposed to the unproductive, one-sided lamentations of the individual who blames his drinking entirely on his nagging or misbehaving spouse (Drewery 1969) or, conversely, blames his own misbehavior, neglect, or infidelity on his partner's drinking. The sincerity of such complaints can always be tested by suggesting that both the drinking and the misbehaving stop for a while, but this usually demonstrates only that the two are playing the kind of game described by Berne (1964), in which the nonalcoholic spouse alternates between savior, persecutor, victim, and bartender, a state of affairs that, while by no means universal, is familiar to anyone who has ever worked with alcoholics. The situation is even more difficult when both partners are alcoholics, for each may fear, and thus try to sabotage, the other's sobriety. The third phase of treatment involves gradual exposure to less supportive *peer groups* like AA's no-holds-barred closed meetings or therapy groups composed of competitive individuals both with and without an alcohol problem. Involvement with groups of this kind, however, should be postponed until the patient has developed confidence in his ability to stay sober and need not fear that some unsettling therapeutic encounter will cause a relapse.

Since both alcohol and sedative prescriptions are easily available, the abuser's access to these drugs can never be blocked entirely. Nevertheless, the abstinent patient's return to drug abuse often hinges on such factors as availability and opportunity, and all measures that *place obstacles in the way of acquiring the drug* will serve to diminish the risk. The patient who is serious about wanting to stop taking sedatives will usually give the psychiatrist permission to apprise his family doctor and his local pharmacy of the situation. The family doctor should be instructed to refer all requests for sedation to the psychiatrist, and the pharmacist should be told to refuse to refill old prescriptions and to call the psychiatrist if new ones appear. Some families even take the trouble of informing each pharmacy in town about the situation, a practice that sometimes reveals in how many places the drugs have been secured in the past. While these preventive measures cannot be employed for the alcoholic, it is helpful, at least until the patient's sobriety is well established, to urge the patient's spouse to refrain from drinking and to suggest to the patient and his family that they keep no alcohol in the house and avoid social engagements at which everyone else will be drinking. If the patient reports that he still craves alcohol or drugs, and states, as many abusers do, that he does not want to stop drinking (or taking drugs) but does "want to *want* to," it is useful to point out that individual episodes of craving usually fade in an hour or less, though for some weeks or months they may recur several times daily. The patient could even be urged to time and record each episode of craving, which would

1/ give him something other than drinking to do while he is experiencing the craving;

2/ encourage him to view the feeling as something observable, objective, and alien; and

3/ demonstrate to him that the episodes of craving are neither overpowering nor likely to last indefinitely and that they gradually become shorter and less frequent.

It can also be of benefit to suggest to the patient that he call someone, a friend, the therapist, or his AA sponsor, when he experiences the urge, for this will give him someone to lean on when he weakens and will at least postpone any other action until the craving wears off.

Occasionally, especially with alcoholics, *conditioned avoidance therapy* with apomorphine or some other nauseant can be helpful, at least for a while. In this procedure, the patient is repeatedly given 2 to 8 mg of apomorphine together with alcohol; the repeated vomiting eventually causes him to become nauseated even when he thinks about alcohol. Succinylcholine-induced apneic paralysis has also been used for the aversion treatment of alcoholics (Madill 1966), as has the playing of video tapes showing the individual's demeanor while drunk (Paredes 1968). Some temporary successes have been reported from giving the patient LSD (Kurland 1967, O'Reilly 1964, Sarett 1966, Smart 1967a), perhaps because this provides him with an extremely "meaningful" experience and thus induces him to reflect on his life style.

While the pharmacopoeia is replete with drug pairs that are

mutually incompatible, the only practical application of such incompatibility to the solution of drug abuse has been the development of disulfiram (Antabuse) (Hald 1948) and calcium carbimide (Temposil) (Mitchell 1958). Disulfiram's effect is to interfere with the enzymatic breakdown of alcohol, thus causing, within 90 minutes after ingestion of 15 to 60 cc of alcohol, an acute *acetaldehyde intoxication* marked by flushing, bloodshot eyes, throbbing headache, nausea, vomiting, palpitations, tachycardia, dyspnea, hyperventilation, sleepiness, and hypotension. Higher doses of alcohol can lead to coma and even to death.

Although some patients taking disulfiram experience little or no discomfort when they drink, those who show the typical reaction and take disulfiram daily will almost certainly not drink on a day they have taken it or for three to four days thereafter, for its effects last at least that long after the drug is discontinued. The patient is thus prevented from drinking on impulse, or at least until he has had a few days to think it over. His rationalizations for discontinuing the use of this agent are, however, remarkably facile; in many cases, he hardly seems to have noticed that he has stopped. The use of disulfiram can thus be of value in helping the therapist to explore the sincerity of the patient's interest in getting well as, no matter how he explains it, the patient's refusal to take disulfiram will expose his apathy or antipathy toward treatment. The same holds true for the alcoholic's spouse who, on being given the responsibility of supervising the patient's disulfiram use, "forgets" to do so, considers its use "no longer necessary" and the patient "cured" after a few weeks, or mislays the drug on the way home from the pharmacy. Discussing errors of this kind without resorting to accusations may be difficult, but will often demonstrate that *both* partners, not just one, are trying to keep the game going.

Disulfiram (Antabuse) therapy should not be started until the patient has had neither alcohol nor paraldehyde for at least 24 hours and is free of significant withdrawal symptoms. On the first day, he is given 2 g; on the second, 1.5 g; on the third, 1.0 g; and from the fourth day on, 0.5 g daily. This dose is continued for four to six weeks, at which time it may be lowered to a maintenance dose of 250 or even 125 mg daily. In order to ascertain whether the drug is effective and to make sure that the patient realizes what will happen if he takes alcohol and thus will refrain from experimenting on his own, an *alcohol-disulfiram reaction* is induced after the patient has been taking the drug for 10 to 14 days. This reaction is set in motion by having the patient drink a shot glass (about 30 cc) of his favorite hard liquor, two cans of his favorite beer, or a waterglass full of his favorite wine every half hour up to four times or until he develops the typical acetaldehyde syndrome. (To waylay the possible suspicion that the reaction is due to the drink's having been "spiked," we have the patient purchase and bring his own liquor for the test.) If the patient's systolic blood pressure begins to fall, he should lie down; if shock develops, an intravenous infusion containing levarterenol (Levophed) should be started and oxygen administered by mask. While these measures generally reverse the hypotension fairly quickly, it may recur soon thereafter and make it necessary to repeat these measures four or five times for several hours. The use of 1,000 mg of intravenous ascorbic acid has also been recommended.

Because of both disulfiram's toxic effects and the dangers of the acetaldehyde syndrome, the drug is contraindicated for patients with psychoses, organic brain syndromes, epilepsy, diabetes, cirrhosis, heart disease, or nephritis, and during pregnancy. Although some patients develop such *side effects* as a sulfurous, metallic, or garlic-like taste in the mouth, acneiform eruptions, gastrointestinal distress, or confusion, these symptoms usually disappear when the daily dose is reduced to the usually still effective level of 125 mg; if the symptoms still persist, the drug should be discontinued. It is often hard to decide, however, whether the patient's complaints about side effects are induced by the drug or by his desire to stop taking it and return to drinking. In many cases, the symptoms are not relieved when a placebo is substituted for the disulfiram; the patient merely develops a new set of symptoms and again demands that the drug be stopped. It is important to warn the patient that ethyl alcohol in any form can cause a reaction and that he must avoid food and sauces prepared with alcohol, medicines with an alcohol base, alcohol rubs, and the concentrated breathing of alcohol fumes (as may occur when shellacking a floor in a poorly ventilated room).

One type of symptom that is rarely dissimulated by patients and, in our experience, occurs far more frequently than the literature suggests is the disulfiram-induced *organic brain syndrome*. The syndrome may be limited to very mild confusion accompanied by lightheadedness, but can progress to dysarthria, ataxia, dysmnesia, disorientation, and paranoid ideation (Von Grage 1952, Macklin 1953, Martensen-Larsen 1951, Smilde 1963), in which case the drug must be discontinued immediately. Once the drug is stopped, the symptoms usually subside within a week or two (Liddon 1967). At this point, lower dose levels (like 125 mg daily) can be tried, but even this may be not tolerated. Substitution with calcium carbimide (Temposil), a somewhat less toxic (but also somewhat less effective) drug with similar properties, might be useful (Ferguson 1956, Levy 1967, Marconi 1961), but this drug is not yet commercially available in the United States.

That the patient taking disulfiram (Antabuse) may eventually arrive at taking the drug by himself makes this technique the most voluntary and thus the most medical of the coercive measures, but it is not the only form of coercion that is used. An alcoholic may agree to take disulfiram only if his spouse threatens to leave him should he refuse, or if his employer permits him to start working only after the plant nurse has seen him take that day's dose. The individual who abuses sedatives may similarly be coerced by a daily urine test (McIsaac 1966) coupled with a threat of dire consequences on any day he fails to deliver a specimen or is found to be using a drug he should avoid. Laws providing for the appointment of a conservator or long-term hospital commitment for alcohol and sedative abusers may also provide some leverage, especially since hospitalization may sever the individual's relationship to his suppliers and give him a protracted period in which to consider his previous behavior while free of both the drug and the craving for it.

Many patients who, after drinking excessively for some time, maintain abstinence for a period of 12 to 24 months are so pleased with their ability to refrain that they make no bid to return; others ask if they are now cured and may once again drink. Some start drinking without discussing the topic with either their families or their physicians, but these almost always run into trouble again. Although such slips should not be taken lightly, they are common and, at times, so brief that they should not cause all concerned to throw up their hands in despair and refuse the patient further support, particularly if the patient has been abstinent long enough to demonstrate that he has some motivation. Repeated slips, particularly by patients who refuse to take disulfiram, must be viewed as evidence of poor motivation, and continuing therapeutic efforts—at least those devoted to the patient's drinking problem—are not warranted.

The patient who asks for permission to resume drinking after some years of abstinence poses a question that is far more complex than the negative answer he usually gets would suggest (Davies 1963, Kendall 1965, Räkköläinen 1969). It is true, of course, that the resumption of drinking is potentially hazardous, especially because those individuals most anxious to return to social drinking are the ones most likely to develop a drinking problem once again. Nevertheless, when the individual's drinking problem has been of relatively short duration, when it seems to have been related to a depression that has subsided in the interim, and when the individual concerned was and remains collaborative, a three-month trial with a prearranged subsequent three-month respite will test his ability to "take it or leave it." Even if this test is successful and the patient thereafter returns to social drinking, it is important that both he and his family understand that the first reversion to problem drinking means that the patient must immediately and permanently return to the earlier path of complete abstinence.

OPIATES AND OTHER ANALGESICS

This category includes opium, as in paregoric; opiates like morphine, heroin, codeine, and dihydromorphinone (Dilaudid); and opioids like meperidine (Demerol), methadone (Dolophine), dextropropoxyphene (Darvon), and to some extent pentazocine (Talwin) (Bellville, 1965, Sandoval 1969, Vandam 1962). While many users start by taking agents of this kind orally, most soon progress to parenteral routes: sniffing, subcutaneous injection, and, finally intravenous administration—the route that provides the greatest pleasure.

The most common, or at any rate most publicized, form of narcotic abuse is the intravenous use of heroin by street addicts. This agent is sold in "trey" (three-dollar) or "nickel" (five-dollar) "bags" of white powder, allegedly containing one or two grains (60-120 mg) of heroin respectively. The buyer usually gets far less than he pays for, however, as it is only the most experienced user who can assess the drug's potency by its effects. Of the drugs seized by police, 10% contain no heroin at all, being composed solely of lactose, baking soda, or some equally inert substance, perhaps with a little quinine added to mimic the bitter taste. Samples seized in New York City in 1965 contained from 14% to 27% heroin (Hess 1965), and, at times of increased police activity, the figure may go down to about 2%. The contents are indeed so variable that a novice may think of himself as addicted when he is in fact using little or no heroin at all (Zinberg 1964). If, by some chance, a user of this kind encounters an inexperienced pusher or one who is new in the business and trying to develop a following, he may be given the drug in unadulterated form and receive what amounts to an overdose in terms of his level of tolerance. This factor is undoubtedly responsible for many of the overdosage fatalities that occur. Such fatalities are extremely common: in the city of New York, there is more than one death from overdosage daily. Indeed, in the 15 to 35 age bracket, diseases related to narcotic abuse cause more death than murder, suicide, or accidents (Helpern 1968).

Acute and Chronic Intoxication

The initial effect of opiates is usually described as a flush or warm glow with a fairly immediate sense of euphoria, relaxation, and freedom from all problems, which, after a brief time, is followed by a light, very pleasant sleepiness called a "nod." The first experiences are not always pleasant, and some people become nauseated or dysphoric. After a few days, however, as use satisfies the developed dependence, these symptoms are displaced by euphoria. Users describe the center of the relaxed feeling as different for different agents, heroin's effects first being felt in the abdomen and then spreading upward; morphine's at the front of the head and in the toes. Meperidine (Demerol) and methadone (Dolophine) are said to produce a peculiar medicinal taste (even when taken intravenously) and do not produce the typical glow. Dextropropoxyphene (Darvon), in doses over 350 mg, can similarly lead to a sensation of well-being, competence, and floating. Codeine, usually taken in cough syrup and only rarely in pill or injectable form, causes effects similar to, but less euphorizing than, those produced by other opiates (Fraser 1960, Murphree 1962, Reynolds 1957, Smith 1962).

Chronic users generally eat poorly, lose weight, and exhibit little sexual interest. Disturbed sleep is common, particularly when the individual takes too little before going to bed and thus awakens in the middle of the night with such withdrawal symptoms as piloerection, sweating, or chills. Experienced users can, to some extent, distinguish one narcotic from another (Lasagna 1955) and usually prefer heroin whenever they have a choice (Martin 1961). Heroin's popularity among users is not readily explainable on the basis of causing greater dependence, for controlled studies (using equivalent doses) have shown that it does not cause dependence or tolerance more rapidly than other narcotics, and that it is not in any other way a more dangerous or pernicious drug (Lasagna 1965). Heroin's reputation for being more pleasurable than other opiates or opioids is, in any case, in the producer's interest, for the drug is two to four times as potent and many times as expensive as the quantity of morphine from which it is made (Reichle 1962). The effect of these agents is so similar and shows such a high degree of cross-dependence that the chronic user, who is unable to obtain the drug he likes best, is usually willing to use any one of the others. If he cannot obtain any opiates at all, he will even turn to a barbiturate or some other CNS depressant, which, though it does not have an identical effect, will at least diminish the discomfort of withdrawal.

Overdosage

The individual who is free of pain and not taking other drugs can develop euphoria and drowsiness on doses of morphine as low as 10 mg, while doses as low as 100 mg may be fatal. Tolerance may increase dramatically after an extended period of use, however, to the point that many hundred times the initial dose is required for an equivalent effect. Some addicts are said to be able to tolerate doses as high as 5 gm (Wikler 1952). The individual who receives an overdose will, within minutes, become increasingly unresponsive and cyanotic; his pulse and respiration will slow, his blood pressure and temperature fall, and his breathing become shallow; eventually coma ensues. Except when the ingested agent is meperidine (Demerol), which causes mydriasis, there is marked pupillary constriction. When such a patient is brought for emergency treatment, needle-marks and blood stains on the shirt sleeves help to clarify the cause, as does inspection of those who accompany the patient. High doses of dextropropoxyphene (Darvon) (Elson 1963) or meperidine (Demerol) produce tremors, twitching, confusion, hallucinations, and sometimes convulsions (Jaffe 1965).

Narcotic intoxication can be reversed rapidly with a competitive antagonist like nalorphine (Nalline) or the ten times more potent levallorphan (Lorfan). As they possess greater affinity for the receptor sites of opiates than the opiates themselves (Woods 1956), narcotic antagonists rapidly displace the previously ingested opiates from their receptors and thus reverse the patient's intoxication. These agents should be used only in severe intoxications (Eckenhoff 1962), as they tend, like the opiates, to depress respiration, and will thus, in a mild intoxication, merely add to the number of occupied receptors and increase the respiratory depression. Moreover, these drugs should be given in small doses (such as nalorphine, 5 to 10 mg intravenously) every 10 to 15 minutes, up to four times, for by displacing the narcotic they unmask the physically dependent patient's latent hyperexcitability and can thus precipitate a severe withdrawal syndrome that cannot be reversed, even with opiates, because of the antagonist's greater affinity to the receptor sites. Nalorphine is so specific and so effective an antagonist to narcotics that the comatose drug user who does not respond to some extent after two to three doses must be suspected of having also ingested another drug, such as a barbiturate, or of being unconscious for some reason unrelated to his drug use.

The Abstinence Syndrome

Withdrawal symptoms start with itching, running of the nose, and yawning, after which the patient develops some or all of the following: lacrimation, dilatation of pupils, polyuria, diaphoresis, diarrhea, chills, and goose flesh; increased temperature, respiration, and blood pressure; tremors, a sense of restlessness and uneasiness, hypersensitivity (particularly in the genitals), spontaneous ejaculation or orgasm, muscle cramps (especially in the legs), nausea, vomiting, insomnia, generalized pains, and the feeling that all his organs are loose (Blachly 1966). These symptoms generally occur in waves; they reach a peak seven to 12 hours after meperidine (Demerol) withdrawal, 24 to 48 hours after dihydromorphinone (Dilaudid) withdrawal, 48 to 72 hours after heroin, morphine, and codeine withdrawal, and about seven to eight days after methadone (Dolophine) withdrawal. Thereafter they diminish in severity and frequency for the next few days. Pure withdrawal syndromes are fairly rare today, for most narcotics users also take some other kind of drug (sedatives in order to cut the dose and thus the expense of the opiates used, or stimulants like amphetamines to enhance the pleasurable effect) (Mitcheson 1970). Increasing tremulousness during the withdrawal period thus leads to the suspicion that the patient has also been taking a barbiturate or some other CNS depressant and must therefore be reintoxicated with and subsequently withdrawn from this agent as well (see p. 299).

It is important to realize that the patient's description of his withdrawal symptoms depends not only on the dose to which he has become accustomed and the length of time he has been taking it but also on the availability of narcotics in the setting where the withdrawal takes place: no matter how mild or severe the objective symptoms of the abstinence syndrome may appear, patients whose withdrawal takes place in a hospital (where descriptions of discomfort can lead to the administration of more drugs) generally report more discomfort than those who withdraw in jail.

The most common *treatment method* is to replace the previously used agent with methadone (Dolophine), which is then gradually withdrawn. The rationale for this method is that methadone can be given orally and, being long-acting, produces less uncomfortable and more gradual withdrawal symptoms (Janssen 1960). When the patient's *previous drug intake is known,* he is given 1 mg of methadone for every 1 to 2 mg of heroin, 3 to 4 mg of morphine, ½ mg of dihydromorphinone (Dilaudid), 30 mg of codeine, 20 mg of meperidine (Demerol), or 7 to 8 cc of paregoric he has been taking. This amount of methadone (divided into four daily doses) is administered for a day or two, reduced by 10% to 30% daily thereafter, and discontinued within five to 10 days (Nyswander 1956). When, as is more commonly the case, the patient's *previous drug intake is unknown,* he is stabilized on just enough methadone to prevent the more severe symptoms of withdrawal, such as vomiting or insomnia (10 to 60 mg daily, in the average case), and thereafter withdrawn in the same fashion. The older the patient is and the poorer his health, the longer the initial stabilization period and the more gradual the withdrawal program should be. Newborn infants whose mothers are using opiates at the time of delivery may have to be given paregoric in gradually decreasing doses over a period of 30 days in order to prevent the development of withdrawal symptoms (Perlmutter 1967, Stern 1966).

When the patient is young and in good health, known to be using only heroin or other opiates, thought to have taken only moderate doses (up to eight or 10 "nickel bags" of heroin or its equivalent daily), and is free of severe symptoms of dehydration, the fastest and perhaps simplest course is *abrupt withdrawal* (Regan 1958, Steele 1957). Emotional support, social stimulation, back and leg massage, and hot baths for cramps should be offered to diminish discomfort, and ample fluid intake should be encouraged. Withdrawal, under these circumstances, is generally quite peaceful and approximates in severity and symptoms a viral infection with gastrointestinal manifestations. If the patient has difficulty in sleeping, 10 to 20 mg of chlordiazepoxide (Librium) may be given every two hours for four days, then reduced over a 10-day period. When extensive observations were made of abrupt withdrawal in a friendly, supportive, but strict setting in which drugs are not available (Synanon), it proved impossible to substantiate the popular view that this method is less humane than gradual withdrawal.

Measures Used to Counter the Abuse of Opiates

Opiates are known to be effective in relieving certain psychological symptoms, at least temporarily, and only half a century ago were prescribed freely for a variety of psychiatric disorders. It is thus especially important that the patient taking opiates be re-evaluated after being withdrawn and, if found to have a hitherto hidden mental illness, be offered more specific treatment. Although therapeutic use of opiates has today fallen largely into disuse and disrepute, occasionally an individual is encountered who is irritable, callous, hedonistic, and in serious conflict with parents, teachers, and the law prior to taking opiates, but becomes more rational and socially acceptable after taking these agents and disturbed once again when such drugs are withdrawn (Gerard 1954). Indeed, the possibility must be considered that such an individual's dependence on drugs reflects aberrant stress responses that at present can be normalized only with narcotics. This may explain the successes reported for both the British method of dealing with addiction and the Dole-Nyswander experiments (Dole 1966b, 1969) in maintaining narcotics users on methadone. The chief characteristic of the British system is that the responsibility for decisions concerning the individual's drug use is placed on his physician rather than on the state; the physician is even permitted, under appropriate safeguards, to administer maintenance opiates (Brain 1965, King 1961, NYAM 1963). The Dole-Nyswander method is similar to the British system, in placing the goal of social rehabilitation above that of abstinence, but differs in being combined with far more stringent safeguards and supportive measures.

In the Dole-Nyswander treatment program, the patient is first hospitalized for a four to six week observation period, during which his immediate health problems are attended to, he is withdrawn from heroin or whatever drug he has been dependent on, and is gradually switched to methadone. The patient is initially given 20 mg of methadone twice daily, and this is increased by 20 mg daily up to a total dose of not more than 200 mg daily until he is comfortable without being sluggish or drowsy. Once the appropriate maintenance dose has been established, the dosage is gradually changed from a twice-a-day to a once-a-day schedule, the morning (or for patients who work at night, the evening) dose being diminished by 5 to 10 mg daily, while the other dose is built up correspondingly. After the patient is discharged from the hospital, his care is transferred to an outpatient clinic, to which he must report daily to receive his dose; in exceptional cases, he will report only twice weekly, receiving each time a supply for three to four days. He will also be given urine tests at appropriate intervals to determine whether he is taking any drugs other than methadone. The climate surrounding this clinical experiment could be best described as a therapeutic community with a good deal of supportive casework. As Nyswander (1967) puts it, the staff tries to do for the patient what a good friend would do: discuss problems, arrange for a home, provide him with work, and promote whatever occupational rehabilitation he requires, while simultaneously helping him to bridge the gap of mutual distrust and alienation that typically exists between himself and the world of the "square."

Although the number of patients who have been treated in this manner is relatively small and includes primarily individuals who *1/* have no medical, neurologic, or psychiatric illness, *2/* are between the ages of 20 and 39, and *3/* were taking no drugs other than opiates, the early results are impressive, particularly when it is realized that patients are admitted to the study only if they have a history of four or more years of heroin abuse and that most of them have a record of repeated arrests. Preliminary observations suggest that patients given enough methadone to keep them comfortable derive little or no pleasure from taking their previous dosage of heroin, do not try to get drugs elsewhere, cease being preoccupied with drugs, have no desire to obtain drugs for intravenous use, show no impairments in pain sensitivity, are capable of handling jobs requiring good motor skills and coordination, and, with the exception of constipation, report no undesirable side effects (Dole 1969).

It is not known to which of the many features of this program the favorable results ought to be attributed. That the majority of individuals involved in this program do not seem, as was feared, to take additional drugs surreptitiously or to ask for increasing doses may be a result of the close controls exerted against cheating, or it may be that, unlike the street addict, the medically legitimized methadone user need not view his behavior as wrong or live with the constant (and dependence-promoting) fear of being separated from his drug supply, without funds to obtain drugs, or arrested for possessing drugs or stealing the wherewithal to procure them. The favorable results may also derive from methadone's pharmacologic characteristics, for, being long-acting, it causes no sudden changes in the patient's level of comfort and none of the severe withdrawal symptoms that cause the user of short-acting opiates to spend his life in a frenzy of activity devoted to avoiding these symptoms by finding more of the drug that relieves them. Since he need not take drugs every few hours, as the user of short-acting agents must, he is not repeatedly exposed to opiate levels that, being far higher than necessary to control his withdrawal symptoms, tend to increase even further his tolerance, dependence, and subsequent drug dosage.

What is even more surprising, at least to those who view a drug's addictiveness as one of its immutable properties, is that the individual given methadone is not only able to work and to resume other obligations but, after some months of use, may even ask to have his dosage lowered or, in some cases, discontinued.

Although this program appears most suitable for those users whose behavior is unequivocally improved while taking opiates and who have not benefited from other pharmacologic, social-rehabilitative, or correctional-punitive measures, Dole and Nyswander's favorable results are not restricted to such users. This suggests that methadone might be a proper treatment approach for not only the anxious, irritable, and impulsive drug user, but also for young psychopaths of any description. There is always the possibility, of course, that some users take the methadone only to supplement the drugs they buy on the street (those given pills to take home even swapping the methadone for heroin, perhaps evading discovery by giving the clinic a friend's urine instead of their own), but if the criterion of success is social rehabilitation rather than abstinence, this need not be a cause for alarm so long as the patient is steadily employed and functioning well.

Experiments with *cyclazocine,* a drug that, taken daily, prevents the user from becoming "high" on other narcotics, suggest a new and promising avenue in the management of drug abuse, that of the drug "inactivator." While the long-term effectiveness of this or other narcotic antagonists is not yet documented, study of a hospital population in which patients who had been abstinent for some time were given 2 mg of cyclazocine twice daily has provided some encouraging results. The patients involved found that subsequent use of opiates did not produce the customary euphoria and did not develop physical dependence (Martin 1966).

Tactical approaches to the *psychotherapy* of the narcotics user vacillate between tough- and tender-mindedness, the differences being largely semantic. Both try to find a way to communicate with the drug user: the tender-minded by teaching the drug user the language of therapy and focusing on the symbolic meaning of self-medication; the tough-minded by learning the language of the addict and focusing on his day-to-day life. The latter's use of the argot of the slums spills over into their scientific works, which are peppered with descriptions of addicts who are "on the nod" because they are "stoned" by the "fix" of "horse" they have obtained from their "connection" while watching out for "the fuzz." Such involvement with the language of the addict reflects the ambivalent nature of professional interest: fascination, a desire to avoid looking "square," and sensationalism on the one hand; a desire to gain the drug user's confidence on the other. Unfortunately, such efforts rarely succeed, for the street addict's alienation from authority figures is so complete that no niceties or unniceties of language are likely to bridge the gap (see Table 51).

Group therapy programs may seem indicated because of the narcotic user's isolation from the mainstream of society, but they are not so successful for ambulatory narcotics users as they are for alcoholics. This is perhaps because the narcotics user always becomes totally involved in and committed to his way of life and, unlike the alcoholic, rarely invests any feeling in a situation not devoted exclusively to the pursuit of drugs. Residential group experiences, however, even when accomplished under duress, may provide the individual with an opportunity for the social learning that he lacks. One of the most interesting of such residential groups is The Synanon Foundation (Casriel 1963, Cherkas 1965, Yablonsky 1962, 1965), an organization composed almost exclusively, both staff and residents, of former drug users. This organization, now 10 years old, provides for its members a group-living experience that stresses appropriate and industrious social functioning within an accepting and autocratically organized small society; makes much use of extremely straightforward and vigorous group therapeutic efforts; and teaches the prevailing social values and norms and acceptable social habits and skills. The day-to-day activities of each resident are subjected to group scrutiny, comment, and criticism; and advancement within the status-conscious hierarchy is dependent on social and communicative skills. Much emphasis is given to "going through the motions" of appropriate social behavior, which, because it is markedly impaired in the majority of residents, is accomplished by instruction and command (Volkman 1963).

Synanon's autocratic control of its formerly sociopathic members, as well as its hostility to researchers and other outsiders, has led some observers to fear that it will eventually conflict with the larger society. This concern and the fact that many of its residents stay within Synanon permanently instead of returning to the community has led to the development by former Synanon members of similar organizations, like Daytop Village in New York, which place greater stress on cooperation with research and governmental authorities and on reintegration of members into the community at large. It will not be known for many years, however, whether such cooperation will compromise the effectiveness of these new organizations by making them seem too closely identified with the "Establishment," with which the sociopathic user feels in conflict, and thus less able to hold onto their members until they are thoroughly prepared to leave. To the extent, however, that such facilities enable users to remain off the streets and free of crime, they should be benevolently observed, as they can provide material with which to understand the dynamics of group interaction. Such information could well be of use in the treatment of other types of drug abuse and in the closely related antisocial and dyssocial personality disorders as well. Persons with such disorders, like the former narcotics user, may find such settings more acceptable because of the absence of medical or correctional personnel, a feature that may be attractive to the community for economic reasons.

Coercive techniques in the treatment of the ambulatory narcotics user include measures that detect drug use and thus help enforce the sanctions placed on it. Periodic nalorphine (Nalline) tests, which unmask opiate dependence by precipitating a withdrawal reaction and causing measurable increase in the patient's pupillary size, can be used to determine whether the former narcotics user continues to abstain (Poze 1962). This agent can produce fairly severe side effects, however, even if the individual is not taking drugs, and quite severe sweating, paresthesias, feelings of unreality, disturbing daydreams, visual hallucinations (Keats 1957), and other withdrawal symptoms, if he is. For this reason and because nalorphine tests are not as reliable as chromatographic urinary determinations (Way 1966), their use has been largely abandoned except by law enforcement agencies that use them to check up on former narcotics users with the (perhaps intended) effect of dissuading their clients from resuming drug use by making them afraid of being thrust into the discomfort of withdrawal.

The questions previously raised concerning the relevance of medical treatment to the problems of drug abuse are underscored by studies from the US Public Health Service Hospital in Lexington, Kentucky (where drug users are admitted either because they request it voluntarily or because they are sentenced to go there upon being convicted of a drug-related crime), that indicate that *enforced abstinence* appears to affect prognosis favorably (Kramer 1968). These studies reveal that, for effective promotion of abstinence, long imprisonment with parole is superior to long imprisonment without parole, that both are superior to short stays, and that the length of both stay and parole correlates positively with the length of abstinence. As long stays are more usual for the sentenced than for the voluntary patient, it is not surprising that 96% of those who were voluntarily hospitalized relapsed within a year of discharge, while 67% of those who stayed for at least nine months and were kept on parole for one year thereafter remained abstinent throughout the period of probation (Vaillant 1966b).

From the standpoint of dissuasion, the superiority of legal coercion over currently available medical treatment can also be detected in the results achieved in the management of that relatively large number of addicts within the health professions who have been shown to respond best to the threat of withdrawal of professional licensure. Indeed, the California system, in which drug-using physicians are placed under the supervision of the State Board of Medical Examiners for a period of five years, is reported to result in 92% freedom from drug use (Jones 1958).

CENTRAL NERVOUS SYSTEM STIMULANTS

This category includes cocaine; amphetamines such as amphetamine sulfate (Benzedrine), dextroamphetamine (Dexedrine), and methamphetamine (Methedrine); and amphetamine congeners like methylphenidate (Ritalin) and phenmetrazine (Preludin). With the exception of cocaine, these agents are readily available by prescription, usually as anorexiants or mood lifters. They are also available on the black market, cocaine and injectable amphetamines being most frequently procured in this manner. They are often used in association with sedatives, which serve both to curb stimulant-induced irritability and to enable the individual to go to sleep at night. Some users combine stimulants and narcotics (especially heroin) to enhance the latter's effects, or take cocaine, amphetamines, narcotics, and sedatives in sequence to create a state of exhilaration followed by relaxation and sleep.

Since the sniffing of cocaine has generally been abandoned in favor of intravenous use, stimulant users may be broadly categorized today into those taking the drugs by mouth and those taking them intravenously. Those taking amphetamines orally generally do so in order to diminish their appetites, enhance their alertness, or improve their mood (Kiloh 1962); they usually take no more than 30 to 40 mg daily and rarely exceed 100 mg daily. Those taking amphetamines (called "speed" by addicts) intravenously generally seek only the immediate pleasure; nowadays they usually take methamphetamine; the individual dose approximates 100 to 500 mg, though as much as 2,500 mg daily may be taken; and in one case 15 gm was taken within 24 hours (Kramer 1967). Users of intravenous stimulants ("speed freaks" in the addict argot) may spend protracted periods doing almost nothing but injecting the drugs, experiencing the pleasures of a 20 to 30 minute "high," and, as they start to feel the discomfort and nervousness of "coming down," injecting another dose. They may repeat this procedure every two hours around the clock for as long as a week to 10 days at a time, until they are exhausted, unbearably irritable, and depressed, at which point they go to sleep for 24 to 36 hours and then begin the process anew.

Acute intoxication with high doses of stimulants, particularly if taken parenterally, will cause the individual to feel alert, energetic, and exhilarated; to be garrulous, gregarious, and hypervigilant; and to believe that his physical and mental competence have increased. Sexual interest is enhanced (presumably less with amphetamines than with cocaine); climax is delayed but, when achieved, said to be more pleasurable than usual (Kramer 1967). More severe intoxication is marked not only by excitement but also by fearfulness, auditory and visual hallucinations, and in some cases, synesthetic experiences. Paresthesias and tactile hallucinations, such as the sensation of small animals crawling on or under the skin (formication), are said to be characteristic of cocaine intoxication (as is a more gradually occurring and receding and thus more comfortable and pleasurable "high"). Paranoid delusions (less organized in acute than in chronic intoxications) may also occur with stimulant abuse and lead to grotesque and impulsive behavior. Increased blood pressure, diaphoresis, and tachycardia are common consequences of stimulant intoxication; convulsions and cardiac arrhythmias, at times with circulatory collapse, are less common. Both the psychological and the somatic symptoms of intoxication can usually be relieved rapidly with intravenous barbiturates or intramuscular chlorpromazine (Done 1961, Espelin 1968); marked hypertension, with a rapid-acting alpha receptor blocking agent like phentolamine mesylate (Regitine).

Protracted use of stimulants is exceptionally dangerous, for, as tolerance increases, larger doses are taken, the patient's sleep and appetite become even worse, his thinking becomes hyperalert, and he develops paranoid delusions and hallucinations. This syndrome is, in many ways, indistinguishable from that seen in paranoid schizophrenics (Angrist 1969, Beamish 1960, Bonhoff 1954, McConnell 1963, Young 1938), with the possible exception that the amphetamine user tends to have more visual hallucinations than the schizophrenic, to retain some insight into the fact that his thinking and perception are disturbed, and to question the validity of his perceptions even after he has become delusional and started to hallucinate (Ellinwood 1967). Some patients develop an anergic, affectless, and almost trance-like state that persists even after the drug's immediate effect wears off. Furthermore, protracted use of high doses seems to leave in its wake certain cognitive and affective disturbances that may interfere grossly with functioning and motivation for many years (Lemere 1963).

The *withdrawal syndrome* consists of lethargy, somnolence, increased appetite, and profound depression, which may last from a few days to a few weeks and prompt the user to want another dose (Connell 1958, Kramer 1967). Although this anergic state is not usually thought of as an abstinence syndrome, it has been conclusively demonstrated that the effects of amphetamine withdrawal on REM activity can be measured as late as eight weeks after withdrawal and, even at this time, can be reversed by readministration of the drug (Oswald 1963).

Clinically, individuals with a propensity to abuse stimulants fall into two distinct categories:

1/ those who initially take them as anorexiants in order to lose weight, but continue to take them for their effect on mood and energy level, despite the negligible effect on their weight; and

2/ those who take them from the beginning solely for the "high" they produce.

The first group is generally introduced to the drugs by a physician and continues to get them from him or from one or more of the burgeoning group of physicians who specialize in giving out stimulants under the guise of scientific weight control; they generally take the drugs in oral form and continue to pursue a legitimate middle-class existence. The second group is usually introduced to stimulants by the dyssocial community in which they live and, though they may start by taking the drugs orally, eventually proceed to intravenous use. The individual who uses stimulants in the belief that they are effective anorexiants will sometimes require no treatment beyond having confirmed what he may already suspect: that the only way to lose weight is to go on a rigorous diet (see p. 479), and that continued stimulant use has long-term deleterious effects. The dyssocial user presents a far greater treatment problem, for he is unlikely to stop taking amphetamines until he is separated from the proselytizing, dependence-promoting, and drug-accessible community of which he is a part. Appropriate coercive measures, combined with detection methods utilizing urine chromatography, may prevent continued drug use but are usually insufficient; thus residential treatment based on the principles outlined for the management of opiate abuse may be required.

PSYCHOTOMIMETICS AND MISCELLANEOUS ABUSED AGENTS

Among the most commonly used psychotomimetic drugs in the United States are cannabis, in the form of marijuana or hashish (Grinspoon 1970, Walton 1938); d-lysergic acid diethylamide, LSD (Stoll 1943); mescaline (Beringer 1927, Mayer-Gross 1951); de-methyltryptamine, DMT; diethyltryptamine, DET (Szara 1957); psilo-cybin (Hollister 1961b); nutmeg (myristica) (Payne 1963); 2, 5-di-methoxy-4-, ethyl-amphetamine, DOM (known to users, however, as STP); and its ethyl homologue, DOET (Snyder 1967, 1969). While many other drugs such as phencyclidine (Sernyl) and JB 329 (Ditran) also have a psychotomimetic effect (Beech 1961, Davis 1964, Luby, 1959), they are disliked by those who take them and almost never abused.

Numerous sources satisfy the demand for these drugs. Marijuana, LSD, DMT, DET, and DOM are increasingly available via misappropria-tion from research facilities, home laboratories and gardens, or the *black markets* that flourish in "hippie" and college circles; mescaline can be procured through *mail-order houses* in Texas and Mexico as "peyote buttons" (Kleber 1965); nutmeg, which contains the hallu-cinogen myristicin, is available in *grocery stores;* and morning glory seeds, known to the Aztecs as ololiuqui and containing lysergic acid derivatives in the Heavenly Blue and Pearly Gate varieties, have been readily available until fairly recently in *garden supply stores.*

There is much similarity between the effects of mescaline, LSD, DMT, DET, psilocybin, and DOM. The apparent differences stem largely from the user's expectations and from variations in their relative potency, onset of action, and duration of effect (Abramson 1960, Isbell 1959, Wolbach 1962). Within an hour, 100 micrograms of LSD, 5 mg of DOM, 15 mg of psilocybin, 50 mg of DMT, or 500 mg of mescaline will produce, first, sympathomimetic effects like pupillary dilatation and a slight rise in temperature, systolic blood pressure, and pulse rate; then, psychotomimetic effects like an alteration in mood (generally in the direction of euphoria, but occasionally mixed with or predominantly depression), distortions of sensory perception (chiefly visual), distortions of body image and of the time sense so that time seems to pass very slowly; depersonalization; increased dis-tractibility; difficulty in expressing thoughts; increased vividness of both real and fantasied sensory perceptions; and sometimes hallu-cinations. Unless excessive doses are taken, the subject usually remains aware of the unreal character of these experiences, and the reaction subsides without complications in four to 16 hours. Administration of LSD, mescaline, or psilocybin for three to five consecutive days produces an almost complete, albeit short-lived, tolerance to the psychotomimetic effects (Isbell 1955, 1956). These drugs also exhibit considerable cross-tolerance. Physical dependence does not seem to occur (Isbell 1961). Few long-term users are faithful to a single drug of this type; most will experiment at one time or another with whatever is available or try combinations of several hallucinogens simultaneously or of hallucinogens together with amphetamines.

The *adverse consequences* of hallucinogen use include:

1/ the possibility of the individual's acting on his altered perceptions in a manner that endangers his life, health, or social reputation;

2/ the kind of unpleasant effects known to users as a "bad trip," by which they mean that the intoxication was marked by a state of discomfort, not by the customary and desired effect. This may result from taking the drugs in an unfamiliar or uncongenial environment, or from being unable to perform in some required way during the phase of intoxication. Users also apply the label of "bad trip" to states of intoxication that, perhaps as a result of excessive dosage, are marked by panic and confusion, last for 12 to 36 hours, and may be followed by partial or complete amnesia;

3/ protracted psychotic reactions marked by fluctuations in awareness, intermittent psychotic ideation, and hallucinatory experiences that would have been called acute undifferentiated schizophrenic episodes had they not immediately followed drug use; and

4/ repeated spontaneous recurrences of the psychedelic experience ("flashbacks") weeks or months after the last use, occurring most frequently in heavy users (Cohen 1960, 1963, Fink 1966, Freedman 1968, Horowitz 1969, Rosenthal 1964, Smart 1967b).

Changes in outlook and personality also occur, in the sense that the individual loses his interest in pursuits he formerly considered important; either embracing new and unaccustomed interests or merely drifting and pursuing no interests other than drugs, he views his drug use, his association with other drug users, and the "insights" he obtains in the intoxicated state as the only meaningful events of his life (Hensala 1967).

Acute intoxication with a psychotomimetic agent generally responds quite rapidly to the administration of phenothiazines like chlorpromazine (Thorazine) (Jacobsen 1963). Reports in the public press that chlorpromazine enhances or fails to diminish the effects of DOM (STP) or that it endangers the user's life have not been confirmed in a controlled study (Snyder 1967). Phenothiazines are also the treatment of choice in the protracted reactions, though in such cases it is hard to know whether the treatment is acting on a drug effect, a schizophrenic episode, or a latent schizophrenia released by the effect of the psychotomimetic. The notion that protracted psychotic reactions are, in reality, not caused but merely released by the drug is underscored by the observation that most of the individuals who experience such complications have had previous psychotic episodes or a history of CNS disturbances, particularly focal cerebral lesions (Korein 1968, McGlothlin 1969), or have at least been somewhat peculiar even before using the drugs (Ditman 1967, Frosch 1965, Ungerleider 1966). The treatment of prolonged LSD reactions is identical with that used in acute schizophrenic episodes (see p. 127): phenothiazine dosage is increased gradually until the patient's symptoms recede (this usually takes two to three weeks); this dosage is maintained for another month or two, then gradually reduced over a period of one to two months. The dosage that originally controlled symptoms should be reinstituted at once if the patient's symptoms recur while the dosage is being lowered.

The most commonly used psychotomimetics in the United States are *marijuana* and *hashish,* which are, respectively, the whole plant and the resin derived from the flowering tops of certain hemp plants. Isomers of the recently synthesized tetrahydrocannabinol (THC) are active ingredients of these drugs (Gaoni 1964, Korte 1965, Taylor 1966), but it is not certain whether they are the only psychoactive agents or whether there are differences between synthetic THC and naturally occurring marijuana (Waskow 1970). Both drugs, but especially marijuana, are widely sold on the black market and are easily obtainable in college and urban communities. Since certain of the hemp plants from which these agents are derived (cannabis sativa, indica, americana, etc.) flourish in any moderate climate, they are often homegrown by amateur botanists with a taste for these agents or a desire to sell them. These drugs may be taken in liquid form or in food, but in the United States are most frequently smoked in cigarettes.

In small doses, the effects resemble those of alcohol: the user may experience either nothing at all or any combination of nausea, drowsiness, exhilaration, impaired judgment, euphoria, slight dryness of the mouth and thirst, slight tremor and ataxia, and markedly increased appetite. There is usually some orthostatic hypotension and a rise in pulse and respiratory rate (Hollister 1968, Weil 1968). Higher doses approximate LSD in effect, but dysphoric or fearful experiences are uncommon. Spatial and temporal distortions occur in which the ground seems many miles away; a leisurely Sunday drive is experienced as a roller coaster ride; and minutes pass like hours. Not infrequently, the user experiences a sense of great insight and makes portentous cryptic statements that even he recognizes as nonsense or banalities once the effect wears off (Isbell 1967). Analgesic and antidepressant effects were reported by Chopra (1939), who, observing marijuana's use in India at a time when it was not prohibited, noted a higher incidence of use among individuals who had previously had insomnia. Under simulated driving conditions, marijuana has been shown to produce less impairment than alcohol (Crancer 1969). Very high doses have effects strikingly similar to those described above for other psychotomimetics, but cross-tolerance has not been demonstrated. Adverse reactions, such as panic states, fear of death, and impulsive behavior, are rare (Keeler 1967). Conjunctival irritation, photophobia, and a characteristic breath that is reminiscent in odor of newmown hay are common, and the user may wear dark glasses and use a breath-sweetener in order to hide these signs. The odor of burning marijuana is, moreover, extremely characteristic and so readily recognizable by anyone who has ever encountered it that marijuana users nowadays usually camouflage their activities by burning incense (see Table 19).

Although some degree of tolerance develops after a week or so of daily use, and some individuals exhibit restlessness, inability to concentrate, insomnia, depression, and anorexia a few days after discontinuing marijuana, there is little evidence that these represent manifestations of physical dependence. Craving as such does not occur, though some individuals do become preoccupied with using it again and again and with finding better, purer, and more exotic kinds of "grass." While heavy users may smoke as many as six to 10 cigarettes daily, most enjoy the drug only now and then and in moderate doses, in which case the dangers do not seem to exceed those of alcohol (McGlothlin 1968). There is, in any case, no evidence for the view that the use of marijuana predisposes an individual to heroin use, except to the extent that marijuana's prohibition may force the user into contact with the same black market sources from which such agents as heroin, hallucinogens, or amphetamines can be obtained (Eddy 1965).

Powdered nutmeg—containing safrole, myristicin, and elemicin in varying amounts (Farnsworth 1968)—is often abused in prison settings where other drugs may be harder to procure. The effects are similar to those of marijuana, characterized by mood fluctuations, sharpened attention, euphoria, and sometimes hallucinations, occurring, however, as long as two to five hours following ingestion (Weil 1967, Weiss 1960). That many of the prisoners who use nutmeg used other agents prior to incarceration shows that some drug abusers are not looking for a *particular* effect, but simply for *any* change in mood or cognition. This fact may explain the ever-increasing, already almost endless list of agents that are being abused, a list that now includes Romilar-CF (Younes 1969), stramonium-containing Asmador, and amyl nitrite, vials of which are broken and sniffed at the moment of orgasm to heighten enjoyment (Goldsmith 1968, Leff 1968).

The inhalation of *gasoline, lighter fluid, airplane glue* (toluene), and *refrigerant* (dichorodifluoromethane) *fumes* is reported to be on the increase among children and adolescents (Ackerly 1964, Brozovsky 1965, Glaser 1966, Massengale 1963). The effects include transient euphoria, exhilaration, and excitement and, in high doses, confusion, headache, nausea, tinnitus, ataxia, tremors, and fasciculations. Hepatic damage, irreversible encephalopathy (Knox 1966) and aplastic anemia with fatal outcome (Gattner 1963, Powars 1965) have been reported, and individuals who inhale the fumes with a plastic bag covering their heads to enhance the effect have even suffocated. Treatment is rarely required for the acute intoxication *per se* since the reaction is usually short-lived and by the time the doctor sees the patient he will be free of symptoms.

Occasional experimentation with hallucinogens on the part of an otherwise well-adjusted individual has not been shown to be a serious hazard to health, to the present; it has even been claimed that such use can heighten the affective resonance and spontaneity of an interpersonally alienated or affectively blocked individual (Bowers 1967, Keniston 1965). But those who go on to more frequent use of these drugs tend to show personality changes incompatible with traditional social functioning and, for this reason, to come to medical attention. Once in treatment, some will feel better without these drugs and will make the decision to refrain from their further use. For others, continued hallucinogen use can be prevented or at least made less rewarding with the administration of phenothiazines or reserpine, drugs that diminish the effect of a subsequently ingested hallucino-

TABLE 19. *Identification of Drug Abuse in Students* *

COMMON SIGNS OF DRUG ABUSE

Changes in school attendance, discipline, and grades
Change in the character of homework
Unusual and apparently unmotivated outbursts of temper
Slovenly or unhealthy physical appearance
Furtive behavior (to conceal drugs and other possessions)
Wearing of sunglasses at inappropriate times (to hide dilated or constricted pupils)
Constant wearing of long-sleeved shirts (to cover needle marks)
Association with known drug abusers
Extensive borrowing of money from other students (to purchase drugs)
Theft of small items from school
Frequenting of such odd places as closets or storage rooms during the school day (to take drugs)
Familiarity with drug user argot (see Table 51)

MANIFESTATIONS OF SPECIFIC FORMS OF DRUG ABUSE

Glue Sniffing

Odor of substance inhaled on breath and clothes
Excess nasal secretions, watering of the eyes
Poor muscular control, drowsiness or unconsciousness
Possession of plastic or paper bags or rags containing dry plastic cement

CNS Depressant Abuse

Symptoms of alcohol intoxication without odor of alcohol on breath
Staggering or stumbling in classrooms or halls
Falling asleep in class
Lack of interest in school activities
Drowsiness and apparent disorientation

Stimulant Abuse

Excessive activity: student is irritable, argumentative, and nervous and has difficulty sitting still in classrooms
Dilated pupils
Dry mouth and nose; bad breath; frequent licking of lips and rubbing and scratching of nose
Chain smoking
Not eating or sleeping for long periods

Narcotic Abuse

Traces of white powder, redness and rawness around the nostrils (caused by inhaling heroin in powder form)
Scars on the inner surface of the arms and elbows (caused by injecting heroin, mainlining); the student therefore wears long-sleeved shirts most of the time
Syringes, bent spoons, cotton, and needles in lockers
Lethargy and drowsiness in the classroom
Pupils that are constricted and fail to respond to light

NOTE: Opiate users are not frequently seen in school; they usually start out by drinking paregoric or cough medicines containing codeine; the presence of empty bottles in wastebaskets or on school grounds is a clue.

TABLE 19. *Identification of Drug Abuse in Students* * (continued)

Marijuana Abuse

Animation and hysteria with rapid, loud talking and bursts of laughter in the early stages

Sleepiness or stupor in the later stages

Distortion of depth perception, which makes driving dangerous

NOTE: Marijuana users are not easily recognized unless they are under the influence of the drug at the time they are being observed. Marijuana cigarettes are rolled in a double thickness of brown or off-white cigarette paper. They are smaller than a regular cigarette with the paper twisted or tucked in at both ends. The contents are greener in color than regular tobacco, and the odor resembles that of burning weeds or rope.

Hallucinogen Abuse

Sitting or reclining quietly in a dream or trance-like state

Fearfulness and an experience of terror which make user attempt to escape from the group

Changes in mood and behavior

Perceptual changes involving sight, hearing, touch, body-image, and time

NOTE: It is unlikely that students who use hallucinogens will do so in school, since they are generally taken in the company of others and under special conditions. The drug is odorless, tasteless, colorless, and may be found in the form of impregnated sugar cubes, cookies, or crackers. LSD is usually taken orally but may be injected. It is often purchased in ampuls of clear blue liquid.

* Adapted from: *Drug Abuse Education . . . A Guide for the Professions* (Second Edition), Amer Pharm Ass, 1968. (The material noted here was originally abstracted by David J. Lehman, M.D., from *Drug Abuse: Escape to Nowhere*, publication of the National Education Association.)

gen. Typically, however, the hallucinogen user considers his experiences to be extremely meaningful and enlightening, and resists efforts to "help" by discontinuing the prescribed tranquilizer fairly quickly. In such a case, the use of a long-acting or "depot" phenothiazine, such as fluphenazine enanthate (Prolixin), may prevent continued drug use. Information concerning the still inconclusive report of chromosomal damage and fetal abnormalities in long-term hallucinogen users (Auerbach 1967, Cohen 1967, Corey 1970, Egozcue 1968, Houston 1969, Judd 1969, Loughman 1967, Roux 1970, Sparkes 1968, Zellweger 1967) may also dissuade some abusers and has already caused many college students to think twice about taking LSD. (For a discussion of possible therapeutic uses of psychotomimetic drugs, see Chapter 16.)

REFERENCES

Abramson, H. A.: Lysergic acid diethylamide (LSD-25): XXX. The questionnaire
technique with notes on its use, J Psychol
49:57-65, 1960.

Achté, K. A., Stenbäck, A., and Terä-
väinen, H.: On suicides committed during
treatment in psychiatric hospitals, Acta
Psychiat Scand 42:272-284, 1966.

Ackerly, W. C., and Gibson, G.: Lighter
fluid "sniffing", Amer J Psychiat 120:1056-
1061, 1964.

Angrist, B. M., et al.: Clinical symptomatology of amphetamine psychosis and its
relationship to amphetamine levels in
urine, Int Pharmacopsychiat 2:125-139,
1969.

Auerbach, R., and Rugowski, J. A.: Lysergic acid diethylamide: Effect on embryos, Science 157:1325-1326, 1967.

Beamish, P., and Kiloh, L. G.: Psychoses
due to amphetamine consumption, J Ment
Sci 106:337-343, 1960.

Beech, H. R., Davies, B. M., and Mor-
genstern, F. S.: Preliminary investigations
of the effects of Sernyl upon cognitive and
sensory processes, J Ment Sci 107:509-513,
1961.

Bellville, J. W., and Green, J.: Respiratory and subjective effects of pentazocine,
Clin Pharmacol Ther 6:152-159, 1965.

Beringer, K.: Der Meskalinrausch: Seine
Geschichte und Erscheinungsweise, Berlin: Springer, 1927.

Berne, E.: Games People Play: The Psychology of Human Relationships, New
York: Grove, 1964.

Bilz, R.: Trinker, Stuttgart: Enke, 1959.

Blachly, P. H.: Procedure for withdrawal
of barbiturates, Amer J Psychiat 120:894-
895, 1964.

——: Management of the opiate abstinence syndrome, Amer J Psychiat 122:
742-745 1966.

Bonhoff, G., and Lewrenz, H.: Über
Weckamine, Berlin: Springer, 1954.

Bowers, M., et al.: Dynamics of psychedelic drug abuse: A clinical study, Arch
Gen Psychiat (Chicago) 16:560-566, 1967.

Brain, L., et al.: Drug addiction. Second
report Interdepartmental Committee, Scot-
tish Home and Health Dept, July 31, 1965,
14 pp.

Brayton, R. G., et al.: Effect of alcohol
and various diseases on leukocyte mobili-
zation, phagocytosis and intracellular bac-

terial killing, New Eng J Med 282:123-128,
1970.

Brotman, R., Meyer, A. S., and Freedman, A. M.: Approach to treating narcotic
addicts based on a community mental
health diagnosis, Compr Psychiat 6:104-
118, 1965.

Brozovsky, M., and Winkler, E. G.:
Glue sniffing in children and adolescents,
New York J Med 65:1984-1989, 1965.

Casriel, D.: So Fair A House: The Story
of Synanon, Englewood Cliffs (NJ), Prentice-Hall, 1963.

Chafetz, M. E.: Consumption of alcohol
in the Far and Middle East, New Eng J
Med 271:297-301, 1964.

Cherkas, M. S.: Synanon Foundation—A
radical approach to the problem of addiction, Amer J Psychiat 121:1065-1068, 1965.

Chopra, R. N., and Chopra, G. S.: Present position of hemp-drug addiction in
India, Indian J Med Res 31:1-119, 1939.

Clemmesen, C., and Nilsson, E.: Therapeutic trends in the treatment of barbiturate poisoning: The Scandinavian method,
Clin Pharmacol Ther 2:220-229, 1961.

Cochin, J.: Analysis for narcotic analgesics and barbiturates in urine by thin-
layer chromatographic techniques without
previous extraction and concentration, Psychopharmacol Bull 3:53-60, 1966.

Cohen, M. M., Marinello, M. J., and
Back, N.: Chromosomal damage in human
leukocytes induced by lysergic acid diethylamide, Science 155:1417-1419, 1967.

Cohen, S.: Lysergic acid diethylamide:
Side effects and complications, J Nerv
Ment Dis 130:30-40, 1960.

Cohen, S., and Ditman, K. S.: Prolonged
adverse reactions to lysergic acid diethylamide, Arch Gen Psychiat (Chicago) 8:475-
480, 1963.

Connell, P. H.: Amphetamine Psychosis,
London: Chapman, 1958.

Corey, M. J., et al.: Chromosome studies on patients (in vivo) and cells (in vitro)
treated with lysergic acid diethylamide,
New Eng J Med 282:939-943, 1970.

Crancer, A., Jr., et al.: Comparison of
the effects of marihuana and alcohol on
simulated driving performance, Science
164:851-854, 1969.

Cutshall, B. J.: The Saunders-Sutton
syndrome: An analysis of delirium tremens,
Quart J Stud Alcohol 26:423-448, 1965.

Davies, D. L.: Normal drinking in recovered alcohol addicts, Quart J Stud Alcohol 23:94-104, 1962.

Davies, D. L., Shepherd, M., and Myers, E.: Two-years' prognosis of 50 alcohol addicts after treatment in hospital, Quart J Stud Alcohol 17:485-502, 1956.

Davis, H. K., et al.: Clinical evaluation of JB-329 (Ditran), Dis Nerv Syst 25:179-183, 1964.

Diskind, M. H., and Klonsky, G.: Second look at the New York State Parole Drug Experiment, Fed Probation 28:34-41, 1964.

Ditman, K. S., et al.: Harmful aspects of the LSD experience, J Nerv Ment Dis 145:464-474, 1967.

Dole, V. P., Kim, W. K., and Eglitis, I.: Extraction of narcotic drugs, tranquilizers, and barbiturates by cation-exchange paper, and detection on a thin-layer chromatogram by a series of reagents, Psychopharmacol Bull 3:45-48, 1966a.

Dole, V. P., and Nyswander, M. E.: Rehabilitation of heroin addicts after blockade with methadone, New York J Med 66:2011-2017, 1966b.

Dole, V. P., et al.: Methadone treatment of randomly selected criminal addicts, New Eng J Med 280:1372-1375, 1969.

Done, A. K.: Clinical pharmacology of systemic antidotes, Clin Pharmacol Ther 2:750-793, 1961.

Drewery, J., and Rae, J. B.: Group comparison of alcoholic and non-alcoholic marriages using the interpersonal perception technique, Brit J Psychiat 115:287-300, 1969.

Duvall, H. J., Locke, B. Z., and Brill, L.: Followup study of narcotic drug addicts five years after hospitalization, Public Health Rep 78:185-193, 1963.

Eckenhoff, J. E., and Oech, S. R.: Effects of narcotics and antagonists upon respiration and circulation in man: A review, Clin Pharmacol Ther 1:483-524, 1962.

Eddy, N. B., et al.: Drug dependence: Its significance and characteristics, Bull WHO 32:721-733, 1965.

Egozcue, J., Irwin, S., and Maruffo, C. A.: Chromosomal damage in LSD users, JAMA 204:214-218, 1968.

Ellinwood, E. H., Jr.: Amphetamine psychosis: 1. Description of the individuals and process, J Nerv Ment Dis 144:273-283, 1967.

Elson, A., and Domino, E. F.: Dextropropoxyphene addiction: Observations of a case, JAMA 183:482-485, 1963.

Espelin, D. E., and Done, A. K.: Amphetamine poisoning, New Eng J Med 278:1361-1365, 1968.

Essig, C. F.: Addiction to nonbarbiturate sedative and tranquilizing drugs, Clin Pharmacol Ther 5:334-343, 1964.

Farnsworth, N. R.: Hallucinogenic plants, Science 162:1086-1092, 1968.

Ferguson, J. K. W., et al.: A new drug for alcoholism treatment, Canad Med Ass J 74:793-798, 1956.

Fink, M., et al.: Prolonged adverse reactions to LSD in psychotic subjects, Arch Gen Psychiat (Chicago) 15:450-454, 1966.

Fort, J.: Use and abuse of alcohol and narcotics around the world, Proc III World Cong Psychiat, vol. 1, 1961, pp. 398-401.

Fraser, H. F., and Grider, J. A.: Treatment of drug addiction, Amer J Med 14:571-577, 1953.

Fraser, H. F., Isbell, H., and Wolbach, A. B.: Addictiveness of new synthetic analgesics, in Minutes of 21st meeting of Committee on Drug Addiction and Narcotics, Appen. 12, NAS-NRC, Washington, DC, 1960.

Fraser, H. F., et al.: Chronic barbiturate intoxication: Further studies, Arch Intern Med 94:34-41, 1954.

Fraser, H. F., et al.: Degree of physical dependence induced by secobarbital or pentobarbital, JAMA 166:126-129, 1958.

Fraser, H. F., et al.: Effects of addiction to intravenous heroin on patterns of physical activity in men, Clin Pharmacol Ther 4:188-196, 1963.

Freedman, D. X.: On the use and abuse of LSD, Arch Gen Psychiat (Chicago) 18:330-347, 1968.

Frosch, W., Robbins, E., and Sterin, M.: Untoward reactions to LSD resulting in hospitalization, New Eng J Med 273:1235-1239, 1965.

Gaoni, Y., and Mechoulam, R.: Isolation, structure and partial synthesis of an active constituent of hashish, J Amer Chem Soc 86:1646, 1964.

Gattner, H.: Blood damage caused by fuel and exhaust fumes, Munchen Med Wschr 105:1160-1168, 1963.

Gerard, D. L., and Kornetsky, C.: Social and psychiatric study of adolescent opiate addicts, Psychiat Quart 28:113-125, 1954.

Gerard, D. L., Saenger, G., and Wile, R.: The abstinent alcoholic, Arch Gen Psychiat (Chicago) 6:83-95, 1962.

Glaser, F. B.: Inhalation psychosis and related states. A review, Arch Gen Psychiat (Chicago) 14:315-322, 1966.

Goldsmith, S. R., Frank, I., and Ungerleider, J. T.: Poisoning from ingestion of a stramonium-belladonna mixture, JAMA *204:*169-170, 1968.

Grinspoon, L.: Marihuana, to be published.

Gross, M. M., *et al.:* Sleep disturbances and hallucinations in the acute alcoholic psychoses, J Nerv Ment Dis *142:*493-514, 1966.

Haizlip, T. M., and Ewing, J. A.: Meprobamate habituation: Controlled clinical study, New Eng Med *258:*1181-1186, 1958.

Hald, J., Jacobsen, E., and Larsen, V.: Sensitizing effect of tetraethylthiuramdisulfide (Antabuse) to ethylalcohol, Acta Pharmacol (Kobenhavn) *4:*285-296, 1948.

Hardison, W. G., and Lee, F. I.: Prognosis in acute liver disease of the alcoholic patient, New Eng J Med *275:*61-66, 1966.

Helpern, M.: Narcotics-related diseases, Quoted in AMA News, August 26, 1968.

Henderson, L. W., and Merrill, J. P.: Treatment of barbiturate intoxication, Ann Intern Med *64:*876-891, 1966.

Hensala, J. D., Epstein, L. J., and Blacker, K. H.: LSD and psychiatric inpatients, Arch Gen Psychiat (Chicago) *16:*554-559, 1967.

Hess, C.: Personal communication, 1965.

Hines, J. D.: Reversible megaloblastic and sideroblastic marrow abnormalities in alcoholic patients, Brit J Haemat *16:*87-102, 1969.

Hollister, L. E., Motzenbecker, F. P., and Degan, R. O.: Withdrawal reactions from chlordiazepoxide (Librium), Psychopharmacologia *2:*63-68, 1961a.

Hollister, L. E.: Clinical, biochemical and psychologic effects of psilocybin, Arch Int Pharmacodyn *130:*42-52, 1961b.

Hollister, L. E., Richards, R. K., and Gillespie, H. K.: Comparison of tetrahydrocannabinol and synhexyl in man, Clin Pharmacol Ther *9:*783-791, 1968.

Horowitz, M. J.: Flashbacks: Recurrent intrusive images after the use of LSD, Amer J Psychiat *126:*565-569, 1969.

Houston, B. K.: Review of the evidence and qualifications regarding the effects of hallucinogenic drugs on chromosomes and embryos, Amer J Psychiat *126:*251-254, 1969.

Hunt, G. H., and Odoroff, M. E.: Followup study of narcotic drug addicts after hospitalization, Public Health Rep *77:*41-54, 1962.

Isbell, H.: Addiction to barbiturates and the barbiturate abstinence syndrome, Arch Intern Med *33:*108-121, 1950.

——: Comparison of the reactions induced by psilocybin and LSD-25 in man, Psychopharmacologia *1:*29-38, 1959.

Isbell, H., *et al.:* Tolerance to diethylamide of lysergic acid (LSD-25), Fed Proc *14:*354, 1955.

Isbell, H., *et al.:* Studies on lysergic acid diethylamide (LSD-25), Arch Neurol Psychiat *76:*468-478, 1956.

Isbell, H., *et al.:* Cross tolerance between LSD and psilocybin, Psychopharmacologia *2:*147-159, 1961.

Isbell, H., *et al.:* Effects of (–) delta⁰-trans-tetrahydrocannabinol in man, Psychopharmacologia *11:*184-188, 1967.

Isselbacher, K. J., and Greenberger, N. J.: Metabolic effects of alcohol on the liver New Eng J Med *270:*351-356 and 402-410, 1964.

Jacobsen, E.: Clinical pharmacology of the hallucinogens, Clin Pharmacol Ther *4:*480-503, 1963.

Jaffe, J. H.: Narcotic analgesics, *in* Goodman, L. S., and Gilman, A., eds.: The Pharmacological Basis of Therapeutics, ed. 3, New York: Macmillan, 1965, pp. 247-284.

Jaffe, J. H., and Kirkpatrick, D.: Use of ion-exchange resin impregnated paper in the detection of opiate alkaloids, amphetamines, phenothiazines and barbiturates in urine, Psychopharmacol Bull *3:*49-52, 1966.

James, I. P.: Blood alcohol levels following successful suicide, Quart J Stud Alcohol *27:*23-29, 1966.

James, I. P., Scott-Orr, D. N., and Curnow, D. H.: Blood alcohol levels following attempted suicide, Quart J Stud Alcohol *24:*14-22, 1963.

Janssen, P. A. J.: Synthetic Analgesics: Part 1, Diphenylproplyamines, London: Pergamon, 1960.

Jones, L. E.: Experience with probation in California, Fed Bull *45:*165-173, 1958.

Jones, T. T.: Gastropancreatic crisis and alcohol intoxication, Quart J Stud Alcohol *26:*498-499, 1965.

Judd, L. L., Brandkamp, W. W., and McGlothlin, E. H.: Comparison of the chromosomal patterns obtained from groups of continued users, former users, and non-users of LSD-25, Amer J Psychiat *126:*626-635, 1969.

Kaim, S. C., Klett, C. J., and Rothfeld, B.: Treatment of the acute alcohol withdrawal state: Comparison of four drugs, Amer J Psychiat *125:*1640-1646, 1969.

Keats, A. S., and Telford, J.: Subjective effects of nalorphine in hospitalized patients, J Pharmacol Exp Ther *119:*370-377, 1957.

Keeler, M. H.: Adverse reaction to marihuana, Amer J Psychiat *124:*674-677, 1967.

Kendall, R. E., Normal drinking by former alcohol addicts, Quart J Stud Alcohol *26:*247-257, 1965.

Kendall, R. E., and Staton, M. C.: Fate of untreated alcoholics, Quart J Stud Alcohol *27:*30-41, 1966.

Keniston, K.: The Uncommitted, New York: Harcourt, 1965.

Kessel, N.: Self-poisoning, *in* Shneidman, E. S., ed.: Essays in Self-Destruction, New York: Science House, 1967, pp. 345-372.

Kiloh, L. G., and Brandon, S.: Amphetamine habituation and addiction, Brit Med J *5296:*40-43, 1962.

King, R.: An appraisal of international, British and selected European narcotic drug laws, regulations, and policies, *in* Drug Addiction, Crime or Disease?, Interim and Final Report of the Joint Committee of the ABA and the AMA on Narcotic Drugs, Bloomington: Indiana Univ Press, 1961, pp. 121-155.

Klatskin, G.: Experimental studies on the role of alcohol in the pathogenesis of cirrhosis, Amer J Clin Nutr *9:*439-445, 1961.

Kleber, H. D.: Student use of hallucinogens, J Amer Coll Health Ass *14:*109-117, 1965.

Knox, J. W., and Nelson, J. R.: Permanent encephalopathy from toluene inhalation, New Eng J Med *275:*1494-1496, 1966.

Korein, J., and Musacchio, J. M.: LSD and focal cerebral lesions. Behavioral and EEG effects in patients with sensory defects, Neurology *18:*147-152, 1968.

Korte, F.: *In* Hashish: Its Chemistry and Pharmacology, Ciba Foundation Study Group #21, Boston: Little, 1965.

Kramer, J. C., Bass, R. A., and Berecochea, J. E.: Civil commitment for addicts: California program, Amer J Psychiat *125:*816-824, 1968.

Kramer, J. C., Fischman, V. S., and Littlefield, D. C.: Amphetamine abuse, JAMA *201:*305-309, 1967.

Kurland, A. A., *et al.:* Psychedelic therapy utilizing LSD in the treatment of the alcoholic patient: Preliminary report, Amer J Psychiat *123:*1202-1209, 1967.

Lasagna, L.: Addicting drugs and medical practice: Toward the elaboration of realistic goals and the eradication of myths, mirages, and half-truths, *in* Wilner, D. M.,

and Kassebaum, G. G., eds.: Narcotics, New York: McGraw-Hill, 1965, pp. 53-67.

Lasagna, L., von Felsinger, J. M., and Beecher, H. K.: Drug-induced mood changes in man: 1. Observations on healthy subjects, chronically ill patients, and "postaddicts", JAMA *157:*1006-1020, 1955.

Leevy, C. M., *et al.:* B-Complex vitamins in liver disease of the alcoholic, Amer J Clin Nutr *16:*339-346, 1965.

Leff, R., and Bernstein, S.: Proprietary hallucinogens, Dis Nerv Syst *29:*621-626, 1968.

Lemere, F.: Amphetamine addiction in Japan, JAMA *185:*414, 1963.

Levin, M.: Bromide psychoses: Four varieties, Amer J Psychiat *104:*798-800, 1948.

———: Bromide hallucinosis, Arch Gen Psychiat (Chicago) *2:*429-433, 1960.

Levy, M. S., Livingstone, B. L., and Collins, D. M.: Clinical comparison of disulfiram and calcuim carbimide, Amer J Psychiat *123:*1018-1022, 1967.

Liddon, S. C., and Satran, R.: Disulfiram (Antabuse) psychosis, Amer J Psychiat *123:*1284-1289, 1967.

Lieber, C. S., and Rubin, E.: Alcoholic fatty liver, New Eng J Med *280:*705-708, 1969.

Lindenbaum, J., and Lieber, C. S.: Hematologic effects of alcohol in man in the absence of nutritional deficiency, New Eng J Med *281:*333-338, 1969.

Loughman, W. D., Sargent, T. W., and Israelstam, D. M.: Leukocytes of humans exposed to lysergic acid diethylamide: damage, Science *158:*508-510, 1967.

Louria, D. B.: Medical complications associated with heroin use, Int J Addict *2:*241-251, 1967.

Luby, E. D., *et al.:* Study of a new schizophrenomimetic drug—Sernyl, Arch Neurol Psychiat *81:*363-369, 1959.

Lundqvist, G.: Delirium tremens, Alkoholfragan *55:*183-185, 1961.

Macklin, E. A., Simon, A., and Crook, G. H.: Psychotic reactions in problem drinkers treated with disulfiram (Antabuse) Arch Neurol Psychiat *69:*415-426, 1953.

Madill, M. F., *et al.:* Aversion treatment of alcoholics by succinycholine-induced apneic paralysis, Quart J Stud Alcohol *27:*483-509, 1966.

Marconi, J., Solari, G., and Gaete, S.: Comparative clinical study of the effects of disulfiram and calcium carbimide 11.

Reaction to alcohol, Quart J Stud Alcohol 22:46-51, 1961

Martensen-Larsen, O.: Psychotic phenomena provoked by tetraethylthiuram disulfide, Quart J Stud Alcohol 12:206-216, 1951.

Martin, W. R., and Fraser, H. F.: Comparitive study of physiological and subjective effects of heroin and morphine administered intravenously in post-addicts, J Pharmacol Exp Ther 133:388-399, 1961.

Martin, W. R., Gorodetzky, C. W., and McClane, T. K.: Experimental study in the treatment of narcotic addicts with cyclazocine, Clin Pharmacol Ther 7:455-465, 1966.

Massengale, O. N., et al.: Physical and psychologic factors in glue sniffing, New Eng J Med 269:1340-1344, 1963.

Mayer-Gross, W.: Experimental psychoses and other mental abnormalities produced by drugs, Brit Med J 2:317-321, 1951.

McConnell, W. B.: Amphetamine substances in mental illnesses in Northern Ireland, Brit J Psychiat 109:218-224, 1963.

McGlothlin, W. H., and West, L. J.: The marihuana problem: An overview, Amer J Psychiat 125:370-378, 1968.

McGlothlin, W. H., Arnold, D. O., and Freedman, D. X.: Organicity measures following repeated LSD ingestion, Arch Gen Psychiat (Chicago) 21:704-709, 1969.

McIsaac, W. M.: Establishment of a new drug addiction program, Psychopharmacol Bull 3:40-44, 1966.

Mendelson, J. H.: Biologic concomitants of alcoholism. I., New Eng J Med 283:24-32, 1970a.

———: Biologic concomitants of alcoholism. II., New Eng J Med 283:71-81, 1970b.

Miller, B. A., Pokorny, A. D., and Hanson, P. G.: Study of dropouts in an inpatient alcoholism treatment program, Dis Nerv Syst 29:91-99, 1968.

Mitchell, E. H.: Use of citrated calcium carbimide in alcoholism, JAMA 168:2008-2009, 1958.

Mitcheson, M., et al.: Sedative abuse by heroin addicts, Lancet 1:606-607, 1970.

Murphree, H. B.: Clinical pharmacology of potent analgesics, Clin Pharmacol Ther 3:473-504, 1962.

New York Academy of Medicine Committee on Public Health: Special report: Report on drug addiction II. Clin Pharmacol Ther 4:425-460, 1963.

Nielsen, J., Juel-Nielsen, N., and Strömgren, E.: Five-year survey of a psychiatric service in a geographically delimited rural population given easy access to this service, Compr Psychiat 6:139-165, 1965.

Nyswander, M.: The Drug Addict as a Patient, New York: Grune, 1956.

———: Methadone treatment of heroin addiction, Hosp Prac 2:27-33, 1967.

O'Reilly, P. O., and Funk, A.: LSD in chronic alcoholism, Canad Psychiat Ass J 9:258-261, 1964.

Oswald, I., and Priest, R. G.: Five weeks to escape the sleeping-pill habit, Brit Med J 2:1093-1095, 1965.

Oswald, I., et al.: Melancholia and barbiturates: A controlled EEG, body and eye movement study of sleep, Brit J Psychiat 109:66-78, 1963.

Parades, A., and Cornelison, F. S., Jr.: Development of an audiovisual technique for the rehabilitation of alcoholics, Quart J Stud Alcohol 29:84-92, 1968.

Payne, R. B.: Nutmeg intoxication, New Eng J Med 269:36-38, 1963.

Perkins, M. E., and Bloch, H. I.: Survey of a methadone maintenance treatment program, Amer J Psychiat 126:1389-1396, 1970.

Perlmutter, J. F.: Drug addiction in pregnant women, Amer J Obstet Gynec 99:569-572, 1967.

Pitts, F. N., and Winokur, G.: Affective disorder. VII. Alcoholism and affective disorder, J Psychiat Res 4:37-50, 1966.

Powars, D.: Aplastic anemia secondary to glue sniffing, New Eng J Med 273:700-702, 1965.

Poze, R. S.: Opiate addiction I. The nalorphine test, II. Current concepts of treatment, Stanford Med Bull 20:1-23, 1962.

Räkköläinen, V., and Turunen, S.: From unrestrained to moderate drinking, Acta Psychiat Scand 45:47-52, 1969.

Regan, P. F.: The psychotherapeutic management of abrupt drug withdrawal, in Hoch, P. H., and Zubin, J. eds.: Problems of Addiction and Habituation, New York: Grune, 1958, pp. 186-201.

Reichle, C. W., et al.: Comparative analgesic potency of heroin and morphine in postoperative patients, J Pharmacol Exp Ther 136:43-46, 1962.

Retterstöl, N., and Sund, A.: Drug addiction and habituation, Acta Psychiat Scand 40 (Suppl 179):9-120, 1964.

Reynolds, A. K., and Randall, L. O.: Morphine and Allied Drugs, Toronto: Univ Toronto Press, 1957.

Ritson, E. B.: Suicide amongst alcoholics, Brit J Med Psychol 41:235-242, 1968.

Rosenthal, S. H.: Persistent hallucinosis following repeated administrations of hallucinogenic drugs, Amer J Psychiat *121:* 238-244, 1964.

Roux, C., Dupuis, R., and Aubry, M.: LSD: No teratogenic action in rats, mice, and hamsters, Science *169:*588-589, 1970.

Sandoval, R. G., and Wang, R. I. H.: Tolerance and dependence on pentazocine, New Eng J Med *280:*1391-1392, 1969.

Saravay, S. M., and Pardes, H.: Auditory elementary hallucinations in alcohol withdrawal psychosis, Arch Gen Psychiat (Chicago) *16:*652-658, 1967.

Sarett, M., Cheek, F., and Osmond, H.: Reports of wives of alcoholics of effects of LSD-25 treatment of their husbands, Arch Gen Psychiat (Chicago) *14:*171-178, 1966.

Schukit, M., *et al.:* Alcoholism. I. Two types of alcoholism in women, Arch Gen Psychiat (Chicago) *20:*301-306, 1969.

Selig, J. W.: Possible oxazepam abstinence syndrome, JAMA *198:*951-952, 1966.

Shapiro, F. L., and Smith, H. T.: Treatment of barbiturate intoxication, Mod Med *37:*104-110, 1969.

Smart, R. G., *et al.:* Lysergic acid diethylamide (LSD) in the treatment of alcoholism, Toronto: Univ Toronto Press, 1967a.

Smart, R. G., and Bateman, K.: Unfavourable reactions to LSD: A review and analysis of the available case reports, Canad Med Ass J *97:*1214-1221, 1967b.

Smilde, J.: Risks and unexpected reactions in disulfiram therapy of alcoholism, Quart J Stud Alcohol *24:*489-494, 1963.

Smith, C. G.: Alcoholics: Their treatment and their wives, Brit J Psychiat *115:* 1039-1042, 1969.

Smith, G. M., Semke, C. W., and Beecher, H. K.: Objective evidence of mental effects of heroin, morphine and placebo in normal subjects, J Pharmacol Exp Ther *136:*53-58, 1962.

Snyder, S. H., Faillace, L., and Hollister, L.: 2,5-Dimethoxy-4-methylamphetamine (STP). New hallucinogenic drug, Science *158:*669-670, 1967.

Snyder, S. H., Faillace, L. A., and Weingartner, H.: New psychotropic agent, Arch Gen Psychiat (Chicago) *21:*95-101, 1969.

Sparkes, R. S., Melnyk, J., and Bozzetti, L. P.: Chromosomal effect in vivo of exposure to lysergic acid diethylamide, Science *160:*1343-1345, 1968.

Steele, G. D. F.: Drug addiction and its management, Brit J Clin Pract *2:*188-192, 1957.

Stenbäck, A., Achté, K. A., and Rimón, R. H.: Physical disease, hypochondria, and alcohol addiction in suicide committed by mental hospital patients, Brit J Psychiat *111:*933-937, 1965.

Stern, R.: The pregnant addict, Amer J Obstet Gynec *94:*253-257, 1966.

Stoll, A., and Hofmann, A.: Partialsynthese von Alkaloiden vom Typus des Ergobasins, Helv Chim Acta *26:*944-965, 1943.

Szara, S.: Comparison of psychotic effect of tryptamine derivatives with effects of mescaline and LSD-25 in self-experiments, *in* Garattini, S., and Ghetti, V., eds.: Psychotropic Drugs, Amsterdam: Elsevier, 1957, pp. 460-467.

Talland, G. A.: Deranged Memory: Psychonomic Study of the Amnesic Snydrome, New York: Acad Press, 1965.

Taylor, E. C., Lenard, K., and Schvo, Y.: Active constituents of hashish—synthesis of dl-delta^6-3,4-trans-tetrahydrocannabinol, J Amer Chem Soc *88:*367, 1966.

Tiebout, H. M.: Direct treatment of a symptom, *in* Hoch, P., and Zubin, J., eds.: Problems of Addiction and Habituation, New York: Grune, 1958, pp. 17-26.

Ungerleider, T., Fisher, D., and Fuller, M.: Dangers of LSD, JAMA *197:*389-392, 1966.

Vaillant, G. E.:Twelve-year follow-up of New York narcotic addicts, I. Relation of treatment to outcome, Amer J Psychiat *122:*727-737, 1966a.

Vaillant, G. E., and Rasor, R. W.: Role of compulsory supervision in the treatment of addiction, Fed Probation *30:*53-59, 1966b.

Vandam, L. D.: Clinical pharmacology of the narcotic analgesics, Clin Pharmacol Ther *3:*827-838, 1962.

Victor, M.: Treatment of alcoholic intoxication and the withdrawal syndrome, Psychosom Med *28:*636-650, 1966.

Victor, M., and Adams, R. D.: On the etiology of the alcoholic neurologic diseases, with special reference to the role of nutrition, Amer J Clin Nutr *9:*379-397, 1961.

Volkman, R., and Cressey, D. R.: Differential association and the rehabilitation of drug addicts, Amer J Sociol *69:*129-142, 1963.

Von Grage, H.: Über die Provokation von Psychosen bei der medikamentösen Behandlung des chron. Alkoholismus (Antabuspsychosen), Psychiat Neurol Med Psychol (Leipzig) *4:*108-111, 1952.

Walton, R. P.: Marihuana. America's New Drug Problem, Philadelphia: Lippincott, 1938.

Waskow, I. E., et al.: Psychological effects of tetrahydrocannabinol, Arch Gen Psychiat (Chicago) 22:97-107, 1970.

Way, E. L.: Detection of narcotic usage by the pupillary method, Psychopharmacol Bull 3:61-63, 1966.

Weil, A. T.: In Ethnopharmacologic Search for Psychoactive Drugs, US Pub Health Service Publication No. 1645, 1967, p. 188.

Weil, A. T., Zinberg, N. E., and Nelson, J. M.: Clinical and psychological effects of marihuana in man, Science 162:1234-1242, 1968.

Weiss, G.: Hallucinogenic and narcotic-like effects of powdered myristica (nutmeg), Psychiat Quart 34:346-356, 1960.

Wikler, A.: Psychodynamic study of a patient during experimental self-regulated readdiction to morphine, Psychiat Quart 26:270-293, 1952.

——: Diagnosis and treatment of drug dependence of the barbiturate type, Amer J Psychiat 125:758-765, 1968.

Winick, W., and Walsh, F. X.: Community hospital industrial rehabilitation program, Ment Hosp 15:147-150, 1964.

Winokur, G., and Clayton, P. J.: Family history studies. IV. Comparison of male and female alcoholics, Quart J Stud Alcohol 29:885-891, 1968.

Winokur, G., et al.: Alcoholism. III. Diagnosis and familial psychiatric illness in 259 alcoholic probands, Arch Gen Psychiat (Chicago) 23:104-111, 1970.

Wolbach, A. B., Jr., Miner, E. J., and Isbell, H.: Comparison of psilocin and psilocybin, mescaline and LSD-25, Psychopharmacologia 3:219-223, 1962.

Woods, L. A.: Pharmacology of nalorphine (N-allylnormorphine), Pharmacol Rev 8:175-198, 1956.

Yablonsky, L.: The anticriminal society: Synanon, Fed Probation 26:50-57, 1962.

——: The Tunnel Back: Synanon, New York: Macmillan, 1965.

Younes, R. P.: Exhilarant cough remedies, New Eng J Med 280:391, 1969.

Young, D., and Scoville, W. B.: Paranoid psychosis in narcolepsy and the possible danger of benzedrine treatment, Med Clin N Amer 22:637-646, 1938.

Zellweger, H., McDonald, J. S., and Abbo, G.: Is lysergic-acid diethylamide a teratogen? Lancet 2:1066-1068, 1967.

Zinberg, N. E., and Lewis, D. C.: Narcotic usage I. A spectrum of a difficult problem, New Eng J Med 270:989-993, 1964.

CHAPTER

TEN

Psychiatric Illness in Childhood

With the collaboration of

DR. GILBERT H. GLASER, *Professor of Neurology*
DR. JONATHAN PINCUS, *Associate Professor of Neurology*
DR. SALLY A. PROVENCE, *Professor of Pediatrics*
Yale University School of Medicine

THE DIFFERENCES BETWEEN THE PSYCHIATRIC ILLNESSES of childhood and those of adulthood are largely a reflection of the natural differences between children and adults. Most important of these, the child's psychobiologic equipment is still developing, and thus his reactions are immature and certain to change. The speed, manner, and evenness with which biologic equipment matures vary greatly from child to child and depend on inherent as well as environmental factors. The environmental forces can obviously operate only within the limits set by the equipment (Knobloch 1960), and are themselves modified by the behavior that the child exhibits as a result of the environment-equipment interaction. The complexity of this closely connected, multiply determined feedback system has engaged man's attention ever since he first tried to unravel how adults come to think and act as they do, and is almost as poorly understood today as it has always been.

The growing-up process can be defined operationally as the acquisition of a particular set of facts and skills; its success is measured by the rapidity with which the individual achieves the goals his environment sets for him. These demands are extremely complex, and their details vary from one culture and subculture to the next, but their outline is universal: the child is expected to master the basic abilities that his environment requires for biologic and social life. In our culture and most others, these abilities include

1/ orderly habits of ingestion and excretion,
2/ regular cycles of sleep and wakefulness,
3/ purposive and coordinated movement,

335

4/ understandable communication and social language,

5/ the acceptance of the prevailing customs and ideas of decency,

6/ well-modulated expression of emotional reactions to the environment,

7/ an orderly pursuit of knowledge and education, and

8/ the integration of these abilities into behavior that is well balanced between the community's expectations and the individual's self-interest.

The community defines "disorder" as that state in which an individual complies poorly or not at all with some or all of these demands; it designates as "pathology" the manner in which the noncompliance becomes manifest. The younger the child, the less the environment expects of him, and the less likely is his unusual behavior to be considered evidence of a disorder. The older he gets, the more is expected, and the wider the variety of "disorders" to which he can be subject. Society's expectations reflect its experience with other children of the same age, but the norms so derived cannot be applied too rigidly. Not only does the overall rate of development vary widely among children, but that for different skills in a given child may be quite uneven.

Since the child's maturation depends on the orderly acquisition of skills and since each new skill becomes a part of the foundation for the next, even a mild slowing or unevenness in development can give the appearance of gross abnormality. The identification of abnormal behavior is further complicated because behavior that is considered pathologic at one age may be common or even universal at another. Headbanging, crying spells, temper tantrums, enuresis, nightmares, echolalia, hyperkinesis, dialogues with imaginary playmates, and refusing to eat, go to bed, greet visitors, or go to school are among the many kinds of behavior that are regarded as normal up to a certain age but indicative of a disorder thereafter. The overt expression of sexual interest, on the other hand, is viewed as normal after puberty but abnormal before.

The stresses to which the environment exposes children are, within broad limits, fairly uniform: the child's physical, intellectual, social, and occupational immaturity make him dependent on others for food, shelter, education, and the satisfaction of such needs as a sense of security and the feeling of being wanted. Since his behavior is thus governed largely by adults, the soundness of their judgment and the consistency of their behavior help to shape his development. Not until he is relatively far along toward maturity is he likely to understand or control his environment sufficiently to avoid its adverse aspects or make it conform to his needs.

Certain other factors common to all children are significant in the assessment of those who are disturbed. The time lag between birth and referral is a matter of years, not—as in adults—of decades. Parental memories of the pregnancy and postnatal period are thus usually sharp enough to supplement data obtained from hospital charts and pediatric records. The almost constant supervision required by the preschool child makes it possible to obtain detailed information about his day-to-day behavior. The degree to which the school-age child conforms to the demands of his teachers will be reflected, at least in broad strokes, in his report card (Thanaphum 1970). Unlike the adult whose relatives, co-workers, and employers may be reluctant or insufficiently trained to provide detailed information, the child is gauged by teachers whose professional responsibility it is to observe and evaluate him. Even if the parents' assessments of the causes of the child's distress are considered of questionable value (Wenar 1963), their reports concerning his birth, development, and current behavior may generally be given credence (Glidewell 1957). The immaturity of the child's cognitive functions and the limitations in his vocabulary make it both harder and easier to examine him. While he tends to have difficulty in putting his feelings into words, he tends also to be less sophisticated and adroit in concealing his views and freer in expressing his feelings through play and dramatization.

EXAMINATION

THE INITIAL INTERVIEW

Unlike the first interview with the adult patient, whose appearance, behavior, and verbal account offer some diagnostic clues, the initial encounter with a child (especially one of preschool age) and his parents may provide little beyond such superficial impressions as that the child is perfectly normal or that he is obviously damaged. The first interview is handicapped somewhat because a child's behavior with strangers can be misleadingly different from his behavior with people he knows; many children will not even talk to outsiders—and especially not to doctors. A child may be afraid of the doctor and insist that his parents remain with him throughout the examination; again, he may separate from them with such ease that he almost seems retarded or autistic. The father and mother, too, may present a misleading first impression by seeming more odd or distraught than they really are, especially if the child's behavior in the doctor's office is so disruptive or bizarre that they must constantly try to make him behave. The situation can become extremely chaotic and the evaluation grind to a halt until the physician is able to restore some semblance of order.

The orderly interview, however, is not always the most productive one: the more comfortable its climate, the more it will reflect the child's maximal capacities and disguise his troubles (Campanelli 1970). A child with an organic brain syndrome, for example, may perform and behave so much better in a simple, well structured examination situation that the physician finds it hard to believe that he is really as disorganized at home and at school as his parents and teachers report.

Since the family's idiosyncrasies need not be the cause of the child's disorder, and since a history of pre- or postnatal complications does not prove that he has an organic deficit (no matter how suggestive the behavioral aberration or the constellation of symptoms), the relative significance and the interplay of organic and functional factors can be determined only after a thorough history has been obtained, the interaction between the parents and the child observed, and the child's examination completed. How detailed such an examination should be and what further studies are required will vary from case to case, but may include

1/ a medical evaluation, including a detailed neurologic examination,
2/ a developmental history and examination, and
3/ specialized studies, such as an EEG, a metabolic assessment, and psychological examinations.

MEDICAL EXAMINATION

While the comprehensive medical evaluation will seek to identify or exclude the myriad medical problems of childhood, particular attention must be paid to history and findings suggestive of a metabolic or CNS disorder. The family history should be explored for evidence of hereditary abnormalities (Knudson 1965) and the health history of the mother during the pregnancy for evidence of infectious illnesses like rubella (Desmond 1967) or metabolic disturbances like diabetes or hypothyroidism (Klosovskii 1963). It is also important to inquire into such perinatal problems as prenatal bleeding, toxemia, prematurity, low birth weight, traumatic delivery, and hypoxia (Chafetz 1965, DeHirsch 1966, Drillien 1967, Moore 1965, Paine 1968, Pasamanick 1956, Prechtl 1967, Scholz 1968, Towbin 1969), for these are commonly associated with organic impairment or developmental retardation. The significance of perinatal complications can be ascertained even when parents are not sure of medical details by simple questions such as, "Did the child need resuscitation? Was he put into an incubator? Was he given oxygen? Did he leave the hospital after his mother did?" A history of kernicterus (Hyman 1969), neonatal convulsions (Tibbles 1965), malnutrition (Chase 1970, Eichenwald 1969), lead intoxication (Moncrieff 1964), head trauma (Fabian 1956), or encephalitis (Greenebaum 1948) is also of great import in the assessment of a given child's psychological difficulties.

It may not be easy to discover whether the child with a behavior disorder has (or has had) a particular illness. If he is febrile and somnolent, shows motor and reflex changes, and has an abnormal spinal fluid, the diagnosis of encephalitis is fairly obvious. The diagnosis is far more difficult if the disorder's psychological manifestations precede the somatic ones, as in Sydenham's chorea (Walker 1948), when the child may be restless, irritable, impulsive, and inattentive for days or even weeks before the more classical picture of choreiform movements, motor awkwardness, and muscular hypotonia appears. The diagnosis may also be difficult when the behavioral disorder is based on some long-past (and almost forgotten) illness or injury. Symptoms or findings that bridge the gap between past illness and present symptoms can usually be discovered, but at times the psychological symptoms are preceded by a totally quiescent period. Such a period, however, may be an artifact: an impairment in adaptive skills that becomes obvious only when the child starts school may well have been present throughout his life, but remained dormant because the demands made on him had been limited. For example, a follow-up study of children who had suffered from lead poisoning many years previously showed that 95% of them subsequently experienced psychological and intellectual difficulties. The majority had intervening problems, but some showed no obvious symptoms until they reached the age at which particular scholastic skills were demanded. (Byers 1943).

The determination of sleep and dream patterns can furnish valuable clues to a child's condition and be as relevant to the assessment of the child as to that of the adult (see pp. 37 ff.). Furthermore,

TABLE 20. *Sleep and*

AGE	AVERAGE HOURS OF NIGHTTIME SLEEP *	FALLING ASLEEP	SOUNDNESS OF SLEEP	WAKING AT NIGHT
4 wk	Almost constant	Gradual, following nursing	Sound	No difficulty
16 wk	11-14	Soon after 6 PM feeding	Sound	No difficulty
28 wk	11-14	Directly after 6 PM feeding without difficulty	Sound	No difficulty
40 wk	11-13	Directly after 6 PM feeding without difficulty; some talk 15-60 min before going to sleep	Sound	Few have wakeful periods of 1 hr or more between 2 and 4 AM
1 yr	12-14	Between 6 and 8 PM	Sound	Some wake from noise and cry
18 mo	12	Between 6 and 8 PM after a brief play period	Intermittent	Frequent, especially after exciting day; easily quieted
2 yr	10½	Difficult; late; 7-9 PM; many bedtime demands after a long play period	Light	Many wake up several times during the night at slightest sound
2½ yr	11	Difficult; late; 6-10 PM, depending some on length of nap; complicated by rituals	Light	Considerable waking during night with crying or demand for toilet or drink
3 yr	11	Less difficult; 7 PM	Light	Frequent, with talking and wandering about house, may wake up after a dream
4 yr	11	No difficulty; 7 PM	Sound	Wake up only to go to toilet, usually need little help from parents
5 yr	11	Almost immediately; 7-8 PM; little presleep activity	Sound	Some wake up after nightmare or to go to toilet either with or without help from parents
5½ yr	11½	Most fall asleep right away; 7-7:30 PM	Sound, even "heavy"	Less trouble from nightmares, toilet without help
6 yr	11	Quick chatty prebed routine; like some companionship; most fall asleep right away; 7-8 PM	Many are "wonderful" sleepers	Some wake up to go to toilet but without help from parents

Dreams in Childhood

REPORTED DREAM ACTIVITY			
NEUTRAL OR PLEASANT	NIGHTMARES	MORNING WAKING	FREQUENCY AND DURATION OF NAPS
—	—	—	4 to 5 in 24 hr
—	—	5-8 AM	3 in 24 hr: early and late morning; afternoon
—	—	—	Fairly wide variety, usually 2 to 3, mid-morning and after-noon most stable
—	—	5-7 AM	Morning after bath; afternoon following play activity
—	—	6-8 AM; most cry; happy after toilet	1 a day, late morning or early afternoon
—	—	6-8 AM; happy after toilet; lie quietly	Usually after noon meal for 1½-2 hr, wake up alert and happy
Some dream activity, esp. about trains	None	6:30-7:30 AM; play happily; easily satisfied	Individualized, some have none
Some; about parents and environment; impersonal in sense that dreamer is not a part of dream	None	8:30-9 AM	Problematical, diffi-culty falling asleep, almost never in crib and sometimes on floor, cross and irri-table on waking up
"	None	6-8 AM; may be whining and fretful	"Play nap," wakes up more pleasantly than at 2½ yr
"	None	7-7:30 AM; play alone quietly	Majority merely have "play naps" or no naps at all
Dreams start to con-cern everyday events, but are still largely impersonal	Troublesome; most about wild animals	7 AM; some play	"
Some pleasant dreams of everyday events	Some, but less disturbing than at age 5	Varies; 6-8 AM	"
Impersonal difficulties such as war, fire, thunder and pleasant dreams of everyday people and play	Some waking from nightmares	7-7:30 AM; most get right up	—

TABLE 20. *Sleep and*

AGE	AVERAGE HOURS OF NIGHTTIME SLEEP *	FALLING ASLEEP	SOUNDNESS OF SLEEP	WAKING AT NIGHT
7 yr	11	Little dawdling; fall asleep immediately or within ½ hr; 7-8 PM	Usually sound; some laughing in sleep	Little waking
8 yr	10½	After some procrastination; 8 PM	Sound	Little waking
9 yr	10	Many dawdle; need reminding; longer period before sleep; 8 PM or later	Usually sound	Usually quiet; some wake up screaming
10 yr	10	Later; 7-9:30 PM; most stall; boys fall asleep quicker; some presleep worry	Usually sound	Usually none but a few wake up or call out during nightmares
11 yr	9½	Many need reminding; presleep thinking and worrying; 7-10 PM	Usually sound; some talking in sleep	Most sleep through
12 yr	9½	Some stalling before going to bed and some dawdling in bed before going to sleep; 9 PM	Sound	Very little
13 yr	9	Less resistance and dawdling; most enjoy bedtime	Usually sound; little talking; individualized	Little waking
14 yr	9	Concept of "need;" many, especially boys, go to sleep at once; 9:30-10 PM	Individual differences as in adulthood	Individual differences as in adulthood. Differentiation between "light," "sound," and "heavy" sleepers becomes manifest as the difference does between those who sleep more and those who sleep less than average
15 yr	8½	"Need" stronger; many fall asleep at once; some lie in bed thinking for awhile; 10-10:30 PM; girls earlier	Sometimes restless	
16 yr	8½	Many drop off to sleep immediately; some thinking and daydreaming in others	Usually sound	

NOTE: — indicates no data available.

    * not counting waking at night.

Reference: Ames, L. B.: Sleep and dreams in childhood, *in* Harms, E., ed.: Problems of Sleep and Dreams in Children, New York, Macmillan, 1964, pp. 6-29.

Dreams in Childhood (Continued)

REPORTED DREAM ACTIVITY			
NEUTRAL OR PLEASANT	NIGHTMARES	MORNING WAKING	FREQUENCY AND DURATION OF NAPS
Chiefly about self and daily events	Fewer, may be last nightmare age	Usually same hour each day; 6:30-7 AM	—
Actual experiences, playmates	Few, uncommon	7 AM; up and dressed without delay	—
Actual experiences, most enjoy dreaming and return to it	Few	"	—
Some good dreams about daily events	More common than neutral or pleasant dreams: dragons, "bad guys," animals, robbers, being chased or killed	7 AM; most get up right away but there are marked individual differences	—
Much dreaming; good dreams predominate; usually about ordinary things: homework, pets, sports, cars	Fewer than at age 10 but still strong and violent	7 AM; most lie in bed, some have to be called, difficult for some	—
Less dreaming; content "mixed up"	Fewer than at age 11	7-7:15 AM; many wake up by themselves; boys earlier	—
Good dreams predominate over nightmares: sports, school, travel; but some "crazy," "funny," or predictive dreams	Few, but more than at age 12	7-7:30 AM; surprisingly large number get right up; some sleepiness	—
Tend to be "weird," "screwy" . . .	Very few	6-8 AM; harder to rouse; seem to need more sleep, esp. on weekends	—
Apparently less dreaming, certainly less reporting of dreams	Almost none	7 AM; up within 15 min, some difficulty, esp. on weekends	—
Nearly all dreams are good: friends, sports, girls, "places I've seen"	Rare	6:45-7:30 AM; nearly all sleep much later during vacation, until 10-11 AM if allowed	—

since approximate norms have been established for each age group, and since these patterns follow other maturational events closely (see Table 20), changes in sleep patterns offer an additional parameter with which to assess the rate and regularity of the child's development (Feinberg 1968, Kohler 1968, Ucko 1965). Minor changes in sleep should not be overvalued, however, as almost any stressful event, even mild infectious illnesses, family turmoil, or a change in the daily routine (missing a nap period or traveling) can cause a transient sleep disturbance. Nightmares and night terrors (*pavor nocturnus*) are common at certain age periods and warrant concern only when they are coupled with disturbed daytime behavior. Unusual rhythmic activities before going to sleep, such as rocking and headbanging, are also common, often appear in several members of the same family, and have little significance unless they continue past the age of three and the child cannot fall asleep without them (Kravitz 1960).

SPECIALIZED STUDIES

EEG *studies* are often helpful, particularly for children with an actual or suspected seizure disorder, but the interpretation of the record presents a number of difficulties (Ritvo 1970, Small 1968). To begin with, children are often uncooperative in this endeavor, and unless an understanding technician is available who can establish a relationship with the child and familiarize him with the procedure, the resulting technical difficulties may produce artifacts. Furthermore, while the EEG becomes increasingly organized in the course of the first decade, the maturation rate varies widely from one child to the next. Slow and sharp wave forms, which are often considered abnormal, may also occur in normal children, especially when they are drowsy, and may well be interpreted erroneously (Demerdash 1968, Scheibel 1964) if the technician fails to take note of the child's drowsiness during the examination. Nor can the EEG be used to establish a relationship between a known cerebral insult and subsequent behavioral symptoms: even when a disturbed child is known to have or have had encephalitis, a head injury, or even epilepsy, his EEG may be within the normal range or equivocal. On the other hand, certain EEG abnormalities may be present in children whose difficulties seem psychogenic (Kennard 1959, Stevens 1968). The value of EEG findings is further limited because a child's EEG may change from abnormal to normal without any improvement in his behavior or intellectual competence (Gibbs 1959). Thus, whatever the EEG results may be, they must be evaluated in the context of other observations and cannot be used in themselves to dictate any particular treatment program.

In addition to the EEG, *other special examinations* may be required. Audiometry is indicated in cases of delayed or defective speech (Holm 1969, Vernon 1968); an ophthalmologic investigation should be performed when the clinical picture includes reading problems or otherwise suggests involvement of the visual system (Smith 1964). Skull x-rays, radioisotopic encephalography, pneumoencephalography, arteriography, and a lumbar puncture may be needed in selected cases, especially when there is reason to suspect progressive deterioration or an intracranial growth. Since illnesses capable of causing mental subnormality can also be present with only the mildest sensory, motor, and mental deficits or ictal manifestations (Paine 1962), a wide variety of etiologic possibilities must be considered even when they are not immediately suggested by the presenting symptoms. *Genetic conditions,* such as chromosomal abnormalities in Klinefelter's or Turner's syndrome (Walzer 1969, Warkany 1964a, 1964b) or in some cases of mongolism (Smith 1970); the ectodermoses; disorders of amino acid, carbohydrate, and lipid metabolism (Carson 1965, Efron 1967, MacBrinn 1969, McMurray 1962, Okada, 1969, Rosenberg 1969); degenerative diseases of gray and white matter; and many others can be diagnosed with certainty only by special studies performed on the patient, and often on the parents and siblings as well. If a child's mother has phenylketonuria, for example, prenatal exposure to elevated phenylalanine levels can result in retardation, even though the child has not inherited the metabolic defect (Mabry 1963). A number of other tests—urine chromatography for amino acids and sugars, estimation of urinary chondroitin sulfate, tests for metachromatic granules, determinations of blood sugar, electrolytes, calcium, phosphorus, uric acid, lead (Greengard 1966) and protein-bound iodine levels, and chromosome analysis (Gordon 1968)—may be indicated by the clinical condition or family history. Even when effective treatment is not available and the tests therefore contribute little to the patient's care, establishing a diagnosis may be essential in order to give the family some idea of what to expect not only from the child in question but from future pregnancies as well. When an Rh incompatibility, inborn error of metabolism, or maternal hypothyroidism is established as the cause, advice may be given for the management of future pregnancies and postnatal periods, and, if indicated, a referral to a birth defect or genetic clinic made (International Directory of Birth Defects Genetic Services 1968).

PSYCHOLOGICAL EXAMINATION

Tests used to gather information about the child's intellectual performance are generally far more reliable than those designed to assess his personality or his unconscious fears and fantasies. The most commonly used intelligence tests are the Stanford-Binet and the Wechsler Intelligence Scale for Children, but it is sometimes preferable to use tests that are less dependent on the child's verbal ability, such as the Kohs' block design, the Kuhlmann, the Porteus Maze, and the Pintner-Patterson performance tests (Taylor 1961).

Unfortunately, even the tests of intellectual performance are most reliable where they are least needed: in the clearly superior and in the obviously impaired (Doris 1963, Herbert 1964). Moreover, the younger the child is at the time of the test, the less its results correlate with his future performance: the first data obtained on a two-year-old would predict his IQ at the age of ten less reliably than an estimate based on his parents' IQ (Bayley 1954). This difficulty comes partly because most tests given to younger children rely more on verbal fluency than on reasoning skills. Thus anything that retards language development tends also to lower the child's test scores, and, conversely, good language skills may raise a child's score even if his reasoning ability is impaired (Taylor 1961). Test scores are also influenced by impairments in the child's hearing, vision, or motor abilities, not only because these affect his ability to perform in the test situation, but also because they diminish his opportunities for academic and social learning (Berko 1954a, b). Tests of overall functioning may have to be supplemented by special tests in arithmetic (Bradley 1951), reading, or speech (Cohn 1961, Rabinovitch 1954), because isolated difficulties in one of these skills can cause the patient to appear grossly impaired and because limitations in the child's ability to hear, speak, read, remember, generalize, classify, and decode communications may, in spiral fashion, augment his problems in learning and life (Faigel 1965, Thelander 1958).

DEVELOPMENTAL EXAMINATION

Maturation entails the progressive mastering of the numerous skills and behavior patterns needed for biologic and social existence.

Biologic factors—like hereditary diseases, fetal anoxia, and post-natal trauma—can retard a child's development and cause behavioral symptoms. Environmental influences (severe under- or overstimulation) and constitutional factors (excessive sensitivity to sensory stimuli) may also have a direct effect on the child's development. The meshing of these forces can cause the child to behave so unusually that his social environment is led to treat him differently from its treatment of most children (as by excluding him from the learning available to his peers) and thus secondarily to retard his development.

While the sequence of steps in the mastery of a particular social, language, motor, or adaptive skill does not vary greatly from one child to the next, there is much variability in the age at which each step is mastered. Moreover, a child may be uniformly slow, average, or fast in his development; slow in only one or a few areas, or slow in most, but average or fast in others. Some children show developmental disturbances from earliest life on; others exhibit normal development up to a certain point and retardation thereafter. Thus thorough assessment involves not only comparing the child's current state of development in each area of functioning with that of his peers, but asking his parents at what age he achieved each of the important landmarks of behavioral development (Rutter 1964). Table 21 details those landmarks of development that are easiest for the clinician to observe and the parents to remember and are also most significant in assessing the individual's course of development.

The questions put to the parents concerning the child's *developmental history* must be fairly precise if the answers are to have significance. It is useless to ask, for example, when the child first sat up unless "without support" (i.e., without propping the child up) is specified. Similarly, asking when the child first started to talk or distinguished word play from words is too ambiguous in itself to have much meaning. Children as young as seven months may start to combine syllables such as "da-da" without really being able to speak. The sound "da-da" quite obviously should be considered a part of communicative speech only when it is used to refer to the father, or is used in his presence, and not when it is merely a part of the child's babble (Illingworth 1966). One must also be sure that the mother's reports are based on her experiences with the child in question: some mothers answer merely in terms of what they think is normal, or if they have other children, they may be confused about the sequence in which different children

TABLE 21. *Landmarks of Normal Behavioral Development* *

AGE	MOTOR BEHAVIOR	ADAPTIVE BEHAVIOR	LANGUAGE	PERSONAL AND SOCIAL BEHAVIOR
Under 4 wk	Makes alternating crawling movements. Moves head laterally when placed in prone position.	Responds to sound of rattle and bell. Regards moving objects momentarily.	Small, throaty, undifferentiated noises.	Quiets when picked up. Impassive face.
4 wk	Tonic neck reflex positions predominate. Hands fisted. Head sags but can hold head erect for a few seconds.	Follows moving objects to the midline. Shows no interest and drops objects immediately.	Beginning vocalization, such as cooing, gurgling, and grunting.	Regards face and diminishes activity. Responds to speech.
16 wk	Symmetrical postures predominate. Holds head balanced. Head lifted 90 degrees when prone on forearm.	Follows a slowly moving object well. Arms activate on sight of dangling object.	Laughs aloud. Sustained cooing and gurgling.	Spontaneous social smile. Aware of strange situations.
28 wk	Sits steadily, leaning forward on hands. Bounces actively when placed in standing position.	One-hand approach and grasp of toy. Bangs and shakes rattle. Transfers toys.	Vocalizes "m-m-m" when crying. Makes vowel sounds, such as "ah," "ah."	Takes feet to mouth. Pats mirror image.
40 wk	Sits alone with good coordination. Creeps. Pulls self to standing position.	Matches two objects at midline. Attempts to imitate scribble.	Says "da-da" or equivalent. Responds to name or nickname.	Responds to social play, such as "pat-a-cake" and "peek-a-boo." Feeds self cracker and holds own bottle.
52 wk	Walks with one hand held. Stands alone briefly.		Uses expressive jargon. Gives a toy on request.	Cooperates in dressing.
15 mo	Toddles. Creeps upstairs.		Says 3 to 5 words meaningfully. Pats pictures in book. Shows shoes on request.	Points or vocalizes wants. Throws objects in play or refusal.

developed a given skill. In this situation, it is often useful to ask the parents to sit down together at home and reconstruct the timing of the developmental landmarks.

The *examination* itself consists of observations made in a well-structured setting in which the child is invited and encouraged to perform certain specified tasks (tests and measurements of various kinds); and in a less structured play setting in which the child interacts either with the examiner or with other children. Test results

TABLE 21. *Landmarks of Normal Behavioral Development* * (continued)

AGE	MOTOR BEHAVIOR	ADAPTIVE BEHAVIOR	LANGUAGE	PERSONAL AND SOCIAL BEHAVIOR
18 mo	Walks, seldom falls. Hurls ball. Walks upstairs with one hand held.	Builds a tower of 3 or 4 cubes. Scribbles spontaneously and imitates a writing stroke.	Says 10 words, including name. Identifies one common object on picture card. Names ball and carries out two directions, for example "put on table" and "give to mother."	Feeds self in part, spills. Pulls toy on string. Carries or hugs a special toy, such as a doll.
2 yr	Runs well, no falling. Kicks large ball. Goes upstairs and downstairs alone.	Builds a tower of 6 or 7 cubes. Aligns cubes, imitating train. Imitates vertical and circular strokes.	Uses 3-word sentences. Carries out four simple directions.	Pulls on simple garment. Domestic mimicry. Refers to self by name.
3 yr	Rides tricycle. Jumps from bottom steps. Alternates feet going upstairs.	Builds tower of 9 or 10 cubes. Imitates a 3-cube bridge. Copies a circle and a cross.	Gives sex and full name. Uses plurals. Describes what is happening in a picture book.	Puts on shoes. Unbuttons buttons. Feeds self well. Understands taking turns.
4 yr	Walks downstairs one step per tread. Stands on one foot for 4 to 8 seconds.	Copies a cross. Repeats 4 digits. Counts 3 objects with correct pointing.	Names colors, at least one correctly. Understands five prepositional directives —"on," "under," "in," "in back of" or "in front of,". and "beside."	Washes and dries own face. Brushes teeth. Plays cooperatively with other children.
5 yr	Skips using feet alternately. Usually has complete sphincter control.	Copies a square. Draws a recognizable man with a head, body, limbs. Counts 10 objects accurately.	Names the primary colors. Names coins: pennies, nickels, dimes. Asks meanings of words.	Dresses and undresses self. Prints a few letters. Plays competitive exercise games.

* Chess, Stella: Psychiatric disorders of childhood. I: Healthy responses, reactive disorders, and developmental deviations, *in* Freedman, A. M., and Kaplan, H. E., eds.: Comprehensive Textbook of Psychiatry, Baltimore, Williams & Wilkins, 1967, pp. 1358-1366.

usually permit fairly accurate inferences regarding the child's progress in such areas as the growth of logical thinking, the capacity to abstract and synthesize, and the awareness of reality. The test situation also reveals some of the relevant characteristics of temperament: degree of interest and energy, pleasure or displeasure, methods of coping with a difficult task, and reaction to fatigue or frustration. (Thomas 1968). The examiner should also note whether the child's feelings are dominated by fear, aggression, excitement, or pleasure. Such traits as orderliness, passivity, curiosity, and shyness may also be observed, and may be quite revealing to the well-trained observer. Not only *what* the child does, then, but *how* he does it is meaningful.

While a single developmental examination can provide evidence that the child's development is abnormal, delineate the areas in which his development is accelerated or retarded, and provide some understanding of why, given the discrepancies in his skills, he behaves as he does, it provides little data concerning his *rate of development*—a most important factor for determining his prognosis. For this purpose, and to assess the effects of environmental changes or therapeutic interventions that might have taken place in the interim, a second or even a third developmental examination some six to 12 months later is imperative (Knobloch 1963, Provence 1968). The *interpretation* of these data is a complicated task of which only a few highlights are given in this chapter. For further information concerning this matter, the reader is referred to specialized texts (Freud 1965, Goodman 1967, Illingworth 1966, Simmons 1969).

In any case, the potential of the apparently retarded child whose life has been marked by *emotional deprivation* or an *impoverishment of sensory stimulation,* as by being neglected or institutionalized (Blodgett 1963, Coleman 1957, Glaser 1956, Krieger 1967, Patton 1962, Provence 1962), may be impossible to assess without offering him a new and more stimulating environment and observing his progress there (Powell 1967, Prader 1963, Talbot 1965). Similarly, the *child who is blind or deaf* and appears retarded or mentally subnormal may show an accelerated development of skills when offered stimulation via the unimpaired sensory channels. The *family history* of the child whose mastery of motor skills, language, or sphincter control lags behind that of his peers is important: evidence that his parents or siblings had similar difficulties but overcame them speaks well for the prognosis. A *recent history of severe illness,* particularly one affecting the CNS, must also be considered in assessing the child's level of development: he may seem hopelessly defective, for example, immediately after such an illness, but return to his premorbid level within a matter of months (Illingworth 1961). Even if the illness has been relatively mild, a cautious assessment is necessary, as the most recently developed skills may be lost temporarily in its wake, and a transient regression thus misinterpreted as a lag in development. Similarly, a child whose development has been satisfactory may, on encountering a stressful situation, discard his most recently acquired modes of behavior and —at least for a time—substitute those he had previously learned (Provence 1968). The assessment of the *premature child's* development ought not to be based on his age from birth but from whatever time his birth would have been due had he not been premature. Finally, even if the child shows definite developmental retardation, his *drive level, personality,* and *perseverance* in overcoming or coping with difficulties will play a major role in determining what level of overall adjustment he will be able to achieve (Chess 1970, Thomas 1968).

GENERAL PRINCIPLES OF TREATMENT

Because many symptoms tend to change spontaneously as the child grows older, real improvement can be said to have taken place only when the patient's original symptoms remit without being replaced by new ones and his achievements come closer to those typical of his particular age group. A hyperkinetic child, for example, can scarcely be viewed as cured if, after he slows down, he is listless and socially awkward (Baumann 1962, Laufer 1957).

THE ROLE OF THE FAMILY

Whatever his presenting problem, a child is inescapably dependent on his family, and its involvement is crucial to the outcome of treatment. The parental attitudes toward, and the timing of, such events in the child's life as weaning and toilet training have been widely assumed to have a major impact on his future. Efforts to demonstrate such interrelationships have not been successful, however. Thus far there is no evidence that—from the standpoint of future mental illness or the development of personality—it makes any difference whether the child is fed by breast or bottle, when or how it is weaned or toilet trained, whether or when a sibling is born or the mother returns to work, or even whether one, both, or neither of the parents lives with the child, unless such events occur in combination with other factors (Casler 1961, Chess 1960, Davis 1965, Yarrow 1964) that would have adverse effects on the child's development (such as institutional placement or other causes of social deprivation). The difficulty in demonstrating what effect these factors may have is to some extent methodologic, yet it underscores the importance of examining the family's transactions in their entirety and casts doubt on theoretic formulations that blame all such difficulties on the child's family, and especially on his much maligned mother (Arajärvi 1964, Beisser 1967, Chess 1964, Rosenberg 1969).

A disturbed child's family may ask the clinician what they have been doing wrong, but it is not his function to tell them how to live, for advice of this kind would be as hard to formulate as to follow. Far more important is that he explain his findings as promptly as he can, help them to recognize the child's limitations, formulate realistic goals for him, and advise them when or whether the child's emotional, intellectual, and motor equipment are sufficient to ready him for the next maturational step (Berg 1969, Blumenthal 1969).

Although most families follow recommendations reasonably well, some sabotage the child's treatment, and others refuse to get involved. If the clinician is unable to obtain the information he needs to assess the child's response to treatment or to modify a potentially noxious environment, he must ask himself if there is anything in his own behavior that has made him unacceptable to the parents. In some cases, their lack of cooperation or hostility to the physician is a reflection of their need to deny the child's illness; in others, of their own psychopathology. In either case, he should meet with both parents at regular intervals. It may even be advisable for him to meet with the patient's siblings or other important members of the household (Grunebaum 1964). Families' group meetings (see p. 498), in which other patients and their families participate, may be helpful and offer the possibility of focusing on the problems of not only the child but also the adults, thus cushioning the child against the demand that he alone give up his unusual behavior (MacNamara 1963).

When the family is unable to tolerate the child's behavior or the therapeutic effort, it may become necessary to hospitalize the child. The profound impact of this decision can be mitigated somewhat by having the mother stay in the hospital with him, an arrangement that has the further advantage of providing the clinician with continuous, direct observation and reports of the parent-child interaction (Brain 1968) and an opportunity for exerting whatever influence on their relationship he may consider indicated (Howells 1963, Mitchell 1966, Solnit 1960).

Pharmacotherapy

The guidelines presented in Chapter 2 for the use of drugs by adults are equally applicable for the treatment of children. Pharmacotherapy is thus indicated for disorders that have a grave effect on the child's social and academic activities and for those that do not usually remit spontaneously. Drugs may also be tried in milder disorders that do not respond to psychotherapy, environmental change, or family treatment.

Obviously, pharmacotherapy introduces certain new elements into the relationship between the doctor, the child, and the family. An initial surge of hope, justified or not, may serve to buoy the family's relationship with the doctor, but the level of trust and confidence will likely recede if such hopes are not rapidly fulfilled. Indeed, many of the changes attributed to drugs—both good and bad—depend as much on the family's expectations as they do on the actual pharmacologic effects (Eisenberg 1964). Because a protracted period of trial and error may be necessary before a satisfactory regimen is found and because the course of drug treatment may be punctuated by transient adverse effects, like further disorganization of the child's behavior, careful preparation of both child and family is essential (Francis 1969). Parents should be given clear instructions concerning the use of the drugs and taught to recognize and report their possible side effects promptly (Eveloff 1966). If the child is old enough to understand, an attempt should be made to explain to him why drug therapy is being used, and he should be encouraged to take his medications at the prescribed times of his own accord. (Fish 1960).

Unless the child is so uncomfortable or his behavior so disruptive that immediate sedation is imperative, it is best to give no more than the minimum daily dose (see Table 22) for a period of 10 to 14 days. Extrapyramidal symptoms, particularly dystonias, may occur when phenothiazines are used, usually within the first 36 hours, but sometimes even after a drug has been well tolerated for weeks or months (often during an infectious illness, but also without any identifiable cause at all) (Shaw 1960). While such symptoms are easily reversible, they can frighten both child and parents so severely that the child is withdrawn from treatment. Concurrent prophylactic administration of an antiparkinsonian agent is advisable, therefore, and the child whose condition is serious enough to warrant high doses of a major tranquilizer should usually be hospitalized until the optimal dose level has been established.

Too little is known about the long-term effects of these agents on growth and development to warrant the use of maintenance medications except in the gravest of circumstances: the potential hazards must in any case be carefully weighed against the disabilities inherent in the child's illness. If it seems necessary to use such drugs

TABLE 22. *Suggested Doses of Psychotropic Agents Useful in Treatment of Children*

DRUG	AGE	MINIMUM DAILY DOSE	MAXIMUM DAILY DOSE
Dextroamphetamine	3-6	2.5 mg	15 mg
	6-12	5.0 mg	40 mg
Methylphenidate (Ritalin)	3-6	5.0 mg	20 mg
	6-12	10 mg	50 mg
Chlordiazepoxide (Librium)	3-6	Not recommended	
	6-12	5.0 mg	50 mg
Meprobamate (Equanil, Miltown)	3-6	Not recommended	
	6-12	200 mg	1,200 mg
Imipramine (Tofranil)	3-6	Not recommended	
	6-12	30 mg	100 mg
Diphenhydramine (Benadryl)	3-6	25 mg	150 mg
	6-12	50 mg	300 mg
* Chlorpromazine (Thorazine)	3-6	0.5 mg/kg	3.0 mg/kg
	6-12	25 mg	600 mg
* Thioridazine (Mellaril)	3-6	0.5 mg/kg	3.0 mg/kg
	6-12	25 mg	600 mg
* Perphenazine (Trilafon)	3-6	0.05 mg/kg	0.1 mg/kg
	6-12	2.0 mg	16.0 mg
* Fluphenazine (Permitil, Prolixin)	3-6	0.01 mg/kg	0.05 mg/kg
	6-12	1.0 mg	8.0 mg
* Haloperidol (Haldol)	3-12	0.01 mg/kg	0.03 mg/kg
	6-12	0.75 mg	6.0 mg

* Psychiatric indications for phenothiazines and butyrophenones (such as haloperidol) below the age of six are limited to childhood psychosis and severe excitement uncontrollable by the traditional CNS depressants.

over an extended period, it is best to avoid the less potent phenothiazines, such as chlorpromazine (Thorazine) and thioridazine (Mellaril), which are reported to have deleterious long-term effects (see p. 589), and to use phenothiazines that are effective at lower dose ranges, such as perphenazine (Trilafon), fluphenazine (Prolixin), and trifluoperazine (Stelazine).

TREATMENT OF SPECIFIC SYNDROMES

ORGANIC BRAIN SYNDROMES AND MENTAL SUBNORMALITY

The Question of "Organicity"

The label "organic," as suggested also in Chapter 11, has a number of different reference points. It may mean that the child's history shows unequivocal evidence of brain damage or dysfunctioning, that his EEG is grossly abnormal, or that his neurologic examination shows such *major (or "hard") signs* of structural damage as hemiplegia, hemianopsia, or pathologic reflexes. The label is sometimes used even if there is no evidence of this kind, but the child's performance and behavior are like those seen in children with demonstrable damage.

The *behavioral manifestations of organicity* include intellectual deficits ranging in scope from a circumscribed impairment like dyslexia or dyscalculia to a global mental subnormality; deviant stress responses ranging from apathy and inattentiveness to hypersensitivity, hyperkinesis, impulsivity, and irritability; and the retarded development of social skills. *Minor (or "soft") neurologic signs,* such as left-right disorientation, disturbances in fine coordination, minor choreathetoid movements or tremor, isolated hyperreflexia, or excessive clumsiness, may also lead to the conclusion that a child's aberrant behavior is organic in origin, as may an impaired memory for shapes and designs, and inability to understand spatial relationships or to integrate auditory and visual information, and a wide discrepancy between verbal and performance IQ, the former sometimes being the higher by as much as 30 points (Birch 1965, Clements 1966, Goldberg 1960, Hertzig 1969, Luria 1961, Paine 1962, Stevens 1967).

Mental Subnormality

The characteristic aspects of the syndromes grouped as mental subnormality are that

1/ the individual's intellectual functioning is significantly below average,
2/ his difficulties were manifest before puberty, and
3/ his adaptive behavior is inadequate (Kidd 1964).

Mild subnormality occurs most frequently in children whose families are socially and culturally deprived and include other members with a low IQ; it is believed to be attributable to genetic factors, the adverse effects of environmental deprivation, and the interaction of the two (Benda 1964, Masland 1958). Other cases, whether mild or severe, respect no class boundaries, but few have an identifiable etiology. The causative factors are many and include all the genetic, intrauterine, perinatal, and postnatal causes of brain damage (JAMA 1965).

The extent of impairment ranges widely and has given rise to certain labeling conventions. An individual's subnormality is called

> *profound* when his mental age is below 3, his IQ below 20, and he is unable to protect himself against common physical dangers ("idiots");
>
> *severe* when his mental age is between 3 and 7, his IQ between 20 and 49, and he cannot manage himself or his affairs or be taught to do so ("imbeciles");
>
> *moderate* when his mental age is between 7 and 8, his IQ between 50 and 69, and he must be cared for or supervised and cannot benefit from instruction in ordinary schools ("low-grade morons"); and
>
> *mild* when his mental age is between 8 and 12, his IQ between 70 and 85, and he needs guidance and assistance when under unusual social or economic stress; while not so impaired that he is unable to achieve any social or vocational skills, he has difficulty in achieving vocational competence ("middle- and high-grade morons") (Eng Ment Def Act 1927, *in* Jervis 1959).

The social problem is immense. Of the total population of 200 million, 3%, or close to six million Americans, have an IQ below 70, and one out of six, or over 30 million, have an IQ below 90. Only the tiniest fraction of the moderately or mildly subnormal and fewer than 20% of the severely subnormal are institutionalized; less than 5% of the institutionalized and even fewer of those in the community have disorders that are even potentially reversible (Paine 1960). The identified mentally defective have traditionally been cared for by educators and institutional personnel. Until recent years, the psychiatrist's major contribution to their treatment has been limited to managing episodes of psychosis or uncontrollable excitement. For these reasons, psychiatrists have generally shown little interest in these patients; nonetheless, the assessment of the patient's intellectual capacities is an important part of every diagnostic evaluation. Not infrequently, a patient whose impaired judgment, delinquent behavior, excessive emotional reactions, or inadequacy in handling life problems appear to derive from environmental stress is found on closer examination to be intellectually limited (Brown 1968). These limitations are not always obvious—especially when the subnormality is mild and the patient is outgoing, verbal, and well-mannered—yet their identification and the correct estimation of the intellectual deficit often determine how helpful the physician can be to the patient and how much guidance he can give the family in their effort to cope with the patient's behavior (Menolascino 1969, Tarjan 1962, 1964).

Treatment and Management

The age at which an organic lesion first affects the patient's mental functioning has two diametrically opposed effects on his prognosis. On the one hand, the nervous system has so great a capacity to adapt (even to relatively severe damage) that the dysfunction tends to diminish with the passage of time. On the other hand, any factor that has a deleterious effect on the child's skills (especially if protracted) impairs the development of subsequent skills; thus the earlier he falls ill, the more diffuse the effects and the smaller the likelihood of full remission (Basser 1962, McFie 1961).

Even though pessimism should be restrained until a developmental lag is demonstrable over a period of years, most illnesses that arise early and severely impair the child have a bleak outlook. Despite the considerable progress that has been made in the treatment of the so-called *inborn errors of metabolism*, less than a third of these syndromes lend themselves to etiologic treatment of any kind (Koch 1965). Even when such disorders as phenylketonuria, galactosemia, maple syrup disease, fructose intolerance, or homocystinuria are identified early enough to offer the appropriate diet, the patient's overall growth pattern is likely to remain relatively slow (Fisch 1969). While there is no direct correlation between intelligence and level of serum phenylalanine, there is now general agreement that the longer the institution of a low-phenylalanine diet is delayed, the more severe the intellectual deficit becomes (Dobson 1968, Knox 1960, 1969).

One recent study (Williamson 1968), in which retarded children were prescreened with the urinary ferric chloride test for phenylketonuria and the positives confirmed by means of urine chromatography and measurement of blood phenylalanine levels, showed that the disease was present in 1% of severely retarded children (IQ under 30), 0.6% of the trainably retarded (IQ 30-50), and 0.13% of the educably retarded (IQ 50-75). There have also been reports of untreated asymptomatic women of normal or even above average intelligence who have phenylketonuria and have given birth to retarded children who do not have the disease (Mabry 1966). Although this finding would suggest that high blood phenylalanine levels damage the developing nervous system, not all such children have been retarded (Bessman 1968, Hackney 1968, Solomons 1966). The nutritional adequacy of the traditional low phenylalanine diet has been questioned on the grounds that a too vigorous application may cause malnutrition and protein deficiency (Mereu 1967) and result in anemia, bone change, hypoglycemia, increased suscepti- bility to infection, unexpected death, and possibly even mental retardation.

While it is hard to demonstrate the effectiveness of *psychosocial or educational measures* (Eisenberg 1961), every effort should be made to offer the child guidance, to retrain the functions he has lost, to teach him to use other abilities, and to help him channel his energies into tasks he can master. Providing him with a social and learning environment that directs his attention away from his im- pairments diminishes the anxiety caused by his handicaps and can thus make him more amenable to retraining. Helping the indi- vidual with mild subnormality to avoid constant confrontation with tasks that he is ill-equipped to master diminishes the likelihood that he will develop a life style oriented toward avoiding failure rather than achieving success (Cromwell 1963, Zigler 1967).

Since specific levels of achievement are demanded of him only during his school years, the person who is mildly retarded is best served by being taught how to function inconspicuously until these years pass and he can go "under cover," in the sense that he takes on some intellectually undemanding job in which his deficits do not come to light. Whether an individual can learn enough to achieve· even this limited goal, however, depends on not only the severity and reversibility of his impairment but also his temperament, physical appearance, and his family's ability to accept him. When the family's economic situation permits them to supervise his behavior and their aspirations do not continually confront him with his incompetence, and when, because his ability to learn is not too greatly impaired and his disposition is amiable, his family accepts and communicates with him, his social difficulties may come to be fairly inconspicuous. If, moreover, his intellectual deficits do not interfere with his school attendance, he will also be exposed to the corrective influences of teachers and peers (Bender 1951).

The *special education program* required for the mentally sub- normal child must take into account that, besides being intellec- tually incompetent, he is likely to feel inadequate, to be gullible and socially awkward, and to suffer from body-image disturbances, problems in equilibrium, disturbed patterning of impulses, and impaired language (Bender 1949, Gallagher 1962). Although there are no statistics on the optimal learning conditions, clinicians and teachers experienced in working with mentally subnormal children tend to agree that the environment must be warm and accepting without being overly permissive; orderly and well-structured in organization; and consistent and firm in discipline. Tasks that are boring or require concentration for more than brief intervals should be avoided and distractions minimized (Brown 1965). To this end, classroom decorations should be plain and simple, and extraneous noises limited (Anderson 1962, Laufer 1962). Specific techniques that attempt to help the child overcome perceptual problems by translating abstract concepts into concrete terms may be useful (Cruikshank 1961). These techniques—including the use of kinesthetic cues to reinforce concept formation —may consist of games involving geometric designs, form boards, puzzles, and Montessori kindergarten materials that facilitate the teaching of spatial relationships. Sticks, beads, and an abacus are useful for teaching numbers (Kaliski 1955), and rhythmic singing can be an effective method for teaching children to count, spell, and follow directions (Antey 1965).

Counseling the parents is frequently as important as training the child. Explaining the child's disability to them and offering them emotional support may halt the spiraling alienation between parent and subnormal child that augments the behavioral deviations (Anderson 1962, Bender 1961a, Clements 1960). The child with organic deficits can of course suffer from neurotic symptoms or a personality disorder as well, contributing factors being his sense of frustration, puzzlement, and inadequacy, and his constant efforts to compensate for his disability (Dudek 1968, Philips 1967). Continued support and resocialization of the kind offered in group or individual psychotherapy can improve both his emotional and intellectual functioning (Kurlander 1965).

Children whose general intelligence is roughly equivalent to that of their age peers, but who exhibit a markedly lower competence in certain academic abilities such as reading, are said to have a *specific learning disability*. The most common or at least the most noticeable of these difficulties (especially in boys, who suffer this condition much more frequently than girls) is reading disability or retardation. This disability has been classified in terms of probable causes as

primary, in the sense that the reading problem reflects a (sometimes genetic) basic disturbed pattern of neurologic organization. The defect is in the ability to deal with letters and words as symbols, with resultant diminished ability to integrate the meaningfulness of written material;

    secondary, in the sense that the capacity to learn to read is intact but, as a result of negativism, anxiety, depression, psychosis, limited schooling, or other external influence, utilized insufficiently to achieve a reading level commensurate with his intelligence; or

    associated with brain injury, in which case clear-cut neurologic deficits and other aphasic difficulties are usually present (Rabinovitch 1954).

The outlook for the child with secondary reading disability is dependent on the treatment or reversibility of the underlying cause; that for the child with a primary disability is more doubtful. The disabilities have been ascribed to such factors as changing the hand with which the child writes from left to right, modern teaching techniques that stress learning words as a whole, "mixed dominance" (being left-eyed and right-handed, left-footed and right-handed, or some other combination of this kind), or the psychodynamic meaning a given letter's external form may have for the child. However, these theories have proved of as little heuristic value as their undoing (by changing back to left-handedness, phonetic learning, orthoptic techniques, or psychoanalysis) has proved of practical value.

The most promising road is in any case the most banal: frequent practice supervised by a tutor; but even this road is unsupported by statistics, and in most cases the child's reading ability will not progress beyond the fourth-grade level. As the child grows into adulthood, vocational training should be emphasized and insistence that he master academic subjects abandoned (Klebanoff 1965). Under these conditions, he may well be enabled to slip into the obscurity of an intellectually undemanding occupation and make a satisfactory contribution to the community.

(The management of the behavioral manifestations associated with seizure disorders and acute brain syndromes is discussed in Chapter 11.)

HYPERKINETIC CHILD SYNDROME
Clinical Picture

The term *hyperkinetic child syndrome* refers to a condition of unceasing hyperactivity with ever-shifting focus. In the typical case, the child is constantly in motion, touching and handling everything he sees, often briefly and without discernible purpose. Seemingly driven by some internal force, he is unable to focus on anything for a sustained period, responds in rapid succession and with equal intensity to every stimulus in his environment, and does not complete the projects or games that he starts. His activity may be so constant that he quickly wears out his toys, clothes, and furniture; if he is at all awkward, he is also highly accident-prone. He may become verbally and physically excited, or even aggressive, and in some cases exhibit socially inappropriate sexual behavior. The hyperkinesis tends to increase when he is anxious, placed in an unfamiliar environment, subjected to a change in his accustomed routine, or exposed to new demands. The condition is three to five times more common in boys than in girls, usually appears between the ages of two and five (Anderson 1963), starts to decline by the age of eight or nine, and has almost invariably subsided by the time puberty is reached (Laufer 1957).

Since this condition can occur in children without clear-cut neurologic or intellectual deficits (Stewart 1965) and is often accompanied by inconsistent parental discipline, many clinicians view it as "functional." Others, noting the frequency with which it occurs in association with demonstrable brain damage or dysfunction such as epilepsy (Ounsted 1955) or in the wake of encephalitis or head injury (Greenebaum 1948), consider the hyperactivity, even when seen by itself, as evidence of "organicity." Needless to say, no final conclusion has been reached.

The child's behavior is bound to have a serious impact on his surroundings. If his mother is not given some respite from him by relatives or babysitters, she will almost surely come to feel severely harassed and eventually may become overtly hostile toward him. His teachers and classmates will also find his behavior disturbing, and his first years in school may be trying for all concerned. For this reason and because certain of his idiosyncrasies may survive the prepubertal diminution of symptoms, the child's long-term adjustment and his ability to concentrate on his work may be permanently affected.

Treatment

Pharmacotherapy is the treatment of choice. Psychotherapy by itself is rarely effective, even when there is evidence that family problems contribute to the child's anxiety and hyperactivity. As a general rule, children showing severe mental subnormality or organic involvement respond best to phenothiazines, while those showing little or no impairment of this kind respond best to stimulants, such as amphetamine or methylphenidate (Ritalin) (Eisenberg 1964, Fish 1968, Knights 1969). Diphenhydramine (Benadryl), an antihistamine with sedative properties, may also be helpful and is so well tolerated that many clinicians start treatment with a seven-to-ten-day trial of 50 to 150 mg daily, turning to other drugs only if the diphenhydramine fails (Fish 1960). .

The child under six should initially receive 2.5 mg of *dextro-amphetamine* or 5.0 mg of *methylphenidate* (Ritalin) daily, after breakfast. If this does not relieve his symptoms within a week, the daily dose is increased by the same amount every week for 12 weeks or until his behavior improves. Children over six are given twice this dosage. These drugs are helpful in 50% to 60% of the patients and, except for causing insomnia if given in late afternoon, are usually well tolerated (Knights 1969). Unless the patient is concurrently suffering from a severe organic brain syndrome or a poorly controlled seizure disorder, his response may far exceed mere diminution of hyperactivity. Not infrequently his sleep, appetite, social behavior, and school performance will also exhibit marked improvement within a very few days (Connors 1967, 1969).

If the child shows little response or becomes tolerant to a stimulant, antidepressants or phenothiazines may be tried. *Amitriptyline* (Elavil), in doses ranging from 20 to 75 mg daily (Krakowski 1965), has been used to combat this hyperactivity, as sedating phenothiazines have also. With *chlorpromazine* (Thorazine) or *thioridazine* (Mellaril), the initial dose is 10 mg b.i.d.; this is then increased by 10 mg daily every three to four days until the symptoms are under control. The sedating phenothiazines have the advantage of causing fewer dystonic and dyskinetic side effects, but are more likley to induce drowsiness. If this effect persists longer than 10 to 14 days, alerting phenothiazines, such as *trifluoperazine* (Stelazine), *fluphenazine* (Permitil), or *haloperidol* (Haldol), should be tried instead (see Table 22; Barker 1968, Garfield 1962, Hunter 1963, Werry 1966). Whatever drug is found helpful, it is best to continue treatment for four weeks or more after satisfactory improvement has taken place. The dosage should then be reduced to the minimum required for keeping the symptoms in check. This maintenance dosage should be given for six months to a year, after which it can be gradually reduced or withdrawn, and reinstated only if symptoms recur.

CHILDHOOD PSYCHOSIS

Descriptively, the term *childhood psychosis* could refer to any gross disturbance of mental functioning arising before puberty, but it is most commonly used as a synonym for childhood schizophrenia. The distinctions between such syndromes as childhood schizophrenia, infantile psychosis, infantile autism, and symbiotic psychosis, however, are so unclear that we prefer to use the term childhood psychosis to describe them all, particularly because it does not imply the unproved relationship to adult schizophrenia (Rutter 1968). However these disorders are defined, they are relatively rare (3.1 cases/10,000 children) and are three times as common in boys as in girls (Treffert 1970).

Symptoms

The variety of symptoms seen in childhood psychosis supports Bender's judgment (1953) that these illnesses represent pathology at every level and in every area of integration and patterning within the central nervous system. The symptoms may be categorized as related to

1/ communicative speech,   4/ perceptual skills,
2/ social behavior,   5/ cognitive functions, and
3/ motor behavior,   6/ affect.
     7/ Demonstrable biologic disturbances are also common.

Communicative speech may fail to develop, develop late, or, having developed, regress (Alanen 1964). The rhythm and tone of the child's voice may lack inflection or be nasal, high-pitched, singsong, wailing, or screeching; the content may resemble the vocal play of infants, marked by echolalia, animal noises, or jargon. Not uncommonly, such children substitute one pronoun for another, using the second-person "you" or the third-person form (own given name) instead of the first person "I." This pronominal confusion has long been thought to represent a specific cognitive defect, but in fact may mean that the child is repeating verbatim sentences that he has heard adults use, saying, for example, "You will go to bed now," to signify his own intention of going to bed (Haworth 1968, Wolff 1964). In addition, his speech is often inhibited and blocked, but this probably represents a more global disturbance, not merely a problem involving the use of language.

The most striking feature of the psychotic child's *social behavior* is his extreme aloneness. He is inclined not only to occupy himself without social stimulation for long periods of time, but to resist strenuously any efforts to change his behavior or environment (Norman 1955). His apparent lack of interest in other children and his inability to relate to them or to adults stands in sharp contrast to his fascination with and skillful handling of objects. The psychotic child often appears unaware of the feelings of others, a blind spot that tends to persist even in those who have achieved some measure of social recovery (Eisenberg 1956a). The child's behavior may be aggressive: he destroys toys, hits, bites, spits at, and verbally abuses adults and other children. He may, in addition, appear unable to distinguish between other people, objects, and himself. On the beach, for example, he may walk a straight line from his family's umbrella to the water, treading relentlessly over chairs, beach blankets, other bathers, and all intervening objects. This behavior can be trying, yet it does not seem malicious, for the child deviates from his path as little to trample on others as to avoid them (Eisenberg 1956b). Even his helplessness and dependency have an impersonal quality, being expressed primarily in physically parasitic or clinging behavior (Norman 1955). Feeding disturbances, such as pica, bulimia, food phobias, or an abnormal preference for certain foods, may occur, as may coprophagia or playing with his own feces. His sexual activity may appear inappropriate and excessive, and he may masturbate openly. Psychotic children also tend to have difficulties in dressing and grooming themselves; some appear totally unable to perform these tasks; others merely seem sloppy. When any of this behavior becomes pronounced, school and social adjustment become well-nigh impossible.

Disturbances in *motor behavior* may appear very early. That the child is somehow different from other children may become obvious in earliest infancy when he fails to exhibit anticipatory postures or to mold himself in his parents' arms as normal children do. Later on, he may look hypoactive, fatigued, apathetic, and lethargic, or appear hyperactive, exhibiting sudden outbursts of vigorous motor behavior, such as jumping, darting, or whirling (Haworth 1968). His motor behavior may seem stereotyped and somewhat bizarre; he may play with his fingers compulsively, twiddle paper or objects in his hands, rock himself back and forth, repeatedly punch his abdomen or bang his head into his pillow or against the wall, or grimace strangely and continually walk on his toes (Ritvo 1968, Shodell 1968). His gross coordination will often be abnormal and his motility patterns distorted in the sense that he looks awkward, controls his limbs poorly, or has an abnormal gait.

Perceptual abnormalities range from general retardation to deviant development of certain sensory and perceptual motor skills (Ornitz 1968). The response to sensory stimulation may appear either as heightened sensitivity (anxiety in the presence of loud sounds or sensitivity to light and color) (Bergman 1949) or diminished attention (apparent deafness or unresponsiveness). Perceptual patterns may lose their boundaries in that the child is unable to integrate details into wholes or distinguish figure ·from ground, and he may have difficulty in spatial orientation.

Cognitive skills may develop slowly, unevenly, or insufficiently (Pollack 1960). IQ scores are often low and frequently display lack of congruence between verbal and performance scores as well as between individual subtests. Islands of normal, near-normal, or exceptional functioning may stand out as exceptions to the general appearance of maldevelopment and retardation. Inhibition, blocking, perseveration, and symbolization are also seen. As the illness progresses, the child's intellectual functions tend to decline further and, even if communicative speech has already developed, the ability to verbalize deteriorates. Phobic, paranoid, hallucinatory, hypochondriacal, and obsessional features are also observed. Phobias often prevent his eating certain foods or playing with certain substances, like clay or finger paint. Obsessional thinking manifests itself in manneristic rituals and in an unusual preoccupation with trifles, with himself, with sex, and with such fears as becoming ill or losing his limbs.

The child's *affect* may be unusual because it is so inappropriate or paradoxical; it may be flat or fluctuating or persevere long past the event to which it pertains. Such children may laugh hollowly or smile in an empty or fatuous way. They are often irritable, but even more often they are diffusely, acutely, and excessively anxious, and their fearfulness may appear illogical and incomprehensible to the observer and seem based almost exclusively on the child's own fantasies. Most striking is the impaired ability to establish emotional rapport with another person.

Physiologic abnormalities of many kinds are common. Many such children have had infantile spasms during their first year of life. About one third have had one or more seizures (Schain 1960), and an even larger number have dysrhythmic EEGs (Creak 1963, White 1964). Abnormal reflexes include deep tendon reflex abnormalities (Gittelman 1967), the persistence of postural and tonic neck reflexes, markedly depressed or absent vestibular responses to caloric or rotational tests (Colbert 1959, Ritvo 1969), inability to dissociate head movements from eye movements, and extreme turning of the head and body in response to optokinetic stimulation. Minor neurologic signs and a history of noxious prenatal, perinatal, and postnatal factors are not uncommon. Pneumoencephalograms may reveal definite though minimal organic involvement. There may be disturbances in the equilibrium of the autonomic nervous system along with such vasomotor abnormalities as flushing, perspiration, a colorless facies, and blue-cold extremities. Irregular sleep patterns are common (Creak 1951), as are abnormalities in weight, height, skeletal maturation, and linear growth (Bender 1947, Simon 1964).

Subtypes

Certain characteristic clinical pictures have been teased out of the broad spectrum of symptoms observed in psychotic children. The most widely studied of these, *early infantile autism,* was first described by Kanner (1943, 1944, 1949). The term refers to children (80% of whom are boys) who, in the first years of life, show an extreme degree of *self-isolation* and an obsessive insistence on the *preservation of sameness* in their environment. The parental attitude toward these children is described as singularly lacking in warmth, but any etiologic significance attached to such observations must be tempered by the parents' report that the children have avoided, rebuffed, and been indifferent to human contact from earliest infancy on. The child's failure to assume an anticipatory posture on nursing, to mold himself to the parent's cradling arms when picked up, to reach out, or to smile responsively are typical examples of this behavior. The parents report: "The minute she could walk she ran away from me"; "She did not want anybody to embrace or kiss her"; and "She never made any personal appeal for help at any time" (Mahler 1952). One of the most characteristic features of these syndromes—and apparently the first hint to the observer that he will be unable to develop a relationship with the child and that he may be autistic—is the avoidance of eye contact. On confronting the observer's gaze, the autistic child tends to avert his eyes, turn his back, or return the gaze in an abnormal fashion, seeming to focus behind the observer's head (Norman 1955, Wolff 1964).

The obsessional behavior described by Kanner as an abnormal "desire for sameness" has been operationally defined as repetitive behavior or insistence on regularity in certain environmental conditions that, when interfered with or denied, leads either to renewed attempts to carry out the act or to manifestations of distress (Wolff 1964). The child may fear new patterns of activity: should a walk not follow the same prescribed course or a particular ritual of words and actions not be repeated at bedtime, he will go into a tantrum. The autistic child's language is also almost invariably disturbed, the disturbances ranging from a failure or delay in the development of useful speech to the use of highly metaphorical language employed with little intent to communicate meaningfully to others (Kanner 1946, 1951). While the child may show little practical understanding of the world and its demands, he may well be skillful and nimble in dealing with objects (Benda 1952), have an intelligent and pensive physiognomy and a phenomenal memory for words or arrangements, even those that are unusually complex. He may be able, for example, to memorize and repeat long lists of names or phrases (though usually in a rote or random fashion and often compulsively) or to reconstruct a complex block design days after first seeing it.

The parents are reported to be sophisticated, intelligent, and so withdrawn and cool that Kanner calls many of them "successfully autistic adults." Compared to the progenitors of adult schizophrenic patients, they are less likely themselves to have been diagnosed as psychotic (Eisenberg 1956b, Kanner 1954), which means either that hereditary factors are of little importance in the development of autism, that the child's autism is but an extreme form of the parents' propensity to cool, withdrawn behavior, or that a child who looks attractive and intelligent and whose family is economically well-situated is more likely to be called autistic than retarded, while the opposite is true of the child with similar symptoms who is unattractive or poor.

In describing children who at the age of three or four become extremely anxious when separated from their mothers and show other bizarre behavior, Mahler (1952) uses the term *symbiotic infantile psychosis*. While the concept of symbiosis may help the clinician understand a given child's psychodynamics, it is not at all clear that this state represents a separate clinical entity. At any rate, very few cases of symbiotic psychosis have been reported, and none of them include follow-up studies that would help in assessing whether, as Mahler implies, the prognosis is different from that of the syndromes labeled *infantile autism* or *childhood schizophrenia*.

The legitimacy of subclassifying the psychoses that arise before the age of 12 has long been a subject for debate; many authors reject the notion that symbiotic psychosis or infantile autism is a separate entity. Reiser (1963), who believes that the most significant clinical fact is the age of onset, proposes that any psychotic illness that arises before the age of five be called an *infantile psychosis,* and that all those that arise thereafter be called *childhood schizophrenia.* Although this view seems reasonable on theoretical (Hirschberg 1954) and prognostic (Eisenberg 1956b) grounds as well, Creak (1951) rejects the idea that there is a qualitative difference between psychoses that arise before the age of five and those that arise thereafter, and prefers to use the single term *childhood schizophrenia* to refer to them all. In her opinion, the psychoses of childhood must be viewed on a continuum of severity. At one end is the child affected by the psychotic process so soon after conception that his illness is already in progress at birth. Next on the continuum comes the child whose development is apparently normal until he reaches the age at which a major developmental step, like talking, should be mastered but is not, so that he remains uncommunicative. Next comes the child whose development is uneventful for an even longer time, so that his speech and other social skills are relatively normal until he develops an illness, becomes mute or withdrawn, or uses distorted and bizarre language, such as ritualistic verbalization or obsessional questioning.

The older the child is at the time he falls ill, the more likely he is to develop clinical features resembling the schizophreniform syndromes of adulthood. After the first decade of life, the picture may be almost indistinguishable from that observed in the full-blown adult schizophrenia, with the exception that until midadolescence such symptoms as derealization, depersonalization, delusions, and true hallucinations are rare (Salfield 1958), and the clinical picture tends instead to be characterized by bizarre speech and motor behavior and by a striking tendency to fluctuate between excitement and complete withdrawal (Leonhard 1960).

Although the behavior of the child with a severe form of mental subnormality, with or without demonstrable organic damage, can be disturbed enough to be called psychotic, the term *childhood psychosis* is generally restricted to disorders in which the qualitative disturbances in intellectual, motor, affective, and social skills are more prominent than the quantitative. This distinction is not intended to suggest that the average psychotic child has normal intellectual abilities (many are subnormal, become subnormal, or are untestable) but only that his intellectual difficulties pale in the face of his social impairments. There is even some question concerning the legitimacy of segregating the childhood psychoses, which De Sanctis (1906) first called *dementia praecocissima,* from other mental subnormalities, for the schizophrenic child's behavior can be strikingly similar to that seen in organic brain syndromes, and sometimes the only difference is the absence of the vacuous facial expression considered typical of the mentally defective.

The distinction between *childhood schizophrenia* and *organic brain syndrome* is thus largely artificial. Distinctions based on the notion that the psychotic child relates more poorly to other people than the one with mental subnormality are equally problematical, for some children whose behavior has been psychotic since early infancy do make efforts to relate to others, and, conversely, some with a demonstrable organic illness do not. Goldfarb (1964), seeking to avoid the confusion caused by indiscriminately grouping all schizophrenias together, differentiated an organic from a nonorganic subtype. He found that, even though both subtypes have many perceptual and cognitive characteristics in common, children with nonorganic disorders, whose EEG or neurologic status is less likely to be abnormal, more often have families showing evidence of psychopathology. However, this view has been questioned by Gittelman (1967), who could find no such relationship.

Prognosis

Long-term studies demonstrate almost uniformly that the outlook for childhood psychosis is bleak. Bashina (1965), reevaluating 123 individuals who had become psychotic during childhood or adolescence, found that 10 to 18 years later 43% of them were incapable of working and that most of those who were working were employed in special shops or as unskilled laborers. Eisenberg's (1957) 10-year study of autistic children shows an equally poor outcome: more than two thirds of the children never emerged from the autistic state at all, but continued to appear severely subnormal or grossly disturbed. More than half were eventually placed in full-time residential settings; fewer than a quarter were able to attend school or have some meaningful contact with people; and fewer than 5% functioned well at the academic, social, and community levels. Interestingly, with a single exception, all the children who did *not* speak in a communicative fashion by age five had a poor outcome, whereas over half of those who *did,* even to a limited extent, had a fairly good outcome. Although there was no evidence that any specific form of treatment affected the outcome, the children who turned out well seemed to have had more effort expended on them by their parents and teachers than those who did poorly; however, this may mean only that those who were least impaired had enough "calling power" to involve the adults. Goldfarb (1966) suggested another fairly good parameter of prognosis: the scorability of the child's *WISC* (Wechsler Intelligence Scale for Children). In the group of children on whom he reported, not one who was unscorable made significant improvements over a three-year period.

The degree of language development, the ability to get adults involved, and the scorability of test results are without question centrally related to the child's level of intelligence, once considered almost irrelevant to the clinical picture and prognosis of childhood psychosis (Fish 1968, Wolff 1965). Even though most psychotic children show some degree of intellectual impairment, those whose IQ is under 70 have a 70% chance of getting worse, while those whose IQ is over 70 have a 70% chance of improving, and when the IQ is over 80, the chance of improving also increases to 80% (Gittelman 1967). Evidence of scatter in the intelligence scores, even if no more than an occasional high subtest or two, once hailed as a harbinger of a good prognosis, has recently come to have less significance, and the patient's highest subtest is no longer considered an adequate measure of his overall potential (Eaton 1966, Lockyer 1969).

Treatment

The thinness of the lines that separate childhood psychoses from the organic syndromes on the one side and from the adult schizophrenias on the other suggests that optimal treatment would combine the individualized educational programs useful in organic syndromes with the somatic treatment modalities found helpful in the schizophrenias. The beneficial effects of educational measures that stress structure, familiarity, and simplicity may be better understood in the light of Kanner's (1958) view that stereotyped behavior in psychotic children functions as a defense against intruding stimuli. This opinion has recently been confirmed by evidence that such behavior increases measurably when an autistic child is confronted with novel or complex environmental stimuli (Hutt 1965). A psychotic child who is assigned too difficult a problem tends to become so disturbed by his failure that his subsequent performance suffers, even when given tasks he has previously been competent enough to perform (Birch 1966), which suggests that he should be assigned only those tasks at which he can succeed, or, at least at first, no tasks at all.

That the psychotic child who develops a social language has a better long-term prognosis (Eisenberg 1956a) could mean that

1/ the child's chance of recovering is improved by learning to talk;

2/ the child whose illness is severe and whose prognosis is bleak becomes ill so early that he has difficulty in developing social language; or

3/ only those children who are not profoundly retarded can learn to speak.

Even if the latter were true and the language-prognosis correlation were not a cause-effect relationship, adult social transactions depend so greatly on the mastery of language that it seems reasonable to expend every effort on developing the child's oral-verbal skills (Colby 1968, Elgar 1966, Wing 1966). Experiments in forcing such children to speak by punishing them each time they do not or using such other measures as offering food, water, or release from physical restraint to reinforce imitative behavior in the proper use of the body and the use of objects and vocalizations have been reported recently (Brawley 1969, Churchill 1969, Hingtgen 1967, Lovaas 1966); but it is too early to determine whether these somewhat unusual methods of *operant conditioning* actually foster the acquisition of communicative language or, if they do, whether this improves the child's long-term prognosis. That such methods are untraditional and superficially abhorrent should not disqualify them from serious consideration, especially as such conventional treatment methods as speech therapy or psychotherapy are of little help in teaching the autistic child to talk. While the psychotic child's hypersensitivity, discomfort, and distrust of interpersonal relationships make it seem reasonable to try to accustom him to human contact, *psychotherapy* can be extremely difficult. In some cases, the child will not even acknowledge the therapist's presence.

The same features of childhood psychosis that guide us in establishing the optimal psychotherapeutic and educational program (his hypersensitivity, distrust, anxiety when confronted with new stimuli, and propensity to perform more poorly following failures) and the similarity of these disturbances to those seen in adult schizophrenics suggest that *drug treatment* may also be helpful. Alerting phenothiazines such as trifluoperazine (Stelazine) (Fish 1961, Freed 1961) and fluphenazine (Prolixin) appear especially useful; children who have been ill for a long time and are unresponsive to phenothiazines may also be tried on reserpine

Lehman 1957). Antidepressants, too, can sometimes be of value, especially if the child is severely withdrawn (Bender 1961b, Feldman 1963, Fish 1963). As in the treatment of adults, the child should initially be given enough phenothiazine (or reserpine) to restore his sleep, which is usually impaired (Creak 1951); and the doses should thereafter be progressively increased as long as his social behavior continues to improve (see Chap. 3). If the child's illness is mild or he is only episodically disturbed, he should be given drugs only during the acute episodes, but if it is severe and protracted, long-term drug administration is needed. Ect is said to be helpful if the child's illness is refractory to drug treatment, has arisen abruptly, or is marked by severe anxiety and disorganization (Bender 1961b). Psychosurgery has also been tried, but the results are disappointing (Freeman 1950).

Parents and other family members are dealt with today very differently from the way they were one or two decades ago. The parents' reactions to the child may seem somewhat strange, but this can be the consequence as easily as the cause of the child's illness (Pitfield 1964), as may be demonstrated by the observations that

1/ most psychotic children are different from earliest infancy onward (Arajärvi 1964, Bergman 1949, Pollin 1966),

2/ many have obvious organic impairments (Rutter 1965, Vorster 1960),

3/ the child's behavior itself may constrain the parents to assume an attitude of emotional distance or overprotective closeness, and

4/ improvements in the child are often followed by improvements in the attitudes of the parents.

The parents' collaboration is necessary, in any case, both in providing the psychotic child with the friendly, well-structured, and corrective environment he requires and in supporting the prolonged and often tedious therapeutic and rehabilitative program. It is important, therefore, that the clinician avoid making the parents feel guilty or angry by suggesting that they are to blame for the child's difficulties (particularly because the etiology of these syndromes is completely unknown). All too often the illness is so severe that it withstands all currently known therapeutic measures, and, if the clinician blames the parents, it is mainly to avoid feeling ineffective. This defense is analogous to the adult psychiatrist's referring to the patient who does not get well as "poorly motivated," "resistant," or "not psychologically minded." Indeed, when a child remains unresponsive, when somatic therapies do not improve his social behavior, and when the prognostic indicators justify pessimism, it might be fairer to explain to his parents that currently available treatment methods are inadequate and to help them accept the child's disability than to involve them in a prolonged, expensive, guilt-provoking, and disappointing treatment program (Kysar 1968).

This defense of the long-maligned parents of psychotic children is not intended to suggest that the child's home environment does not occasionally worsen his difficulties or provide too little structure, stimulation, or warmth to help him improve. In such situations, or when the child's impairment or behavioral disturbance is so severe that he requires the full-time supervision and training in self-care offered only by experienced personnel, full-time residential treatment may be necessary.

FUNCTIONAL DISORDERS OF CHILDHOOD

Having concluded our discussion of those childhood disorders in which intellectual deficits, developmental retardation, or other organic factors are prominent and those in which the child's behavior is so bizarre, autistic, or poorly integrated that it may be labeled psychotic, we move now to disorders that, for want of a better generic term, are called "functional" on the grounds that

1/ identifiable organic or developmental impairments are either absent or at least not the most prominent feature; and
2/ the child's cognitive functioning seems generally intact.

Functional disorders include

1/ such relatively harmless but socially obnoxious *habits* as bed-wetting, nailbiting, and thumbsucking,
2/ disturbances, such as excessive aggressiveness or shyness, that in adults would be called *personality disorders,* and
3/ *the neurotic disorders,* including depressive, anxiety, conversion, obsessive-compulsive, and phobic neuroses.

Because it is usually not the child but his parents (or some community agency) who request the physician's help, it may be assumed that the referral is as often occasioned by their discomfort as it is by his (Shepherd 1966). Since their discomfort is in turn a function of their attitudes toward the child's difficulties, it is not surprising that aggressive children are seen more commonly than shy ones and that those with functional disorders are seen far less frequently than those with organic or psychotic disorders. Because children tend not to be seen until their behavior disturbs their environment, the time of referral does not necessarily coincide with either the beginning of the disorder or its peak. In many cases, the symptoms have long been in progress and are not themselves the reason for the referral so much as the child's reaching an age at which this particular type of behavior interferes with the social functioning now required of him.

That children under four are rarely referred to psychiatrists for symptoms of anxiety is not because they are never anxious, but because the mother considers such symptoms as poor sleep, feeding problems, and inadequate control of bladder and bowels to lie within the pediatrician's domain. That enuretic boys are not usually referred to a psychiatrist at age five, the age by which most boys become dry, but around the age of eight is because enuresis causes few social difficulties until the child is old enough to go to camp or stay overnight at the home of a friend. The excessively shy or aggressive child will not be brought to a psychiatrist until he has started school, for it is only at this time that his personality traits are likely to affect his performance. Many psychological difficulties are overlooked by a child's parents until they are pointed out by his teacher, who, because she is more objective and has seen far more children than they, has a better opportunity to notice any disturbance that may exist. The socially inadequate child and the one with a deficit in his learning skills are also most likely to be confronted with their flaws for the first time on entering school and at this time to become distressed, behaviorally disturbed, or phobic about school attendance.

Similarly, that most of the aggressive and antisocial children seen in guidance clinics are adolescents is not because of some sudden age-linked change in the child's life style or attitudes, but because sexual delinquency requires sexual maturation, assaultiveness requires physical strength, car theft requires motor coordination, and truancy requires a place to go. Moreover, it is only after he reaches puberty that the community considers the child socially and legally responsible for his behavior rather than naughty, and only then puts pressure on his parents to initiate treatment.

Habit Disturbances

Certain repetitive activities that are esthetically displeasing or offensive to others, such as nailbiting, thumbsucking, tics, enuresis, and stuttering, are called *habit disturbances*. Such "habits" may impair a child's ability to communicate with his environment by disturbing those around him. Moreover, some evidence indicates that children with other behavioral disorders and those who later become delinquent often have or have had habit disturbances (Mulligan 1963). However, there is no reason to believe that such habits are prima facie evidence of childhood maladjustment or that the child will, if he does not already have them, develop more serious symptoms (Ballinger 1970, Corbett 1969, Mensh 1959, Tapia 1960). Most of these habits disappear as the child grows older, and even if they recur at times of stress, they invariably disappear again once the stress is relieved. Although *tics* and *stuttering* are often thought to be caused by unconscious psychological conflicts and may sometimes occur in imitation of some person with whom the child is familiar, they can also be a manifestation of delayed or faulty development or of an occult neurologic disorder. Thus, in addition to supportive or exploratory psychotherapy, it may be useful to have the child seen by a neurologist or (in the case of stuttering) a speech therapist. Cases of stuttering that persist into adulthood are highly refractory to any current form of treatment (Karlin 1950).

The venerable but rare *Gilles de la Tourette's* syndrome is a disorder of unknown etiology that begins in childhood and is characterized by violent muscular jerks, facial grimacing, and remarkable spasmodic articulations, which, though initially unintelligible, later develop into that explosive uttering of foul expletives known as coprolalaia (Feild 1966). Alerting phenothiazines and haloperidol (Haldol), 1-6 mg daily, are very effective in these syndromes (Kelman 1965, Shapiro 1968, Stevens 1966).

Enuresis nocturna or bedwetting past the age of five is a symptom that can occur both independently of and together with any other behavioral disorder. Parental beliefs that the bedwetting is caused by some genitourinary difficulty (Jarecki 1961) can be confirmed in only 10% of the cases (Pierce 1967), and in these there is generally some daytime wetting as well. Daytime wetting, however, is not firm evidence for a genitourinary cause, as occasional daytime lapses occur in more than 40% of nightime enuretics. Of enuretic children, 85% have never had prolonged periods of dry nights (*primary* enuresis); the remainder establish control of nocturnal micturition, but then, some months or even years later, perhaps after being unduly excited or fatigued or having had some surgical or medical illness, start to wet their beds once again (*secondary* enuresis). Patients who are enuretic despite adequate efforts on the part of their parents to train them often have a significantly reduced bladder capacity (Starfield 1967), a family history of bedwetting (Illingworth 1961), or a past and a family history of somnambulism (Pierce 1963). Abnormal EEG findings have been reported (Lempp 1965), but enuresis is rarely caused by nocturnal seizures (Saint-Laurent 1963).

Because enuresis seems to be connected to specific non-REM stages of sleep (Gastaut 1964, Pierce 1961), it is interesting that imipramine (Tofranil), an agent that not only modifies sleep (Whitman 1961) but has an anticholinergic action as well, seems to help in both primary and secondary enuresis (Mariuz 1963, Tec 1963). Given in doses of 25 to 75 mg nightly, both imipramine and amitriptyline (Elavil) are relatively well tolerated, increase the patient's bladder capacity (Hägglund 1965), and lessen or eliminate the enuresis in 40% to 90% of the cases (Maclean 1960, Miller 1968, Poussaint 1965, 1966). Many children relapse after the drug is withdrawn, and the length of treatment required cannot be predicted from the outset. Sometimes the patient will require the drug until he reaches puberty, at which time the disorder usually remits spontaneously (Oppel 1968). It is generally best to withdraw the drug for a three-to-four week period every six months to see if it is still needed, taking care, however, not only to make the withdrawal gradual, so that the patient does not develop such symptoms of abstinence as irritability or gastrointestinal distress, but also to time the withdrawal so as not to coincide with a period during which renewed bedwetting might embarrass the child, such as just before he goes off to summer camp. Treatment successes have also been achieved with a conditioning technique that has been in use for over 60 years (Pfaundler 1904). The method is quite simple: the child's bed is equipped with an electric sheet that, on becoming wet, closes a circuit and activates a buzzer that awakens the child (Coote 1965, Forsythe 1970, Mowrer 1938, Werry 1965). Regardless of which method is used, the social consequences of success are almost universally favorable: the child feels freer to join in peer-group activities that involve sleeping away from home; "symptom substitution," the bugbear of former times, has not been reported (Bindelglas 1968, Elliott-Binns 1964).

Patients whose enuresis persists past adolescence are rare and usually show other kinds of psychopathology as well (Rosenthal 1969). Indeed, a triad consisting of fire setting, cruelty to animals, and enuresis persisting past puberty is associated with a delinquent career and aggressive antisocial behavior in over half the cases (Hader 1965, Hellman 1966, Michaels 1961, Vandersall, 1970).

Encopresis, or fecal soiling, is not so common as enuresis nocturna and, except in the mentally subnormal, is usually secondary in that it develops after normal bowel habits have been established. Although many encopretic children are enuretic by night, soiling is more common in the daytime. Parental attitudes toward toilet training are said to be relevant in some cases, and it is not uncommon to find psychological disturbances of other kinds: mental subnormality, sleep and feeding disturbances, temper tantrums, and fire setting (Vaughan 1954). Psychotherapy and parental counseling is recommended, but no controlled studies of outcome are. available. Behavior modification techniques using positive reinforcement have been successful in some cases (Barrett 1969), and, as in enuresis, imipramine has produced improvement (Abrahams 1963).

Personality Disorders

Although there is a wide variety of personality disorders, those that come to medical attention tend to fall within a relatively narrow range (Rutter 1964, Sabot 1969). They can be categorized into two major subgroups of characteristic behaviors:

1/ overanxious, inhibited, shy, withdrawn, or depressed;
2/ aggressive, truant, stealing, or sexually delinquent.

As in other functional illnesses, factors extraneous to the disorder itself help to determine whether and when the child will be referred. That the parents of shy and inhibited children brought to psychiatric clinics tend to be guilt-ridden and overprotective, while those of aggressive children tend to be absent, rejecting, or anti-social (Jenkins 1964), could be interpreted to mean that familial attitudes determine the nature of the disorder. It could also mean, however, that shy children are brought not because they need it, but because their parents, being overprotective, are simply more likely to see trouble where little or none exists.

That the average shy and inhibited child brought to a guidance clinic is no more disturbed than the one not brought is borne out by studies showing that such behavior is quite common in normal children (Ryle 1965) and little cause for alarm. By the time the shy child reaches adulthood, his adjustment level is equal to that of his less shy peers; he may show a few neurotic symptoms, but is unlikely to become psychotic (Michael 1957, Morris 1954, Sundby 1968). The aggressive child's prognosis is by no means so good:

fewer than 20% of such children become well-adjusted adults; a full 20% are psychotic by the time they are 18 years old; and 40% continue to behave asocially throughout their lives (Morris 1956, O'Neal 1960).

Referral practices rather than any sex-linked propensity to behavioral difficulties may account for the 2½:1 preponderance of boys in clinic populations. This ratio *is not* found in randomly selected school children (Ryle 1965), but *is* found in children with postencephalitic behavioral disorders (Morris 1956). Their preponderance in clinics is probably because even normal boys in our culture, once they have passed the age of three, tend to be more rebellious and negativistic than girls (Johnson 1940), so that, all things being equal, a girl will be easier to tolerate than a boy even when she does become less manageable than she has been in the past (Baldwin 1968). That boys are referred more readily than girls leads to the conclusion that girls seen by clinics tend to be far more disturbed than the boys, a conclusion that finds support in long-term follow-up studies, which demonstrate that girls who have been referred to clinics for aggressive behavior are, by the time they are 18, three times as likely to have become psychotic as boys (37% as compared to 13%), and three times less likely than boys (11% and 28%) to have to have adjusted well (Morris 1956). Moreover, women who have had behavioral difficulties during childhood are more likely to have marital difficulties and divorce than men with similar histories (O'Neal 1960). Clearly, it is not justifiable to consider all adolescents with symptoms of an antisocial or other personality disturbance merely persons in "adolescent turmoil," for many are likely to remain psychiatrically disabled (Masterson 1966).

The *treatment of the child with a personality disorder* entails establishing a psychotherapeutic relationship geared to the teaching of alternate patterns of relating to the world. The mode of treatment used depends on the age of the child: until he is old enough to express his conflicts and fears in words, play therapy (Levy 1939, Lowrey 1955) will provide the best interactional forum. Increasingly, however, especially in the child over eight (and long before in some children), words will and should become a significant part of the exchange.

For optimal effect, *treatment of the child with an antisocial personality disorder* must begin as soon as the disorder is recognized: occasionally the symptoms are manifest from earliest childhood onward. Hyperactivity, difficulties in getting along with other children, unusually frequent temper tantrums, stealing, and sexual provocativeness may be in evidence throughout his life; destructiveness and unmotivated lying may begin before puberty, and sexual promiscuity soon thereafter. Such antisocial behavior may appear to be a response to a corrupt or otherwise disturbed and disturbing environment, or it may seem to come out of the blue (see also p. 252). Longstanding patterns of this kind are much harder to influence than recent ones, but in either case the outcome may depend more on the child's luck in avoiding disasters until the disorder "matures out" than on the nature, or even the provision, of treatment (McCord 1959).

An outpatient treatment program can have no effect unless it attracts and involves the child. In some cases, the therapist himself will be able to capture the child's loyalty and imagination sufficiently to motivate him to make some changes in his life. More commonly, the patient and therapist do not have enough time together, and even when they do, the child may prefer being with an older child to being with an adult. For these reasons, we try, whenever possible, to involve some nonprofessional companion, a few years the child's senior, with whom the child can spend a good deal of time and whom he can adopt as a hero and role-model. The companion is urged to look for the child's potential skills and to help him channel them into some form of achievement that his peers can admire. Ideally, the child will be able to achieve legitimate recognition in some form of competitive activity, preferably some athletic activity, in which he can express his unresolved hostility in a structured and peaceful way. Outpatient treatment cannot continue if the child's antisocial behavior continually threatens his safety or freedom: if, after some months, he remains severely disruptive, he should be placed in a residential treatment center of the kind described for adults (see p. 255), but modified in accordance with the activities and socialization patterns of the child (Shaw 1966).

Neurotic Disorders

The nature, duration, and development of the neurotic symptoms seen in childhood depend in large measure on the child's age. Neurotic symptoms seen in the child under four, for example, include generalized anxiety, temper tantrums, protracted crying spells, and fleeting phobias. Excessive clinging to adults or to some inanimate, comforting object like a blanket or a toy, reluctance to go to sleep, nightmares, night terrors (*pavor nocturnus*), finicky eating or refusal to eat, abdominal pain, nausea, or vomiting will also be seen in the neurotic child (Adam 1964, Lo 1969, Schachter 1964, Vernon 1966). The child exhibiting several of these symptoms simultaneously is viewed as having a *gross stress reaction*. Symptoms of this kind in a child who has recently been separated from one or both parents are usually considered *separation anxiety*, particularly if the new environment is unable to meet his needs for affection, warmth, and sensory stimulation. Symptomatically similar reactions can occur, however, in the wake of other environmental stresses (even fairly mild ones, if the child is the type that overresponds) and as the prodromata, concomitants, and sequelae of a wide variety of other disorders, both organic and functional.

Most of the neurotic symptoms seen during early childhood recede on their own within a few weeks, especially those arising around the age of four and those that arise soon after puberty (Förster 1955a, 1955b, Kennell 1966). If not, a more detailed exploration of the family dynamics ought to be undertaken. In some cases, the patient's family seems so disturbed that it soon becomes obvious that it is they rather than he who should be treated. That they fight among themselves or even argue with or nag the child does not necessarily mean that their behavior is the sole cause of his difficulties; not infrequently, their behavior, especially toward the child, is both an effect and a cause of the child's symptoms. If, for example, a child should develop a sleep disorder that awakens him every night and causes him to get out of bed and wander about the house, his parents, both because their own sleep is disturbed and because they confuse his insomnia with recalcitrance, may permit an escalating series of punishments and demands to replace what had previously been a fairly normal relationship. In such cases, it can be helpful to explain to the family that the child's problem is not disobedience but insomnia, and to give the child a mild sedative like diphenhydramine (Benadryl) or chlordiazepoxide (Librium) in the expectation that the family's irritation will subside as soon as his sleep is restored.

Between the ages of four and seven, a child may have episodes of apparently unmotivated tearfulness, withdraw from his parents and peers, voice irrational fears, or have nightmares or other sleep difficulties. If he later develops a *depressive episode*, these symptoms can be viewed as the first manifestations of his illness, but children under seven rarely develop affective disorders at all like those seen in adults (Prugh 1963). After this age, the child may exhibit many of the symptoms seen later in life, such as circumscribed phobias, ruminations about dying or about the death of the parents, difficulty in school adjustment, gastrointestinal complaints, anorexia, weight loss, apathy, anergia, difficulty in concentration, slowed motor activity, vacillation between clinging to and unreasonable hostility toward parents, low self-esteem and self-deprecation, and complaints about loneliness or feeling unwanted (Frommer 1967, Hollon 1970, Toolan 1969). Suicidal preoccupation and even suicide attempts may also occur, but the latter are rarely successful (Glaser 1965, Gould 1965, Lukianowicz 1968, Mattsson 1969, Winn 1966). With the onset of adolescence, girls show a marked increase of somatic symptoms and boys of rebellious, negativistic behavior (Collins 1962).

Similarly, cyclical mood changes, such as episodes of unmotivated elation and hyperactivity alternating with more sedate behavior, have been observed before puberty, but *manic episodes* similar to those seen in adults are decidedly rare (Anthony 1960, Harms 1951). During and after puberty, however, such episodes are not at all infrequent in the typical case. Hyperactivity and antisocial behavior alternate with anergia and periods of depression. Unlike the affective disorders seen in preschool children, which tend to be brief, those seen in children of school age may last for several months. The majority respond fairly well to a friendly environment and supportive psychotherapy; those that do not may require some form of somatic treatment. Chlordiazepoxide (Librium) or some other minor tranquilizer should be used first, but if this is not helpful, the child should be given the drugs that are used in the affective disorders of adulthood (see p. 174), albeit with appropriate modifications of dosage (see Table 22). Clinicians are often reluctant to hospitalize a child with a depression because of the chance that this will further disturb his self-image and add to his fear of being separated from his parents, but such conservatism is justified only when there is clear evidence that the parents are capable of supervising the child closely. If, however, the child is preoccupied with suicide or has made a suicide attempt, or if he keeps running away from home or getting into accidents, he should be hospitalized, for such symptoms are indexes of either the depth of the depression, the lack of support from the environment, or both (Seiden 1969, Shaw 1965). It is always important to assess the parents' mood, as the child may be responding to or imitating the suicidal preoccupations of his parents.

Nausea, vomiting, abdominal pain, headache, and other somatic symptoms are common reactions to stress during childhood, but *conversion symptoms* involving the voluntary musculature are seldom seen before the end of the first decade. Shortly before puberty, however, a child may feel unable to stand or to walk (astasia-abasia) or as if he has a lump in his throat; he may swallow and belch air involuntarily, overbreathe, and develop muscular weakness or paralysis (Prugh 1963). Functional back pain, interestingly, is extremely rare before the age of 16. Just as in adults, the patient's nervousness, histrionic style, blandness, or use of secondary gain may cause him to be suspected of overacting, but should not disqualify him from further investigations (Apley 1967, Robins 1953). Appetite disturbances, phobias about particular foods, and obstinate refusals to eat are also common throughout childhood (Brandon 1970), although the typical constellation of symptoms seen in *anorexia nervosa* (see p. 474) has not been reported in children under 10.

Obsessive preoccupations are common throughout childhood, but persistent and clearly defined *obsessive-compulsive syndromes* are infrequent before the age of eight (Judd 1965, Warren 1960). In the typical case, the child is exceptionally clean and orderly, engages in such stereotyped activities as repeatedly touching or moving toys or doorknobs, and asks the same question again and again. Answering the child's questions is of temporary benefit at best, for he almost inevitably doubts the answers he gets. A complete history of the illness' prior course may help in making a well-educated guess about the future: symptoms that are mild at the beginning and progress so slowly that they have little effect on the child's functioning for months or years tend to persist in one form or another; syndromes that arise suddenly and progress rapidly, on the other hand, tend to remit within a few months (even if left untreated), although episodic recurrences throughout the patient's life are not uncommon (see p. 232). Whatever the prior course, patients whose symptoms persist or progress should be given antidepressants, either alone or in combination with phenothiazines.

Fleeting *phobias* of various kinds are a natural part of development; crippling and protracted ones, however, are rare until the eighth or ninth year of life (Anthony 1967). The single exception, and the one that we shall discuss at somewhat greater length because of its frequency, is the reluctance to attend school known as *school phobia*. Upon first entering school, children are often understandably apprehensive and dislike attending until they get used to it. They may also be reluctant to go if they are bullied by one or more of the other children, have difficulty in adjusting to a new teacher, or dislike participating in some required activity. The most typical example of this is the physical education class, in which the child must change his clothes or display his lack of skill before others (Moore 1966). If the child's reluctance is mild or transient, it is not usually considered pathologic; but if he refuses to go to school for a prolonged period of time, engages in extreme or unusual behavior in order to avoid going, explains his refusal in a way that his environment considers irrational, and his parents consider his attendance essential, he may be referred to a psychiatrist.

Although the desire to stay home from school has, for reasons of parsimony, been given the single label of *school phobia*, it has a number of different causes, ranging from emotional lability to intellectual dysfunctioning. In some cases, a child may find the standard school experience unbearable from the outset; in others, such as a child with a specific learning deficit like dyslexia, he may not feel uncomfortable or reluctant to go until he has reached the third or fourth grade and finds himself unable to cope with the increased reading demands (Hermann 1959, Tjossem 1962). If their difficulties are not too severe, some organically impaired or intellectually subnormal children are able to reach the same level of school achievement as their peers simply by being more industrious. Others can cope with the scholastic tasks only by making "shifts" (Boshes 1964) in their behavior, such as developing compulsive work habits. These shifts, which are chiefly attempts to avoid facing up to a feeling of incompetence and inadequacy, may become so time-consuming and uncomfortable that the child eventually refuses to attend school. The amount of intellectual dysfunction that makes school intolerable for a given child is not absolute: even a normal child whose parents have standards that he cannot or does not wish to live up to, or one who has been placed in a class with intellectually superior children, may fear and dislike school.

The clinical picture is relatively uniform: it begins with the child's simply voicing a disinclination to go to school without giving any reason for it. When the parents try to force him to go, he counters with temper tantrums or by refusing to dress, leave the house, climb on the school bus, or enter the school building. If his parents insist that he explain his behavior, he will offer such "reasons" as difficulties with a particular teacher, classmate, or subject. If they reject his reasons and insist he attend, he may start to display physical symptoms that would prevent his going, such as abdominal pain, nausea, headache, and the like. As soon as it is too late to go, or his parents agree to his staying home for the day, the symptoms recede; almost invariably, however, they reappear the following morning. Although the child's refusal to go to school is the most dramatic event that takes place, it is not always the first symptom to appear. In many cases, a thorough history will reveal that the child has been suffering from sleep disturbance, anorexia, temper tantrums, and somatic complaints for weeks or months before expressing the desire to remain home from school.

The child's obvious difficulty in handling separation from his parents strongly suggests that his behavior is exclusively psychogenic, but this need not be the whole story. That the child's difficulties become manifest in the morning and subside by the afternoon, that depressed adults often reveal a past history of school phobia, and that school phobic children often have a family history of depressive illness (Agras 1959) all suggest that such phobic syndromes may be akin to, perhaps the childhood equivalent of, depression. The longer the child is absent from school and the more used he gets to staying home, the more difficult it becomes for him to return (Eisenberg 1958, Rodriguez 1959). If the child's distress is so conspicuous and so touching that the parents find it hard to insist that he go, the physician may need to help them overcome their desire to protect him. In some cases, they will be unable to come to terms with their feelings until the child's symptoms subside (Millar 1961).

Close collaboration between doctor, teacher, and guidance counselor is essential in managing the school phobic child (Roll 1964). Discussions with the child will sometimes reveal just how the school situation can be made more tolerable: a change of teachers, placement in a class geared to his ability and not just his age, transfer to a noncoeducational school for an adolescent so self-conscious with the other sex that he or she is unable to concentrate, and the like. Instruction at home during the most acute phase may prevent the child from falling behind in his classwork and thus feeling even less prepared to return, but this is a double-edged sword, as it may perpetuate the child's phobia. A psychotherapeutic relationship in which the child is permitted to ventilate his concerns and encouraged to overcome them is also important, but it should not be allowed to substitute for his return to school. Some children appear to be constantly just on the verge of understanding and changing their behavior, but if this state of maneuvering goes on for too long, further exploration should be postponed until the child is back in school. A mild sedative such as chlordiazepoxide (Librium), 5-10 mg, b.i.d., should be tried for a week or two. If this is not effective, or if the child's sleep and appetite are also disturbed, an antidepressant like imipramine (Tofranil), 11 to 25 mg, 2 to 3 times daily, should be added. If successful, drug therapy should be continued for a few weeks or months after the child's symptoms remit; thereafter, he may remain free of symptoms, even after the drug is reduced or withdrawn.

The clinical picture of *truancy*, adolescent avoidance of school, is usually quite different from that seen in the typical case of school phobia, even among those children who have experienced an episode of school phobia during earlier years (Warnecke 1964), for it is merely one of many ways in which the adolescent demonstrates a generalized rebelliousness. Some children are openly and provocatively truant; others are so secretive about their behavior that their parents do not learn of it until the school authorities advise them of the many months of absenteeism and repeated forging of parental excuses. Parents who feel unable to handle a rebellious adolescent may tacitly support his truancy by ignoring it, in the hope that the crisis will subside. This attitude is not necessarily so harmful as it might appear, for rigid insistence on school attendance, often of value in the younger child, is less effective in adolescents, and can even reinforce the offender's recalcitrance. It is often physically impossible, moreover, to force an adolescent to return to school. When his attitude is simply one facet of a posture of antiauthoritarian defiance, excessive coercion can needlessly lock him into a position of obdurate refusal. It may thus be preferable to permit an adolescent to stay away from school for six to twelve months on the condition that he take a job in the meantime. This will provide him with an opportunity for further maturation, allow him to escape an uncomfortable situation, and, if he remains in psychotherapy, give him the time and opportunity to explore his attitude toward school and to begin determining what sort of life route he wants to pursue.

REFERENCES

Abrahams, D.: Treatment of encopresis with imipramine, Amer J Psychiat *119*:891-892, 1963.

Adam, R.: Two aspects of the pathology of sleep in children: 1. Personality features in children with sleep disturbances, *in* Harms, E., ed.: Problems of Sleep and Dream in Children, New York: Macmillan, 1964, pp. 116-122.

Agras, S.: Relationship of school phobia to childhood depression, Amer J Psychiat *116*:533-536, 1959.

Alanen, Y. O., Arajärvi, T., and Vitamäki, O.: Psychoses in childhood, Acta Psychiat Scand *40*(Supp 174):1-93, 1964.

Anderson, C. M., and Plymate, H. B.: Management of the brain damaged adolescent, Amer J Orthopsychiat *32*:492-500, 1962.

Anderson, W. W.: The hyperkinetic child: A neurological appraisal, Neurology (Minneap) *13*:968-973, 1963.

Antey, J. W.: Sing and Learn—Simple Songs and Rhythms that Retarded Children Can Enjoy While Learning Basic Lessons, New York: Day, 1965.

Anthony, E. J.: Psychiatric disorders of childhood. II: Psychoneurotic, psychophysiological, and personality disorders, in Freedman, A. M., and Kaplan, H. I., eds.: Comprehensive Textbook of Psychiatry, Baltimore: Williams & Wilkins, 1967.

Anthony, J., and Scott, P.: Manic-depressive psychosis in childhood, J Child Psychol Psychiat 1:53-72, 1960-61.

Apley, J.: Child with recurrent abdominal pain, Pediat Clin N Amer 14:63-72, 1967.

Arajärvi, T., and Alanen, Y. O.: Psychoses in childhood I. A clinical, family and follow-up study, Acta Psychiat Scand 40:(Suppl 174)5-32, 1964.

Baldwin, J. A.: Psychiatric illness from birth to maturity: Epidemiological study, Acta Psychiat Scand 44:313-333, 1968.

Ballinger, B. R.: Prevalence of nail-biting in normal and abnormal populations, Brit J Psychiat 117:445-446, 1970.

Barker, P., and Fraser, I. A.: Controlled trial of haloperidol in children, Brit J Psychiat 114:855-857, 1968.

Barrett, B. H.: Behavior modification in the home: Parents adapt laboratory-developed tactics to bowel-train a 5½-year-old, Psychother Psychosom 6:172-176, 1969.

Bashina, V. M.: Work capacity and social adaptation of schizophrenic patients who became ill in childhood and adolescence, Int J Psychiat 1:248-252, 1965.

Basser, L. S.: Effects of hemispherectomy on speech, Brain 85:422-460, 1962.

Baumann, M. C., et al.: Five Year Study of Brain-damaged Children, Springfield (Ill): The Mental Health Center, 1962.

Bayley, N.: Some increasing parent-child similarities during the growth of children, J Educ Psychol 45:1-21, 1954.

Beisser, A. R., Glasser, N., and Grant, M.: Psychosocial adjustment in children of schizophrenic mothers, J Nerv Ment Dis 145:429-440, 1967.

Benda, C. E., et al.: Development Disorders of Mentation and Cerebral Palsies, New York: Grune, 1952.

Benda, C. E., et al.: Relationship between intellectual inadequacy and emotional and sociocultural privation, Compr Psychiat 5:294-313, 1964.

Bender, L.: Childhood schizophrenia: Clinical study of one hundred schizophrenic children, Amer J Orthopsychiat 17:40-56, 1947.

———: Psychological problems of children with organic brain disease, Amer J Orthopsychiat 19:404-441, 1949.

———: Psychological treatment of the brain damaged child, Quart J Child Behav 3:123-132, 1951.

———: The brain and child behavior, Arch Gen Psychiat (Chicago) 4:531-547, 1961a.

Bender, L., and Faretra, G.: Organic therapy in pediatric psychiatry, Dis Nerv Syst 22:110-111, 1961b.

Bender, L., and Helme, W. H.: Quantitive test of theory and diagnostic indicators of childhood schizophrenia, Arch Neurol (Chicago) 70:413-427, 1953.

Berg, J. M., Gilderdale, S., and Way, J.: On telling parents of a diagnosis of mongolism, Brit J Psychiat 115:1195-1196, 1969.

Bergman, P., and Escalona, S. K.: Unusual sensitivities in very young children, Psychoanal Stud Child 3:333-352, 1949.

Berko, M. J.: Some factors in the perceptual deviations of cerebral palsied children, Cereb Palsy J 15:3-4, 1954a.

———: Measurement of behavioral development in cerebral palsy, Cereb Palsy J 15:16-17, 1954b.

Bessman, S. P.: PKU—some skepticism, New Eng J Med 278:1176-1177, 1968.

Bindelglas, P. M., Dee, G. H., and Enos, F. A.: Medical and psychosocial factors in enuretic children treated with imipramine hydrochloride, Amer J Psychiat 124:1107-1112, 1968.

Birch, H. G., and Belmont, L.: Auditory-visual integration in brain-damaged and normal children, Develop Med Child Neurol, 7:135-144, 1965.

Birch, H. G., and Walker, H. A.: Perceptual and perceptual-motor dissociation: Studies in schizophrenic and brain-damaged psychotic children, Arch Gen Psychiat (Chicago) 14:112-118, 1966.

Blodgett, F. M.: Growth retardation related to maternal deprivation, in Solnit, A. J., and Provence, S. A., eds.: Modern Perspectives in Child Development, Part II, New York: Internat Univ Press, 1963.

Blumenthal, M. D.: Experiences of parents of retardates and children with cystic fibrosis, Arch Gen Psychiat (Chicago) 21: 160-171, 1969.

Boshes, B., and Myklebust, H. R.: Neurological and behavioral study of children with learning disorders, Neurology (Minneap) 14:7-12, 1964.

Bradley, C.: Behavior disturbances in epileptic children, JAMA 146:436-441, 1951.

Brain, D. J., and Maclay, I.: Controlled study of mothers and children in hospital, Brit J Med 1:278-280, 1968.

Brandon, S.: An epidemiological study

of eating disturbances, J Psychosom Res *14*:253-257, 1970.

Brawley, E. R., *et al.:* Behavior modification of an autistic child, Ment Health Dig *1*:23-25, 1969.

Brown, B. S., and Courtless, T. F.: Mentally retarded in penal and correctional institutions, Amer J Psychiat *124*:1164-1170, 1968.

Brown, R. I.: Distractibility and some scholastic skills, J Child Psychol Psychiat *6*:55-62, 1965.

Byers, R. K., and Lord, E. E.: Late effects of lead poisoning on mental development, Amer J Dis Child *66*:471-494, 1943.

Campanelli, P. A.: Sustained attention in brain damaged children, Exceptional Child *36*:317-323, 1970.

Carson, N. A. J., *et al.:* Homocystinuria: Clinical and pathological review of ten cases, J Pediat *66*:565-583, 1965.

Casler, L.: Maternal deprivation: Critical review of the literature, Monogr Soc Res Child Develop *26*:(No. 2), 1961.

Chafetz, M. D.: Etiology of cerebral palsy: Role of reproductive insufficiency and the multiplicity of factors, Obstet Gynec *25*:635-647, 1965.

Chase, P. H., and Martin, H. P.: Undernutrition and child development, New Eng J Med *282*:933-939, 1970.

Chess, S.: Mal de Mère, Amer J Orthopsychiat *34*:613-614, 1964.

Chess, S., and Korn, S.: Temperament and behavior disorders in mentally retarded children, Arch Gen Psychiat (Chicago) *23*:122-130, 1970.

Chess, S., *et al.:* Implications of a longitudinal study of child development for child psychiatry, Amer J Psychiat *117*:434-441, 1960.

Churchill, D. W.: Psychotic children and behavior modification, Amer J Psychiat *125*:1585-1590, 1969.

Clements, S. D.: Child with minimal brain dysfunction. A multidisciplinary catalyst, J Lancet *86*:121-123, 1966.

Clements, S. D., and Peters, J. E.: Minimal brain dysfunctions in the school age child, Arch Gen Psychiat (Chicago) *6*:185-197, 1960.

Cohn, R.: Delayed acquisition of reading and writing abilities in children: A neurological study, Arch Neurol (Chicago) *4*:153-164, 1961.

Colbert, E. G., Koegler, R. R., and Markham, C. H.: Vestibular dysfunction in childhood schizophrenia, Arch Gen Psychiat (Chicago) *1*:600-617, 1959.

Colby, K. M.: Computer-aided language development in nonspeaking children, Arch Gen Psychiat (Chicago) *19*:641-651, 1968.

Coleman, R. W., and Provence, S.: Environmental retardation (hospitalism) in infants living in families, Pediatrics *19*: 285-292, 1957.

Collins, L. F., Maxwell, A. E., and Cameron, K.: Factor analysis of some child psychiatric clinic data, Brit J Psychiat *108*: 274-285, 1962.

Conners, C. K., Eisenberg, L., and Barcai, A.: Effect of dextroamphetamine on children: Studies on subjects with learning disabilities and school behavior problems, Arch Gen Psychiat (Chicago) *17*:478-485, 1967.

Conners, C. K., *et al.:* Dextroamphetamine sulfate in children with learning disorders, Arch Gen Psychiat (Chicago) *21*: 182-190, 1969.

Coote, M. A.: Apparatus for conditioning treatment of enuresis, Behav Res Ther *2*:233-238, 1965.

Corbett, J. A., *et al.:* Tics and Gilles de la Tourette's Syndrome: Follow-up study and critical review, Brit J Psychiat *115*: 1229-1241, 1969.

Creak, M.: Psychoses in childhood, Brit J Psychiat *97*:545-554, 1951.

———: Childhood psychosis: Review of 100 cases, Brit J Psychiat *109*:84-89, 1963.

Cromwell, R. L.: A social learning approach to mental retardation, *in* Ellis, N. R., ed.: Handbook of Mental Deficiency; Psychological Theory and Research, New York: McGraw-Hill, 1963, pp. 41-91.

Cruickshank, W. M., *et al.:* Teaching Method for Brain-injured and Hyperactive Children: A Demonstration-pilot Study, Syracuse: Syracuse Univ Press, 1961.

Davis, R. E., and Ruiz, R. A.: Infant feeding method and adolescent personality, Amer J Psychiat *122*:673-678, 1965.

DeHirsch, K., Jansky, J., and Langford, W. S.: Comparisons between prematurely and maturely born children at three age levels, Amer J Orthopsychiat *36*:616-628, 1966.

Demerdash, A., Eeg-Oloffson, O., and Petersen, I.: The incidence of 14 and 6 per second positive spikes in a population of normal children, Develop Med Child Neurol *10*:309-316, 1968.

De Sanctis, S.: Dementia praecocissima, Riv Sper Freniat *32*:14-23, 1906.

Desmond, M. M., *et al.:* Congenital rubella encephalitis, J Pediat *71*:311-331, 1967.

Dobson, J., *et al.:* Cognitive development and dietary therapy in phenyl-ketonuric children, New Eng J Med *278:* 1142-1144, 1968.

Doris, J.: Evaluation of the intellect of the brain-damaged child: Historical development and present status, *in* Solnit, A. J., and Provence, S. A., eds.: Modern Perspectives in Child Development, New York: Internat Univ Press, 1963, pp. 162-205.

Drillien, C. M.: Incidence of mental and physical handicaps in school age children of very low birth weight, Pediatrics *39:* 238-247, 1967.

Dudek, S. Z., and Lester, E. P.: The good child facade in chronic underachievers, Amer J Orthopsychiat *38:*153-160, 1968.

Eaton, L., and Menolascino, F. J.: Psychotic reactions of childhood: Experiences of a mental retardation pilot project, J Nerv Ment Dis *143:*55-67, 1966.

Efron, M. L., and Ampola, M. G.: Aminoacidurias, Pediat Clin N Amer *14:* 881-903, 1967.

Eichenwald, H. F., and Fry, P. C.: Nutrition and learning, Science *163:*644-648, 1969.

Eisenberg, L.: Autistic child in adolescence, Amer J Psychiat *112:*607-612, 1956a.

——: Course of childhood schizophrenia, Arch Neurol (Chicago) *78:*69-83, 1957.

——: School phobia: Diagnosis, genesis, and management, Pediat Clin N Amer *5:* 645-666, 1958.

——: Role of drugs in treating disturbed children, Children *2:*167-173, 1964.

Eisenberg, L., and Gruenberg, E. M.: Current status of secondary prevention in child psychiatry, Amer J Orthopsychiat *31:*355-367, 1961.

Eisenberg, L., and Kanner, L.: Childhood schizophrenia: Symposium 1955. 6. Early infantile autism 1943-1955, Amer J Orthopsychiat *26:*556-566, 1956b.

Elgar, S.: Teaching autistic children, *in* Wing, J. K., ed.: Early Childhood Autism, New York: Pergamon, 1966.

Elliott-Binns, C. P.: Electric-buzzer treatment of enuresis in general practice, Practicioner *192:*546-549, 1964.

Eveloff, H. H.: Psychopharmacological agents in child psychiatry, Arch Gen Psychiat (Chicago) *14:*472-481, 1966.

Fabian, A. A.: Prognosis in head injuries in children, J Nerv Ment Dis *123:*428-431, 1956.

Faigel, H. C.: Language disability, Amer J Dis Child *110:*258-264, 1965.

Feild, J. R., *et al.:* Gilles de la Tourette's syndrome, Neurology (Minneap) *16:* 453-462, 1966.

Feinberg, I.: Eye movement activity during sleep and intellectual function in mental retardation, Science *159:*1256, 1968.

Feldman, H.: Place du Niamid en neuro-psychiatrie infantile, Ann Pediat (Paris) *201:*(Suppl)1-21, 1963.

Fisch, R. O., *et al.:* Twelve years of clinical experience with phenylketonuria, Neurology (Minneap) *19:*659-666, 1969,

Fish, B.: Drug therapy in child psychiatry: Psychological aspects, Compr Psychiat *1:*55-61, 1960.

——: Influence of maturation and abnormal development on the responses of disturbed children to drugs, Proc III World Cong Psychiat, vol. 2, 1961, pp. 1341-1348.

——: Pharmacotherapy in children's behavior disorders, Curr Psychiat Ther *3:* 82-90, 1963.

Fish, B., *et al.:* Classification of schizophrenic children under five years, Amer J Psychiat *124:*1415-1423, 1968.

Förster, E.: Der Einfluß des Lebensalters auf den Verlauf kindlicher Neurosen, Acta Paedopsychiat (Basel) *22:*117-122, 1955a.

Förster, E.: Über den spontanen Verlauf neurotischer Storungen im Kindesalter, Der Nervenarzt *26:*285-287, 1955b.

Forsythe, W. I., and Redmond, A.: Enuresis and the electric alarm: Study of 200 cases, Brit Med J *1:*211-213, 1970.

Francis, V., Korsch, B. M., and Morris, M. J.: Gaps in doctor-patient communication: Patients' response to medical advice, New Eng J Med *280:*535-540, 1969.

Freed, H., and Frignito, N.: Tranquilizers in child psychiatry: Current status on drugs, particularly phenothiazines, Penn Psychiat Quart *1:*39-48, 1961.

Freeman, W. F., and Watts, J. W.: Psychosurgery, Springfield (Ill): Thomas, 1950.

Freud, A.: Normality and Pathology in Childhood, New York: Internat Univ Press, 1965.

Frommer, E. A.: Treatment of childhood depression with antidepressant drugs, Brit Med J *1:*729-732, 1967.

Gallagher, J. J.: Changes in verbal and nonverbal ability of brain-injured mentally retarded children following removal of special stimulation, Amer J Ment Defic *66:*774-781, 1962.

Garfield, S. L., *et al.:* Effects of chlorpromazine on emotionally disturbed children, J Nerv Ment Dis *135:*147-154, 1962.

Gastaut, H., and Broughton, R. J.: Conclusions concerning the mechanisms of enuresis nocturna, Electroenceph Clin Neurophysiol *16:*626, 1964.

Gibbs, F. A., *et al.:* Electroencephalographic abnormality in "uncomplicated" childhood diseases, JAMA *171*:1050-1055, 1959.

Gittelman, M., and Birch, H. G.: Childhood schizophrenia: Intellect, neurologic status, perinatal risk, prognosis, and family pathology, Arch Gen Psychiat (Chicago) *17*:16-25, 1967.

Glaser, K., and Eisenberg, L.: Maternal deprivation, Pediatrics *18*:626-642, 1956.

Glaser, K.: Attempted suicide in children and adolescents: Psychodynamic observations, Amer J Psythother *19*:220-227, 1965.

Glidewell, J. C., Mensh, I. N., and Glider, M. C. L.: Behavior symptoms in children and the degree of sickness, Amer J Psychiat *114*:47-53, 1957.

Goldberg, H. K.: Role of brain damage in congenital dyslexia, Amer J Ophthal *50*:586-590, 1960.

Goldfarb, W.: Investigation of childhood schizophrenia: A retrospective view, Arch Gen Psychiat (Chicago) *11*:620-634, 1964.

Goldfarb, W., Goldfarb, N., and Pollack, R. C.: Treatment of childhood schizophrenia: A three-year comparison of day and residential treatment, Arch Gen Psychiat (Chicago) *14*:119-128, 1966.

Goodman, J. D., and Sours, J. A.: Child Mental Status Examination, New York: Basic, 1967.

Gordon, R. R.: Indications for chromosome analysis as an aid to the clinician, Clin Pediat *7*:83-87, 1968.

Gould, R. E.: Suicide problems in children and adolescents, Amer J Psychother *19*:228-246, 1965.

Greenebaum, J. V., and Lurie, L. A.: Encephalitis as a causative factor in behavior disorders of children: An analysis of seventy-eight cases, JAMA *136*:923-930, 1948.

Greengard, J.: Lead poisoning in childhood: Signs, symptoms, current therapy, clinical expressions, Clin Pediat *5*:269-276, 1966.

Grunebaum, H. U., and Strean, H. S.: Some considerations on the therapeutic neglect of fathers in child guidance, J Child Psychol Psychiat *5*:241-249, 1964.

Hackney, I. M., *et al.*: Phenylketonuria: Mental development, behavior, and termination of low phenylalanine diet, J Pediat *72*:646-655, 1968.

Hader, M.: Persistent enuresis, Arch Gen Psychiat (Chicago) *13*:296-298, 1965.

Hägglund, T. B., and Parkkulainen, K. V.: Enuretic children treated with imipramine (Tofranil): A cystometric study, Ann Paediat Fenn *11*:53-59, 1965.

Harms, E.: Differential patterns of manic-depressive disease in childhood, Nerv Child *9*:326-356, 1951.

Haworth, M. R., and Menolascino, F. J.: Some aspects of psychotic behavior in young children, Arch Gen Psychiat (Chicago) *18*:355-359, 1968.

Hellman, D. S., and Blackman, N.: Enuresis, fire setting and cruelty to animals: a triad predictive of adult crimes, Amer J Psychiat *122*:1431-1435, 1966.

Herbert, M.: The concept and testing of brain-damage in children: A review, J Child Psychol Psychiat *5*:197-216, 1964.

Hermann, K.: Reading Disability, Copenhagen: Ejnar Munksgaard, 1959.

Hertzig, M. E., Bortner, M., and Birch, H. G.: Neurologic findings in children educationally designated as "brain-damaged," Amer J Orthopsychiat *39*:437-446, 1969.

Hingtgen, J. N., Coulter, S. K., and Churchill, D. W.: Intensive reinforcement of imitative behavior in mute autistic children, Arch Gen Psychiat (Chicago) *17*:36-43, 1967.

Hirschberg, J. C., and Bryant, K. N.: Problems in the differential diagnosis of childhood schizophrenia, *in* Neurology and Psychiatry in Childhood, Baltimore: Williams & Wilkins, 1954, pp. 454-461.

Hollon, T. H.: Poor school performance as a symptom of masked depression in children and adolescents, Amer J Psychoth *25*:258-263, 1970.

Holm, V. A., and Kunze, L. H.: Effect of chronic otitis media on language and speech development, Pediatrics *43*:833-839, 1969.

Howells, J. G.: Child-parent separation as a therapeutic procedure, Amer J Psychiat *119*:922-926, 1963.

Hunter, H., and Stephenson, G. M.: Chlorpromazine and trifluoperazine in the treatment of behavioral abnormalities in the severely subnormal child, Brit J Psychiat *109*:411-417, 1963.

Hutt, C., and Hutt, S. J.: Effects of environmental complexity upon stereotyped behaviors in children, Anim Behav *13*:1-4, 1965.

Hyman, C. A., *et al.*: CNS abnormalities after neonatal hemolytic disease or hyperbilirubinemia, Amer J Dis Child *117*:395-405, 1969.

Illingworth, R. S.: Predictive value of developmental tests in the first year, with special reference to the diagnosis of mental subnormality, J Child Psychol Psychiat *2*:210-215, 1961.

———: Development of the Infant and

Young Child, ed. 3, Baltimore: Williams & Wilkins, 1966.

International Directory of Birth Defects Genetic Services: The National Foundation—March of Dimes, 1968.

JAMA: Mental retardation: A handbook for the primary physician. Report of the AMA conference on mental retardation, Chicago 1964. *191*:183-222, 1965.

Jarecki, H. G.: Maternal attitudes toward child rearing Arch Gen Psychiat (Chicago) *4*:340-356, 1961.

Jenkins, R. L., and Cole, J. O.: Diagnostic classification in child psychiatry, Psychiat Res Rep Amer Psychiat Ass *18*: 1-152, 1964.

Jervis, G. A.: The mental deficiencies, *in* Arieti, S., ed.: American Handbook of Psychiatry, vol. 2, New York: Basic, 1959, pp. 1289-1314.

Johnson, W. B., and Terman, L. M.: Some highlights in the literature of psychological sex differences published since 1920, J Psychol *9*:327-336, 1940.

Judd, L. L.: Obsessive compulsive neurosis in children, Arch Gen Psychiat (Chicago) *12*:136-143, 1965.

Kaliski, L.: Educational therapy for brain injured retarded children, Amer J Ment Defic *60*:71-77, 1955.

Kanner, L.: Autistic disturbances of affective contact, Nerv Child *2*:217-250, 1943.

———: Early infantile autism, J Pediat *25*:211-217, 1944.

———: Irrelevant and metaphorical language in early infantile autism, Amer J Psychiat *103*:242-246, 1946.

———: Problems of nosology and psychodynamics of early infantile autism, Amer J Orthopsychiat *19*:416-426, 1949.

———: Conception of wholes and parts in early infantile autism, Amer J Psychiat *108*:23-26, 1951.

———: To what extent is early infantile autism determined by constitutional inadequacies?, Res Publ Ass Res Nerv Ment Dis *33*:378-385, 1954.

———: Specificity of early infantile autism, Acta Paedopsychiat (Basel) *25*:108-113, 1958.

Karlin, I. W.: Stuttering—A problem today, JAMA *143*:732-736, 1950.

Kelman, D. H.: Gilles de la Tourette's disease in children: A review of the literature, J Child Psychol Psychiat *6*:219-226, 1965.

Kennard, M. A.: Characteristics of thought disturbances as related to electroencephalographic findings in children and adolescents, Amer J Psychiat *115*:911-921, 1959.

Kennell, J. H., and Bergen, M. E.: Early childhood separations, Pediatrics *37*:291-298, 1966.

Kidd, J. W.: Toward a more precise definition of mental retardation, Ment Retard *2*:209-212, 1964.

Klebanoff, L. B.: Community-oriented program for the retarded, Psychiatric Opinion, Summer, 1965.

Klosovskii, B. N.: The Development of the Brain and its Disturbance by Harmful Factors, New York: Macmillan, 1963.

Knights, R. M., and Hinton, G. G.: Effects of methylphenidate (Ritalin) on the motor skills and behavior of children with learning problems, J Nerv Ment Dis *148*:643-653, 1969.

Knobloch, H., and Pasamanick, B.: Environmental factors affecting human development before and after birth, Pediatrics *26*:210-218, 1960.

———: Developmental behavioral approach to the neurologic examination in infancy, Child Develop *33*:182-198, 1962.

———: Predicting intellectual potential in infancy, Dis Child *106*:43-51, 1963.

Knox, W. E.: Evaluation of the treatment of phenylketonuria with diets low in phenylalanine, Pediatrics *26*:1-11, 1960.

———: Inherited enzyme defects, Hosp Practice *4*:33-41, 1969.

Knudson, A. G., Jr.: Genetics and Disease, New York, Blakiston, 1965.

Koch, R., et al.: Nutritional therapy of galactosemia, Clin Pediat *4*:571-576, 1965.

Kohler, W. C., Coddington, R. D., and Agnew, H. W., Jr.: Sleep patterns in 2-year-old children, J Pediat *72*:228-233, 1968.

Krakowski, A. J.: Amitryptyline in treatment of hyperkinetic children: A double-blind study, Psychosomatics *6*:355-360, 1965.

Kravitz, H., et al.: Study of head-banging in infants and children, Dis Nerv Syst *21*:203-208, 1960.

Krieger, I., and Sargent, D. A.: A postural sign in the sensory deprivation syndrome in infants, J Pediatrics *70*:332-339, 1967.

Kurlander, L. F., and Colodny, D.: "Pseudo-neurosis" in the neurologically handicapped child, Amer J Orthopsychiat *35*:733-738, 1965.

Kysar, J. E.: Reactions of professionals to disturbed children and their parents, Arch Gen Psychiat (Chicago) *19*:562-570, 1968.

Laufer, M. W.: Cerebral dysfunction and behavior disorders in adolescents, Amer J Orthopsychiat *32*:501-507, 1962.

Laufer, M. W., Denhoff, E., and Solomons, G.: Hyperkinetic impulse disorder in children's behavior problems, Psychosom Med *19*:38-49, 1957.

Lehman, E., Haber, J., and Lesser, S. R.: Use of reserpine in autistic children, J Nerv Ment Dis *125*:351-356, 1957.

Lempp, R.: Enuresis nocturna und Epilepsie, Z Kinderheilk *92*:324-329, 1965.

Leonhard, K.: Uber Kindliche Katatonien, Psychiat Neurol Med Psychol (Leipzig) *12*:1-12, 1960.

Levy, D.: Release therapy, Amer J Orthopsychiat *9*:713, 1939.

Lo, W. H.: Aetiological factors in childhood neurosis, Brit J Psychiat *115*:889-894, 1969.

Lockyer, L., and Rutter, M.: Five- to fifteen-year follow-up study of infantile psychosis. III. Psychological aspects, Brit J Psychiat *115*:865-882, 1969.

Lovaas, O. I., *et al.*: Acquisition of imitative speech by schizophrenic children, Science *151*:705-707, 1966.

Lowrey, L. G.: Therapeutic play techniques (Symposium), Amer J Orthopsychiat *25*:574 and 747, 1955.

Lukianowicz, N.: Attempted suicide in children, Acta Psychiat Scand *44*:415-435, 1968.

Luria, A. R.: Study of the abnormal child, Amer J Orthopsychiat *31*:1-16, 1961.

Mabry, C. C., Denniston, J. C., and Coldwell, J. G.: Mental retardation in children of phenylketonuric mothers, New Eng J Med *275*:1331-1336, 1966.

Mabry, C. C., *et al.*: Maternal phenylketonuria: Cause of mental retardation in children without the metabolic defect, New Eng J Med *269*:1404-1408, 1963.

MacBrinn, M., *et al.*: Beta-galactosidase deficiency in the Hurler syndrome, New Eng J Med *287*:338-343, 1969.

MacLean, R. E. G.: Imipramine hydrochloride (Tofranil) and enuresis, Amer J Psychiat *117*:551, 1960.

MacNamara, M.: Helping children through their mothers, J Child Psychol Psychiat *4*:29-46, 1963.

Mahler, M. S.: On child psychosis and schizophrenia: Autistic and symbiotic infantile psychosis, Psychoanal Stud Child *7*:286-305, 1952.

Mariuz, M. J., and Walters, C. J.: Enuresis in non-psychotic boys treated with imipramine, Amer J Psychiat *120*:597-599, 1963.

Masland, R. L., Sarason, S. B., and Gladwin, T.: Mental Subnormality: Biological, Psychological, and Cultural Factors, New York: Basic, 1958.

Masterson, J. F., Jr., and Washburn, A.: Symptomatic adolescent: Psychiatric illness or adolescent turmoil?, Amer J Psychiat *122*:1240-1248, 1966.

Mattsson, A., Seese, L. R., and Hawkins, J. W.: Suicidal behavior as a child psychiatric emergency, Arch Gen Psychiat (Chicago) *20*:100-109, 1969.

McCord, W., and McCord, J. with Zola, I. K.: Origins of Crime, New York: Columbia Univ Press, 1959.

McFie, J.: Effects of hemispherectomy on intellectual functioning in cases of infantile hemiplegia, J Neurol Neurosurg Psychiat *24*:240-249, 1961.

McMurray, W. C.: Genetic errors and mental retardation, Canad Med Ass J *87*:486-490, 1962.

Menolascino, F. J.: Emotional disturbances in mentally retarded children, Amer J Psychiat *126*:168-176, 1969.

Mensh, I. N., *et al.*: Children's behavior symptoms and their relationships to school adjustment, sex, and social class, J Soc Issues *15*:8-15, 1959.

Mereu, T.: Adequacy of low-phenylalanine diet, Amer J Dis Child *113*:522-523, 1967.

Michael, C. M., Morris, D. P., and Soroker, E.: Follow-up studies of shy, withdrawn children. II. Relative incidence of schizophrenia, Amer J Orthopsychiat *27*:331-337, 1957.

Michaels, J. J.: Enuresis in murderous aggressive children and adolescents, Arch Gen Psychiat (Chicago) *5*:94-97, 1961.

Millar, T. P.: The child who refuses to attend school, Amer J Psychiat *118*:398-404, 1961.

Miller, P. R., Champelli, J. W., and Dinello, F. A.: Imipramine in the treatment of enuretic school children. A double-blind study, Amer J Dis Child *115*:17-20, 1968.

Mitchell, N., and Turton, C.: Children under five in an adult psychiatric ward, Brit J Psychiat *112*:1117-1118, 1966.

Moncrieff, A. A., *et al.*: Lead poisoning in children, Arch Dis Child *39*:1-13, 1964.

Moore, B. C.: Relationship between prematurity and intelligence in mental retardates, Amer J Ment Defic *70*:448-453, 1965.

Moore, T.: Difficulties of the ordinary child in adjusting to primary school, J Child Psychol Psychiat *7*:17-38, 1966.

Morris, D. P., Soroker, E., and Burruss, G.: Follow-up study of shy, withdrawn children. I. Evaluation of later adjustment, Amer J Orthopsychiat 24:743-754, 1954.

Morris, H. H., Escoll, P. J., and Wexler, R.: Aggressive behaviour disorders of childhood—a follow-up study, Amer J Psychiat 112:991-997, 1956.

Mowrer, O. H., and Mowrer, W. M.: Enuresis—A method for its study and treatment, Amer J Orthopsychiat 8:436-459, 1938.

Mulligan, G., et al.: Delinquency, Proc Roy Soc Med 56:1083-1086, 1963.

Norman, E.: Affect and withdrawal in schizophrenic children, Brit J Med Psychol 28:1-17, 1955.

Okada, S., and O'Brien, J. S.: Tay-Sachs Disease: Generalized absence of a Beta-D-N-acetylhexosaminidase component, Science 165:698-700, 1969.

O'Neal, P., et al.: The relation of childhood behavior problems to adult psychiatric status: A 30-year follow-up study of 262 subjects, in Gottlieb, J. S., and Tourney, G.: Scientific Papers and Discussion Division Meeting 1959, Detroit: Amer Psychiat Ass, 1960, pp. 99-117.

Oppel, W. C., Harper, P. A., and Rider, R. V.: Age of attaining bladder control, Pediatrics 42:614-626, 1968.

Ornitz, E. M., and Ritvo, E. R.: Perceptual inconstancy in early infantile autism, Arch Gen Psychiat (Chicago) 18:76-98, 1968.

Ounsted, C.: Hyperkinetic syndrome in epileptic children, Lancet 2:303-311, 1955.

Paine, R. S.: Evaluation of familial biochemically determined mental retardation in children, with special reference to aminoaciduria, New Eng J Med 262:658-665, 1960.

———: Minimal chronic brain syndromes in children, Develop Med Child Neurol 4:21-27, 1962.

———: Prenatal and perinatal factors affecting the central nervous system, Clin Proc Child Hosp DC 24:277-293, 1968.

Pasamanick, B., Rogers, M. E., and Lilienfeld, A. M.: Pregnancy experience and the development of behavior disorder in children, Amer J Psychiat 112:613-618, 1956.

Patton, R. G., and Gardner, L. I.: Growth Failure in Maternal Deprivation: With an introduction by Julius B. Richmond, Springfield (Ill): Thomas, 1962.

Pfaundler, M.: Demonstration eines Apparates zur selbsttaetigen Signalisierung, Verh Ges Kinderh 21:219-220, 1904.

Philips, I.: Psychopathology and mental retardation, Amer J Psychiat 124:29-35, 1967.

Pierce, C. M.: Dream studies in enuresis research, Canad Psychiat Ass J 8:415-419, 1963.

———: Enuresis, in Freedman, A. M., and Kaplan, H. I., eds.: Comprehensive Textbook of Psychiatry, Baltimore: Williams & Wilkins, 1967.

Pierce, C. M., et al.: Enuresis and dreaming, Arch Gen Psychiat (Chicago) 4:166-170, 1961.

Pitfield, M., and Oppenheim, A. N.: Child rearing attitudes of mothers of psychotic children, J Child Psychol Psychiat 5:51-57, 1964.

Pollack, M.: Comparison of childhood, adolescent and adult schizophrenias: Etiologic significance of intellectual functioning, Arch Gen Psychiat (Chicago) 2:652-660, 1960.

Pollin, W., et al.: Life history differences in identical twins discordant for schizophrenia, Amer J Orthopsychiat 36:492-509, 1966.

Poussaint, A. F., and Ditman, K. S.: A controlled study of imipramine (Tofranil) in the treatment of childhood enuresis, J Pediat 67:283-290, 1965.

Poussaint, A. F., Ditman, K. S., and Greenfield, R.: Amitriptyline in childhood enuresis, Clin Pharmacol Ther 7:21-25, 1966.

Powell, G. F., Brasel, J. A., and Blizzard, R. M.: Emotional deprivation and growth retardation simulating idiopathic hypopituitarism. I. Clinical evaluation of the syndrome, New Eng J Med 276:1271-1278, 1967.

Prader, A., Tanner, J. M., and Harnack, G. A. von: Catch-up growth following illness or starvation: Example of developmental canalization in man, J Pediat 62:646-659, 1963.

Prechtl, H. F.: Neurological sequelae of prenatal and perinatal complications, Brit Med J 4:763-767, 1967.

Provence, S.: On predicting mental development, Conn Med 32:575-578, 1968.

Provence, S., and Lipton, R.: Infants in Institutions, New York: Internat Univ Press, 1962.

Prugh, D. G.: Toward an understanding of psychosomatic concepts in relation to illness in children, in Solnit, A. J., and Provence, S. A., eds.: Modern Perspectives in Child Development, New York: Internat Univ Press, 1963, pp. 246-367.

Rabinovitch, R. D., et al.: A research

approach to reading retardation, *in* McIntosh, R., and Hare, C. C., eds.: Neurology and Psychiatry in Childhood, Baltimore: Williams & Wilkins, 1954, pp. 363-387.

Reiser, D. E.: Psychosis of infancy and early childhood as manifested by children with atypical development, New Eng J Med *269:*790-798, 844-850, 1963.

Ritvo, E. R., Ornitz, E. M., and La Franchi, S.: Frequency of repetitive behaviors in early infantile autism and its variants, Arch Gen Psychiat (Chicago) *19:* 341-347, 1968.

Ritvo, E. R., *et al.:* Decreased postrotatory nystagmus in early infantile autism, Neurology (Minneap) *19:*653-658, 1969.

——: Correlation of psychiatric diagnoses and EEG findings: Double-blind study of 184 hospitalized children, Amer J Psychiat *126:*988-996, 1970.

Robins, E., and O'Neal, P.: Clinical features of hysteria in children, with a note on prognosis: A two to seventeen year follow-up study of 41 patients, Nerv Child *10:*246-271, 1953.

Rodriguez, A., Rodriguez, M., and Eisenberg, L.: The outcome of school phobia: A follow-up study based on 41 cases, Amer J Psychiat *116:*540-544, 1959.

Roll, M.: Discussion: synthesis of the research conference, *in* Jenkins, R. L., and Cole, J. O., eds.: Diagnostic Classification in Child Psychiatry, Psychiat Res Rep Amer Psychiat Ass *18:*142-146, 1964.

Rosenberg, C. M.: Determinants of psychiatric illness in young people, Brit J Psychiat *115:*907-915, 1969.

Rosenberg, L. E.: Inherited aminoacidopathies demonstrating vitamin dependence, New Eng J Med *281:*145-153, 1969.

Rosenthal, S. H., and Richmond, L. H.: Adult enuretics and imipramine, Compr Psychiat *10:*147-150, 1969.

Rutter, M.: Classification and categorization in child psychiatry, J Child Psychol Psychiat *6:*71-83, 1965.

——: Concepts of autism: Review of research, J Child Psychol Psychiat *9:*1-25, 1968.

Rutter, M., *et al.:* Temperamental characteristics in infancy and the later development of behavioural disorders, Brit J Psychiat *110:*651-661, 1964.

Ryle, A., Pond, D. A., and Hamilton, M.: The prevalence and patterns of psychological disturbance in children of primary age, J Child Psychol Psychiat *6:*101-113, 1965.

Sabot, L. M., Peck, R., and Raskin, J.: Waiting room society: A study of families

and children applying to a child psychiatric clinic, Arch Gen Psychiat (Chicago) *21:*25-32, 1969.

Saint-Laurent, J. C., *et al.:* Polygraphic study of nocturnal enuresis in the epileptic child, Electroenceph Clin Neurophysiol *15:*904-905, 1963.

Salfield, D. J.: Depersonalization and allied disturbances in childhood, J Ment Science *104:*472-476, 1958.

Schachter, M.: Rhythmic patterns of sleep rocking in children, *in* Harms, E., ed.: Problems of Sleep and Dream in Children, New York: Macmillan, 1964, pp. 135-142.

Schain, R. J., and Yannet, H.: Infantile autism: An analysis of 50 cases and a consideration of certain relevant neurophysiologic concepts, J Pediat *57:*560-567, 1960.

Scheibel, M. E., and Scheibel, A. B.: Some neural substrates of postnatal development, *in* Hoffman, M. L., and Hoffman L. W., eds.: Review of Child Development Research, vol. 1, New York: Russell Sage Foundation, 1964, pp. 481-519.

Scholz, B., *et al.:* Physical and mental development of children of mothers with toxemia of pregnancy, German Med Monthly *13:*487, 1968.

Seiden, R. H.: Suicide among youth, Nat Clearinghouse Mental Health Information, Suppl Bulletin of Suicidology, 1969, pp. 1-62.

Shapiro, A. K., and Shapiro, E.: Treatment of Gilles de la Tourette's Syndrome with haloperidol, Brit J Psychiat *114:*345-350, 1968.

Shaw, C. R.: The Psychiatric Disorders of Childhood, New York: Appleton, 1966.

Shaw, C. R., and Schelkun, R.: Suicidal behavior in children, Psychiatry *28:*157, 1965.

Shaw, E. B.: Side reactions from tranquilizing drugs, Pediat Clin N Amer *7:* 257-268, 1960.

Shepherd, M., Oppenheim, A. N., and Mitchell, S.: Childhood behaviour disorders and the child-guidance clinic: Epidemiological study, J Child Psychol Psychiat *7:*39-52, 1966.

Shodell, M. J., and Reiter, H. H.: Self-mutilative behavior in verbal and nonverbal schizophrenic children, Arch Gen Psychiat (Chicago) *19:*453-455, 1968.

Simmons, J. E.: Psychiatric Examination of Children, Philadelphia: Lea, 1969.

Simon, G. B., and Gillies, S. M.: Some physical characteristics of a group of psychotic children, Brit J Psychiat 110:104-107, 1964.

Small, J. G.: Epileptiform electroencephalographic abnormalities in mentally ill children, J Nerv Ment Dis 147:341-348, 1968.

Smith, G. F.: Analysis of clinical features of Down's syndrome in relation to chromosomal changes, Ann NY Acad Sci 171:587-601, 1970.

Smith, J. L.: Pediatric neuro-ophthalmology, in Smith, J. L., ed.: The University of Miami Neuro-ophthalmology Symposium, Springfield (Ill): Thomas, 1964, pp. 344-384.

Solnit, A. J.: Hospitalization: An aid to physical and psychological health in childhood, Amer J Dis Child 99:155-163, 1960.

Solomons, G., Keleske, L., and Opitz, E.: Evaluation of the effects of terminating the diet in phenylketonuria, J Pediat 69:596-602, 1966.

Starfield, B.: Functional bladder capacity in enuretic and nonenuretic children, J Pediat 70:777-781, 1967.

Stevens, D. A., et al.: Presumed minimal brain dysfunction in children. Relationship to performance on selected behavioral tests, Arch Gen Psychiat (Chicago) 16:281-285, 1967.

Stevens, J. R., and Blachly, P. H.: Successful treatment of the maladie des tics. Gilles de la Tourette's syndrome, Amer J Dis Child 112:541-545, 1966.

Stevens, J. R., Sachdev, K., and Milstein, V.: Behavior disorders of childhood and the electroencephalogram, Arch Neurol (Chicago) 18:160-177, 1968.

Stewart, M. A., et al.: The natural history of the hyperactive child syndrome, Presented at the annual meeting of the APA, New York, 1965.

Sundby, H. S., and Kreyberg, P. C.: Prognosis in Child Psychiatry, Baltimore: Williams & Wilkins, 1968.

Talbot, N. B.: Pediatric frontiers in developmental medicine: Overview, Amer J Dis Child 110:287-290, 1965.

Tapia, F., Jekel, J., and Domke, H. R.: Enuresis: An emotional symptom? J Nerv Ment Dis 130:61-66, 1960.

Tarjan, G.: Research and clinical advances in mental retardation, JAMA 182:617-621, 1962.

——: Rehabilitation of the mentally retarded, JAMA 187:867-870, 1964.

Taylor, E. M.: Psychological Appraisal of Children with Cerebral Defects, Cambridge: Harvard Univ Press, 1961.

Tec, L.: Unexpected effects in children treated with imipramine, Amer J Psychiat 120:603, 1963.

Thanaphum, S., Costello, J., and Hirsch, J. G.: Assessment of individual functioning through classroom observation. The clinician in the preschool setting, Arch Gen Psychiat (Chicago) 23:16-19, 1970.

Thelander, H. E., Phelps, J. K., and Kirk, E. W.: Learning disabilities associated with lesser brain damage, J Pediat 53:405-409, 1958.

Thomas, A., Chess, S., and Birch, H. G.: Temperament and Behavior Disorders in Children, New York: NY Univ Press, 1968.

Tibbles, J. A. R., and Prichard, J. S.: Prognostic value of the electroencephalogram in neonatal convulsions, Pediatrics 35:778-786, 1965.

Tjossem, T. D., Hansen, T. J., and Ripley, H. S.: An investigation of reading difficulty in young children, Amer J Psychiat 118:1104-1113, 1962.

Toolan, J. M.: Depression in children and adolescents, in Caplan, G., and Lebovici, S., eds.: Adolescence: Psychosocial Perspectives, New York: Basic, 1969.

Towbin, A.: Cerebral hypoxic damage in fetus and newborn, Arch Neurol (Chicago) 20:35-43, 1969.

Treffert, D. A.: Epidemiology of Infantile Autism, Arch Gen Psychiat (Chicago) 22:431-438, 1970.

Ucko, L. E.: Comparative study of asphyxiated and non-asphyxiated boys from birth to five years, Develop Med Child Neurol 7:643-657, 1965.

Vandersall, T. A., and Wiener, J. M.: Children who set fires, Arch Gen Psychiat (Chicago) 22:63-71, 1970.

Vaughan, G. F., and Cashmore, A. A.: Encopresis in childhood, Guy Hosp Rep 103:360-370, 1954.

Vernon, D. T., Schulman, J. L., and Foley, J. M.: Changes in children's behavior after hospitalization. Some dimensions of response and their correlates, Amer J Dis Child 111:581-593, 1966.

Vernon, M., and Rothstein, D. A.: Prelingual deafness. Experiment of nature, Arch Gen Psychiat (Chicago) 19:361-369, 1968.

Vorster, D.: An investigation into the part played by organic factors in childhood schizophrenia, Brit J Psychiat 106:494-522, 1960.

Walker, E. R. C.: Treatment of Sydenham's chorea, Med Press (London) 220:445-448, 1948.

Walzer, S., Breau, G., and Gerald, P. S.:

Chromosome survey of 2,400 normal newborn infants, J Pediat *74:*438-448, 1969.

Warkany, J., *et al.:* Chromosome analyses in a children's hospital. Selection of patients and results of studies, Pediatrics *33:*290-305, 1964a.

———: *Ibid.,* pp. 454-465, 1964b.

Warnecke, R.: School phobia and its treatment, Brit J Psychol *37:*71-79, 1964.

Warren, W.: Some relationships between the psychiatry of children and of adults, Brit J Psychiat *106:*815-826, 1960.

Wechsler, D.: Wechsler Intelligence Scale for Children, New York: Psychological Corporation, 1949.

Wenar, C.: The reliability of developmental histories: Summary and evaluation of evidence, Psychosom Med *25:*505-509, 1963.

Werry, J. S., and Cohrssen, J.: Enuresis —an etiologic and therapeutic study, Pediatrics *67:*423-431, 1965.

Werry, J. S., *et al.:* Studies on the hyperactive child. 3. Effect of chlorpromazine upon behavior and learning ability, J Amer Acad Child Psychiat *5:*292-312, 1966.

White, P. T., DeMyer, W., and DeMyer, M.: EEG abnormalities in early childhood schizophrenia: Double-blind study of psychiatrically disturbed and normal children during promazine sedation, Amer J Psychiat *120:*950-958, 1964.

Whitman, R. M., *et al.:* Drugs and dreams. II. Imipramine and prochlorperazine, Compr Psychiat *2:*219-226, 1961.

Williamson, M., Koch, R., and Henderson, R.: Phenylketonuria in school age retarded children, Amer J Ment Defic *72:* 740-747, 1968.

Wing, J. K., and Wing, L.: Clinical interpretation of remedial teaching, *in* Wing, J. K., ed.: Early Childhood Autism, New York: Pergamon, 1966.

Winn, D., and Halla, R.: Observations of children who threaten to kill themselves, Canad Psychiat Ass J *11:*S283-S294, 1966.

Wolff, S., and Chess, S.: A behavioral study of schizophrenic children, Acta Psychiat Scand *40:*438-466, 1964.

———: Analysis of the language of fourteen schizophrenic children, J Child Psychol Psychiat *6:*29-41, 1965.

Yarrow, L. J.: Separation from parent during early childhood, *in* Hoffman, M. L., and Hoffman, L. W., eds.: Review of Child Development Research, vol. 1, New York: Russell Sage Foundation, 1964, pp. 89-136.

Zigler, E.: Familial mental retardation: A continuing dilemma, Science *155:*292-298, 1967.

CHAPTER
ELEVEN

Organic Brain Syndromes

THE CONCEPT OF "ORGANICITY"

THE TERM *organic brain syndrome* refers to impairments in mental functioning that are believed to be caused by structural or functional abnormalities of brain tissue. The patient's impairments may be labeled organic because they

1/ are associated with symptoms or signs indicative of neurologic dysfunction on clinical, neuroradiologic, or electroencephalographic examination;

2/ developed in the wake of an intoxication, infectious illness, head injury, or other event that is known to have injured or at least to be capable of injuring the central nervous system; or

3/ are associated with dysmnesia, disorientation, or episodic disturbances of awareness, symptoms so commonly linked with neurologic changes or postmortem evidence of brain damage that they are considered pathognomonic of organic disease (Bini 1959).

That mental syndromes coupled with direct or indirect evidence of brain involvement are labeled *organic* does not of course mean that those without such evidence are nonorganic (or, as the psychiatric phrase goes, "functional"). If the discoveries of the past few decades are any guide, it is safe to predict that more and more disorders currently viewed as cryptogenic will in the future be shown to have biologic causes or correlates and that the dichotomy implied by the very term *organic* will thus gradually lose its significance.

Regardless of the possible reservations concerning the classification, there are decided advantages in discussing the so-called "organic" syndromes together. Foremost is that many of the illnesses labeled organic, if not checked, can endanger the patient's life and cause further brain damage. Thus the label alerts the clinician to the gravity of the patient's condition and the urgency of undertaking appropriate diagnostic studies and treatment measures (Guze 1967).

Organic disorders, moreover, are the only mental syndromes for which in some cases a probable cause can be found and a specific, rather than empiric, treatment applied. Finally, regardless of cause, those organic syndromes that cannot be reversed tend after a variable period of time to have a common outcome, namely dementia, and thus give rise to similar management problems.

Diseases that affect brain functioning can produce an almost infinite number of clinical pictures, depending on their severity and duration, the brain area they affect, the environment in which they occur, and the age, physiologic state, and premorbid personality pattern of the individual involved. Yet, despite the diversity of theoretical possibilities, most of the syndromes customarily called organic fall into one of three somewhat overlapping patterns. According to the clinical picture seen when the disorder is full-blown, these patterns can be designated dementiform, deliriform, and epileptiform.

The first group is characterized by dysmnesia, disorientation, personality changes, and such other impairments of intellectual functioning and adaptation as are associated with *dementia.*

The second is characterized not only by dysmnesia and disorientation but also by dysattention and such other symptoms of *delirium* as delusions, hallucinations, excitement, or apathy.

The third group, characterized by episodic disturbances of consciousness, includes the psychological disorders that are associated with grand mal, petit mal, or psychomotor *seizures.* The syndromes of *narcolepsy* and *somnambulism,* though not strictly speaking epileptiform, share with this group the *paroxysmal* occurrence of symptoms.

DEMENTIFORM SYNDROMES

DESCRIPTION

The cardinal symptoms of the dementiform syndrome are dysmnesia, disorientation, and difficulty with abstract reasoning. These symptoms may also be present in deliriform syndromes and depressions but, in the former, occur in association with and are usually overshadowed by dysattention and a fluctuating level of awareness and in the latter, by apathy, anergia, and sadness. The most prominent of the dementiform symptoms is *dysmnesia*—an impairment in the ability to retain and recall information. The mildest (and thus in progressive dementias the earliest) type of memory disturbance consists of diminished efficiency at absorbing and retaining new information. This may be so mild at the outset that it seems like mere *absent-mindedness.* In more severe cases, the individual will have difficulty in remembering the events of the *recent past.* Things learned and events experienced before the period of memory failure began may still be recalled at this stage, but as the dysmnesia becomes more severe, it invades the patient's memory of the time period before he fell ill, then extends further and further into the *remote past* until it is finally *global,* in the sense that he neither understands the present nor remembers any part of the past.

Disorientation, often described as if it were independent of dysmnesia, is in fact closely related: knowing what time it is, being able to tell where one is, and identifying the person one is dealing with are not functions of some internal radar equipment but of the individual's memory. Disorientation is thus rare without an appreciable memory impairment and, like dysmnesia, shows characteristic gradations of severity. The mildest (and thus in progressive dementias the earliest) type of disorientation consists of an impaired *time* sense. Initially, the patient will be unable to recall when or in what order the current or previous day's events occurred, though he will still be able to describe them; thereafter he may be unable to tell the day of the month, month of the year, day of the week, or year. As his temporal disorientation becomes more severe, he will begin to lose his orientation to *place:* at the outset, he will have difficulty in locating or identifying a particular place only if he has never been there before; in more severe cases, he will even have difficulty identifying familiar surroundings; in the most severe form, he will be unable to remember his own address or, if at home or at a hospital, to identify it as such. As these manifestations of disorientation mount, he will begin to have difficulty in identifying the *persons* around him, forgetting first their names and thereafter their relationship to him. Not until almost every other intellectual function is impaired, however, will he have difficulty identifying himself or remembering his own name, a fact that can be important when the differential diagnosis includes a simulated amnesia or dissociative state.

Other impairments in intellectual functioning found in dementiform syndromes include *difficulty in abstract reasoning* (testable by asking the patient to explain or rephrase a proverb or to explain the difference between objects having certain similarities, such as a dwarf and a child) and an *inability to bear several factors in mind simultaneously* (testable by asking him to repeat five numbers in reverse order or to serially and continuously subtract sevens from 100).

There is, then, some measure of uniformity in the order in which the patient's memory, orientation, and other intellectual abilities wane. At first, such deficits may be so *mild and uneven* that they are erroneously attributed to the stress of the examination rather than organic disease. Even after the individual's impairments are sufficiently pronounced to be *demonstrable on testing,* he may be so lucid and remain so competent in his performance of familiar tasks that he can *continue to function at his job.* The more his job depends on his ability to make decisions or to gauge and deal with sensitive interpersonal situations, however, the sooner his *impairments become manifest* to those around him, as he may overlook the most obvious factors, to the point that his *judgment becomes unreliable* and his decisions and behavior inappropriate. Eventually, whatever his occupational responsibilities, there will be no mistaking the *generalized diminution and slowing of intellectual functioning* (and even impoverishment of speech) characteristic of this disorder. As the dysmnesia and disorientation come to affect more and more of his interpersonal and social transactions, his grooming, eating, personal hygiene, and ability to manage his financial affairs decline until he is finally *unable to take care of himself* at all.

The clinical picture is far more complex, however, than the foregoing list of intellectual and social deficits would suggest. Fully as important as the intellectual deficits are the *emotional reactions, adaptive efforts,* and *personality changes* that the disease and its consequences bring in their wake. While these dimensions of the clinical picture generally mesh with the intellectual deficits, they may also be colored, especially at the outset, by the patient's *premorbid personality,* the *rate of deterioration* caused by the particular illness involved, the *environmental demands, stresses, and supports* to which he is exposed, and his *state of health,* including whatever *physical impairments* he may have (Busse 1967).

The most common manifestation of emotional disturbance seen in the patient with a dementiform syndrome is an *inability to modulate his emotional response.* The patient may initially react in a somewhat dull manner to stimuli that would in the past have interested him, but once aroused, is unable to dampen his reactions

and appears unduly excited or tearful. At first, he may show no symptoms other than *diminished vitality,* increasingly constricted and shallow responsiveness, and progressively *declining interest* in his environment. Either simultaneously or somewhat later (and often before
his intellectual impairments are noticed), he may develop *irritability, depression, affective lability, euphoria,* and *diffuse somatic
complaints without identifiable cause,* and thus be considered to have
an affective or psychosomatic disorder (Nicol 1968, Surridge 1969).

The clinical picture is also affected by the patient's efforts to
adapt to his impairments and the distress he experiences when he
is unable to do so. In considering the kinds of efforts that are
labeled "adaptive," those that help the individual to *circumvent his
impairments* are obviously of greater advantage than those that
merely help him *avoid becoming upset* by them. The patient who,
by becoming compulsively orderly or continually writing himself
little notes and reminders, prevents himself from misplacing his
belongings or forgetting his tasks may, if his dementia is stable or
progresses so slowly that some measure of learning is still possible,
be able to take on a different and simpler kind of job. Even if he
keeps the same job, he can usually avoid inflicting his difficulties
on his co-workers by laying aside those portions of his work that
have become too complex or require more memory functions than
he commands. His explanation for his behavior, however, may be
an example of the second type of adaptive effort. The senile business
executive who has delegated most of his functions to his subordinates
may defend himself against recognizing his deterioration by claiming that his memory has gotten better, not worse, and say with real
conviction: "Now that I have learned to let other people take care
of all the unimportant little details, I can concentrate on the larger
issues of my business—those that really require my personal
attention."

The kinds of adaptive efforts the patient makes both to improve
his poor performance and to avoid noticing it and indeed the way
he handles his impairments are determined at first by his *premorbid
personality.* Given an equal degree of impairment, the patient who
has always been unusually orderly may be able to perform better
than the one with less organized habits, but he is also more likely
to become disturbed by his inability to perform with his accustomed
precision. As the disorder progresses, *personality changes* start to
appear. Unlike the maturation process, however, which, by smooth-
ing rough edges and adding to the individual's repertoire of adaptive
skills, can improve his disposition, progressive brain disease tends

to make him rely on those coping mechanisms he knows best and, by limiting him to their use, brings out the worst in him. Thus, while interpersonal and occupational difficulties are often the first signs of a brain disorder, they do not always derive from the intellectual deterioration itself nor even the resultant increase in social ineptitude, but from an apparent intensification of premorbid personality traits and the personality caricaturization that this process induces (Vispo 1962). Individuals with preexisting personality disturbances, particulary those who have always been isolated, withdrawn, suspicious, or otherwise socially inept, are even more vulnerable to such difficulties (Fisch 1968, Kay 1959, Lange 1964). As Agnes Royden has said, "If you want to be a dear old lady at 70, you must begin early, say about 17" (Zeman 1965).

Although the individual's defenses may at first be effective at hiding his intellectual impairments, the way he handles them tends to become increasingly inefficient and maladaptive. Such socially acceptable coping mechanisms as sublimation, repression, and denial are gradually replaced by more primitive ones, such as the assumption of a *paranoid attitude*. The denial of impairment that once functioned to protect the patient against being confronted with and thus made anxious by his cerebral incompetence can degenerate to a *negativistic* refusal to collaborate with his environment in any way at all. Finally, "with progressive functional cerebral impairment, the role of personality factors recedes as a determinant of behavior, and the residual capacities shape the response in greater and greater measure" (Ullman 1961).

The patient's efforts to circumvent and hide his impairments help him to maintain his equilibrium. When these efforts fail, when his impairments prevent him from achieving what he wants or conforming to his environment's demands, or when his intellectual difficulties cause him to misinterpret or be frightened by events he does not understand, he may react with *catastrophic anxiety*, profound depression, or apparently unmotivated aggressiveness. Such reactions may in turn affect his sleep and appetite and, in addition, cause those around him to act differently and even more puzzlingly toward him. Thus, unless his environment is structured so that he is not faced with demands he cannot satisfy or forced in some other way to confront his own incompetence, his anxiety will mount and his performance decline even further.

The efficiency of the patient's own adaptive efforts, and thus both the ease with which his illness can be diagnosed and the degree of environmental structuring he needs, depend not only on the extent but also on the *rate of intellectual deterioration.* The milder the dementia and the slower its progress, the more use he can make of his usual defenses against stress and the more compensatory mechanisms he can develop. Since the earliest and most obvious symptoms in such cases are personality changes, it is very likely that for some time the disorder may be considered characterologic rather than organic in origin. The mild or slowly progressing dementia may therefore be harder to identify than the one that develops suddenly and produces an abrupt and far more obvious change in the patient's life style. The clinical picture and course of the senile dementia (in which the deterioration may take years or even decades to progress from absentmindedness and mild concreteness to global dysmnesia and disorientation) thus differ greatly from that seen in degenerative encephalopathies like Jakob-Creutzfeldt's disease (in which the degenerative process may take no more than a few months) or febrile deliria (in which the process takes but a few hours or days).

The extent to which the patient's performance is affected by his deterioration—and thus the likelihood of his being confronted and discomfited by it—depends also on the demands, stresses, and supports to which his *environment* exposes him. The individual who has a repetitive simple job that requires little interpersonal skill and a family that is unsophisticated and demands little emotional attention may function quite adequately despite fairly massive deterioration. This balance, however, is often tenuous. For example, despite some forgetfulness, a patient may appear quite stable within his environment but, after an apparently trivial event, suddenly become much more forgetful and confused, and be at least temporarily unable to maintain an independent existence. One way of explaining this is that the brain-damaged individual's intellectual, emotional, and biologic reserves are so marginal that almost any stressful event can aggravate his symptoms and cause subclinical impairments to become manifest. Particularly stressful for the brain-damaged patient (and thus especially likely to cause such a decline) are events that decrease, overload, or distort his sensory input. ECT, cataract surgery, the use of barbiturates or other psychotropic agents, and physical illnesses that interfere with the patient's sleep, otherwise dampen his alertness, or cause him to be placed in an unfamiliar environment (like a hospital) are for this reason among the most common antecedents of accelerated deterioration (Locke 1964, Ziskind 1963).

The kind of environmental event that can confuse or excite the brain-damaged patient enough to cause a sudden decline varies from one individual to the next. The patient who has always been shy and whose most intimate relationship was with his wife may become suddenly worse at the time of her death; one who was deeply involved with his job, soon after his retirement. Deterioration in the wake of such losses should not be routinely attributed to the resultant sadness, loneliness, or loss of self-esteem (Post 1966), as the patient's deterioration can also be accelerated by environmental changes that could be expected to please him. Most clinicians are familiar with the situation in which a couple's grown children proudly buy their parents a modern and comfortable home only to find that one or the other has such difficulty in becoming accustomed to the new house or is so pleased and excited by it that he develops insomnia and anorexia. This reaction compounds whatever difficulty in orientation the parent might previously have experienced, and the well-meant gesture is thus met with decompensation rather than gratitude.

The clinical picture is also affected by the patient's physical disabilities and their practical and emotional consequences (Von Werssowetz 1966). The *tremor* of parkinsonism and the patient's concern about it, the *aphasia* that can follow a cerebrovascular accident and the resultant effect on interpersonal relationships, and the generalized *physical deterioration* associated with aging or arteriosclerosis and the dependency it engenders can handicap an individual far more than the intellectual deterioration itself (Blenkner 1969).

The senile patient's decline in social functioning tends to be aggravated by a number of other factors that are not a direct result of his intellectual deterioration. If, as often the case, his *hearing or vision is impaired,* his sensory input may be so reduced or distorted that his environmental feedback system no longer helps him to determine whether his behavior is appropriate (Corso 1968). If he lives alone and shops and cooks for himself, is edentulous and unable to chew, or is uninterested in food and poorly supervised, he is likely to eat poorly and develop *nutritional deficiencies* that can accelerate his deterioration. Such physical problems as poor vision or hearing, missing teeth, constipation, or arthritis may in addition make so many *demands on his time and energy* that his vitality and his ability to function and care for himself are impaired. The elderly patient suffering from physical ailments or disabilities, may also experience a disturbance in his *body image,* a decline in his *sense of self-worth,* and an exaggerated *fear of death.* Furthermore, because he is apathetic, poorly behaved, or abandoned, he may have little contact with his family or any other source of sensory and social stimulation, and thus become increasingly unable to understand the world around him' or function adaptively to the point that his behavior becomes irrelevant to his situation and finally appears grossly disturbed.

EXAMINATION

A comprehensive assessment of the patient with dysmnesia, disorientation, and difficulty in abstract reasoning begins with an attempt to determine whether he is suffering from an organic dementia, whether the factors that have caused it are still operative, and what these factors may be. Because such neurologic impairments as aphasia, apraxia, and agnosia impede the patient's ability to perform as requested, they also mimic organic dementia, but can usually be distinguished by a few simple tests. For a review of such tests and their interpretation, the reader is referred to specialized texts (DeMyer 1969, Logothetis 1970). Severe dysmnesia and disorientation without fluctuations in awareness are characteristic findings in organic dementias, but such symptoms may also be seen, albeit in milder form, in depressions (especially involutional ones) and late schizophrenias (Eaton 1969). Since patients with any of these three syndromes may also exhibit anergia, retardation, hypochondriasis, and mildly paranoid ideation, it is often impossible to make a firm diagnosis without obtaining a thorough history, following the course of the symptoms for a number of months, or trying an antidepressant regimen (Butler 1967, Colbert 1966, Davies 1969, Gibson 1961, Kay 1964, Walton 1958).

Such mimicry is by no means one-sided, for dementia in its early stages can wear any number of diagnostic masks, including that of perfect health. Whether such difficulties or the mild memory defects described above should be ascribed to illness or to low intelligence cannot be decided, however, unless the patient's prior level of functioning is known and the deficits clearly represent a change for the worse. While the presence and, to some extent, the severity of the average patient's dementia can be determined by tests as simple as the Ten-Question Mental Status (Kahn 1960; see Table 23), the patient whose premorbid intelligence was good and whose social facade is well-developed may require thorough and repeated psychological testing to determine whether and what degree of deterioration has taken place and how rapidly it is progressing. The

TABLE 23. *Ten-Question Mental Status Examination*

1. What is the name of this place?	6. How old are you?
2. Where is it located (address)?	7. When were you born (month)?
3. What day of the week is it?	8. When were you born (year)?
4. What is the month now?	9. Who is the President of the United States?
5. What is the year?	10. Who was the President before him?

Kahn, R. L., *et al.*: Brief objective measures for the determination of mental status in the aged, Amer J Psychiat *177*:326-328, 1960.

diagnostic problems become even more complex when the basic cause of the patient's dementia is known but the dementia unexpectedly starts to accelerate in the wake of some superimposed environmental or physical stress, such as a job change, a depressive syndrome, or an intercurrent illness.

Once the clinician has decided that the patient's symptoms do in fact represent an organic dementia, he must try to determine *whether the causative factors are still operative.* This judgment is easiest when the causative factors have been identified, but even when they have not, it is possible to decide whether they are still active by scrutinizing the patient's history and observing his course, with particular attention to his intellectual functioning, behavioral patterns, and transactional style.

Clinical or historical evidence that the patient's symptoms have not progressed for some time or, better yet, have partly subsided suggest that the underlying *disorder is quiescent,* but months or years of observation may be needed before it is certain that the symptoms have not merely come to a temporary halt. While this wait is often inevitable, certain clues may enable the clinician to arrive somewhat earlier at a well-educated guess about the patient's prognosis. If the clinical history should reveal that, some days, weeks, or months earlier, the patient had experienced *an acute insult to the* cns (such as an encephalitis, head injury, or cerebrovascular accident), had then become comatose, stuporous, or delirious, and had thereafter exhibited the characteristic symptoms of dementia, it would be reasonable to assume that the causative factor is no longer operative. Such an assumption would also be justified if the dementia were caused by a clearly identifiable *medically or surgically reversible disease* (like hypothyroidism, chronic intoxication, or a benign tumor) that in the interim had been treated and relieved. If, on the other hand, the patient has a *family history of heredodegenerative disease* or exhibits *increasing neurologic impairment,* severe *arteriosclerosis,* or intractable *hypertension,* the dementia may be expected to progress.

The most obvious evidence that the *causative factors are still operative* is that the patient's *intellectual deterioration is progressive*. Once these factors have come to a halt, whether spontaneously or as a result of treatment, viable brain tissue gradually recovers, and the patient's intellectual functioning shows some measure of improvement for the next 12 or 24 months and, in exceptional instances, longer (LaBaw 1969). By the end of this period, the patient's *intellectual impairment is stable* in the sense that it has either subsided or resulted in a residual defect, which, though unlikely to improve, is also unlikely to extend any further.

The behavioral patterns seen in the course of the diagnostic interview and psychological examination provide additional data with which to assess the severity of the brain disorder. The greater the physician's experience with such patients, the less credence he will give to the popular fiction that brain-damaged or senile patients behave in a random and incomprehensible fashion, are apathetic, withdrawn, unresponsive, willful, irritable, negativistic, or unmotivated to perform well. Kurt Goldstein (1942) called attention to the ways in which such patients

1/ deny their defects,
2/ refuse to perform certain tasks,
3/ perform substitute tasks with which they can cope,
4/ are compulsively orderly, and
5/ simplify their environment.

These mechanisms, more common in moderate than in mild or severe cases, are believed to be intended to stave off the *catastrophic reaction* of massive fear, anxiety, and discomfort that occurs when the patient's mental incompetence or failure in a given task becomes obvious. The particular way in which a patient employs these mechanisms provides additional clues to the extent of his impairment.

Some patients acknowledge their incapacitated condition realistically, be it an impairment of intellectual functioning or a physical disability (such as the paresis of a limb). Others, incapable of adopting the abstract attitude that would link whatever defects they have to the rest of their existence, deal with them on a concrete level by ordering their external environment so as to avoid reference to their defects, and exhibit a transactional style that seems dedicated to warding off such confrontations (Ullmann 1961). Some do this by attempting to *control the situation*—refusing to answer the examiner's questions, feigning deafness, or diverting the discussion toward their physical symptoms. Other patients try to *gain time* to think, as by answering a question different from the one asked and later going back to the original question. Substitute responses may also be used: when asked his age, the patient may say "I was born in 1882"; asked how many months there are in a year, he may name them individually; asked about the immediate past, he may give a detailed description of an event that took place long ago. Rationalizations, such as "We didn't study that in school," or "I've got such a bad headache that I can't remember right now," are also common, as are outright confabulations, as when the patient describes yesterday's menu so spontaneously and in such detail that the listener finds it hard to believe that it bears no resemblance whatsoever to what was really served. Responses like these generally mean that the patient's dementia is not too far advanced, for they show that he has appraised the interview situation realistically, has accepted its rules, and is making an effort to operate within them. Patients whose dementia is more severe tend to respond in ways that are not really responsive but merely efforts to *bind anxiety*. For example, a patient may pretend that the situation is social rather than medical and, acting as if the examiner were a guest rather than a doctor, flatter him, make friendly conversation, try to flirt with him, and tell long-winded anecdotes about the past, especially those that demonstrate his physical or sexual prowess, his family's high social status, and his children's good jobs and wealth. A reaction that demonstrates an even more compromised intellectual competence is that of *projection,* in which the patient accuses the examiner of trying to get him upset with his questioning. When all these mechanisms fail and the confrontation cannot be avoided, the patient will exhibit a catastrophic reaction, by which is meant that he responds to questions he cannot answer by abruptly becoming angry or bursting into tears.

The patient's disturbed perception is a fertile field for the development of *delusional symptoms.* The more his intellectual functioning deteriorates, the more likely he is to become delusional, and the less cohesive his delusions are likely to be. Characteristically, the more cohesive delusions reflect the patient's real life situation and everyday irritations, particularly his feelings of helplessness, loneliness, and abandonment. For example, when a patient in a home for the aged complains that his food is being poisoned, the clinician, by asking other residents, may discover that the word "poisoned" is in that particular home merely a delusionally elaborated euphemism for oversalted, undercooked, or burned. The individual who mislays his things may accuse those around him of stealing them. The one whose heirs are already discussing his estate may accuse them of trying to kill him. Not surprisingly, accusations containing a kernel of truth tend to make the individual's relatives, companions, and medical attendants feel guilty and irritated and thus deal with him in an angry, defensive, or even punitive fashion. The physician must therefore explore the feelings of such persons, so that these accusations can be placed in the proper perspective and thus either ignored or responded to good naturedly.

If the patient's dementia is caused by a reversible medical illness, his chance for full or even partial rehabilitation depends on the rapidity with which the disease is identified and treated. Therefore, when there is evidence that the causative factors are still operative, it is essential to obtain as thorough and as rapid a medical evaluation as needed to establish the illness' cause. Although most *progressive dementias* are due to degenerative senile, presenile, and arteriosclerotic encephalopathies and are thus untreatable and irreversible, the search for a reversible causative factor should not be abandoned until each possibility has been excluded individually, no matter how old the patient may be or how impaired he appears (Wang 1969).

Among the dementias that can be partially or even fully reversed, if the underlying disorder is identified and treated before permanent brain damage results, are those caused by hypoxia (and/or CO_2 intoxication) secondary to cardiovascular or pulmonary insufficiency (Austen 1957, Dalessio 1965, Dulfano 1965); chronic intoxication with such agents as alcohol, barbiturates, bromides, (see p. 292) or anticholinergics (Korolenko 1969, Longo 1966); hypothyroidism, hyperthyroidism, and other endocrine disorders (Bleuler 1954, Hossain 1970, Petersen 1968, Sheehan 1939, Whybrow 1969); brain tumor; subdural hematoma (Gal 1958, Hunter 1968, Ommaya 1969); spirochetal, viral, and other infectious illnesses affecting the central nervous system (Himmelhoch 1969, Schwab 1969, Shearer 1964); Parkinson's and Wilson's disease (Asso 1969, Calne 1969, Cotzias 1969, Goldstein 1968, Sternlieb 1968); nutritional deficiencies such as pellagra or vitamin B_{12}, folic acid, thiamine, or protein deficiency (Brain 1969, Sandstead 1969, Strachan 1965); hepatic disease (Read 1967); chronic renal insufficiency (Tyler 1968); periarteritis and other collagen disorders (DuBois 1964, Tseitlin 1963); or occult hydrocephalus of whatever cause (Adams 1965, Benson 1970). Even when the patient is known to have a degenerative encephalopathy, the road of diagnostic exclusion must be traveled to the very end, especially if his deterioration suddenly accelerates, for this may represent a superimposed and perhaps treatable disease. One frequently overlooked cause of accelerated deterioration is the infectious illness that is superimposed on mild senility, probably because infections tend to be less acute in the elderly. The source of the patient's intellectual deterioration may be hard to determine if he is suffering from a medical disease that can produce such deterioration and is treated with an agent that can also have this effect, as with the cardiac patient treated with digitalis (Sodeman 1965), the patient with a collagen disease treated with steroids (Ford 1965, O'Connor 1966), or the patient with an infectious disease treated with antimicrobial agents (Medical Letter 1968).

Management

The physician's task in the rehabilitation and management of the patient with a dementiform syndrome depends largely on the prognosis. If the dementia is *progressive but caused by a treatable disease,* rehabilitative efforts will usually be postponed until the disease itself has been treated. If it *persists even after the causative factor is no longer operative*—whether a head injury, an encephalitis, a cerebrovascular accident, or even one of the treatable illnesses referred to above—the primary therapeutic task consists of teaching the patient new ways of doing things, encouraging him in their use, and helping him and his relatives adapt to whatever impairments remain. If the dementia is *progressive and irreversible,* the clinician's task consists of helping the patient to avoid noticing his failing abilities while helping his relatives to stop denying them, that is, helping them to accept the inevitability of his decline and the necessity of making adequate provisions for his (and their) long-term well-being.

Relevant as the distinction between stable, progressive, reversible, and treatable dementia may be from the standpoint of treatment planning, there is much overlap between them. When the patient's dementia is due to an injurious event or to a disease that is treatable but was so severe or prolonged that it has caused extensive brain damage, the management follows the principles outlined for the stable dementia. If the patient's impairment is very severe or his family is unable to supervise him, he may need the same kind of custodial arrangements as those required in the final stages of the progressive dementia of unknown or irreversible cause.

If the patient's dementia is subsiding or stable but not sufficiently severe to prevent him from absorbing new ideas, both the rate of his recovery and its eventual extent will be favorably affected by a comprehensive rehabilitation program. The effectiveness of such efforts may be hard to define precisely but, even when the achievements seem very modest, can be of major significance to the individual involved. If, for example, the patient has had a stroke that has left him aphasic and paralyzed and after a long course of speech and physical therapy finally becomes able (even if with some difficulty) to talk well enough to be understood and to walk well enough to move a few paces by himself, the casual observer might consider the results fairly meager and wonder whether they have been worth the time and expense. The benefits cannot be measured in such terms as size of vocabulary or distance walked independently, however, but in less tangible ones, like resocialization and improved self-esteem (Hodgins 1964, Rusk 1969). Since retraining proceeds best when the patient is comfortable and emotionally stable, the tasks assigned to him, at least initially, should be tasks that he is capable of performing; the setting in which he is domiciled should be simple and well-structured so that he has little opportunity to confront or to be upset by his incompetence; if he is too upset to benefit from the rehabilitation program, he should be given psychotropic agents that, by moderating his discomfort, can help him use his limited resources more effectively and thus facilitate his retraining (Zane 1962).

As long as the patient's dementia is improving, retraining should have first priority. Once the improvement slows and the patient remains at the same stage for so long that it seems unlikely that he will improve further, the emphasis should shift to helping him to accept, and to gear his expectations to, his level of functioning. Regardless of what he did in the past, he must assume tasks he can perform, lest he become so dissatisfied with himself and so anxious about his impairments that he is unable to work at all. In some cases, he can be trained for and placed in a job that requires simple mechanical or repetitive manipulations or is in some other way less complex than his previous work. While this may disappoint him and his family, they will soon discover that he can obtain more satisfaction from performing a simple job well—even if it is in a sheltered workshop—than from returning to his former occupation unsuccessfully or, even worse, doing nothing at all.

The management of the *progressively dementing or already severely demented* patient offers neither the hope implicit in the treatment of the underlying disease nor the satisfaction implicit in retaining residual faculties, and is therefore a badly neglected field of endeavor. Those who devote themselves to it, however, discover that much good can be accomplished by seeing to the patient's well-being, keeping him mentally active for as long as possible, diminishing his discomfort, assuaging his relatives' guilt, and in general making his decline dignified and human. This group is composed to a large extent of the aged senile, who generally have a broad variety of physical impairments as well and therefore require careful and continued medical observation, especially because they often fail to report their physical symptoms. The treatment goals may be summarized as: keeping them interested and active, monitoring their physical condition, and preventing their becoming disturbed by their difficulties.

Although each brain-damaged individual has unique psychological problems, certain difficulties shared by the entire group are amenable to a particular psychotherapeutic approach. Such patients should be encouraged to obtain as much gratification as they can on their own and to rely on others as little as possible. They should not be encouraged to explore their feelings about their condition but should rather be safeguarded from insight into their situation, for such insight generally serves only to damage the patient's self-image even further and to heighten his puzzlement about what is happening to him. For this reason, it is by no means an error to support his efforts to ignore or deny his life difficulties. Even if his abstractive ability were not so impaired as to prevent him from understanding psychodynamic subtleties, he is far less likely to benefit from recognizing such feelings as hating the son who evicted, institutionalized, and abandoned him than from being permitted to wax enthusiastic about this son's accomplishments, even if they are fantasies. In order to support this type of denial, it is good for the patient in a nursing or old-age home to have pictures and news of his family. The more abandoned he really is, the more the therapist must do to replace the significant figures in his former environment. The physician may thus be most helpful by engaging the patient in a verbal flirtation or holding discussions that avoid topics that might make him become aware of his incompetence

(Goldfarb 1954, 1956). The same principle obtains in other areas: if, for example, the patient continually wanders away from his home and gets lost in the community, it is better to arrange for another person to accompany him on his walks than to prevent them and thereby magnify his feeling of inadequacy and incarceration.

Recommendations concerning the patient's care must take into account his total circumstances, and, in the case of the aged patient, this includes the extent of family support he receives and the severity of whatever other disabilities he may have (Gaitz 1969). If his physical condition permits him to remain independent and he desires to live by himself, provision for some degree of supervision and, perhaps equally important, some measure of social stimulation must be made. In many cases, however, the physician's task lies not in sustaining a dangerously marginal extramural adjustment, but in assuring the family and the patient that a supervised group-living experience may be safer and more entertaining for the patient than living alone.

Quite apart from their favorable effect on the patient's emotional potential for rehabilitation, psychotropic agents, though of no benefit for the underlying illness, can be valuable in relieving such symptoms as anxiety, impulsivity, hyperkinesis, depression, and paranoid ideation. Sedatives and other CNS depressants are contraindicated, for they tend to increase the brain-damaged patient's confusion and excitement (Bender 1964, Seidl 1966). The disastrous consequences of "routine" postoperative sedative orders for older, immobilized, or sensory deprived persons may be seen on many urologic and eye surgery wards, which may, when inundated with sedatives, seem more disturbed than the acute admission wards of psychiatric hospitals.

More frequent than pure anxiety states or depressions are mixed syndromes, which tend to respond remarkably well to alerting phenothiazines such as fluphenazine (Permitil) in doses as small as 0.25-0.5 mg, 3-4 times daily. Patients with postencephalitic or posttraumatic disturbances in impulse control tend to respond well to amphetamines or small doses of nonsedating phenothiazines, such as perphenazine (Trilafon), 4 mg, or trifluoperazine (Stelazine), 2 mg, 3-4 times daily (Ayd 1960). Brain-damaged children with symptoms of hyperkinesis, agitation, anxiety, and antisocial behavior may respond favorably to stimulants, phenothiazines, or antidepressants (see p. 361).

When the dementia is associated with psychomotor retardation and a depressed mood, the administration of an antidepressant like imipramine (Tofranil), 10-25 mg t.i.d., may improve the patient's intellectual and social performance (Bowers 1969, Lawson 1969). Imipramine may also benefit some cases of parkinsonism, especially those associated with depression and other psychological disturbances (Strang 1965), and may even have a favorable effect on the patient's hypomotility. Psychotropic agents may also be of value in certain other neurological syndromes with behavioral manifestations. Patients with Gilles de la Tourette's syndrome may achieve remission when given moderate doses of major tranquilizers such as 6-8 mg fluphenazine (Prolixin, Permitil), or 10-12 mg of haloperidol, daily (see p. 375). The gains produced in Huntington's chorea are more modest but still worthy of trial: depression, irritability, and impulsivity, which may precede the appearance of extrapyramidal symptoms by as much as five to ten years or be the predominant symptoms early in the course, can be also mitigated by alerting phenothiazines, and there may be a reduction of choreiform movements as well (Cohen 1962, Mersky 1961, Oliphant 1960, Whittier 1968).

When given at their usually effective dose levels, these drugs produce remarkably few problems. Many of them, notably phenothiazines, benztropine mesylate (Cogentin), and imipramine (Tofranil), have anticholinergic properties, however, and must be given with caution to the elderly, in order to avoid prostatic obstruction, constipation, glaucoma, and hypotension (see p. 602). Medication schedules, in any case, should be as simple as possible, because of the increased possibility of patient error (Ley 1967). If this danger seems excessive, it may be necessary to mobilize the patient's relatives, neighbors, or even a visiting nurse to supervise the drug intake.

DELIRIFORM SYNDROMES

DESCRIPTION AND EXAMINATION

We use the term *deliriform syndromes* to refer to a number of illnesses of organic origin that are characterized by *dysmnesia, disorientation,* and such disturbances of sleep-wakefulness regulation as *insomnia, somnolence, fluctuating awareness,* and *dysattention.* (Dysattention may be defined as a failure to focus attention on those elements of the environment that are most relevant to the tasks at hand, and ranges in severity from distractibility to complete inattention to, or indeed loss of contact with, the environment.) Patients showing only these symptoms are said to be suffering from a *predelirious state*, which may, but need not, develop into a full-blown delirium, by which we mean that the patient also harbors *illusions, hallucinations* (particularly visual ones), and poorly organized *delusions* of rapidly changing content. He may misidentify spots on the wall as insects and thereafter hallucinate that they are crawling around; or exhibit *illusive pseudo-recognition,* misidentifying relative strangers (such as the doctor or nurse) as persons he has known in the past. Whether a predelirious state will develop into a full-blown delirium cannot be predicted from the outset. It is not necessary, however, to wait very long to find out, for the process generally takes no more than a few hours or days.

Neurologic findings in deliriform syndromes include headache, dysarthria, an EEG dominated by the development of *slow waves,* initially in theta but then also in delta ranges, and such abnormalities of motor activity as coarse and irregular 8-10 per second *tremor;* bilateral asynchronous *asterixis* (an involuntary jerking movement that can be elicited best in the fingers and hands by asking the patient to dorsiflex his wrists and spread his extended fingers); and *multifocal myoclonus* (sudden, nonrhythmic, nonpatterned gross muscle contractions, which can occur in a resting person) (Posner 1967).

While there is some regularity to the way the patient's symptoms develop and recede (see Table 24), no two illnesses develop in quite the same way. In some, the patient appears fairly drowsy from the outset and eventually becomes stuporous or even comatose; in others, he initially appears very excited and becomes drowsy only after he is exhausted. In still others, the only consistent feature of the clinical picture is that it continually fluctuates, the patient at one moment appearing calm and lucid or at most mildly perplexed, at the next grossly excited and massively confused, and then, soon after, quite lucid again. Whatever the preceding picture, shortly before recovery many patients drift into a 12 to 18 hour period of deep sleep known as a "terminal sleep."

One of the most valuable tools for evaluating the patient's current condition, for deciding whether and when to intervene, and for assessing the effectiveness of any treatment measures used is the *mental status examination.* This examination is much like that used in dementiform syndromes (see p. 404), with the exception that it

TABLE 24. *Symptoms in Deliriform Syndromes*

	STAGE I	STAGE II	STAGE III	STAGE IV — EXCITED DELIRIUM	STAGE IV — STUPOROUS DELIRIUM
SLEEP	Difficulty falling asleep	Intermittent and irregular		Total insomnia	Somnolence
PSYCHOMOTOR ACTIVITY	Restlessness	Overactivity that appears purposive	Purposeless hyperactivity	Purposeless thrashing, rubbing, trembling, muttering, or impulsive violence	Hypoactivity (sometimes with bizarre or primitive motions)
SPEECH	Talkativeness	Incoherence, slurring	Paraphasias, iterations, and perseverations	Screaming and shouting	Slowed speech and mutism
ATTENTION AND CONCENTRATION	Increased sensitivity to stimuli	Inability to concentrate	Easy distractibility	Complete inability to focus attention, sometimes overreaction even to insignificant stimuli	
ORIENTATION	Disorientation for time	Disorientation for time and place	Global disorientation	Untestable	
MEMORY	Difficulty in retaining new material	Disturbance in recent memory	Global dysmnesia (with or without confabulation)	Untestable	
PERCEPTION	Distortions in sense of time and space	Olfactory and auditory hallucinations	Somatic and elementary visual hallucinations; Single visual hallucinations	Vivid visual hallucinations (in scenes or extended sequences) or hypnoidal imagery	
REALITY TESTING	Mild suspiciousness	Misinterpretations of environment	Delusions that explain hallucinations and feeling state	Unsystematized fleeting delusions	
MOOD	Elation, moroseness, irritability, or bewilderment	Apathy or lability	Depression or fearfulness	Excitation and fearfulness	Constriction and dullness
EEG *	Small amount of regular and irregular slow frequencies (5-7 cps); some decrease of activity in normal frequency range	Further decrease of regularity; increase of low-voltage fast activity and irregular slow rhythms (4-7 cps)	Predominant low-voltage fast activity with some irregular slow rhythms (3-6 cps); little activity in normal frequency range	Disorganized irregular record with dominant slow frequency (2-7 cps), small amounts of low-voltage fast activity, groups of high-voltage very slow waves (1-3 cps). Fairly regular, moderately high-voltage slow activity (3-7 cps) with few or no normal frequencies	

* Romano, J., and Engel, G. L.: Delirium: I. EEG data, Arch Neurol Psychiat (Chicago) 51:356-485, 1944.

must be repeated far more frequently. Following head injuries or other events leading to loss of consciousness, the patient's clinical course can be best monitored by determining the extent of retrograde and anterograde amnesia, and carefully recording the degree of impairment or deterioration from one examination to the next (Welch 1968). The patient may be so mute, incoherent, or obtunded, however, that his mental functioning can be evaluated only in terms of his spontaneous behavior or of the intensity of stimulation required to evoke a response. When it is otherwise impossible to tell whether his unresponsiveness is of psychological or organic origin, it may be useful to assess his oculovestibular response to cold stimulation, the so-called cold caloric test (Nathanson 1966).

Whatever the characteristics of the clinical picture, both delirium and the predelirious state must be considered grave medical emergencies. In the first place, the patient's behavior can become dangerous and unmanageable. In addition, many of the illnesses that give rise to delirium, if unchecked, can cause permanent brain damage and endanger the patient's life (Guze 1964, Unterberger 1969). Finally, depending on the nature and severity of the underlying illness, stupor, coma, convulsions, or even status epilepticus may occur. In order to prevent these consequences, the contributing factors must be identified as rapidly as possible, but there are innumerable conditions—indeed as many as there are illnesses that disturb body chemistry and brain functioning—to be considered (see Table 25). The delirium itself offers few clues to its cause, not even such general ones as are embodied in the long-held but recently discredited notions that the delirium marked by excitement is likely to be caused by an illness of more acute onset than the one marked by stupor, or that specific ailments lead to particular kinds of delirium (Stenbäck 1967). Uremia and hypothyroidism, for example, both of which are commonly believed to produce only stuporous deliria, may also lead to excited ones, perhaps with equal frequency. To establish the delirium's cause, then, the same sources of information must be relied on as are used to identify other medical illnesses: the history, the physical examination, and the laboratory findings. Among the most useful diagnostic criteria are the patient's ventilatory status and acid-base balance (see Table 26).

MANAGEMENT

Unless the dysmnesia, delusions, and hallucinations 1/ are the patient's only symptoms, 2/ so vastly overshadow any other symptoms he may have as to make him appear "insane," or 3/ develop in an individual who is already in psychiatric treatment (such as an addict in withdrawal or a patient taking psychotropic drugs that are likely to produce a toxic psychosis), the delirious patient will in all likelihood be seen by the psychiatrist at the behest of another physician. In the typical case, the attending physician will have tried to control the patient's excitement with sedatives or mechanical restraint. The psychiatrist tends thus to come on the scene after these measures have not only failed but have further reduced the patient's sensory input and increased his fearfulness. The patient's struggle to remove his restraints and his efforts to cope with his dampened sensorium may make him appear even more excited than he would if he were not being "helped."

Under these circumstances, then, the psychiatrist is rarely asked to identify the etiologic factors or to make a prognosis, but simply to quiet the patient. Knowing that there are probably two or three fairly quiet delirious patients (for whom no psychiatrist is called) to every one that is excited, the psychiatrist may indeed count himself lucky if his attendance has not been requested solely to legitimize transferring the patient to a mental hospital. But the delirious patient is medically ill and thus far more likely to receive proper attention in a general hospital, where the diagnostic problems can best be resolved and superior overall care is easier to provide, than in a psychiatric hospital. It is therefore of vital importance to relieve the patient's psychomotor agitation and confusion rapidly enough to enable him to collaborate in his treatment or at the very least to render him manageable in the general hospital setting.

To some extent, the *treatment* of the deliriform syndrome is that *of the underlying medical illness.* In the interim, the emphasis is on maintaining the patient's fluid, electrolyte, and nutritional balances, and protecting him against such complications as infection, cardiac embarrassment, and hyperthermia. While these measures are not generally the psychiatrist's responsibility, he must see to it that the patient's agitation and obstreperousness do not cause the need for *supportive care* to be overlooked. In some cases, the delirious patient's anxiety and agitation can be relieved with *psychological measures* alone. In mild confusional states, for example, simple reassurance may suffice to relieve the individual's anxiety. When his anxiety is aggravated by confusion, it is of value to simplify and add structure to his environment. Such simple measures as providing him with a night light or having someone stay with him—particularly someone he knows, like a family member—may

TABLE 25. *Causes of Delirium, Stupor, and Coma*

I. SUPRATENTORIAL MASS LESIONS

Epidural hematoma
Subdural hematoma
Intracerebral hematoma
Cerebral infarct
Brain tumor
Brain abscess

II. SUBTENTORIAL LESIONS

Brainstem infarct
Brainstem tumor
Brainstem hemorrhage
Cerebellar hemorrhage
Cerebellar abscess

III. INTRINSIC DISEASES OF THE NEURONS OR NEUROGLIAL CELLS
(Primary Metabolic Encephalopathy)

A. *Gray Matter Diseases:*
Jakob-Creutzfeldt disease
Pick's disease
Alzheimer's disease and senile dementia
Huntington's chorea
Progressive myoclonic epilepsy
Lipid storage diseases

B. *White Matter Diseases:*
Schilder's disease
Marchiafava-Bignami disease
The leukodystrophies

IV. DISEASES EXTRINSIC TO NEURONS AND GLIA
(Secondary Metabolic Encephalopathy)

A. *Deprivation of Oxygen, Substrate, or Metabolic Cofactors*

1. Hypoxia (interference with oxygen supply to the entire brain—cerebral blood flow normal)

   a. Decreased oxygen tensions and content of blood
      Pulmonary disease
      Alveolar hypoventilation
      Decreased atmospheric oxygen tension

   b. Decreased oxygen content of blood—normal tension
      Anemia
      Carbon monoxide poisoning
      Methemoglobinemia

   c. Normal oxygen content and tension of blood—brain oxygen needs increased
      Seizures and postictal states

2. Ischemia (diffuse or widespread multifocal interference with blood supply to brain)

   a. Decreased cerebral blood flow resulting from decreased cardiac output
      Stokes-Adams; cardiac arrest; cardiac arrhythmias
      Myocardial infarction
      Congestive heart failure
      Aortic stenosis

   b. Decreased CBF resulting from decreased peripheral resistance in systemic circulation
      Syncope: orthostatic vasovagal
      Carotid sinus hypersensitivity
      Low blood volume

TABLE 25. *Causes of Delirium, Stupor, and Coma* (continued)

    c. Normal oxygen content and tension of blood-brain oxygen needs increased
        Hypertensive encephalopathy
        Hyperventilation syndrome
        Increased blood viscosity (polycythemia)
  3. Hypoglycemia
      Resulting from exogenous insulin
      Spontaneous (endogenous insulin, liver disease, etc.)
  4. Cofactor deficiency
      Thiamine (Wernicke's encephalopathy)
      Niacin
      Pyridoxine
      B_{12}

B. *Diseases of Organs Other Than Brain*
  1. Diseases of nonendocrine organs
      Liver (hepatic coma)
      Kidney (uremic coma)
      Lung (CO_2 narcosis)
  2. Hyperfunction and/or hypofunction of endocrine organs
      Pituitary
      Thyroid (myxedema-thyrotoxicosis)
      Parathyroid (hyper- and hypoparathyroidism)
      Adrenal (Addison's disease, Cushing's disease, pheochromocytoma)
      Pancreas (diabetes, hypoglycemia)
  3. Other systemic diseases
      Cancer
      Porphyria

C. *Exogenous Poisons*
  1. Sedative drugs
      Barbiturates
      Nonbarbiturate hypnotics
      Tranquilizers
      Bromides
      Ethanol
      Anticholinergics
      Opiates
  2. Acid poisons or poisons with acidic breakdown products
      Paraldehyde
      Methyl alcohol
      Ethylene glycol
  3. Enzyme inhibitors
      Heavy metals
      Organic phosphates
      Cyanide
      Salicylates

D. *Abnormalities of Ionic or Acid-Base Environment of CNS*
  1. Water and sodium (hyper- and hyponatremia)
  2. Acidosis (metabolic and respiratory)
  3. Alkalosis (metabolic and respiratory)
  4. Potassium (hyper- and hypokalemia)
  5. Magnesium (hyper- and hypomagnesemia)
  6. Calcium (hyper- and hypocalcemia)

E. *Diseases Producing Toxins or Enzyme Inhibition in CNS*
  Meningitis
  Encephalitis
  Subarachnoid hemorrhage

F. *Traumatic Neuronal Dysfunction without Structural Change (Concussion)*

Plum, Fred, and Posner, Jerome B.: The Diagnosis of Stupor and Coma, Philadelphia, Davis, 1966.

TABLE 26. *A Differential Analysis of Hyperventilation and Hypoventilation in Delirious Patients*

CLINICAL AND LABORATORY FINDINGS	PROBABLE DIAGNOSIS
I. Hyperventilation:	
A. Serum pH $<$ 7.30, serum HCO_3^- $<$ 10 mEq./1 (if pH $<$ 7.30 and HCO_3^- $>$ 20 mEq./1, see respiratory acidosis)	*Metabolic acidosis*
1. BUN $>$ 60 mg. per 100 ml.	Uremic encephalopathy
2. Hyperglycemia (blood sugar $>$ 250 mg. per 100 ml.)	Diabetic coma
a. 4+ Serum acetone	Diabetic ketoacidosis
b. No acetonemia	Diabetic lactic acidosis
3. Cyanosis (pO_2 $<$ 50 mm. Hg), shock	Anoxic lactic acidosis
4. BUN, sugar, oxygen, blood pressure—normal	Exogenous poisoning
a. Paraldehyde odor on breath	Acidosis secondary to paraldehyde ingestion
b. Hyperemic optic discs, dilated sluggish pupils	Methyl alcohol poisoning
c. Oxalate crystals in urine	Ethylene glycol poisoning
5. None of the abnormal findings above	Spontaneous lactic acidosis
B. Serum pH $>$ 7.45, serum HCO_3^- $>$ 10 but $<$ 20 mEq./1 (if pH $>$ 7.45, and HCO_3^- $>$ 30, see metabolic alkalosis)	*Respiratory alkalosis*
1. Serum HCO_3^- $<$ 15, hyperthermia, positive urine $FeCl_3$ test	Salicylate poisoning
2. Serum HCO_3^- $>$ 15, hepatomegaly, serum NH_3 elevated	Hepatic encephalopathy
3. Serum HCO_3^- $>$ 15, cyanosis (pO_2 $<$ 50 mm. Hg)	Cardiopulmonary disease
a. Rales, elevated venous pressure, cardiomegaly	Pulmonary edema
b. No heart disease	Pneumonia, alveolar-capillary block
4. Serum HCO_3^- $>$ 15, absent pupillary and oculovestibular responses, decerebrate rigidity	Central neurogenic hyperventilation
5. Serum HCO_3^- $>$ 15, nystagmus on caloric testing, normal examination	Psychogenic hyperventilation

be of great help. It will also make sense to protect him from excessive stimulation, as by shading his lights, restricting the number of nurses in attendance, and in other ways providing an environment that is peaceful yet not so monotonous that he becomes excited in an effort to combat sensory deprivation (Lipowski 1967).

When psychological measures do not suffice, *pharmacologic treatment* is indicated. Whether and what kind of drug regimen should be given the delirious patient depends on whether

TABLE 26. *A Differential Analysis of Hyperventilation and Hypoventilation in Delirious Patients* (continued)

CLINICAL AND LABORATORY FINDINGS	PROBABLE DIAGNOSIS
II. Hypoventilation:	
A. Serum pH $<$ 7.35, serum HCO_3^- $>$ 20 mEq./l	*Respiratory acidosis*
1. Serum HCO_3^- $>$ 20 mEq./l but $<$ 30 mEq./l	
a. Normal lungs	Depressant drug poisoning
b. Rales, emphysema, pO_2 $<$ 40 mm. Hg	Chronic pulmonary disease with acute CO_2 retention
2. Serum HCO_3^- $>$ 30 mEq./l	
a. Normal lungs	
(1) obesity	Pickwick's syndrome
(2) not obese	"Central alveolar hypoventilation"
b. Rales, emphysema, pO_2 $<$ 40 mm. Hg	Chronic pulmonary disease with slowly developing CO_2 retention
B. Serum pH $>$ 7.45, serum HCO_3^- $>$ 30 mEq./l	*Metabolic alkalosis*
a. Vomiting, hypotension, hypovolemia	Gastric HCl depletion
b. Edema, heart disease	Diuretic therapy
c. Hypokalemia, moon face, truncal obesity	Cushing's syndrome secondary to adrenal hyperfunction, steroid therapy, hormone-secreting lung neoplasms
d. Hypertension, hypokalemia	Primary hyperaldosteronism
e. Renal disease	Hypokalemic alkalosis
f. Peptic ulcer	$NaHCO_3$ ingestion alkalosis

Plum, Fred, and Posner, Jerome B.: The Diagnosis of Stupor and Coma, Philadelphia: Davis, 1966.

1/ his delirium is making him so disruptive to his environment that it is interfering with his diagnostic work-up and the management of the underlying medical illness;

2/ the diagnostic studies required to identify the causative factors are still in progress;

3/ his vital signs and neurologic condition are stable;

4/ seizures have or may be expected to occur (as in CNS depressant withdrawal, encephalitides, or patients with a past history of seizures); and

5/ the underlying illness (if known) is more likely to produce brief or protracted delirious states.

Since almost all the drugs used to calm delirious patients can mask, modify, or dissimulate organic signs (Pevehouse 1960) and are unpredictable in their effects until the patient's condition is stable, any patient who is not so disruptive as to make immediate action mandatory should be given nothing beyond supportive care until the diagnostic studies are completed and his vital signs and neurologic condition are stable. If the patient is very disruptive and something must be done immediately, low doses of phenothiazines, such as 0.5-1.0 mg of fluphenazine (Prolixin), 1-2 mg of perphenazine (Trilafon), or 10-20 mg of chlorpromazine (Thorazine) may be used. In all but CNS depressant withdrawal syndromes, phenothiazines are preferable, as CNS depressants often increase rather than diminish the patient's confusion and excitement, and may make him so ataxic, dysarthric, and drowsy that the underlying illness is erroneously thought to have worsened. Barbiturates are in any case contraindicated for patients with severe renal disease, pulmonary insufficiency, or acute intermittent prophyria (Levere 1970, Sharpless 1965). Low doses, just enough to diminish the excitement but not enough to suppress the delirium, should be administered. The goal at this point is merely to keep the symptoms sufficiently in check to permit the patient's diagnostic work-up and medical treatment to proceed. Since phenothiazines can facilitate seizures, each dose should be covered with a low dose of a CNS depressant such as 2-4 mg of diazepam (Valium), particularly if the patient is tremulous, has previously taken high doses of CNS depressants, or there is some other reason to anticipate the occurrence of seizures.

As soon as the patient's vital signs and neurologic condition are stable and the diagnostic work-up has been completed, more vigorous treatment may be pursued. If the delirium is caused by some factor that can be rapidly relieved with appropriate treatment or, though untreatable, is expected to remit rapidly, no psychotropic agents need be given. If, on the other hand, the disorder's cause remains unknown or, though known cannot be relieved rapidly, the patient may be given a course of phenothiazines even if he is not disruptive (here again covered with CNS depressants if a seizure danger exists). In this event, the phenothiazine dosage should initially be identical to the levels listed above, but gradually increased to whatever level is required to diminish the patient's delusions and thus reverse his delirium.

Because baroceptor reflexes are impaired in many brain syndromes, especially those with a cerebrovascular component (Appenzeller 1964), and because some phenothiazines can produce hypotension, patients with cardiovascular or cerebrovascular illnesses should be given phenothiazines with little hypotensive effect (such as fluphenazine, trifluoperazine, or perphenazine) or, better yet, a butyrophenone like haloperidol (Haldol), starting with doses of 0.5-1 mg, 3-4 times daily. In thyrotoxic crises, reserpine, 5 mg i.m., followed by 5-10 mg p.o. daily, seems to be a fast and effective adjunct to other treatment measures (Canary 1957, Ingbar 1966).

After the appropriate agent has been chosen, the dose schedule should be built up cautiously lest fluctuations in the delirious patient's condition lead to an excessive drug effect at dose levels that previously appeared safe. Drugs should therefore be initiated in small doses at long intervals, so that the tranquilization effect is minimal. Parenteral administration is preferable for the first three or four days because it is more precise, and should be continued until the patient is free of all factors (such as dysphagia, malabsorption, or uncooperativeness) that might impede adequate oral drug intake or render it unreliable.

Occasionally, after the diagnosis has been firmly established and the associated disease process has improved or remitted fully, the remnants of a delirious state will require a further course of phenothiazines. If the patient's delirium is exceptionally refractory to psychopharmacologic management or he is so toxic, emaciated, or otherwise debilitated that the drug dosage required to reverse his symptoms may be hazardous, one or two electroshock treatments may be helpful and in some cases even life-saving (Blachly 1967, Kalinowsky 1969, Weinstein 1967).

SYNDROMES FOLLOWING HEAD INJURY

That the line between delirium and dementia cannot be so finely drawn as the foregoing might indicate is best illustrated by the disorders in mental functioning that follow head injuries, when almost identical pathologic processes may lead to

a delirium that looks like a toxic encephalopathy and, like it, clears up after a few days,

a delirium that initially looks toxic, then clears, but leaves a residual dementia that may either itself clear up after some weeks or months or persist, or

a period of unconsciousness followed immediately by symptoms of dementia.

The exact course of the symptoms cannot be predicted on the basis of the type of injury suffered. Whether the eventual impairment will be mild, moderate, or severe can be predicted to some extent on the basis of such findings as how long the individual was unconscious after the injury and the length of the period for which he is amnesic (Whitty 1966). Syndromes in which the patient was not unconscious or was unconscious for less than an hour are labeled *mild:* usually he is slightly confused for a few hours or days, exhibits amnesia for the incident and for a brief time before it, and recovers fully within a few days or weeks. In *moderate* cases, the unconsciousness may last for several hours. When it ends, the patient experiences a clouding of consciousness (sometimes in the form of a severely agitated hallucinating and delusional delirium) that may last for a number of days and then slowly remit. He may forget as much as a week of the period around his accident and exhibit some general impairments in his intellectual ability. If these impairments recede, they generally do so gradually. In the first stage of improvement, only the memory disturbances remain; thereafter even these fade, but it is usually several months before the patient can return to work. In *severe* cases, consciousness is lost for many hours, days, or even weeks, and as this period lengthens, the likelihood of irreversible brain damage increases (Lishman 1968). On becoming conscious, the patient may be amnesic for a protracted period, and exhibit moderate to severe intellectual impairments. Many develop posttraumatic psychoses, often of the Korsakoff type, and almost a third develop seizures (Achté 1969, Evans 1962, Russell 1952, 1953, 1955, Symonds 1935). Full recovery is relatively rare in severe cases, although some measure of occupational rehabilitation may occur over a period of six to 24 months (Cairns 1942, Guttman 1946, Russell 1933, Symonds 1949, Welch 1968). Moreover, for the rest of the patient's life, his risk of becoming psychotic is markedly increased (Achté 1969).

A common complication of head injury, and one that is of unique importance because of the ease with which it is confused with psychoneurotic syndromes and even with malingering is the *postconcussion syndrome,* which also bears some resemblance to the psychological disturbances following *whiplash injuries* (Schutt 1968, Torres 1961). Typically, within hours or days after the injury, the patient develops a throbbing headache, dizziness, difficulty in concentrating, irritability, anxiety, depression, hypochondriacal-appearing concern with a wide variety of physical and psychological symptoms and a high sensitivity to loud noises and intervening stresses (Modlin 1967).

While these complaints sometimes become chronic, and may even progress insidiously to a state of advanced dementia (Corsellis 1959, Critchley 1957), they usually remit within three to six months. That the patient manifests no objective symptoms means that in the interim he may be subjected to searching inquiries into his motives for presenting his complaints. Although preexisting personality problems (at least in retrospect) lead some clinicians to consider these and the prospect of compensation to be important determinants, nonlitigants and those without previous personality disturbances show as high an incidence of such complaints as litigants. It seems probable, therefore, that the theorized relationship between the complaints and the potential compensation is an unwarranted interpretation, not a reasoned conclusion. It is important that the patient be protected against such accusations and discouraged from returning to work prematurely in order that his irritability not be stimulated. The affective lability can to some extent be moderated with minor tranquilizers like diazepam (Valium), 1-2 mg, 2-3 times daily, or if this is not successful within a few days, with imipramine (Tofranil), 10-25 mg, 3-4 times daily.

PAROXYSMAL DISORDERS

Seizure Disorders

Description

The clinical manifestations of seizure disorders, like those of other organic syndromes, are the result of brain tissue dysfunction, in this case the origination and spread of abnormal electrical discharges. This situation is in many ways analogous to what occurs in the heart when the discharge of an ectopic focus spreads and causes contractions. In both instances, the abnormal discharge is modulated by the individual's physiologic state and may be caused by scarring, necrosis, tumor, or biochemical changes in the affected tissue itself, or by a variety of other changes elsewhere in the body. Diphenylhydantoin (Dilantin), as if in confirmation of such an analogy, has even been used to block certain cardiac arrhythmias (Harris 1950). The analogy falters in two important respects, however, the first being that the spread of excitation is usually more generalized in the heart than in the brain; the second that, irrespective of where in the heart the discharge travels, the heart muscle's only response is contraction whereas each area of the brain has functions of its own and abnormal discharge thus comes to clinical attention in a far wider variety of ways.

The clinical features of the individual seizure depend on the site at which the abnormal discharge originates, the areas to which it spreads, and the routes by which it travels. In most cases, it originates in and spreads to the same general area on each occasion, so that the clinical manifestations are similar in each episode. In others, the site or route of the discharge, and consequently the seizure manifestations seen, vary from one seizure to the next. Under these circumstances, and when the site of origin or the route of spreading are unusual, syndromes appear that, because they are atypical, are often (erroneously) considered psychogenic. Finally, there are abnormal discharges that are limited in their spread or affect only "silent" areas of the brain; in these the individual may exhibit no clinical symptoms at all, despite EEG evidence of cerebral dysrhythmia.

Many factors affecting the central nervous system, both intrinsic and extrinsic, are known to produce abnormal discharges. When the seizure disorder seems secondary to some identified illness, it is called *symptomatic;* when a specific structural or biochemical cause cannot be found, it is called *idiopathic,* by far the more common of the two. In both types, propensity to seizures is related to genetic endowment, as is demonstrated by the observations that monozygotic twins show a 20% concordance for idiopathic epilepsy, while individuals who develop a seizure disorder in the wake of a head injury have six times as many epileptics in their families as nonepileptics do (Hedenström 1969, Metrakos 1960, 1961, Ounsted 1952). Whether a given trauma or illness will lead to a seizure disorder or a given event cause a seizure depends, then, not only on the severity of the illness and the magnitude of the event but on the individual's susceptibility as well. As Russell (1952) has said: "It is simpler to think of all people as epileptics and regard the matter as one of threshold."

In the normal person, seizure activity develops only after such *major stresses* as ECT, electrolyte imbalance, hypoglycemia, hypocalcemia, infection, hyperpyrexia, or CNS depressant withdrawal. A more susceptible person may have a seizure with *less severe provocations,* such as sleeplessness (Bennett 1963), fatigue (Weinberg 1945), or psychological stress (Pond 1965). The nature of the stimulus, too, varies from one person to the next, some even being provoked to seizures by such otherwise *innocuous activities* as listening to music (Critchley 1937); reading (Baxter 1961, Bickford 1956); performing a mathematical task (Ingvar 1962); being touched without warning (Calderon-Gonzales 1966); or watching television, a chess game, flickering lights, or passing cars (Bower 1963, Davidson 1956). That the individual's unusual response is at least in part determined by his emotional reaction to the event in question is suggested by experiments that have conditioned subjects to respond to formerly neutral stimuli with electroencephalographically demonstrable "startle effects" and have extinguished such responses in individuals who have previously had them (Booker 1965). Naturally, the convergence of several potentially ictogenic factors or the presence of a structural lesion that gives rise to abnormal electrical discharge increases the propensity.

The propensity represents, then, an organic substrate of abnormal function or structure that affects the facilitation or inhibition of discharge and spreading. The functional disturbances may be extrinsic to the CNS, as in electrolyte imbalance, or intrinsic to the CNS, as in disturbances of the "pacemaker" functions that regulate the rhythmicity of spontaneous electrical activity in the brain. Structural abnormalities (such as a tumor or scarring) may be reflected both in the focus at which the abnormal electrical discharge is initiated and in the route by which it spreads.

Classification

Although the traditional distinctions between grand mal, petit mal, and focal or partial seizures facilitate the establishment of an investigative plan, a therapeutic program, and a prognostic formulation, these categories are by no means mutually exclusive or sharply defined, and several types of seizures may occur in a single patient (Gibbs 1952, O'Brien 1959). Not only do patients with petit mal seizures tend to develop other types of seizures as they grow older, but patients with grand mal seizures may in the pre-, post-, or interictal period show symptoms of focal seizures (Dongier 1959).

The distinction between one type of seizure disorder and another, indeed the diagnosis of a seizure disorder itself, cannot be based on the EEG alone, for this diagnostic tool is sensitive to so wide a variety of external factors that it may show abnormalities where none exist. Moreover, those that do exist may be overlooked or modified, as the EEG detects only those abnormal discharges that are of sufficient voltage to be measured through the scalp or from other extracranial leads; it is incapable of reproducing in their original form rhythms that arise in deeper layers of the brain and have thus been altered by the time they reach the cortex (Brazier 1968, Glaser 1963). In many cases, special EEG techniques are required to reveal an occult cerebral dysrhythmia. Quite apart from *hyperventilation* and *photic stimulation,* which should be included in every EEG, it may be of value to obtain a sleep EEG, either by depriving the patient of sleep the night before the examination (Mattson 1965, Pratt 1968), or by administering a short-acting sedative. The administration of drugs that *activate epileptogenic foci* such as pentylenetetrazol (Metrazol) or bemegride (Megimide) may also be helpful, as may the use of nasopharyngeal, sphenoidal, or other *special leads* (Arellano 1949, Jones 1951, Maclean 1949). Even with these techniques, however, single recordings are often insufficient to establish a diagnosis, and *repeated examinations* may be needed (Strobos 1968).

The clinical characteristics, the electrophysiologic events, and, as a consequence, the diagnostic category to which the patient's disorder is assigned are to some extent determined by the individual's age (see Table 27; Busse 1965, Cohn 1958, Dekaban 1960, Gibbs 1953, 1963). *The effect of age on the seizure's clinical characteristics* is shown by the course of petit mal epilepsy, which almost invariably arises in childhood or early adolescence and tends either to remit or to convert to grand mal or psychomotor epilepsy as the child grows older (Charlton 1967, Currier 1963). Similarly, patients who, during childhood, displayed such symptoms of psychomotor-temporal-limbic seizures as paroxysmal vomiting, abdominal pain, headache, aimless wandering, fear, anger, or gesture automatisms, on approaching adolescence, may develop more complex sequences of behavioral disorder together with anxiety attacks, depressions of sudden onset, or schizophreniform psychoses (Vizioli 1962). *The effect of age on the electrophysiologic events* is reflected in the EEG findings as well: the most common site of spike discharge in children under five is the occipital area, while in older children and adults spiking is most common in the temporal area. Such forward wandering of seizure activity has been revealed by annually repeated EEGs of children with abnormal electric activity in the occipital lobe, which showed that spiking activity tended to shift to the temporal areas as they grew older.

The most dramatic and therefore most easily diagnosed type of seizure is the *grand mal,* which is marked by loss of consciousness and

TABLE 27. *Age Characteristics of Various Types of Spike Discharge*

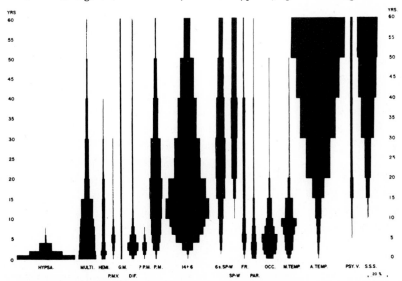

Age characteristics of various types of spike discharge. This figure is based on 19,350 consecutive cases with spike discharges, classified by age and type of discharge. The percentage incidence of each type in all age groups gives the *age characteristic* of that type of discharge. This is represented graphically as a segment of the total incidence of spikes at a given age; the segment is separated and moved so as to center over the corresponding segment showing the percentage incidence of that type of discharge in other age groups.

The contour of the area above each designated type of discharge shows how the incidence of a particular pattern waxes or wanes with age. The 20% calibration at the lower right margin allows the width of the column to be read as percentage incidence of a particular type of discharge in a given age group. For example, 60% of persons with spikes who are under one year of age have hypsarrhythmia; 65% of persons with spikes who are 60 years of age or over have anterior temporal spikes; and 50% of children between 10 and 15 years of age who have spikes have 14- and 6-per-second positive spikes, and so on.

Abbreviations are as follows:

HYPSA—hypsarrhythmia

MULTI—multiple foci of spike seizure activity

HEMI—spikes limited to one hemisphere

PMV—discharge of the petit mal variant type

GM—discharge of the grand mal type

DIF—diffuse irregular spike and wave

?PM—discharge of the pseudo petit mal type

PM—discharge of the petit mal type

14 + 6—14- and 6-per-second positive spikes

6s SP-W—6-per-second spike and wave

SP-W—spike and wave

FR—spike focus in the frontal area

PAR—spike focus in the parietal area

OCC—spike focus in the occipital area

M TEMP—spike focus in the midtemporal area

A TEMP—spike focus in the anterotemporal area

PSY V—psychomotor variant type of discharge

SSS—small sharp spikes

Gibbs, F. A., Rich, C. L., and Gibbs, E. L.: Psychomotor variant type of seizure discharge, Neurology *13*:991-998, 1963.

generalized tonic and clonic movements. It is usually preceded by a brief aura during which, depending on the seizure's locus of origin, the patient may experience such sensations as fear; a peculiar epigastric sensation welling up into the throat; or olfactory, auditory, or visual hallucinations. At the conclusion of the motor fit, the patient may regain consciousness immediately; more commonly, he falls into a heavy sleep that may last anywhere from a few minutes to several hours. When he awakens, he is often confused and usually amnesic for the seizure and, temporarily, for the events immediately preceding it. At times, the seizure is followed by a marked clouding of consciousness and, on rare occasions, by excitability and assaultiveness of psychotic proportions. During the grand mal episodes, the EEG usually shows high amplitude, fast spiking, or mixed activity. Between attacks, the EEG often contains paroxysms of bilateral, essentially synchronous 4-7 and 8-12 cps discharges from all areas, interspersed with nonspecific patterns of high amplitude spikes and slow waves. About a fourth of such patients, however, show no EEG abnormality between seizures (Glaser 1967).

The typical *petit mal* attack, also called an *absence,* is a brief episode of unconsciousness that is not preceded by an aura or accompanied by any motor manifestations other than staring, 3-per-second blinking of the eyelids, a slight turning to one side of the eyes and head, or brief almost imperceptible movements of the lips and hands. Such episodes usually last from two to 30 seconds and may occur 20, 30, or occasionally as often as several hundred times a day. Episodes of severe confusion may occur in the postictal period, but excitement is relatively rare (Jaffe 1962). Both during and between seizures a characteristic 3 cps spike and wave complex may be seen in the EEG.

Grouped with the petit mal seizures, partly because of similarities in the electrocortical patterns and partly because of their equally poor response to the anticonvulsants that are effective in grand mal seizures, are: *akinetic seizures,* in which the patient falls to the floor and may briefly lose consciousness; and *myoclonic jerks* or seizures, in which the patient exhibits sudden involuntary contractions either of a single muscle or of several muscle groups, may or may not fall, and does not usually lose consciousness. These syndromes form the so-called *petit mal triad* and are seen almost exclusively in children and young adolescents. They are often hereditary (particularly the myoclonic jerks), and both akinetic seizures and myoclonic jerks are remarkably unresponsive to treatment (Yahr 1959). While they are rarely seen after the age of 20, their prognosis is by no means benign. Almost 40% of the children with petit mal seizures eventually develop grand mal attacks; those most likely to escape this consequence are the children who show average or above average intelligence and a good response to treatment before the age of ten (Charlton 1967, Currier 1963). Akinetic seizures are often associated with severe brain damage and intellectual retardation; myoclonic jerks with such illnesses as subacute inclusion body encephalitis and Unverricht's myoclonus epilepsy.

In contrast to the grand and petit mal types of epilepsy, which are generalized, *focal or partial seizures* may also occur. Although these are typical of acquired epilepsy, it is not always possible to demonstrate definite morphologic lesions. The EEG is marked by slow waves, spikes, and sharp and slow complexes localized over the particular cerebral region involved. The abnormalities are often bilateral but asynchronous, representing transmission and diffusion of the abnormal discharge from one hemisphere to its mirror point on the other. If the lesion is deeply situated, standard scalp leads may show little or nothing at all without some type of activation.

The classic example of the partial seizure is the *Jacksonian motor seizure,* which is caused by a sharply localized lesion in the motor cortex and begins as a repetitive movement at the distal portion of an extremity that proceeds to spread upward toward the trunk. More relevant from the psychiatric standpoint are the focal sensory, autonomic, and psychomotor seizures. *Sensory seizures* are caused by a lesion involving the sensory cortex and may produce a march of abnormal sensations, such as tingling or numbness of an extremity, or paroxysmally occurring visual, auditory, olfactory, gustatory, or vertiginous sensations. *Autonomic seizures* are attributable to lesions in the deep temporal, limbic, and diencephalic areas and are characterized by such symptoms as paroxysmal abdominal pain, piloerection, sweating, incontinence, salivation, and even fever. One type of partial seizure, characteristically seen in children and young adults, is the so-called "abdominal epilepsy," manifested by bouts of acute abdominal pain that are associated with hunger, nausea, or vomiting, usually occur in the morning, rarely last longer than fifteen minutes, and are often followed by headaches, drowsiness, and markedly labile affect (Chao 1964, Glaser 1967, Sheeby 1960).

Psychomotor, temporal, or limbic seizures are attributable to seizure activity involving the temporal lobe, its deeper nuclear masses, and their associated limbic system structures; they may manifest themselves by abrupt alterations of consciousness and behavior and a wide variety of changes in affective and cognitive processes (Daly

1958). The patient may appear quite normal and then suddenly become successively confused, angry, and paranoid, start to mutter incomprehensibly, engage in odd bits of behavior, such as arising from his chair, overturning a wastebasket, and then sitting down again, and just a few seconds or minutes later, once more appear lucid and calm. Stereotyped gesture automatisms, such as lipsmacking, swallowing, or aimless twisting of the arms and legs may precede or accompany the seizures. Déjà vu phenomena, dreamy states, forced thinking, sexual arousal, ideational blocking, paranoid ideation, hallucinations, micropsia, and macropsia may also occur. The attacks are frequently ushered in by an aura of visceral symptoms, anxiety, irritability, and a peculiar feeling tone, usually a mixture of sadness and fearfulness (Margerison 1961). The patient's behavior is often bizarre or even aggressive; may appear to have sexual overtones; and seems in some measure to be affected by the environment in which it takes place (Aggernaes 1965). Although the attacks tend to be stereotyped, in the sense that the same symptoms occur in the same sequence on each occasion, the behavior displayed may create the impression of being volitional because of its complexity (Gibbs 1951, Mulder 1952). While episodes in which the patient seems to remain in contact with his environment may pose a continuing diagnostic problem, their ictal character can usually be established by

1/ the aura;
2/ the stereotyped sequence of events;
3/ the presence of characteristic EEG abnormalities in the midst of the episode;
4/ concomitant motor manifestations (even if fairly mild); and
5/ a previous history of other types of seizures.

It is unclear whether there is a link between temporal lobe epilepsy and the development of psychosis, but there is some evidence that epilepsy of the nondominant temporal lobe is associated with affective symptoms, while that of the dominant temporal lobe is associated with schizophreniform symptoms. It is claimed, moreover, that individuals with a high frequency of temporal fits are less likely to exhibit psychosis than those with a lower frequency (Flor-Henry 1969).

Sexual deviations also appear to be more common among such patients, and, to our astonishment, we have been able to confirm the existence of four cases of the incestuous father-daughter relationship described as an integral part of "Main's syndrome" (Bourne 1960, Main 1957), in which there is

1/ massive conflict between family members and even between professionals involved with a

2/ female patient between 15 and 25 who suffers from

3/ motor and psychomotor seizures that are so atypical that a dispute emerges between the professionals involved in the case over whether the patient should be censured for obviously feigning illness or protected from so unfair an accusation, and

4/ exhibits EEG findings characteristic of temporal lobe epilepsy.

Patients who develop temporal lobe epilepsy in middle age (as true of all who develop seizure disorders past the age of 20) must be carefully examined for the possibility of a neoplasm (Preston 1964). In patients under 20 who develop seizures, the cause is usually a head injury or unknown; between 20 and 29, most likely a head injury; between 30 and 39, most commonly a head injury or brain tumor; and after the age of 40, most commonly cerebrovascular disease or a brain tumor (Juul-Jensen 1964).

Management

SOMATIC TREATMENT

Although there is no unanimity among epileptologists concerning the order and manner in which the various anticonvulsants should be tried, increased, or combined, it is possible to formulate certain general guidelines for treatment in terms of the classical models of grand mal, petit mal, and psychomotor seizures. Patients with *grand mal and focal motor epilepsy* usually respond favorably to hydantoins and/or barbiturates; those with *petit mal absences* are treated with succinimides and oxazolidines; patients with *psychomotor epilepsy* should be given first some combination of hydantoins and barbiturates, but if this is ineffective, oxazolidines and succinimides (especially methsuximide) should be tried. The most commonly used *hydantoin* is diphenylhydantoin (Dilantin); when this is ineffective or poorly tolerated, mephenytoin (Mesantoin) and the less toxic but also less effective ethotoin (Peganone) may be substituted for all or part of the diphenylhydantoin. The most commonly used *barbiturates* are phenobarbital, primidone (Mysoline, strictly speaking a barbiturate congener), mephobarbital (Mebaral), and (in myoclonic seizures) metharbital (Gemonil). The most commonly used of the *succinimides* (indeed the drug of choice in petit mal epilepsy) is ethosuximide (Zarontin); but phensuximide (Milontin) and methsuximide (Celontin) may be added or substituted if the former is ineffective. The most commonly used *oxazolidine* is trimethadione (Tridione), but when this is poorly tolerated, the less toxic but also less effective paramethadione (Paradione) may be used. *Phenacemide* (Phenurone), a hydantoin analog, may be effective in all types of seizures but is potentially so toxic that its use is largely restricted to resistant cases of psychomotor epilepsy.

Although the patient should initially be given but a single anticonvulsant (diphenylhydantoin for grand mal and psychomotor, ethosuximide for petit mal epilepsy), by the time the trial-and-error technique of finding the optimal drug regimen is completed, one or more other drugs may have been added to or substituted for the original drug. Except when the patient's seizures are life-threatening and immediate control is essential, the road to the right combination generally starts with giving him fairly low doses of the drug considered most likely to work (Abbott 1950). Since the effective dose range is often quite close to the toxic one, the dosage is increased only gradually. If, in the course of these increases, the patient's symptoms come under control, the dosage is held constant at whatever level this occurs. Should symptoms of toxicity arise, the dose is gradually reduced (or even discontinued) to the point at which the toxic symptoms disappear, while a second drug of the same type is initiated, in gradually increasing doses. It is preferable not to exceed the lower of the moderate therapeutic dose ranges listed in Table 39, and when this (usually nontoxic) dose has been reached, to add another of the drugs that is effective in the disorder in question. If the second drug is also ineffective in bringing the disorder under control, it may be necessary to use a third drug or to exceed the lower dose ranges.

There are several commonly used adjuvants to anticonvulsant treatment. *Acetazolamide* (Diamox) is of greatest benefit in petit mal epilepsy and in those seizure disorders that become more severe just before the menstrual period; because tolerance can develop, intermittent use is indicated. *Dextroamphetamine* (Dexedrine) is used when the patient's seizures seem to be related to drowsiness or respond only to an anticonvulsant regimen that makes the patient excessively drowsy. Minor tranquilizers, such as *Diazepam* (Valium) and *chlordiazepoxide* (Librium), may be used in small doses to control the anxiety and tension experienced by the epileptic; diaze-

pam is also a very effective anticonvulsant and may be used intra
venously for the treatment of status epilepticus (Parsonage 1967).
Bromides, while effective in grand mal epilepsy, are rarely prescribed today because of their toxicity. Cortisone and ACTH preparations may be used in infantile spasms, akinetic spells, and myoclonic seizures.

Major tranquilizers (phenothiazines, thioxanthenes, and butyrophenones) and *antidepressants* are also used in seizure disorders,
especially in those manifested by or associated with behavioral
abnormalities. Although high or rapidly increasing doses of these
agents can initially provoke seizures in some patients (Logothetis
1967, Mauceri 1956, Merlis 1955), low or slowly increasing doses
often have a beneficial effect on the behavioral manifestations and
sometimes even diminish the frequency of the patient's motor seizures (Bonafede 1957, David 1953, Detre 1963, Frain 1960, Itil 1970,
Winkelman 1954).

As in the case of the anticonvulsants, the proper use of psychotropic agents is established by trial and error. Some patients respond
best to anticonvulsants alone, some to psychotropic agents alone;
others require a carefully chosen combination of the two. Patients
with behavioral symptoms, cloudy and dysphoric states, or low stress
tolerance generally respond best to alerting phenothiazines like
fluphenazine (Prolixin); those with motor excitement, to sedating
phenothiazines like thioridazine (Mellaril). When the seizure disorder has dysphoric features that are refractory to the administration of phenothiazines, a small dose of an antidepressant like
imipramine (Tofranil), 25-75 mg daily, may be tried.

Decisions concerning the effectiveness of anticonvulsant-psycho-
tropic agent combinations must be based on the patient's overall
condition before and after treatment. The appearance of slow EEG
rhythms following the administration of phenothiazines is in itself
of no clinical significance (Steiner 1965). If, however, the patient's
seizures increase in frequency and it becomes necessary to choose between withdrawing the phenothiazines or "covering" them by increasing the dosage of anticonvulsants, the decision must take into
consideration

1/ the dangers to which increased seizure activity would expose
him in his environment;
2/ the severity of his pretreatment behavioral manifestations;
and
3/ the extent of the behavioral improvement already achieved.

For example, if a hospitalized patient with psychomotor seizures responds to phenothiazines with marked behavioral improvement but more frequent seizures, the effort to find the proper level of phenothiazines may be continued because his seizures are unlikely to pose a grave danger as long as he is hospitalized. However, if the increased seizure frequency does not subside within one or two weeks, the phenothiazines must be "covered" with a slightly increased dose of anticonvulsant, but if this does not help, may have to be withdrawn. In the case of a phenothiazine-produced increase in grand mal seizures, more anticonvulsant must be given without delay; if this does not reduce the frequency to the prephenothiazine baseline within three to four days, the phenothiazine dose must be reduced or withdrawn. Once a phenothiazine that is helpful has been found and the optimal dosage determined, it should be continued for at least six months. The dose may then be gradually lowered, but some patients will need small doses indefinitely.

Other types of somatic treatment have also been used. Prolonged twilight states unresponsive to anticonvulsants can sometimes be brought to a halt by the administration of ECT (Pond 1957). When a seizure disorder that is severely disabling cannot be controlled with anticonvulsants, and the presence and location of an abnormal discharge focus have been established, *surgical excision* of the area in question may be considered. Such measures have been of great benefit in some cases, but the results, on the whole, have been disappointing. Thus, even though temporal lobectomy may diminish seizures and improve behavior in patients with otherwise uncontrollable psychomotor seizures (Serafetinides 1962), surgical measures are generally considered the very last resort. The principal reasons for this are that 1/ the vast majority of seizure disorders can be managed pharmacologically (Aird 1967); 2/ the surgical trauma itself can produce additional foci for abnormal discharges; and 3/ such operations can have deleterious psychological aftereffects much like those described with leucotomies (see p. 663), and may aggravate paranoid and depressive elements of psychomotor seizures (James 1960).

There is no way, moreover, to be sure that the focus has been localized correctly. The cortical area believed to be the focus because of the patient's symptoms or the EEG findings, in reality, may be nothing but a projection of

1/ an underlying subcortical focus,
2/ a cortical focus in a different area, or

3/ the combined irradiations of other cortical and subcortical foci.

4/ It has also been suspected that the original focus can produce a mirror focus on the opposite side, thereafter become inactive (Fischer-Williams 1963, Hughes 1966, Proctor 1966), and leave the mirror focus as the only active one.

In some cases, the problems involved in selecting the appropriate site for excision have been overcome by surgically implanting electrodes into the suspected area of the brain and repeatedly stimulating them to determine whether the typical seizure develops, in which case the area chosen is probably the one involved in the attack (Driver 1969).

THE ROLE OF THE PSYCHIATRIST

Recognized Seizure Disorders. The patient with recognized grand mal, petit mal, or focal motor seizures is usually referred to a psychiatrist only when *1/* he also has psychological symptoms or *2/* his seizures are not satisfactorily controlled with anticonvulsants and the referring physician attributes this to emotional factors. Since in either of these cases the patient is probably taking some combination of anticonvulsants, the psychiatrist's first job is to determine whether the psychological symptoms reflect

a/ the psychotoxic effects of anticonvulsants;
b/ focal seizures that have not been controlled (or may even have been aggravated) by anticonvulsants;
c/ the seizure disorder's effect on his personality; or
d/ a mental illness that, as far as can be judged, is unrelated to the seizure disorder.

Any and all of these factors may be operative simultaneously, and the psychiatrist's task is to piece together their relative significance.

The most common *psychotoxic effects* of anticonvulsants are drowsiness, depersonalization, and dysmnesia. While these symptoms can occur even at moderate dose levels, the more anticonvulsants the individual takes, the more likely he is to suffer such symptoms. If the dosage is not decreased, he may eventually become delirious, develop disturbances in impulse control, or be so blunted or drowsy that his perception and judgment are impaired. Depressions, conversion symptoms, and dissociative states may also be seen but do not usually develop until the patient has been taking anticonvulsants for several weeks (Buchthal 1960, Gowers

1888, Kimura 1964, Kokenge 1965, Kutt 1964, Patel 1968, Roseman 1961, Swerdlow 1965); even seizure frequency may be increased as a result of anticonvulsant overdosage (Levy 1965). The psychological symptoms caused by anticonvulsants can usually be distinguished from those caused by the seizure disorder itself in that the former *1/* develop in the first weeks or months after anticonvulsant treatment is initiated or the dose increased, *2/* are continuous rather than intermittent, and *3/* are associated with drowsiness, dysarthria, nystagmus, and ataxia.

While a patient's seizure disorder is occasionally so severe that he must pay for his freedom from seizures with a moderate amount of drowsiness, most psychotoxic effects can be reversed by diminishing the dosage or using a different combination of drugs. Drug changes must be undertaken very cautiously, however, especially if the patient has previously had grand mal seizures, lest seizure manifestations that have been quiescent escape control or the patient develop status epilepticus (Hunter 1959). If the patient is already taking large doses of anticonvulsants at the time he becomes toxic, it is necessary to decide whether or not to substitute another anticonvulsant while the previous dosage is reduced. If he is taking large doses because lower ones did not control his seizures, the anticonvulsant dosage should be reduced by 10% to 15% weekly, while an equivalent amount of another drug of the same or (if this is unsuccessful) a different group is substituted. If, however, the current anticonvulsant dosage was arrived at so rapidly that it is not known whether the patient might have fared equally well on a lower dosage, or, as sometimes occurs, the dosage was increased even after the motor seizures were under control because the patient exhibited psychological symptoms of some kind, it may be safe to reduce the dosage by 10% to 15% weekly, without substituting another anticonvulsant, until the lowest effective dose level listed in Table 39 or the one at which he previously had no symptoms of toxicity is reached. If at this point he is still toxic, or if seizures develop during the course of this change, another anticonvulsant should be substituted.

In some cases, the anticonvulsant regimen relieves the patient's motor symptoms or episodes of unconsciousness but fails to relieve certain focal components of seizure activity that are manifested in affective, cognitive, or behavioral disturbances. These symptoms are called *psychomotor-temporal-limbic, sensory,* or *autonomic seizures* when they appear independent of other types of seizures; if they arise soon after the dose of anticonvulsant has been decreased, they can usually be brought under control by raising the dose again. If this makes the patient toxic or, as may occur, psychological symptoms characteristic of focal seizures become manifest as the generalized ones subside (Levy 1965), the entire anticonvulsant regimen may need to be modified until a regimen that controls all components of the seizure disorder is found. If increasing or changing the patient's anticonvulsant regimen does not relieve the behavioral and psychological components of the seizure, the anticonvulsant dosage should again be reduced to the level required to keep the motor seizures in check and an alerting phenothiazine added (Stevens 1966). Commonly used for this purpose is fluphenazine, which is started at a daily dose of 0.5 mg and increased by 0.5 mg every week until the patient's symptoms improve or he is receiving 6 mg daily. Higher doses should be avoided, however, for phenothiazines are potentially ictogenic; even the low doses can lead to an increase in the frequency or severity of the patient's seizures, and in this case must be discontinued or "covered" with additional anticonvulsants. The possibility has been considered that the antifolic acid effects of diphenylhydantoin (Dilantin), phenobarbital, and primidone (Mysoline) are responsible for the psychotoxic effects, including the dementiform changes that follow use of these agents (Gordon 1968, Reynolds 1967), but the relationship has not been conclusively demonstrated (Jensen 1969, Snaith 1970).

In addition to, and often more important than, the psychological symptoms that reflect seizure activity or anticonvulsant toxicity are the *long-term sequelae* of the many changes that the disorder imposes on the patient's entire life. That these changes have a deleterious effect on the individual's personality, and that epileptics have more than their share of personality problems and mental disorder, is today generally agreed. Not agreed, indeed widely disputed, is the once common notion that there is a specific "epileptic personality," manifested by dependency, irritability, interpersonal "stickiness," and attempts at ingratiation. To be sure, the individual whose life is punctuated by episodes of fits and unconsciousness and who experiences impairments in brain functioning even during the periods between seizures may feel that he is constantly walking on eggs and, because he is dependent on the helpfulness and good will of those around him, must act as ingratiatingly as he can. His view of himself, moreover, is gravely affected by his inability to carry out his plans with much continuity and by the fact that most people are repelled by the sight of seizures, consider epileptics to be strange, and treat him accordingly. Body image changes (Ionasescu 1960) and word-finding difficulties, difficulties in concentration, and inconstancy in perceptual accuracy are also common and may affect the patient's ability to deal with his surroundings (Geller 1970). The individual with petit mal epilepsy who suffers from frequent episodes of "absence" during his school years may learn so little that he appears mentally defective; if his seizures interfere greatly with his learning of social, intellectual, or occupational skills, he may well appear severely maladjusted. Seizures may also cause the patient to lose confidence in his own judgment and emotional stability and lead him to develop a generalized distrust of the world around him. Add to these problems the many limitations that the illness' dangers impose on such day-to-day activities as driving and engaging in sports, and the constant threat of being acutely embarrassed at crucial moments (even in the midst of sexual intimacies), and it is a wonder that some epileptics are as well-adjusted as they are.

The epileptic's personality difficulties do not, of course, occur in a vacuum, but affect and are affected by his relationship to his immediate environment. The patient may exaggerate the extent of his disability, treat himself as an invalid, terrorize his family into acceding to his every demand by threatening to become sicker if they do not comply, prevent his family from expressing their resentment and anger by claiming that they are "blaming" him for his illness, be encouraged in his invalidism (even in his refusal to take pills) by an overindulgent family, and, in short, participate in all the other (often deadly) games that emerge whenever patients and families are struggling with a chronic disease that responds poorly to treatment and is coupled with subtle changes in awareness.

Thus, if the drug therapy that is essential in the treatment of seizure disorders is to have a lasting effect, it must be combined with measures that promote social rehabilitation and enable the patient to acquire the social and intellectual skills that he needs and lacks. Psychotherapy, especially family and group therapy, can relieve these intrapsychic, interpersonal, and intrafamilial difficulties to some extent, especially if the patient's seizures can be controlled. In some cases, however, the patient and his family deal with each other and with the illness in a manner that makes medical supervision and seizure control impossible without hospitalizing the patient (Livingston 1969). If, even after the seizures are under control, the family continues to relate in a controlling, dependent, overindulgent, or hostile manner or, by "forgetting" the patient's medications, prompts a new bout of seizures, it is evident that these patterns are firmly entrenched and cannot be altered without separating the patient from his family. In this case, the patient may benefit from exposure to a therapeutic community or residential treatment program.

When the epileptic's psychological symptoms are attributable to a completely *unrelated mental illness,* his treatment should follow a suitable modification of the principles outlined in the chapter on the particular mental disorder involved. The patient who has both a seizure disorder and a mental illness tends (almost regardless of the illness involved) to have a more agitated and confusion-prone course and may be so obstreperous, negativistic, uncollaborative, or retarded that he cannot be relied on to take his anticonvulsants or avoid hazardous situations, and he must therefore be supervised more closely than the patient who has either disorder alone. Another important difference is that the psychological stress or fatigue that may come in the wake of the mental disorder may cause the seizures to increase in frequency or severity, in which case the anticonvulsant dose must be increased. Finally, since most of the drugs used in severe mental illnesses have ictogenic effects, it is necessary to start with as low a dose as possible, increase it as gradually as the patient's condition allows and, as stated earlier, if seizures occur or higher dose ranges of major tranquilizers or antidepressants are required, "cover" it with additional anticonvulsants.

Sometimes the patient with a recognized seizure disorder is referred to a psychiatrist not so much because of associated psychological or behavioral symptoms but because *the referring physician believes that the patient's seizures are triggered by emotional factors.* Although few neurologists would subscribe to a psychogenic causation of the propensity to seizures, it is generally agreed that individuals with this propensity may have more seizures during a period of emotional distress or develop a seizure in response to an upsetting event (Freedman 1968, Gottschalk 1956, Groethuysen 1957). Furthermore, while most patients are extremely anxious to avoid seizures, some, having learned how to provoke them, tend to do so on purpose when it suits their needs (Andermann 1962, Green 1968, Liddell 1965, Robertson 1954, Sherwood 1962). A patient might stop taking anticonvulsants in order to escape a conflict-ridden situation. Similarly, a socially inhibited patient, who has learned that hyperventilation changes his level of consciousness, may overbreathe when he wishes to rid himself of his inhibitions and express strong feelings (Mahl 1964, Penfield 1952, 1960). Some patients (even nonepileptics) may go so far as to simulate seizures when under pressure.

Patients who provoke or simulate seizures, however, are far rarer than those who, because their seizures are atypical, are accused of such maneuvers and considered to have hysteroepilepsy or pseudo-seizures. The distinction is, in any case, most difficult and rarely possible by observing a single seizure or assessing single (or even repeated) EEGs (Ajuriaguerra 1951). In contradistinction to the commonly accepted stereotype, patients with a bona fide seizure disorder may

1/ have normal EEGs,
2/ remain conscious while having bilateral convulsive movements (Walker 1960), or
3/ remember much of what happened during the seizure (Ziegler 1967).

The mistake of taking the epileptic to be a hysteric is thus much commoner than its converse (Slater 1969).

Ictogenic factors of an emotional nature can occasionally be modified by psychotherapy. When the patient's seizures have in the past been triggered by emotionally charged events, their frequency can sometimes be reduced by identifying the kinds of events to which he is likely to overrespond and teaching him how to cope with or avoid them. Seizures triggered by the fatigue that comes in the wake of continual family struggle may diminish when the participants understand their cause and are taught other ways of resolving· their disagreements (see Chap. 13). Since family treatment repeatedly confronts the individual with the situation to which he overreacts, it may be considered a form of conditioning therapy. The previously described experiments in extinguishing startle responses with conditioning therapies suggest that more formal conditioning therapies may also be helpful (Booker 1965, Pond 1965).

"Occult" Seizure Disorders. When an internist, neurologist, or family physician refers a patient with an already identified seizure disorder to the psychiatrist, he is not asking for help with the diagnosis but with certain related or unrelated psychological symptoms or with the patient's complete or partial unresponsiveness to anticonvulsants. Not all epileptics have their label so neatly pinned on their chests, however. The patient with *petit mal,* for example, may be sent to the psychiatrist because he is thought to "daydream" too much or to be inattentive to his schoolwork. The patient with autonomic, sensory, or psychomotor-temporal-limbic seizures may be sent to the psychiatrist with a diagnosis of hysteria, depersonaliza-

tion, dissociation, schizophrenia, or explosive or antisocial personality (Niedermeyer 1961). Any patient, therefore, whose symptoms develop and recede abruptly must be suspected of having an *"occult" seizure disorder,* especially when

1/ his symptoms are similar or identical from one episode to the next;

2/ he has a family or personal history of seizure disorder, motor fits, or unexplained episodes of unconsciousness;

3/ he describes a sense of premonition or "aura" that precedes each episode;

4/ he exhibits focal motor manifestations, particularly stereotyped ones, during the episodes;

5/ he seems vague and confused for a brief time after the episode subsides; and

6/ at the conclusion of the episode, he is unable to remember what his behavior was like during its course.

Even when a patient showing the behavioral abnormalities described above has an EEG suggestive of seizure disorder, the diagnosis must be held in abeyance, since psychological symptoms arising in the wake of exciting events are often associated with substantial sleep loss, and this factor alone can cause a previously normal EEG to become dysrhythmic. Thus, before coming to a definite diagnostic conclusion, it is necessary to restore the patient's sleep. This can usually be accomplished with phenothiazines, which have the added advantage that they may well relieve the symptoms that led to psychiatric referral. If, after the patient's sleep has been restored, the clinical and EEG findings remain suggestive of a seizure disorder, and especially if the EEG abnormalities become more pronounced during or immediately before the periods of behavioral disturbance, he should be given anticonvulsants. Should the symptoms prove refractory or get worse after an adequate trial, low doses of phenothiazines should be added, then gradually increased; if this too is unsuccessful, the anticonvulsant regimen must be modified in accordance with the principles outlined on page 433.

NARCOLEPSY

The term *narcolepsy* is used to describe a syndrome of unknown etiology characterized by repeated attacks of drowsiness and sleep (Gélineau 1880, Yoss 1960). While these episodes may last for as long as a few hours, the majority subside within 10 to 15 minutes. At their conclusion, that is to say, when the patient awakes, he will usually feel alert and refreshed. This feeling does not usually last for long, though, and the patient may soon have a fresh attack. Although some patients experience dozens of these episodes daily, most have no more than two or three in a day. The attacks may arise without provocation but are most common when the patient is engaged in boring, repetitive, or monotonous activities that might make even a normal person feel slightly drowsy. The syndrome usually arises during the second or third decade of life, and there is often a family history of similar disorders. If one counts the attenuated forms, the disorder is not so rare as was thought at the time it was first reported: one out of 8,670 patients admitted to the psychiatric service of the Mayo Clinic was diagnosed as having narcolepsy (Yoss 1957).

The narcoleptic patient's difficulties are not limited to the sleep attacks, however. Even when he is not struggling against sleep, he tends to be drowsy, anergic, and irritable. His constant efforts to remain awake may cause him to appear anxious, fatigued, and hypochondriacal, and he may develop somatic symptoms of various kinds. Thirty percent are quite obese (some remarkably so). After a number of years, marked personality changes, usually of a passive-aggressive character, may develop. Psychotic states may also occur: a full 10% of such patients eventually exhibit schizophrenic psychosis (Sours 1963).

In the majority of cases, the patient will experience certain other characteristic disturbances of alertness. Among these are *cataplexy* (attacks during which the patient remains awake but suddenly becomes akinetic and falls down), *hypnagogic or hypnopompic hallucinations* (episodes in which, just before falling asleep or just after awaking, the patient sees or hears things that he later realizes did not exist but seem so real to him at that time that he acts as if they were), and *sleep paralysis* (episodes in which, just before falling asleep or just after awaking, the patient considers himself fully awake but feels unable to move). While each of these disturbances can occur independently, they are so frequently seen in patients who also have sleep attacks that they are grouped with narcolepsy itself as components of a *narcoleptic tetrad*. Thorough questioning of large randomly selected populations and detailed introspective studies (Oswald 1962) have shown sleep paralysis and hypnagogic hallucinations to be the most common of these phenomena, but these symptoms are rarely disturbing enough to be brought to medical attention. As a result, the most frequently reported clinical pictures are the combinations of narcolepsy and cataplexy (37%) and narcolepsy alone (19%). Less common are the combination of narcolepsy, cataplexy, and hypnagogic hallucinations (12%); narcolepsy, cataplexy, and sleep paralysis (12%); and the full tetrad (11%). All the other possible combinations, including the occurrence of cataplexy alone, are rare (Bowling 1961, Sours 1963).

During the narcoleptic attack, the EEG has the features of normal light sleep (low voltage, irregular, relatively fast patterns containing slow components in the 4 to 6 cps range); between attacks, it is usually normal, with the exception that some patients show Stage I sleep patterns even while they appear behaviorally alert. The narcoleptic patient's sleep patterns also differ: unlike normal individuals, who show no REM sleep patterns until they have been asleep for 60 minutes or more, narcoleptics, especially those who also have cataplexy, tend to show such patterns within minutes of falling asleep (Rechtschaffen 1963). One other remarkable feature of these disorders, again most true of the patient with cataplexy, is that such episodes can develop in response to emotionally charged events.

The diminished muscle tone in cataplexy or sleep paralysis and the experience of dreaming while half-awake that occurs in hypnagogic and hypnopompic hallucinations are not pathologic phenomena when they appear in the proper relationship to falling asleep and awakening, but normal components of this process. In narcolepsy, these components come to clinical attention or cause discomfort because their temporal harmony is disrupted and thus they appear in abnormal proportions and combinations (Hishikawa 1965). The physiologic road toward sleep consists of the individual's gradually becoming drowsy, lying down, losing awareness of his surroundings, developing muscular flaccidity, and dreaming. As he awakes, the process is reversed. When the muscular flaccidity occurs before the patient has become drowsy enough to lie down and go to sleep and he falls atonic to the ground while fully awake, he is said to be having a cataplectic attack. In some cases, only single muscle groups are affected: when the eye muscles are affected, the patient may develop diplopia, ptosis, or blurred vision (Dale 1964). If the generalized flaccidity occurs after he lies down but before he loses consciousness or persists after he awakes, he experiences sleep paralysis, which, though it rarely lasts for more than 30 or 40 seconds, may be quite frightening. Similarly, if he goes to bed and starts to dream before losing awareness of his surroundings, he is said to be having a hypnagogic hallucination; if he continues to dream after he awakens, he is said to have hypnopompic hallucinations.

The *differential diagnosis* of excessive sleepiness ,includes encephalitis, lead poisoning, concussion, and taboparesis. That of sleepiness coupled with obesity includes hypothyroidism, hyperinsulinism, the depressed phase of manic-depressive disease, chronic schizophrenia, and the Pickwickian syndrome, in which obesity leads (perhaps mechanically) to alveolar hypoventilation and thence to polycythemia, hypercapnia, cerebral hypoxia, and somnolence (Sours 1963). Because of the associated somnolence, patients with these disorders are often said to have *symptomatic* or *secondary narcolepsy,* but the term is a misnomer, as their drowsiness tends to be constant rather than episodic. The differential diagnosis rarely presents much difficulty, however; only narcolepsy manifests

   1/ brief and recurrent attacks of sleep followed by a feeling of alertness;

   2/ one or more of the other symptoms of the tetrad (particularly cataplexy);

   3/ a history dating back to adolescence;

   4/ a family history of similar disorders (Daly 1959, Gelardi 1967); and

   5/ the absence of identifiable causative factors.

A very rare syndrome said to have a certain relationship to narcolepsy is the *Kleine-Levin syndrome* of episodic hypersomnia and bulimia. This disorder, generally seen in adolescent males, is characterized by episodes of sleep that last for days or weeks at a time and are punctuated by brief episodes of awaking during which the patient eats ravenously, with a particular hunger for sweets. While the patient with a Kleine-Levin syndrome is (as the narcoleptic may be) obese, frequently tired, yawning, thick-tongued, dysmnesic, and confused, this syndrome may be distinguished from primary narcolepsy by the length of the attacks and the tendency to subside as the patient reaches adulthood (Critchley 1962, Garland 1965, Kleine 1925, Levin 1929, 1936).

The treatment of narcoleptic syndromes consists primarily of the administration of stimulants. In some cases, daily doses of 5 to 15 mg of dextroamphetamine or 20 to 80 mg of methylphenidate (Ritalin) will suffice, but doses as high as 40 or 200 mg, respectively, may be required. The high doses of amphetamine do not appear to cause the excessive stimulation noted in normal subjects; it is possible, however, that the paranoid syndromes sometimes seen in narcoleptic patients (Young 1938) are caused by their prolonged exposure to high doses of stimulants rather than by the disease itself (Coren 1965). Imipramine (Tofranil), 50 to 75 mg daily, appears to have a favorable effect on the cataplectic components but little effect on the sleep attacks (Akimoto 1960). While the reason for the favorable response to antidepressants is unknown, it is interesting that many syndromes with similar features (such as conversion neurosis and fugue states) also respond to antidepressants or stimulants; that some narcoleptic syndromes respond to agents used in petit mal epilepsy; and that it is as difficult on the basis of the symptoms alone to determine whether one patient's syncope represents a conversion symptom, an akinetic seizure, or a cataplectic attack as it is to decide whether another patient's confused drowsiness represents a fugue state, an epileptic dysphoria, or an attack of narcolepsy.

SOMNAMBULISM

In contrast to narcolepsy, in which behavior usually associated with sleep intrudes into the waking state, somnambulism (sleepwalking) and such closely related symptoms as somniloquy (speaking while asleep) consist of behavior typical of the alert state that intrudes into the time of sleep. During a somnambulistic episode, the patient's eyes are open; initially, he may appear somewhat confused; and his motor activities are simple and repetitive. As the episode continues, he becomes increasingly aware of his environment and may even engage in complex and apparently goal-related sequences. Spontaneous speech is common, though not always coherent or understandable. The patient usually answers questions in one or two words when spoken to, although it is difficult to maintain his attention or awaken him (Arkin 1966). When he awakens in the morning, he generally has little or no recollection of the night's events (Jacobson 1965).

Like enuresis nocturna, somnambulistic activity usually begins in Stage III or IV sleep (slow-wave sleep) and not during REM (Kales 1966). That somnambulism and enuresis are in some way related is also suggested by the high familial incidence of somnambulism among patients with enuresis nocturna (Broughton 1968). Moreover, the two symptoms are often seen together; in children, they are frequently joined by *pavor nocturnus,* a term used to refer to night terror in which the patient responds to a nightmare by screaming and crying so loudly that he awakens everyone in the house but himself. Various forms of psychotherapy and drugs have been tried for somnambulism and pavor nocturnus, but their effectiveness remains to be documented.

REFERENCES

Abbott, J. A., and Schwab, R. S.: Serious side effects of the newer antiepileptic drugs: Their control and prevention, New Eng J Med *242*:943-949, 1950.

Achté, K. A., Hillbom, E., and Aalberg, V.: Psychoses following war brain injuries, Acta Psychiat Scand *45*:1-18, 1969.

Adams, R. D., *et al.:* Symptomatic occult hydrocephalus with "normal" cerebrospinal fluid pressure: treatable syndrome, New Eng J Med *273*:117-126, 1965.

Aggernaes, M.: Differential diagnosis between hysterical and epileptic disturbances of consciousness or twilight states, Acta Psychiat Scand *41*: (Suppl 185) 1-101, 1965.

Aird, R. B.: Drug treatment of epilepsy, Mod Med, Aug. 14, 1967, pp. 30-40.

Ajuriaguerra, J.: Le problème de l'hystérie, L'Encéphale *40*:50-87, 1951.

Akimoto, H., Honda, Y., and Takahashi, Y.: Pharmacotherapy in narcolepsy, Dis Nerv Syst *21*:704-706, 1960.

Andermann, K., *et al.:* Self-induced epilepsy. A collection of self-induced epilepsy cases compared with some other photoconvulsive cases, Arch Neurol (Chicago) *6*:49-65, 1962.

Appenzeller, O., and Descarries, L.: Circulatory reflexes in patients with cerebrovascular disease, New Eng J Med *271*: 820-832, 1964.

Arellano, A. P.: A tympanic lead, Electroenceph Clin Neurophysiol *1*:112-113, 1949.

Arkin, A. M.: Sleep-talking: review, J Nerv Ment Dis *143*:101-122, 1966.

Asso, D., *et al.:* Psychological aspects of the stereotactic treatment of Parkinsonism, Brit J Psychiat *115*:541-553, 1969.

Austen, F. K., Carmichael, M. W., and Adams, R. D.: Neurologic manifestations of chronic pulmonary insufficiency, New Eng J Med *257*:580-590, 1957.

Ayd, F. J., Jr.: Tranquilizers and the ambulatory geriatric patient, J Amer Geriat Soc *8*:909-914, 1960.

Baxter, D. W., and Bailey, A. A.: Primary reading epilepsy, Neurology *11*: 445-449, 1961.

Bender, A. D.: Pharmacologic aspects of aging: Survey of the effect of increasing age on drug activity in adults, J Amer Geriat Soc *12*:114-134, 1964.

Bennett, D. R.: Sleep deprivation and major motor convulsions, Neurology *13*: 953-958, 1963.

Benson, D. F., *et al.:* Diagnosis of normal-pressure hydrocephalus, New Eng J Med *283*:609-615, 1970.

Bickford, R. G., *et al.:* Reading epilepsy: Clinical and electroencephalographic study of a new syndrome, Trans Amer Neurol Ass *81*:100-102, 1956.

Bini, L., and Bazzi, T.: Trattato di Psichiatria, Milano: Casa Editrice Dottor Francesco Vallardi, vol. 1, Psicologia Medica, 1959.

Blachly, P. H., and Semler, H. J.: Electroconvulsive therapy of three patients with aortic valve prostheses, Amer J Psychiat *124*:233-236, 1967.

Blenkner, M.: Normal dependencies of aging, Ment Health Dig *1*:36-38, 1969.

Bleuler, M.: Endokrinologische Psychiatrie, Stuttgart, Thieme, 1954.

Bonafede, V. L.: Chlorpromazine (Thorazine) treatment of disturbed epileptic patients, Arch Neurol (Chicago) *77*:234-246, 1957.

Booker, H. E., Forster, F. M., and Klove, H.: Extinction factor in startle (acoustico-motor) seizures, Neurology *15*: 1095-1103, 1965.

Bourne, H.: Main's syndrome and a nurse's reaction to it, Arch Gen Psychiat (Chicago) *2*:576-581, 1960.

Bower, B. D.: Television flicker and fits, Clin Pediat (Phila) *2*:134-138, 1963.

Bowers, M. B., Jr.: Clinical aspects of

depression in a home for the aged, J Amer Geriat Soc *17:*469-476, 1969.

Bowling, G., and Richards, N. G.: Diagnosis and treatment of the narcolepsy syndrome: Analysis of seventy-five case records, Cleveland Clin Quart *28:*38-45, 1961.

Brain, M.: Miscellaneous advances. Neurological manifestations of folate deficiency, *in* Brain, L., and Wilkinson, M., eds.: Recent Advances in Neurology and Neuropsychiatry, ed. 8, London: Churchill, 1969, pp. 129-146.

Brazier, M. A. B.: Electrical activity recorded simultaneously from the scalp and deep structures of the human brain, J Nerv Ment Dis *147:*31-39, 1968.

Broughton, R. J.: Sleep disorders: disorders of arousal? Science *159:*1070-1078, 1968.

Buchthal, F., and Svensmark, O.: Aspects of the pharmacology of phenytoin (Dilantin) and phenobarbital relevant to their dosage in the treatment of epilepsy, Epilepsia (Amst) *1:*373-384, 1960.

Busse, E. W.: Geriatrics today—An overview, Amer J Psychiat *123:*1226-1233, 1967.

Busse, E. W., and Obrist, W. D.: Presenescent electroencephalographic changes in normal subjects, J Geront *20:*315-320, 1965.

Butler, R. N.: Aspects of survival and adaptation in human aging, Amer J Psychiat *123:*1233-1243, 1967.

Cairns, H.: Discussion on rehabilitation after injuries to the central nervous system, Proc Roy Soc Med *35:*299-301, 1942.

Calderon-Gonzalez, R., Hopkins, I., and McLean, W. T.: Tap seizures: Form of sensory precipitation epilepsy, JAMA *198:*521-523, 1966.

Calne, D. B., *et al.*: L-dopa may alleviate idiopathic parkinsonism, Lancet *2:*973-976, 1969.

Canary, J. J., *et al.*: Effects of oral and intramuscular administration of reserpine in thyrotoxicosis, New Eng J Med *257:*435-442, 1957.

Chao, D., Sexton, J. A., and Davis, S. D.: Convulsive equivalent syndrome of childhood, J Pediat *64:*499-508, 1964.

Charlton, M. H., and Yahr, M. D.: Long-term follow-up of patients with petit mal, Arch Neurol (Chicago) 595-598, 1967.

Cohen, N. H.: The treatment of Huntington's chorea with trifluoperazine (Stelazine), J Nerv Ment Dis *134:*62-71, 1962.

Cohn, R., and Nardini, J. E.: Correlation of bilateral occipital slow activity in the human EEG with certain disorders of behavior, Amer J Psychiat *115:*44-54, 1958.

Colbert, J., and Harrow, M.: Depression and organicity, Psychiat Quart *40:*96-103, 1966.

Coren, H. Z., and Strain, J. J.: A case of narcolepsy with psychosis (paranoid state of narcolepsy), Compr Psychiat *6:*191 199, 1965.

Corsellis, J. A. N., and Brierley, J. B.: Observations on the pathology of insidious dementia following head injury, J Ment Sci *105:*714-720, 1959.

Corso, J. F.: Sensory effects of aging in man, Scientia *103:*675-676, 1968.

Cotzias, G. C., Papavasiliou, P. S., and Gellene, R.: Modification of Parkinsonism—chronic treatment with L-dopa, New Eng J Med *280:*337-345, 1969.

Critchley, M.: Musicogenic epilepsy, Brain *60:*13-27, 1937.

———: Medical aspects of boxing, particularly from a neurological standpoint, Brit Med J *1:*357-362, 1957.

———: Periodic hypersomnia and megaphagia in adolescent males, Brain *85:*627-656, 1962.

Currier, R. D., Kooi, K. A., and Saidman, L. J.: Prognosis of "pure" petit mal: A follow-up study, Neurology (Minneap) *13:*959-967, 1963.

Dale, R. T., and Langworthy, O. R.: Narcoleptic tetrad with spontaneous diplopia and strabismus, Neurology (Minneap) *14:*773-775, 1964.

Dalessio, D. J., Benchimol, A., and Dimond, E. G.: Chronic encephalopathy related to heart block, Neurology (Minneap) *15:*499-503, 1965.

Daly, D.: Ictal affect, Amer J Psychiat *115:*97-108, 1958.

Daly, D. D., and Yoss, R. E.: Family with narcolepsy, Mayo Clin Proc *34:*313-319, 1959.

David, M., Benda, P., and Klein, F.: Traitement de l'état de mal épileptique par la chloropromazine, Société Médicale des Hopitaux de Paris, June 26, 1953, pp. 691-697.

Davidson, S., and Watson, C. W.: Hereditary light sensitive epilepsy, Neurology (Minneap) *6:*235-261, 1956.

Davies, G. V.: Differential diagnosis of the mental disorders of late life, Med J Aust *1:*242-245, 1969.

Dekaban, A.: Idiopathic epilepsy in early infancy, Amer J Dis Child *100:*181-188, 1960.

Dement, W., Rechtschaffen, A., and Gulevich, G.: Nature of the narcoleptic sleep attack, Neurology (Minneap) *16:* 18-33, 1966.

DeMyer, W.: Technique of the Neurologic Examination. A Programmed Text, New York: Blakiston, 1969.

Detre, T., and Feldman, R. G.: Behavior disorder associated with seizure states: Pharmacological and psychosocial management, *in* Glaser, G. H., ed.: EEG and Behavior, New York: Basic, 1963, pp. 366-376.

Dongier, S.: Statistical study of clinical and electroencephalographic manifestations of 536 psychotic episodes occurring in 516 epileptics between clinical seizures, Epilepsia (Amst) *1:*117-142, 1959.

Driver, M. V.: Electroencephalography in the study of epilepsy, *in* Brain, L., and Wilkinson, M., eds.: Recent Advances in Neurology and Neuropsychiatry, ed. 8, London: Churchill, 1969, pp. 175-213.

Dubois, E. L., and Tuffanelli, D. L.: Clinical manifestations of systemic lupus erythematosus: Computer analysis of 520 cases, JAMA *190:*104-111, 1964.

Dulfano, M. J., and Ishikawa, S.: Hypercapnia: Mental changes and extrapulmonary complications, Ann Intern Med *63:*829-841, 1965.

Eaton, M. T., Jr.: Mental health of the older executive, Geriatrics *24:*126-134, 1969.

Evans, J. H.: Post-traumatic epilepsy, Neurology (Minneap) *12:*665-674, 1962.

Fisch, M., *et al.:* Chronic brain syndrome in the community aged, Arch Gen Psychiat (Chicago) *18:*739-745, 1968.

Fischer-Williams, M., and Cooper, R. A.: Depth recording from the human brain in epilepsy, Electroenceph Clin Neurophysiol *15:*568-587, 1963.

Flor-Henry, P.: Psychosis and temporal lobe epilepsy, A controlled investigation, Epilepsia (Amst) *10:*363-395, 1969.

Ford, R. G., and Siekert, R. G.: Central nervous system manifestations of periarteritis nodosa, Neurology (Minneap) *15:*114-122, 1965.

Frain, M. M.: Preliminary report on Mellaril in epilepsy, Amer J Psychiat *117:*547-548, 1960.

Freedman, D. A., and Adatto, C. P.: On the precipitation of seizures in an adolescent boy, Psychosom Med *30:*437-447, 1968.

Gaitz, C. M.: Functional assessment of the suspected mentally ill aged, J Amer Geriat Soc *17:*541-548, 1969.

Gal, P.: Mental symptoms in cases of tumor of temporal lobe, Amer J Psychiat *115:*157-160, 1958.

Garland, H., Sumner, D., and Fourman, P.: The Kleine-Levin syndrome, Neurology (Minneap) *15:*1161-1167, 1965.

Gelardi, J. M., and Brown, J. W.: Hereditary cataplexy, J Neurol Neurosurg Psychiat *30:*455-457, 1967.

Gélineau: De la narcolepsie, Gazette des Hopitaux, Paris 1880, pp. 626-628.

Geller, M., and Geller, A.: Brief amnestic effects of spike-wave discharges, Neurology *20:*1089-1095, 1970.

Gibbs, E. L., and Gibbs, F. A.: Electroencephalographic evidence of thalamic and hypothalamic epilepsy, Neurology (Minneap) *1:*136-144, 1951.

Gibbs, F. A., and Gibbs, E. L.: Atlas of Electroencephalography, ed. 2, vol. 2, Cambridge: Addison-Wesley Press, Inc., 1952.

——: Changes in epileptic foci with age, Electroenceph Clin Neurophysiol Suppl *4:* 233-234, 1953.

Gibbs, F. A., Rich, C. L., and Gibbs, E. L.: Psychomotor variant type of seizure discharge, Neurology (Minneap) *13:*991-998, 1963.

Gibson, A. C.: Psychosis occurring in the senium: Review of an industrial population, Brit J Psychiat *107:*921-925, 1961.

Glaser, G.: Limbic epilepsy in childhood, J Nerv Ment Dis *144:*391-397, 1967.

Glaser, G. H.: Normal electroencephalogram and its reactivity, *in* Glaser, G. H. ed.: EEG and Behavior, New York: Basic, 1963, pp. 3-23.

Goldfarb, A. I.: Psychotherapy of the aged: The use and value of an adaptational frame of reference, Psychoanal Rev *43:*68-81, 1956.

Goldfarb, A. I., and Sheps, J.: Psychotherapy of the aged: 3. Brief therapy of interrelated psychological and somatic disorders, Psychosom Med *16:*209-219, 1954.

Goldstein, K.: Aftereffects of Brain Injuries in War, New York: Grune, 1942.

Goldstein, N. P., *et al.:* Psychiatric aspects of Wilson's disease (hepatolenticular degeneration): Results of psychometric tests during long-term therapy, Amer J Psychiat *124:*1555-1561, 1968.

Gordon, N.: Folic acid deficiency from anticonvulsant therapy, Develop Med Child Neurol *10:*497-504, 1968.

Gottschalk, L. A.: Relation of psychologic state and epileptic activity, Psychoanal Stud Child *11:*352-380, 1956.

Gowers, W. R.: Manual of Diseases of the Nervous System, Philadelphia: Blakiston, 1888.

Green, J. B.: Seizures on closing the eyes, Neurology (Minneap) *18:*391-396, 1968.

Groethuysen, U. C., *et al.:* Depth electrographic recording of a seizure during a structured interview, Psychosom Med *19:*353-362, 1957.

Guttman, E.: Late effects of closed head injuries: Psychiatric observations, Brit J Psychiat *92:*1-18, 1946.

Guze, S. B., and Cantwell, D. P.: Prognosis in "organic brain" syndromes, Amer J Psychiat *120:*878-881, 1964.

Guze, S. B., and Daengsurisri, S.: Organic brain syndromes, Arch Gen Psychiat (Chicago) *17:*365-366, 1967.

Harris, A. S., and Kokernot, R. H.: Effect of diphenlhydantoin sodium (Dilantin Sodium) and phenobarbital sodium upon ectopic ventricular tachycardia in acute myocardial infarction, Amer J Physiol *163:*505-516, 1950.

Hedenström, I. V.: Sensitivity to photic stimulation in the relatives of epileptics, J Amer Med Wom Ass *24:*227-229, 1969.

Himmelhoch, J., *et al.:* Subacute encephalitis: behavioral and neurological aspects, Brit J Psychiat, *116:*531-538, 1970.

Hishikawa, Y., *et al.:* H-reflex and EMG of the mental and hyoid muscles during sleep, with special reference to narcolepsy, Electroenceph Clin Neurophysiol *18:*487-492, 1965.

Hodgins, E.: Episode: Report on the Accident Inside My Skull. New York: Atheneum, 1964.

Hossain, M.: Neurological and psychiatric manifestations in idiopathic hypoparathyroidism: response to treatment, J Neurol Neurosurg Psychiat *33:*153-156, 1970.

Hughes, J. R.: Bilateral EEG abnormalities on corresponding areas, Epilepsia (Amst) *7:*44-52, 1966.

Hunter, R. A.: Status epilepticus: History, incidence and problems, Epilepsia (Amst) *1:*162-188, 1959.

Hunter, R., Blackwood, W., and Bull, J.: Three cases of frontal meningiomas presenting psychiatrically, Brit Med J *3:*9-16, 1968.

Ingbar, S. H.: Management of emergencies, IX. Thyrotoxic storm, New Eng J Med *274:*1252-1254, 1966.

Ingvar, D. H., and Nyman, G. E.: Epilepsia arithmetices: New psychologic trigger mechanism in a case of epilepsy, Neurology (Minneap) *12:*282-287, 1962.

Ionasescu, V.: Paroxysmal disorders of the body image in temporal lobe epilepsy, Acta Psychiat Scand *35:*171-181, 1960.

Itil, T. M.: Convulsive and anticonvulsive properties of neuro-psycho-pharmaca, *in* Niedermeyer, E., ed.: Modern Problems of Pharmacopsychiatry, vol. 4, Epilepsy, Basel and New York: Karger, 1970, pp. 270-305.

Jacobson, A., *et al.:* Somnambulism: All-night electroencephalographic studies, Science *148:*975-977, 1965.

Jaffe, R.: Ictal behavior disturbance as the only manifestation of seizure disorder, J Nerv Ment Dis *134:*470-476, 1962.

James, I. P.: Temporal lobectomy for psychomotor epilepsy, J Ment Sci *106:*543-558, 1960.

Jensen, O. N., and Olesen, O. V.: Folic acid and anticonvulsive drugs, Arch Neurol (Chicago) *21:*208-215, 1969.

Jones, D. P.: Recording of the basal electroencephalogram with sphenoidal needle electrodes, Electroenceph Clin Neurophysiol *3:*100, 1951.

Juul-Jensen, P.: Epilepsy: Clinical and social analysis of 1020 adult patients with epileptic seizures, Acta Neurol Scand *40:*(Suppl 15)1-148, 1964.

Kahn, R. L., *et al.:* Brief objective measures for the determination of mental status in the aged, Amer J Psychiat *117:*326-328, 1960.

Kales, A., *et al.:* Somnambulism: Psychophysiological correlates, Arch Gen Psychiat (Chicago) *14:*586-594, 1966.

Kalinowsky, L. B., and Hippius, H.: Pharmacological, Convulsive and Other Somatic Treatments in Psychiatry, New York: Grune, 1969.

Kay, D.: Observations on the natural history and genetics of old age psychoses: Stockholm material 1931-1937, Proc Roy Soc Med *52:*791-794, 1959.

Kay, D. W., Beamish, P., and Roth, M.: Old age mental disorders in Newcastle upon Tyne, Brit J Psychiat *110:*668-682, 1964.

Kimura, D.: Cognitive deficit related to seizure pattern in centrencephalic epilepsy, J Neurol Neurosurg Psychiat *27:*291-295, 1964.

Kleine, W.: Periodische Schlafsucht, Mschr Psychiat Neurol *57:*285-298, 1925.

Kokenge, R., Kutt, H., and McDowell, F.: Neurological sequelae following Dilantin overdose in a patient and in experimental animals, Neurology (Minneap) *15:*823-829, 1965.

Korolenko, C. P., Yevseyeva, T. A., and Volkov, P. P.: Data for a comparative account of toxic psychoses of various aetiologies, Brit J Psychiat *115:*273-279, 1969.

Kutt, H., *et al.:* Diphenylhydantoin and phenobarbital toxicity, Arch Neurol (Chicago) *11:*649-656, 1964.

LaBaw, W.: Diary of a doctor's recovery from brain trauma, Resident and Staff Physician, December, 1969, pp. 61-67.

Lange, E., and Poppe, G.: Social isolation preceding syndromes of paranoid interference in old age, Nervenarzt *35:* 194-200, 1964.

Lawson, I. R., and MacLeod, R. D. M.: Use of imipramine ("Tofranil") and other psychotropic drugs in organic emotionalism, Brit J Psychiat *115:*281-285, 1969.

Levere, R. D., and Kappas, A.: Porphyric diseases of man, Hosp Practice *5:* 61-73, 1970.

Levin, M.: Narcolepsy (Gelineau's syndrome) and other varieties of morbid somnolence, Arch Neurol Psychiat *22:* 1172-1200, 1929.

———: Periodic somnolence and morbid hunger: A new syndrome, Brain *59:*494, 1936.

Levy, L. L., and Fenichel, G. M.: Diphenylhydantoin activated seizures, Neurology (Minneap) *15:*716-722, 1965.

Ley, P., and Spelman, M. S.: Communicating with the Patient, St. Louis: Warren H. Green, Inc., 1967.

Liddell, D. W.: Uses of epilepsy, J Psychosom Res *9:*21-23, 1965.

Lipowski, Z. J.: Delirium, clouding of consciousness and confusion, J Nerv Ment Dis *145:*227-255, 1967.

Lishman, W. A.: Brain damage in relation to psychiatric disability after head injury, Brit J Psychiat *114:*373-410, 1968.

Livingston, S.: When to hospitalize the epileptic child, Hosp Practice *4:*77-86, 1969.

Locke, S.: The neurological concomitants of aging, Geriatrics *19:*722-724, 1964.

Logothetis, J.: Spontaneous epileptic seizures and electroencephalographic changes in the course of phenothiazine therapy, Neurology (Minneap) *17:*869-877, 1967.

———: Guide to a systematic neurologic clinical examination, Behav Neuropsychiat *1:*14-21 (Feb-Mar) 1970.

Longo, V. G.: Behavioral and electroencephalographic effects of atropine and related compounds, Pharmacol Rev *18:* 965-996, 1966.

Maclean, P. D.: A new nasopharyngeal lead, Electroenceph Clin Neurophysiol *1:* 110-112, 1949.

Mahl, G. F., *et al.:* Psychological responses in the human to intracerebral electrical stimulation, Psychosom Med *26:* 337-368, 1964.

Main, T. F.: The ailment, Brit J Med Psychol *30:*129-145, 1957.

Margerison, J. H., and Liddell, D. W.: Incidence of temporal lobe epilepsy among a hospital population of long-stay female epileptics, J Ment Sci *107:* 909-920, 1961.

Mattson, R. H., Pratt, K. L., and Calverly, J. R.: Electroencephalograms of epileptics following sleep deprivation, Arch Neurol (Chicago) *13:*310-315, 1965.

Mauceri, J., and Strauss, H.: Effects of chlorpromazine on the electroencephalogram with report of a case of chlorpromazine intoxication, Electroenceph Clin Neurophysiol *8:*671-675, 1956.

The Medical Letter 10 (September 20), 1968.

Merlis, S.: Discussion comment, *in* Chlorpromazine and Mental Health, Philadelphia, Lea, 1955.

Merskey, H., Rice, T., and Troupe, A.: Investigation of some therapeutic and physiological effects of perphenazine in Huntington's chorea, Psychopharmacologia *2:*436-445, 1961.

Metrakos, J. D., and Metrakos, K.: Genetics of convulsive disorders, I. Introduction, problems, methods, and base lines, Neurology (Minneap) *10:*228, 1960.

Metrakos, K., and Metrakos, J. D.: Genetics of convulsive disorders, II. Genetic and electroencephalographic studies in centrencephalic epilepsy, Neurology (Minneap) *11:*474-483, 1961.

Modlin, H. C.: Postaccident anxiety syndrome: psychosocial aspects, Amer J Psychiat *123:*1008-1012, 1967.

Mulder, D. W., and Daly, D.: Psychiatric symptoms associated with lesions of temporal lobe, JAMA *150:*173-176, 1952.

Nathanson, M.: The "unresponsive" state—organic versus psychogenic, J Hillside Hosp *15:*43-47, 1966.

Nicol, C. F.: Depression as viewed through neurologic spectacles, Psychosomatics *9:*252-254, 1968.

Niedermeyer, E., and Knott, J. R.: Psychiatric implications of the 14 and 6 positive spike pattern of the EEG, Proc III World Cong Psychiat, vol. 1, 1961, pp. 436-439.

O'Brien, J. L,. Goldensohn, E. S., and Hoefer, P. F. A.: Electroencephalographic abnormalities in addition to bilaterally synchronous 3 per second spike and wave activity in petit mal, Electroenceph Clin Neurophysiol *11:*747-761, 1959.

O'Connor, J. F., and Musher, D. M.: Central nervous involvement in systemic lupus erythematosus, Arch Neurol (Chicago) *14:*157-164, 1966.

Oliphant, J., Evans, J. I., and Forrest, A. D.: Huntington's chorea: Some biochemical and therapeutic aspects, Brit J Psychiat *106:*718-725, 1960.

Ommaya, A. K., and Yarnell, P.: Subdural hematoma after whiplash injury, Lancet *2:*237-239, 1969.

Oswald, I.: Sleeping and Waking: Physiology and Psychology, Amsterdam: Elsevier, 1962.

Ounsted, C.: Factors of inheritance in convulsive disorders in childhood, Proc Roy Soc Med *45:*865-868, 1952.

Parsonage, M. J., and Norris, J. W.: Use of diazepam in treatment of severe convulsive status epilepticus, Brit Med J *3:*85-88, 1967.

Patel, H., and Crichton, J. U.: Neurologic hazards of diphenylhydantoin in childhood, J Pediat *73:*676-684, 1968.

Penfield, W.: Memory mechanisms, Arch Neurol Psychiat *67:*178-198, 1952.

———: A surgeon's chance encounters with mechanisms related to consciousness, J Roy Coll Surg Edinb *5:*173-190, 1960.

Petersen, P.: Psychiatric disorders in primary hyperparathyroidism, J Clin Endocr *28:*1491-1495, 1968.

Pevehouse, B. C., Bloom, W. H., and McKissock, W.: Ophthalmologic aspects of diagnosis and localization of subdural hematoma, Neurology (Minneap) *10* (11):1037-1041, 1960.

Pond, D. A.: Psychiatric aspects of epilepsy, J Indian Med Prof *3:*1441-1443, 1957.

———: The influence of psychophysiological factors on epilepsy, J Psychosom Res *9:*5-20, 1965.

Posner, J. B.: Delirium and exogenous metabolic brain disease, *in* Beeson, P. B., and McDermott, W., eds.: Cecil-Loeb Textbook of Medicine, Philadelphia: Saunders, 1967, pp. 1437-1444.

Post, F.: Somatic and psychic factors in the treatment of elderly psychiatric patients, J Psychosom Res *10:*13-19, 1966.

Pratt, K. L., *et al.:* EEG activation of epileptics following sleep deprivation: Prospective study of 114 cases, Electroenceph Clin Neurophysiol *24:*11-15, 1968.

Preston, D. N., and Atack, E. A.: Temporal lobe epilepsy: Clinical study of 47 cases, Canad Med Ass J *91:*1256-1259, 1964.

Proctor, F., Prince, D., and Morrell, F.: Primary and secondary spike foci following depth lesions, Arch Neurol (Chicago) *15:*151-162, 1966.

Read, A. E., *et al.:* Neuropsychiatric syndromes associated with chronic liver disease and an extensive portal-systemic collateral circulation, Quart J Med *36:* 135-150, 1967.

Rechtschaffen, A., *et al.:* Nocturnal sleep of narcoleptics, Electroenceph Clin Neurophysiol *15:*599-609, 1963.

Reynolds, E. H.: Schizophrenia-like psychoses of epilepsy and disturbances of folate and vitamin B_{12} metabolism induced by anti-convulsant drugs, Brit J Psychiat *113:*911-919, 1967.

Robertson, E.: Photogenic epilepsy: Self-precipitated attacks, Brain *77:*232-251, 1954.

Roseman, E.: Dilantin toxicity: clinical and electroencephalographic study, Neurology (Minneap) *11:*912-921, 1961.

Rusk, H.: How far can we take the brain-damaged patient? Med Opin Rev *1:*13-17, 1965.

Russell, W. R.: After-effect of head injury, Trans Med Chir Soc Edin *41:*129-144, 1933.

Russell, W. R., and Whitty, C. W. M.: Studies in traumatic epilepsy; 1. Factors influencing the incidence of epilepsy after brain wounds, J Neurol Neurosurg Psychiat *15:*93-98, 1952.

———: Studies in traumatic epilepsy; 2. Focal motor and somatic sensory fits: Study of 85 cases, J Neurol Neurosurg Psychiat *16:*73-97, 1953.

———: Studies in traumatic epilepsy; 3. Visual fits, J Neurol Neurosurg Psychiat *18:*79-96, 1955.

Sandstead, H. H., Carter, J. P., and Darby, W. J.: How to diagnose nutritional disorders in daily practice, Nutr Today *4:*20-25, 1969.

Schutt, C. H., and Dohan, F. C.: Neck injury to women in auto accidents. A metropolitan plague, JAMA *206:*2689-2692, 1968.

Schwab, J. J.: Psychiatric illnesses produced by infections, Hosp Med, Oct., 1969, pp. 98-108.

Seidl, L. G., *et al.:* Studies on the epidemiology of adverse drug reactions; II. Reactions in patients on a general medical service, Bull Hopkins Hosp *119:*299-315, 1966.

Serafetinides, E. A., and Falconer, M. A.: Effects of temporal lobectomy in epileptic patients with psychosis, J Ment Sci *108:* 584-593, 1962.

Sharpless, S. K.: Hypnotics and sedatives. I. The barbiturates, *in* Goodman, L. S., and Gilman, A., eds.: The Pharmacological Basis of Therapeutics, ed 3, New York, Macmillan, 1965, pp. 105-128.

Shearer, M. L., and Finch, S. M.: Periodic organic psychosis associated with recurrent herpes simplex, New Eng J Med 271:494-497, 1964.

Sheeby, B. N., Little, S. C., and Stone, J. J.: Abdominal epilepsy, J Pediat 56: 355-363, 1960.

Sheehan, H. L.: Simmonds's disease due to postpartum necrosis of the anterior pituitary, Quart J Med 8:277-309, 1939.

Sherwood, S. L.: Self-induced epilepsy: collection of self-induced epilepsy cases, Arch Neurol (Chicago) 6:49-65, 1962.

Slater, E., and Roth, M.: Mayer-Gross Clinical Psychiatry, ed. 3, Baltimore: Williams & Wilkins, 1969.

Snaith, R. P., Mehta, S., and Raby, A. H.: Serum folate and vitamin B_{12} in epileptics with and without mental illness, Brit J Psychiat 116:179-183, 1970.

Sodeman, W. A.: Diagnosis and treatment of digitalis toxicity, New Eng J Med 273:35-37, 1965.

Sours, J. A.: Narcolepsy and other disturbances in the sleep-waking rhythm: Study of 115 cases with review of the literature, J Nerv Ment Dis 137:525-542, 1963.

Steiner, W. G., and Pollack, S. L.: Limited usefulness of EEG as a diagnostic aid in psychiatric cases receiving tranquilizing drug therapy, in Himwich, W. A., and Schade, J. P., eds.: Progress in Brain Research, vol. 16, Amsterdam: Elsevier, 1965.

Stenbäck, A., and Haapanen, E.: Azotemia and psychosis, Acta Psychiat Scand 43:9-65, 1967.

Sternlieb, I., and Scheinberg, I. H.: Prevention of Wilson's disease in asymptomatic patients, New Eng J Med 278:352-359, 1968.

Stevens, J. R.: Psychiatric implications of psychomotor epilepsy, Arch Gen Psychiat (Chicago) 14:461-471, 1966.

Strachan, R. W., and Henderson, J. G.: Psychiatric syndromes due to avitaminosis B_{12} with normal blood and marrow, Quart J Med 34:303-317, 1965.

Strang, R. R.: Imipramine in the treatment of Parkinsonism: double-blind placebo study, Brit Med J 2:33-34, 1965.

Strobos, R. J., and Kavallinis, G. P.: Changes in repeat electroencephalograms in epileptics, Neurology (Minneap) 18:622-633, 1968.

Surridge, D.: Investigation into some psychiatric aspects of multiple sclerosis, Brit J Psychiat 115:749-764, 1969.

Swerdlow, B.: Acute brain syndrome associated with sodium diphenylhydantoin intoxication, Amer J Psychiat 122:100-101, 1965.

Symonds, C. P.: Traumatic epilepsy, Lancet 2:1217-1220, 1935.

——: Concussion and contusion of the brain and their sequelae, in Brock, S., ed.: Injuries of the Brain and Spinal Cord and Their Coverings, ed. 3, Baltimore: Williams & Wilkins, 1949, pp. 71-115.

Torres, F., and Shapiro, S. K.: Electroencephalograms in whiplash injury: Comparison of electroencephalographic abnormalities with those present in closed head injuries, Arch Neurol (Chicago) 5:28-35, 1961.

Tseitlin, V. L.: Psychic disorders in disseminated lupus erythematosus, Soviet Psychol Psychiat 2:58-61, 1963.

Tyler, H. R.: Neurologic disorders in renal failure, Amer J Med 44:734-748, 1968.

Ullman, M., and Gruen, A.: Behavioral changes in patients with strokes, Amer J Psychiat 117:1004-1009, 1961.

Unterberger, H., and Reynolds, A. S.: Study of chronic organic brain disorders in a psychiatric hospital, Behav Neuropsychiat 1:18-22, 1969.

Vispo, R. H.: Pre-morbid personality in the functional psychoses of the senium. A comparison of ex-patients with healthy controls, J Ment Sci 108:790-800, 1962.

Vizioli, R.: Clinical and EEG study on infantile and childhood epilepsy, Epilepsia (Amst) 3:1-13, 1962.

Von Werssowetz, O. F.: Mental and emotional readjustment of the hemiplegic patient, Psychiat Dig 27:24-37, 1966.

Walker, A. E.: State of consciousness in focal motor convulsions, Epilepsia (Amst) 1:592-599, 1960.

Walton, D.: Diagnostic and predictive accuracy of the modified word learning test in psychiatric patients over 65, Brit J Psychiat 104:1111-1117, 1958.

Wang, H.-S.: Organic brain syndromes, in Busse, E. W., and Pfeiffer, E., eds.: Behavior and Adaptation in Late Life, Boston: Little, 1969, pp. 263-287.

Weinberg, M. H.: Fatigue as a precipitating factor in latent epilepsy, J Nerv Ment Dis 101:251-256, 1945.

Weinstein, M. R., and Fischer, A.: Electroconvulsive treatment of a patient with artificial mitral and aortic valves, Amer J Psychiat 123:882-884, 1967.

Welch, L. K.: Head injury, a clinical perspective, Aerospace Med 39:1231-1235, 1968.

Whittier, J. R., and Korenyi, C.: Effect

of oral fluphenazine on Huntington's chorea, Int J Neuropsychiat *4:*1-3, 1968.

Whitty, C. W. M., and Zangwill, O. L.: Traumatic amnesia, *in* Whitty, C. W. M., and Zangwill, O. L., eds.: Amnesia, London: Butterworth, 1966, pp. 92-108.

Whybrow, P. C., Prange, A. J., and Treadway, C. R.: Mental changes accompanying thyroid gland dysfunction, Arch Gen Psychiat (Chicago) *20:*48-63, 1969.

Winkelman, N. W.: Chlorpromazine in the treatment of neuropsychiatric disorders, JAMA *155:*18-21, 1954.

Yahr, M. D.: Drug therapy of convulsive seizures, Int J Neurol *1:*76-82, 1959.

Yoss, R. E., and Daly, D. D.: Criteria for the diagnosis of the narcoleptic syndrome, Mayo Clin Proc *32:*320-328, 1957.

————: Narcolepsy, Med Clin N Amer *44:* 953-968, 1960.

Young, D., and Scoville, W. B.: Paranoid psychosis in narcolepsy and the possible danger of benzedrine treatment, Med Clin N Amer *22:*637-646, 1938.

Zane, M. D.: Therapeutic process and behavior—as observed in physical rehabilitation, Amer J Psychiat *119:*246-250, 1962.

Zeman, F. D.: Myth and stereotype in the clinical medicine of old age, New Eng J Med *272:*1104-1106, 1965.

Ziegler, D. K.: Neurological disease and hysteria—differential diagnosis, Int J Neuropsychiat *3:*388-396, 1967.

Ziskind, E., *et al.:* Hypnoid syndrome in sensory deprivation, Recent Advances Biol Psychiat *5:*331-346, 1963.

CHAPTER

TWELVE

The Psychiatrist as Consultant

THE EXIGENCIES OF THE MODERN WORLD have forced man to come to grips with the reality that his behavior falls short of the ideals of logic, reason, and humanitarianism to which he aspires. This realization has led him increasingly to seek advice about all manner of problems as well as mental illness from the professional whose business is pathologic irrationality—the psychiatrist. Judges consult him about criminal responsibility and testamentary competence; educators ask for help in improving pedagogic techniques for the slow or the fast learner; correctional workers enlist his aid in looking for effective ways to help a man go straight; industrial managers turn to him for shortcuts to improved productivity and morale. Lawmakers, city planners, even leaders of the nation ask the psychiatrist to help with the planning and implementation of social engineering programs intended to solve the age-old problems of injustice, poverty, greed, and war. Whether the psychiatrist is more competent or knows more about these matters than the well-informed layman is a question too broad to discuss in a text devoted to treatment. We shall therefore confine our discussion of his consultative functions to those he performs for colleagues in other branches of medicine in conjunction with patient care.

THE PSYCHIATRIST'S ROLE IN THE MANAGEMENT OF MEDICAL, SURGICAL, AND OBSTETRIC PATIENTS

The psychiatrist's role as a consultant is most clearly defined when the referring physician is satisfied with his own assessment of the patient's medical condition but has specific questions regarding the patient's psychological well-being or psychosocial management. When mental symptoms develop in the course of a medical condition, the psychiatrist may be asked whether they are somehow related to the condition or the treatment the patient is receiving for it, or are independent of both. Similarly, when a mentally ill patient must undergo surgery, the psychiatrist may be asked

1/ how the operation will affect the patient's psychological condition,

2/ how the drugs he has been using (whether prescribed or purchased illicitly) will affect his operative course, and

3/ how competently he will collaborate with the surgeon in the postoperative period.

Again, when a woman who is pregnant develops a mental illness or a woman who is or has been mentally ill becomes pregnant, he may be consulted regarding her psychiatric management or the advisability of a therapeutic abortion or sterilization.

Psychiatric Aspects of Medical and Surgical Illnesses

When a patient develops anxiety, depression, agitation, confusion, or massive denial during the course of a medical illness, the psychiatrist must try to distinguish between 1/ the effect of the patient's illness or treatment on the functioning of his central nervous system (see p. 404), 2/ the effect of his attitude toward his illness or treatment on his social and psychological functioning, and 3/ the effect of the many stresses inherent in being ill on his adaptive skills. Pain, respiratory distress, and a host of other symptoms can disturb the patient's sleep and, with it, his psychological well-being. Anemia, hypercapnia, and acidosis, as well as radiation therapy, innumerable drugs, and even the enforced bed rest common to most hospital regimens can all lead to fatigue, apathy, and confusion. The patient's response to his illness can also be significantly shaped by such consequences of the illness as uncertainty about the future, separation from his family, concern about financial arrangements, the physical and mental discomfort of being subjected to a multitude of diagnostic procedures about which he knows little except that their outcome may be vital to his health, and the need to depend on the competence and kindness of others in an unfamiliar and sometimes impersonal environment.

While the demands made on the patient's adaptive skills vary from one illness to the next, they are obviously greatest when his life is in jeopardy. Psychiatric problems are thus particularly common in patients with terminal illnesses, those with renal insufficiency severe enough to require periodic hemodialysis, and those who require transplantation of some vital organ (Abram 1969, Kemph 1969). The stresses are also considerable when the illness forces the individual to adopt entirely new attitudes and living patterns (Lesse 1967): a woman who has built her life around her goods looks thus reacts more strongly to a mastectomy or a masculinizing tumor than one who has largely ignored them. Prior experience with the illness in question also affects the patient's way of dealing with it: the individual with a family member who died of diabetic gangrene will obviously be more upset about developing diabetes than one who has had no such experience (Lipowski 1967b).

Even in the presence of such sensitizing factors, most patients cope fairly well with serious illness (Hackett 1968, Patterson 1963). Those who do not are often found to have a history of psychiatric illness or at least enough premorbid symptoms to suggest a preexistent subclinical disorder that has erupted under the stress of the current illness (Knox 1961). Whatever its cause, emotional turmoil can impede the treatment of medical illness. If, in response to the news that he must undergo surgery, a patient becomes anxious, dissociates, despairs of getting well, or denies that he is ill and thus is unable or unwilling to provide a valid consent for an operation, his psychological difficulties may need to be explored before the operation can proceed.

Since the patient's fantasies and conjectures about his illness often add to his fear and discomfort, it is important to keep him as informed as practicable about what to expect (Janis 1958, 1964). Explaining the planned diagnostic and therapeutic procedures generally has a far more salutary effect than any tranquilizer could. Even such somatic symptoms as postoperative nausea and pain can be lessened if the patient is warned about them in advance (Egbert 1964). The explanations, of course, must be geared to the patient's current level of comprehension. When he is too confused, frightened, or intellectually limited to benefit from a full explanation of his disorder, he should nonetheless be repeatedly reassured and told just what is likely to happen next.

How much of the truth the critically ill or the *dying patient* should be told is a question that has long engaged medical attention. All too often the answer reflects the physician's moral convictions rather than his concern to keep the patient comfortable, functioning, and collaborative for as long as possible. The question becomes even more crucial when the patient's family tries to reassure him (and themselves) and to avoid painful or embarrassing scenes by plying him with lies, distortions, and unbelievable explanations of his symptoms. After a few days of this, the relatively astute patient starts to feel like a fragile fool and, recognizing that his family has come to regard him as an object and not as a person, feels increasingly isolated (Ellard 1968).

We do not mean to suggest that the patient must be confronted with the realization that he may die on the operating table or that his disease is fatal, but only to point out how excessive efforts to conceal the worst may make him feel more anxious than the news itself would (Mozden 1969). Indeed, to insist on principle that the patient has a right to know that his disease is fatal can be as inhumane and nonsensical as denying him anesthetics on the ground that he has the right to know he is in pain (Ravitch 1969). Fortunately, the patient usually makes it clear that he does not want to know how grave his condition is and, if told of it, is apt to forget it. More important than a knowledge of the gravity of his situation is the knowledge that some friend or relative will be nearby throughout the illness or operation. Even the patient who is estranged from his family (perhaps after face-saving protestations of not wanting to see them) will be glad to have family members nearby.

No matter how effective the family's or even the doctor's support has been, its impact can be vitiated by such unexpected or threatening experiences as the patient's awakening from an operation to discover that the procedure has been more extensive or disfiguring than he expected; finding himself surrounded by others who are disabled or dying, as in an intensive care unit (Bruhn 1970); or suddenly developing symptoms when the physician he knows best is not around. Anticipating and, whenever possible, avoiding such experiences is imperative.

DECISIONS CONCERNING THE ADVISABILITY OR TIMING OF SURGERY

When a patient who is slated for surgery seems excessively anxious or otherwise disturbed, the psychiatrist may be asked whether the procedure should be postponed. The question must be answered by weighing the seriousness and the type of mental disturbance against the urgency of attending to the surgical condition. If the procedure is elective and the patient's dread of the surgery is not the prime cause of his symptoms, it might be best to arrange a brief postponement during which a vigorous attempt can be made to alleviate the patient's psychiatric symptoms. Even if the procedure is elective, however, it is usually not advisable to postpone it for long, especially if there is a chance that the surgery will improve the patient's social functioning. If, for example, a middle-aged paranoid and depressed patient requires aural fenestration or cataract surgery but asks to postpone the procedure until he feels "up to it" or "more like myself," the decision must take into account that any improvement in the patient's perceptual apparatus is likely to have a salutary effect on his psychological symptoms. When the surgical procedure is not elective but mandatory, the patient's psychological condition should not be considered grounds for postponing the procedure and the psychiatrist's role is to make recommendations concerning the kind of supervision the patient is likely to need in the pre- and postoperative period. If the patient is expected to require close supervision or is considered likely to benefit from continuous interpersonal contacts, it may be advisable to have a psychiatric nurse in attendance, even on the surgical division. This course is preferable in any event to transferring the patient to a psychiatric service, where he is less likely to obtain the intensive medical care he needs.

With the increase in *cardiac surgery* and *organ transplants*, psychiatrists are often asked whether the patient is a good candidate for such a procedure. While the patient's postoperative psychosocial adjustment depends to some extent on his preoperative level of functioning (Kennedy 1966, Kimball 1969), it depends even more on the extent to which his biologic functioning can be restored and the degree of support available to him in the recovery phase (Greene 1969).

The psychiatrist may also be asked to see the patient who desires *cosmetic surgery,* especially if there is current or past evidence of mental illness. Because the patient's satisfaction with the outcome depends largely on the realism of his expectations for change, he must be made to understand that the improvement in his looks, by itself, will not enhance his social acceptability, job performance, or romantic pursuits. If such warnings appear to be falling on deaf ears, if the procedure required seems disproportionate to the severity of the disfigurement, or if the patient has a history of psychiatric disorder or a long series of prior cosmetic operations for minor disfigurements, the surgeon should be alerted to the possibility that the patient may be disappointed by the outcome and become seriously and overtly disturbed afterward (Taylor 1966).

The Question of Abortion

Seldom is the psychiatrist's role as a consultant to his medical colleagues so complex and beset with nonmedical issues as when his advice is sought in the psychological problems of unwanted pregnancy. Ostensibly, he is asked only to render an objective judgment concerning the effect that continued pregnancy would have on the patient's safety and psychological well-being; in reality, however, he is often under pressure—both external and internal—to evaluate the situation in terms of its psychosocial consequences (D. H. Russell 1967). In many states, he is used as a safety valve by which repressive abortion laws can be mitigated, especially for the affluent (Gold 1965, Hall 1967). In others, the law has been liberalized to allow for psychosocial factors, and the psychiatrist is assigned the job of assessor (Schur 1968).

Unfortunately, most studies intended to investigate objectively the dangers to mother or child of the mother's mental illness during or immediately after pregnancy tend to stray far beyond the realm of psychiatry and delve into such moral issues as woman's right to make decisions regarding her own body, the need for population control, and the possibility that the community's moral standards might be jeopardized by freeing the sexually active woman from the inhibiting fear of impregnation (Gap 1969, Sloane 1969).

To simplify the discussion, let us state the case *against* the psychiatric recommendation of abortion:

1/ on the basis of a patient's current condition or her past history, it cannot be predicted with any precision whether she will become psychotic in a subsequent pregnancy;

2/ there is no evidence that psychotic illness remits more rapidly if the patient is aborted;

3/ in almost all cases, patients whose mental illnesses arise during pregnancy can be as well or better safeguarded against the dangers of suicide or further deterioration by means other than abortion (Arén 1961);

4/ patients who visit a psychiatrist for the first time during an unwanted pregnancy do not, despite their stated desire for help, tend to continue in treatment (Bolter 1962).

Factors *in favor* of recommending abortions are that

1/ the woman who develops a mental illness during pregnancy may be undertreated out of concern for the fetus and thus unduly exposed to the dangers of her illness;

2/ a mentally ill mother, even if able to function, is not likely to be able to give proper care to either the newborn or her other children;

3/ there is little likelihood that abortion will be followed by severe guilt or psychosis (Clark 1968, Niswander 1966, Patt 1969, Peck 1966, Simon 1967);

4/ the frequently cited statistic that the suicide rate of pregnant women is low is irrelevant for the depressed patient;

5/ the incidence of fantasied, attempted, or actual infanticide is remarkably high among women suffering from a postpartum psychosis (Bratfos 1966), and the guilt associated with these events, even if they have been only fantasied, may be a source of self-torture for years; and

6/ women who have had an affective disorder in the puerperium are ten times as likely as the general population to develop another.

Taking the foregoing considerations into account, we recommend a therapeutic abortion if the woman desires it and has had a prior episode of psychotic illness that *1/* occurred during or immediately after a previous pregnancy, *2/* was accompanied by impulse control disturbances (suicidal or aggressive concerns or behavior), *3/* required hospitalization for several months or *4/* disabled her so that she could not care for her children or house for more than two months. Abortion may also be indicated if *5/* the patient is currently psychotic, her socioeconomic status and personal relationships are unsatisfactory or unsupportive, and it is impossible to provide full-time supervision, *6/* the pregnancy is a result of rape or incest, or *7/* the patient is unable to care for the children she currently has.

Even when, on the basis of the patient's history and the clinical impressions gained in the interview, a therapeutic abortion seems advisable, the sincerity of the patient's desire to terminate pregnancy must be probed. Not infrequently, she is yielding to the wishes and pressures of others. This might be the case when young unmarried women want an abortion in order to protect the family name or to spare the boyfriend embarrassment. Catholic wives in religiously mixed marriages may similarly mute their scruples in order to demonstrate to their husbands that they are sophisticated enough to disregard their own value systems. The patient's wish to terminate her pregnancy can be rooted in delusional self-derogation: she may consider herself "bad," a poor mother, or incurably sick. When there is any question concerning the patient's motives (or the husband's desires, if she is married), an attempt must be made to clarify the issues in the presence of the spouse or other significant relatives. Both in these meetings and in those with the patient alone, the psychiatrist must guard against the intrusion of his own moral views.

Just as the desire for an abortion can be irrational, so can the desire to become pregnant. A classic example (and one in which a psychiatrist is often consulted about the merits of abortion) is the woman who, since adolescence or since her first delivery, has had a chronic depression that lifts only when she becomes pregnant but recurs after delivery. Once she has noticed how much better she feels when pregnant, she may try desperately, in the midst of depression, to become pregnant again. Because this is a short-term solution at best, and a dangerous one, she must be dissuaded from taking this road to recovery. Traditional antidepressant regimens are usually effective; in some cases, the symptoms may be relieved by continuous administration of estrogens in doses that are increased whenever breakthrough bleeding occurs.

The surest way to avoid the problems inherent in pregnancy and the fear of pregnancy is to give the patient advice on contraception. The choice between mechanical devices, contraceptive drugs, tubal ligation, or vasectomy should be left to the gynecologist and the couple, though the psychiatrist must advise whether the patient is rational and efficient enough to assume the responsibility of inserting a diaphragm, taking a pill, or checking the position of an intrauterine device. The psychotoxic effects of contraceptive drugs are not yet fully known. Some patients seem to feel better when taking them, while others seem to feel worse. Contraceptive-induced aggravation or development of a depression (Kane 1968) is particularly common in patients with a prior or family history of depression (Kimball unpublished data) or when the progestin content is of high proportion, and it is reasonably well documented that such adverse effects persist even after the patient has been taking oral contraceptives for some time (Behrman 1969, Lewis 1969, Nilsson 1968.) While these drugs are known to have a wide range of organic effects, including EEG changes (Matsumoto 1966), both the favorable and the unfavorable effects on the patient's mood may be psychological in origin and related to her freedom from the fear of impregnation, her feeling that she is behaving immorally or is no longer a "complete woman," or her husband's displeasure over her "infertility" (Lidz 1969).

Psychotropic Agents in the Management of Medical, Surgical, and Obstetric Patients

We have emphasized before (see Chapters 2, 4, 10, and 11) that, in prescribing a psychotropic agent, the psychiatrist must take into account its total systemic effect and its compatibility with the patient's medical condition as well as his current treatment. For example, a patient immobilized while recovering from a fracture ought not be given a phenothiazine that is liable to produce akathisia or dyskinesia. Similarly, as he begins to walk, he should not be given an agent that causes hypotension or ataxia. It is also important to remember that

1/ a wide variety of apparently unrelated drugs can be potentiated by MAO inhibitors (see p. 605),

2/ many tranquilizing and antidepressant drugs produce electrocardiographic and electroencephalographic changes and thus lead to diagnostic confusion (see pp. 435 and 584),

3/ cardiac arrhythmias and hypotension have been observed following the administration of imipramine and its congeners (see p. 603), and

4/ reserpine is contraindicated in patients with a history of peptic ulcer (see p. 595).

A patient's response to a psychotropic agent, moreover, can be altered by both psychological and biologic stress. Like the epileptic taking anticonvulsants, the diabetic taking insulin, or the cardiac patient taking digitalis, the psychiatric patient may react differently to the psychotropic agent he is taking after being exposed to an unsettling event or a medical illness. A dosage level that has previously controlled his symptoms satisfactorily may prove to be inadequate or excessive, thus aggravating the original symptoms or causing the drug's side effects to become intolerable.

To avoid such complications, the patient's psychological distress should be relieved, whenever possible, with environmental support alone. If sedation is needed, a rapidly acting sedative may be preferable to a tranquilizer. If the patient is already taking tranquilizers or antidepressants, their suspension may be indicated until after the medical diagnosis has been established, the surgical procedures have been completed, or the clinical course has stabilized. This is not always feasible, especially if the patient is so delirious or disorganized that he cannot be managed without phenothiazines, or he is so dependent on their continued use that without them he is likely to decompensate within hours or days. Discontinuing phenothiazines at the time of a medical or surgical emergency, moreover, is seldom of practical significance, for their effects persist in some degree for days or weeks. In addition, almost all of their deleterious effects during surgery can be avoided by informing the anesthesiologist just what drugs have previously been used (Alper 1963, Elliott 1962).

Although there is no evidence that psychotropic agents increase the incidence of malformations in the newborn (Ayd 1964, Kris 1962, Vorster 1965), the tragic consequences that followed the widespread use of thalidomide serve as a reminder that conservatism is warranted in administering any new drug to a pregnant woman. This is particularly true for psychotropic agents, as the majority pass the placental barrier (Baker 1960) and thereby affect the fetus and newborn. Infants whose mothers have been given phenothiazines or reserpine in the days or weeks prior to delivery may exhibit prolonged respiratory distress, abnormal muscle activity, lethargy, and anorexia (Budnick 1955, Hill 1964, 1966); those born to mothers taking reserpine may also suffer from nasal congestion and, as a result, feeding difficulties.

Since such complications are not encountered with the use of succinylcholine-modified electroshock therapy, this treatment is to be preferred to high doses of psychotropic drugs whenever a pregnant patient is agitated, impulsive, or suicidal (Impastato 1964, Sobel 1960) (see p. 647). If her condition is refractory to ECT and there is no choice except to give her a psychotropic agent, it should be administered in as low dosage as possible during the first trimester and, if feasible, reduced or discontinued altogether 10 to 14 days before the baby is due.

When the patient has been using a drug that produces physical dependence, the psychiatrist may be called in to manage the withdrawal schedule. In general, the principles outlined in Chapter 9 for the management of drug abuse are applicable to medical, surgical, and obstetric patients as well. With the exception of alcohol, which cannot be titrated with sufficient precision and is therefore replaced with a minor tranquilizer, it is usually best to give the patient the same drug to which physical dependence has developed. Withdrawal should proceed somewhat more slowly, and be extended over a period of two to three weeks rather than the 10 days that are sufficient for patients without a concomitant disease. When a patient who has used drugs that produce withdrawal syndromes goes into labor, both the obstetrician and the pediatrician should be alerted to the possibility that the baby, too, may show withdrawal symptoms (Nichols 1967, Van Leeuwen 1965) and that both baby and mother may need to be placed on a withdrawal schedule (Hill 1963). Because the patient addicted to sedatives is often depressed and tends to become more so after delivery, it is usually best to transfer her to a psychiatric service both to complete the withdrawal schedule and to reevaluate her in a drug-free state.

DISTURBANCES IN THE
DOCTOR-PATIENT-FAMILY RELATIONSHIP

Consultation requests are not always clear-cut, however, especially when they are based on some entanglement in the skein of relationships between the referring doctor, the patient, and the patient's family. Such entanglements are particularly apt to occur when the diagnosis is uncertain or the patient's illness is prolonged; under these circumstances, both patient and family may feel dissatisfied with the treating physician, the family may feel excessively burdened by the patient, and the physician may feel puzzled and frustrated by both (Coles 1969). As a result, the physician's ability to provide adequate medical care may suffer, the patient's symptoms worsen, and the family's willingness to take care of the patient or collaborate with the doctor deteriorate (Lipowski 1967a).

Among the most common of such disturbances is *conflict between the patient and his family* that arises in relation to his illness. Such problems occur when the patient's symptoms, physical or mental, disrupt the family's traditional way of functioning, or the patient makes demands quite beyond those he requires to achieve symptom relief. However his requests are expressed, their general tenor is likely to be: "Stay with me," "Don't upset me," or "Do it for me." Which of these demands the patient makes and how he expresses it depends to some extent on his personality, but is also determined by the nature of his illness and the manner in which his symptoms lend themselves to communicative purposes. If he has an illness (such as asthma) that can cause him to need help rapidly, he is most likely to ask that he not be left alone. If the illness (like heart disease) can be aggravated by psychological stress, he may want his physical environment to remain stable. If the illness is one that has immobilized him (such as multiple sclerosis or a hemiplegia following a stroke), he may expect those around him to assume tasks that would otherwise have been his.

While such demands can be burdensome for any family, they are most likely to provoke conflict when the family considers them illegitimate, feels that the patient has become inordinately dependent or passive, or believes that he is using his symptoms to control their lives. The mother who gasps, clutches her chest, and tells her son that his marriage will kill her is so common as to have become a caricature. The diabetic child who refuses his insulin or breaks his prescribed diet whenever his parents quarrel differs from the blackmailing mother only in that his maneuvers are less direct and more likely to help him avoid the difficulties by escape from the combat zone to the quiet and safety of the hospital.

Even when the patient's illness is genuine and the resulting disability severe enough to legitimize his requests, his family may be too busy, too anxious, or too poor to tolerate the extra burdens. This can lead them to feel guilty and, in turn, to deny that his illness is genuine or his requests legitimate. In other cases, either to assuage a sense of guilt or to keep the patient dependent on them, the family complies with all such demands, even those that are unreasonable and have nothing to do with relieving his symptoms; they may even insist that the doctor follow their example and are offended if he refuses. Under any of these circumstances, the referring doctor, caught in the middle, may turn for assistance to the psychiatrist in the hope that his expertise in interpersonal relationships will shed light on the problems and help solve them.

Less common, but equally problematic, is a *disturbance in the doctor's relationship with the patient or his family.* The most clear-cut expression of this kind of difficulty is the refusal to follow the doctor's orders. Minor derelictions, such as the failure to stop smoking or to diet, will not usually come to the psychiatrist's attention, but he may well be consulted about more serious ones, like a brittle diabetic's refusal to take insulin or follow the prescribed diet, a neurologically impaired patient's refusal to submit to a lumbar puncture, or a family's insistence that a critically ill patient leave the hospital. Reluctance to follow medical advice may be rooted in some unfounded fear that they cannot discuss with the physician in charge (Pasternack 1969), like a patient's belief that a hysterectomy will dampen her sexual interest or attractiveness, but usually the causes are far deeper than mere misinformation. For example, a family may become jealous of the patient's dependence on and fondness for the physician, and insist (usually covertly) that he demonstrate his loyalty to them by ignoring the doctor's recommendations or by changing doctors. These situations are by no means uncommon, but the psychiatrist is rarely involved early enough to be of much help: he is generally called just before the patient signs out of the hospital, when it is useless to find out why they are all angry with the patient's physician, and all he can do is suggest that they get advice from another doctor before taking any precipitous and potentially harmful step (Himmelhoch 1970).

A patient may also be sent to a psychiatrist because he is so hostile, complaining, or dependent that the doctor finds it difficult to make a diagnosis or provide care. Although the referring physician may be frank in acknowledging his irritation with the patient, the referral more commonly sails under false colors, and the psychiatrist is told that the patient's symptoms are illogical, devoid of physical causation, psychogenic, imaginary, self-inflicted, indicative of a mental illness, or that they reflect a desire to get attention or to be difficult. Whatever the acknowledged reason for referral, the psychiatrist must bear in mind that it could be related to some unspoken disturbance in the patient-family-doctor axis (Schwab 1968). That the patient's symptoms are unusual or obscure in origin or that his personality is irritating is no evidence that his disorder is psychogenic or that his complaints are "all in his mind." Thus, when the psychiatrist is asked to evaluate a patient whose symptoms are puzzling, whose response to treatment is unsatisfactory or unusual, or whose behavior is obnoxious, he must note the referring physician's frustration and dissatisfaction (Astrachan 1966). He should not become, however, so fascinated with the interpersonal dynamics that he ignores the unusual features of the patient's behavior and the need for a proper diagnosis. One risk a patient runs when a psychiatrist is consulted is that his complaints will come to be "understood" and thus not investigated or treated. The psychiatrist must therefore decide whether there has been an adequate medical work-up, and if he has any doubts, suggest that another consultant be called to help complete the diagnostic evaluation. Once he is satisfied that the problems for which he is being consulted are not due to some undiagnosed mental or physical illness, but to the relationship between the individuals involved, he is ready to formulate a treatment plan.

While it is usually sufficient to encourage the participants to discuss their interpersonal difficulties with each other, this kind of intervention would not seem to require the services of a psychiatrist. There are several reasons, however, why he is better equipped than the referring doctor to explore the psychological difficulties that might have contributed to the patient's illness, affected his response to treatment, or disturbed his relationship to the doctor. First, the patient may experience less embarrassment in talking to a stranger about his feelings toward his family or physician than he would in telling them directly (Lipsitt 1969). The psychiatrist, moreover, has learned to protect himself against the impact of such feelings as anger or dependence by considering them manifestations of transference rather than personal attacks or demands (Szasz 1963). For this reason and because of his special training, he is likely to be more alert than the referring physician to the patient's indirect responses—his nonverbal behavior and psychological stance. The psychiatrist may be able to use his own relationship with the patient as the context within which to explore the patient's traditional mode of relating to doctors or other authority figures, and thus to clarify for the referring physician why and how the patient's relationships to his family and doctor are disturbed. He may also find it useful to invite the referring physician to participate in family meetings to observe how intrafamilial stresses contribute to the obstacles he faces in managing the patient. In most cases, however, neither the family nor the treating physician need be involved, for the patient wants nothing more than an opportunity to talk about his fears with impunity.

PSYCHIATRIC MANAGEMENT OF SYNDROMES WITH PRIMARILY SOMATIC SYMPTOMS AND SIGNS

Psychiatric consultations are increasingly initiated by the referring physician's belief that the patient's somatic symptoms or illness are caused or aggravated by his psychological problems. This view is especially likely when the patient's symptoms

1/ respect no anatomic or physiologic boundaries,

2/ cannot be accounted for by concomitant physical findings,

3/ are described by the patient in so metaphoric or histrionic a manner that they appear inconsistent with any known nonpsychiatric disease (Walters 1961),

4/ suggest that the patient is suffering from a mental illness (as when they are delusionally elaborated, associated with a depressed mood, or show diurnal exacerbation), or

5/ are based on the patient's persistence in practices that are obviously harmful to his health (as in the case of anorexia nervosa or obesity).

SOMATIC COMPLAINTS OF UNKNOWN ORIGIN

The patient who complains of pain or other somatic disturbances and whose examination reveals no organic basis for his complaints may be labeled in several different ways. Which label he receives depends less on his symptoms than it does on his general demeanor, his attitude toward his symptoms, or his doctor's attitude toward him. When he appears depressed and his mood disturbance is as conspicuous as his somatic complaints, his disorder will probably be called a *somatized depression*. When the physical complaints are dominant and the depression absent or of lesser impact, his disorder is likely to be labeled *hypochondriasis* (Kenyon 1964, 1965). When his discomfort is less conspicuous than his dysfunction, and especially when he appears indifferent to his disturbances or behaves histrionically, his disorder is commonly termed a *conversion neurosis*. That the patient with a headache whose complaints are considered genuine or respond to biologic treatment (like ergotamine) is said to be suffering from a *psychophysiologic disorder,* while the one whose personality is difficult or whose headaches are frustratingly unresponsive to treatment is said to be suffering from *hysteria,* demonstrates not only that the labeling process is as arbitrary as the categories are poorly defined but also that the labels serve pejorative as well as descriptive purposes.

The label given a patient's disorder might be irrelevant were it not for the dangers inherent in assuming complaints to be psychogenic merely because no organic cause can be found or because the patient's behavior is odd. Once his symptoms have been called psychogenic, he is ever after likely to find a prejudiced medical audience that assumes him to be "converting" anxiety and tends to ignore other alternatives. Personality changes, severe anxiety, or a depressed mood, however, can be the first, and for some months or even years the only, signs of such serious illnesses as presenile dementias, pernicious anemia, or carcinoma of the pancreas (Fras 1967, Mitchell 1967). That out of a group of 85 patients labeled as "hysteric" in a university hospital only 22 could still be given the same label 10 years later, the remainder having died, become psychotic, or shown themselves to be suffering from some unmistakable organic disease (Slater 1965), illustrates the dangers in using this term and the need to remain alert to alternative explanations of the patient's symptoms. Similarly prejudicial labels are used for patients who, after suffering a head injury, start to complain of headaches, irritability, easy fatigability, dizziness, difficulty in concentration, insomnia, decreased libido, and lowered tolerance to alcohol. If an automobile or industrial accident involves them in litigation or entitles them to compensation or sick leave, they may suddenly come to be labeled as suffering from a *compensation neurosis* or even to be *malingering*. The foregoing concatenation of symptoms, however, is so commonly associated with head injuries that its genuineness can scarcely be doubted (Fellner 1964) (see p. 424).

In the foregoing observations, we do not intend to ignore the numerous individuals who come to physicians' offices with so little organic pathology and so deep and painful a sense of loneliness that it is obvious that they want a meaningful personal relationship far more than the treatment for which they allege to have come (Balint 1957, 1970). Recognizable by a long list of symptoms, doctors, and operations and a demand for immediate action, the patient will sometimes be rescued from further diagnostic procedures by being sent to a psychiatrist. In extreme cases, the individual's desire to be "doctored" is so strong that he spends a good part of his life wandering from hospital to hospital, seeking treatment for obscure, fictitious, and unusual self-induced symptoms such as pyrexia, hematuria, or hemoptysis, willing to submit to painful, even crippling, surgery to remain at the center of some physician's interest. These patients are described as having *Münchausen's syndrome* (Asher 1951, Barker 1962, Bursten 1965, Ireland 1967) because of their *pseudologia phantastica;* they have an interesting counterpart in another group of hospital addicts with whom, in some ironic paradise, they might well be matched: the *medical imposters*—individuals with little or no medical training who are so fascinated by the medical scene and so dominated by their desire to participate in it that they don white coats in hospital corridors and cafeterias or even forge medical credentials in an attempt to practice.

By the time a psychiatrist is asked to evaluate and treat a patient with an undiagnosed somatic complaint, the patient is likely to be discouraged with his previous treatment and may well be querulous, negativistic, and accustomed to doctor-hopping. He may have become addicted to analgesics or soporifics and, despite warnings that these can mask, mimic, or aggravate his symptoms, be unwilling to stop using them (Murray 1970). The psychiatrist must therefore obtain as much information as he can about the previous course of the illness and its management. Then he must obtain a clear mandate from the patient or the family to proceed with the psychiatric investigation on his own terms, making it clear that for the time being he alone will decide what additional consultants are needed and what diagnostic or therapeutic plan is to be initiated. This approach will in some cases require hospitalizing the patient for the initial phase of evaluation.

Once the psychiatrist has accepted the patient for treatment, he should gradually withdraw him from all drugs that are not of obvious benefit and attempt to engage him in psychotherapy. In its simplest form, this consists of explaining that tension, depression, and conflict can cause or aggravate pain. All too often, however, the patient —who tends to consider himself an expert on his symptoms and illness

—feels that by such explanations the doctor is implying that his pain is imaginary. If he assumes this viewpoint, he may eventually provoke the physician into accusing him—directly or by implication—of inventing his symptoms. There is of course no such thing as imaginary pain (Klein 1967, Merskey 1967): either the patient has the pain he reports, or he is lying. It is thus more useful in psychotherapy to focus on the effect that the patient's complaints have on the doctor-patient relationship and, by extension, on his other relationships as well.

The response to consistent, firm psychotherapeutic management and the gradual reduction of sedatives or narcotic drugs can be most gratifying. Even after their entire life style has been dominated by their symptoms and a never-ending search for new doctors and new treatments, some patients can learn to cope with physical discomfort and show marked improvement in social functioning (Tumulty 1960). For others, the withdrawal of sedatives and analgesics clarifies the delusional proportions of the somatic complaints or reveals other symptoms that demonstrate an affective disorder or a schizophrenia (Lesse 1968). Still other patients, though they might not have evidenced sadness or fatigue even at the height of their illness, improve markedly on a regimen of either antidepressants alone or antidepressants together with phenothiazines (see p. 163). A favorable response to antidepressants is particularly common in the disorders called *depressive equivalents* because they resemble typical depressions in that:

1/ no organic basis for the symptoms can be found;

2/ a mood disorder precedes, accompanies, or follows the onset of symptoms;

3/ the symptoms show a diurnal pattern, being worse in the morning and improving as the day proceeds;

4/ the symptoms are associated with a sleep disturbance, especially middle-of-the-night or early morning awakening;

5/ the symptoms recur periodically;

6/ paranoid querulousness coexists with somatic complaints;

7/ the symptoms of discomfort include nausea, dizziness, or pain that is not shifting or diffuse but relatively well localized, as in the head, neck, back, face, chest, or stomach; and

8/ the patient fixes his attention primarily on his pain or discomfort, ignores anything not immediately related to his suffering, and becomes withdrawn from and indifferent to the world around him (Bradley 1963, Cleghorn 1959, Dowling 1964, Lascelles 1966, Lindberg 1965, Spear 1967).

Whether the antidepressant-induced improvement in syndromes show-ing these features means that the somatic complaints are in reality the symptoms of an occult depression, secondary to the symptoms of chronic depression, or merely imipramine-responsive is not known and, at least to the patient whose symptoms respond, is in any case of little moment.

"PSYCHOPHYSIOLOGIC" AND "PSYCHOSOMATIC" DISORDERS

Some referrals, although fewer than the wealth of literature would indicate, are based on the assumption that certain illnesses with demonstrable organic lesions (peptic ulcer, bronchial asthma, and ulcerative colitis, to name a representative few) are linked in some special way to psychological factors and particularly respon-sive to psychiatric treatment. Such disorders are often called psychophysiologic or psychosomatic, but there are in reality no psychosomatic illnesses, only psychosomatic points of view about illness and illnesses to which these views have been applied (Prugh 1963). It is thus important to understand these points of view. Ob-viously, they go well beyond recognizing the necessity of studying an individual's psychological makeup in order to understand his illness, for this would be just as important in ailments that would not be considered psychosomatic, such as accidents, infections, or congenital deformities. How much additional meaning is included by the individual using the label psychosomatic depends on his background and orientation, the diversity of which is readily apparent in that those who adhere to psychosomatic views rarely agree on definitions (Graham 1969). Nevertheless, most adherents of the psychosomatic viewpoint would accept the following formulation: circumstances or events that are stressful to an individual because of their meaning to him can cause, precipitate, or aggravate certain symptom-pro-ducing, anatomic or physiologic changes in one or more organs or systems.

Principal support for this viewpoint is derived from the observa-tion that individuals subjected to psychological stress may exhibit certain biologic changes that, were they to remain operative for extended periods, could lead to demonstrable lesions. It has not been demonstrated, however, that the physiologic correlates of emo-tion in and of themselves are ever of sufficient magnitude or dura-tion to produce the lesions observed in the illnesses termed *psychosomatic* (Reiser 1968). Whenever an explanation of psychosomatic illness on the basis of psychological stress is attempted, the conclusion is almost always similar to that of Kessel (1964), who in writing about peptic ulcer concluded: "A wealth of observation and experiment has demonstrated that emotional factors influence the state of the gastric mucosa and the degree of gastric acidity. But it has not been satisfactorily demonstrated that personality factors, environmental stresses, or psychological illnesses are etiologically associated with peptic ulceration." (Altschule 1969, Brandes 1967, Cochrane 1969, Hinkle 1968, Mendeloff 1970, O'Connor 1967, Pedder 1969, Rubenstein 1969, Stavraky 1968).

There is, then, no reason to believe, and much practical experience to justify doubt, that psychological exploration helps with the understanding of these illnesses or that the symptoms of which the patient complains most can be alleviated by psychiatric treatment. Just as in any other syndrome—whether diabetes, cancer, or poliomyelitis—the psychiatrist can make a significant contribution to the patient's management, provided that the illness and its consequences significantly affect or are affected by the patient's mood and cognition, or the patient uses his symptoms as a tool in transacting with his environment (Lipowski 1968).

DISORDERED REGULATION OF FOOD INTAKE AND WEIGHT

The patient who eats too little or too much is referred to a psychiatrist only when his behavior

1/ cannot be explained in terms of an identifiable organic illness
or
2/ does not change in the desired direction with traditional treatment measures.

Anorexia Nervosa

CLINICAL PICTURE

Among the most striking of such food intake disturbances is the anorexia nervosa syndrome, characterized by the patient's adamantly starving himself (or more commonly herself) to the point of emaciation (Gull 1874). Such a patient's weight loss can be distinguished from that in other psychiatric syndromes by its severity and the fact that it is not associated, at least at the outset, with any lack of appetite. That it is not a volitional whim, mere stubbornness, or an isolated symptom, but a syndrome, is suggested by numerous other similarities found among patients showing such behavior. Typically, the patient is female and between the ages of 12 and 25; her history often reveals one or more periods of obesity, especially prior to puberty (Kay 1967); amenorrhea is common when the syndrome reaches its peak and may even precede the patient's aversion to food; in many cases, the patient exhibits a fine hairy growth all over her body (Arnsø 1966). Sometimes these patients heighten their emaciated, cadaver-like appearance with bizarre makeup, such as exaggerated use of white face powder and dark eyeshadow and an unusual hair style. Early in the course, the self-imposed starvation may alternate with episodes of uncontrollable eating, during which the patient raids the icebox and gorges on whatever she finds there, raw food, leftovers, or used cooking fat; in extreme cases, she will even raid the garbage pail (King 1963). These episodes of compulsive eating, and even such therapeutic measures as forced feeding, are often followed by self-induced vomiting and the use of laxatives and enemas. Rationalizations for this behavior are as odd as the behavior itself: weighing less than 70 pounds, she may express a fear of becoming "too fat." Remarkably enough, the patient is not generally weak or debilitated but may remain vigorous, possibly even overactive, until her emaciation is far advanced.

Apart from weight loss, the disorder has a number of features in common with *pituitary insufficiency:* amenorrhea, hypotension, low basal metabolism rate, flat glucose tolerance curve, and (in patients in their early teens) stunted physical development. The differential diagnosis rarely presents any difficulty, however. Unlike anorexia nervosa, pituitary insufficiency is often preceded by a severe infection or a difficult delivery, and is usually associated with anergia, diminished sexual drive, pubic and axillary hair loss, and atrophy of the sexual organs. In anorexia nervosa, urinary 17-keto-steroids and in some cases corticosteroids are low, but plasma cortisol levels and their response to ACTH administration is normal (Christy 1967). The differential diagnosis between a *malabsorption syndrome* and anorexia nervosa may be problematic, particularly early in the course or when the clinical picture is atypical, because of the patient's idiosyncratic reaction to food. However, profound anemia and hypoproteinemia are always present in malabsorption syndromes, are infrequent even in emaciated anorexia nervosa patients, and, when present, are easily corrected by refeeding (G. F. M. Russell 1967, Sleisinger 1969).

TREATMENT

In most other illnesses associated with anorexia, the patient is troubled by his lack of interest in food and eager to obtain help, even if (as in depressions) he is skeptical about the results or (as in paranoid illnesses) distrustful of the doctor's motives. The patient with anorexia nervosa, however, wants nothing to do with the doctor and seeks to frustrate treatment at every turn. She may assume a superficial and falsely compliant stance at the outset, but this is soon superseded by negativism and stubborn defiance. This behavior is often in striking contrast to the family's description of the patient as a heretofore unusually obedient, circumspect, clean, eager-to-please, helpful-at-home, and precociously dependable child.

Keeping the patient alive depends on recognizing the therapeutic relationship for what it is: a struggle with a person who means to resist being fed at any cost and will not shrink from the most fraudulent means of achieving this goal. Patients who are weighed at regular intervals may avoid urinating for hours or days beforehand or drink enormous quantities of water just before they are weighed. Others may eat and pretend to enjoy it, but secretly vomit immediately afterwards. They may go so far as to set family members against each other in an effort to avert the possibility of medical intervention (and the resultant forced feeding) and, upset though a patient's family may be by her weight loss and cadaverous appearance, they remain indecisive, continue to believe her assurance that she will soon start eating, and fail to consult a psychiatrist until the situation is extremely advanced.

Supervision of eating habits is diffcult on the outside, and hospitalization is mandatory whenever the patient's weight falls below 75% of the minimum weight expected of persons of like sex, height, build, and age. The first step in treatment is of course to *initiate proper food intake*. Should the patient refuse to eat, feeding by nasogastric tube must begin without delay. Such feedings should be fairly small at first, then increased gradually over an eight to 10 day period, and continued until the patient weights more than 80% of the normal expected weight. If at any point the patient prefers to eat unassisted, she should be permitted to do so, but it should be made clear that the forced feeding will be resumed whenever she stops gaining weight. Persuasion, cajolery, promises, or threats on the part of the staff are contraindicated, for these only serve to reactivate the power struggle. Once the patient's food intake reaches 2,500 to 3,000 calories daily, she should, unless she is secretly vomiting, gain about four or five pounds weekly. Some degree of refeeding edema usually develops after the first 10 to 14 days; as a result, weight gains of six or eight pounds may occur within 24 hours (Berkman 1930). The edema usually recedes during the next seven to fourteen days and requires no treatment beyond reassurance. It can be confusing, however, for the disappearance of the edema can cause the patient to lose weight even though she is eating as she is supposed to.

A psychological exploration of the patient's motives is of little value at the outset, because the patient's only reason for cooperating is to maneuver changes in her overall management. She might pretend to be learning a good deal about herself in psychotherapy or to be forming a close relationship with her therapist, but only as a means of postponing the demand that she eat. *Psychotherapy*, therefore, should be directive and supportive at first and the question of motivation delayed until her weight is restored (Frazier 1965). Psychoanalytically oriented psychotherapy is, in any case, less valuable than an exploration of the patient's self-image, the blandness with which she denies the bizarreness of her behavior or physical appearance, and the feelings she has about the social feedback she receives (Bruch 1962, 1965, 1969, Crisp 1965, Frazier 1965, Giffin 1957, Thomä 1961). Whether problems in becoming autonomous or the family's reluctance to let go are of etiologic significance or are merely effects of the illness is not known, but the theme of autonomy is a central one that often predates the anorexia by months or years. The refusal to eat thereby looms as an important transactional tool with which an individual can protest her real or imagined subjugation (Amdur 1969). Thus as soon as a patient's weight approaches the norm, an investigation of her relationship to her family is indicated. Only after she has learned to communicate verbally rather than by manipulating her food intake should a psychotherapeutic matrix independent of family treatment be considered. At this time a combination of peer group and individual psychotherapy may be of value.

Drugs also have a place in the treatment of anorexia nervosa. In the first phase of treatment, as the patient's food intake increases, she may complain about abdominal distention and cramps, symptoms that can be relieved by an anticholinergic agent like propantheline bromide, in doses of 15 mg tid. Phenothiazines and CNS depressants may also be used, both to reduce the patient's hyperactivity and to stimulate appetite. In view of the starved patient's low weight, precarious metabolic balance, and tendency to hypotension and circulatory collapse, the dose ranges are identical to those used in children. Typical starting doses are fluphenazine (Permitil), 0.25 mg, tid or qid, alone or together with chlordiazepoxide (Librium), 5 mg, tid or qid. The doses may then be increased gradually until the patient is taking 4 to 5 mg of fluphenazine or 30 to 40 mg of chlordiazepoxide daily. If she becomes hypotensive at any point, the dosage is decreased, and increased only after she has gained additional weight. If, as a result of such complications as infection or shock, the patient requires intravenous fluids, the greatly reduced muscle mass and body weight must be taken into account in calculating the fluid and electrolyte requirements. Anabolic steroids, such as nandrolone decanoate (Deca-Durabolin) (Tec 1963) and insulin have been used, but are considered dangerous (Berczeller 1962), and evidence for their value is inconclusive (Kay 1954).

As the patient's bizarre eating habits subside and she begins to approximate her normal weight, she may develop such symptoms as crying, sleep disturbances, or increased anxiety. At this time, small doses of antidepressants, such as imipramine (Tofranil), 10 to 20 mg, tid or qid, may be used either alone or in combination with the fluphenazine-chlordiazepoxide regimen outlined above. The patient's menstrual period may not return for a year of more after normal or near-normal weight has been achieved (Dally 1967); estrogen preparations can be used to hasten this process.

Given the patient's single-minded efforts to sow dissension in the ranks of her doctors and family, the establishment of regular meetings between all concerned is of utmost importance. The family must understand from the first that the patient will not be discharged until her weight has been normal for three weeks (which can take six months or more); that she will complain bitterly about the inhumane treatment she is receiving; and that, if they value her life, they must resist the urge to rescue her. After discharge, both patient and family must remain in regular contact with the therapist. Even more important is the continuing coercion exerted by the therapist in weighing the patient during each visit and warning her that she will immediately be rehospitalized if her weight goes below 90% of the norm.

The only available *follow-up data* are based on earlier studies, in which no phenothiazines were used, treatment was terminated on hospital discharge, and family involvement was not considered an essential component of the program. While reported improvement rates vary, in most studies 30% of the patients showed marked improvement, 40% marginal improvement, and 30% were unchanged or deteriorated. The gravity of the problem is underlined by the death rate: follow-up studies ranging from two to 25 years have shown that as many as one out of five patients died from the illness or its complications (Farquharson 1966, Kay 1953). Relapse is common, particularly during the first year, but of little prognostic significance (Dally 1967) if rehospitalization is promptly arranged.

Obesity

Americans place such emphasis on maintaining a trim and youthful appearance that, at any given time, vast numbers of them are on some kind of reducing diet. Not all who diet have a good reason for doing so, but the culture is at once so sedentary and food-oriented, that even the average individual's weight is 10% to 15% above that which correlates with the greatest longevity (Society of Actuaries 1959). As overweight increases, mortality and morbidity increase even more rapidly; an individual's obese appearance may come to endanger his social and occupational success (Solomon 1969). As a result, many obese persons seek medical assistance for losing weight. Some consult a psychiatrist for this purpose, but there is little evidence that he is better equipped than the nutritionist or family doctor to propagate and explain the banal requirement for weight loss: diminished food intake (Fazekas 1962). The rare patient with a treatable endocrine disorder should of course be referred to and managed by an internist.

From a therapeutic standpoint, the current situation is bleak. While it is true that almost anyone who can be moved to stop eating, whether by despair, faith, suggestion, or infatuation, can lose weight, it is also true that the obese individual tends to stop dieting before achieving much weight loss and, even if he continues to diet, usually reaches a plateau not more than 5% to 6% below his initial weight. Once the dieting stops, his weight tends to increase to the initial level. As a result, individuals who have achieved a major weight loss and successfully maintained it over a period of years are extremely rare (Stunkard 1959).

Constitutional factors probably play a significant role in obesity. The odds against an obese child becoming an adult of normal weight are more than 4:1, and against those who do not reduce by the time they reach adolescence, more than 28:1. The individual who is anxious or depressed is even less likely than the average person to succeed in his attempts to lose weight. There is no evidence, however, to support the common belief that dieting increases the individual's psychological symptoms, and what statistics exist suggest the reverse (Holland 1970, Shipman 1963, Silverstone 1965).

At present, then, the most favorable treatment for the obese person is involvement with a person or group that provides hope, encouragement, frequent supervision of diet and weight, and nutritional education, and that emphasizes realistic rather than "quick weight loss" programs. Self-help groups such as Weight Watchers (London 1966, Spargo 1966, Wagonfeld 1968), which combine these ingredients with a sense of belonging and frequent exhortation, have benefited some patients, but such programs have been in existence for too short a time to assess their long-term effects (Solomon 1969). In many cases, the kindest thing to do is to help the patient adapt to being overweight, to accept himself for what he is, and to compensate for it by developing other attributes and skills that make him attractive (Stunkard 1967). It is certainly no unkindness to remind these patients that their temperaments are often more likable than those of persons with a "lean and hungry look" and that the final word on the relationship between mortality and obesity has not yet been spoken.

REFERENCES

Abram, H. S.: The psychiatrist, the treatment of chronic renal failure, and the prolongation of life: II., Amer J Psychiat 126:157-167, 1969.

Alper, M. H., Flacke, W., and Krayer, O.: Pharmacology of reserpine and its implications for anesthesia, Anesthesiology 24:524-542, 1963.

Altschule, M. D.: Physiology of some so-called "psychosomatic" disorders, Curr Med Digest, 36:577-588, 1969.

Amdur, M. J., et al.: Anorexia nervosa: Interactional study, J Nerv Ment Dis 148: 559-566, 1969.

Arén, P., and Åmark, C.: The prognosis in cases in which legal abortion has been granted but not carried out, Acta Psychiat Scand 36:203-278, 1961.

Arnsø, F.: Anorexia nervosa illustrated by a psychotherapeutic casuistry, Acta Psychiat Scand 42:107-123, 1966.

Asher, R.: Münchausen's syndrome, Lancet 1:339-341, 1951.

Astrachan, B. M., and Bowers, M.: Transfers to a psychiatric service within a general hospital, Compr Psychiat 7:118-125, 1966.

Ayd, F. J., Jr.: Children born of mothers treated with chlorpromazine during pregnancy, Clin Med 71:1758-1763, 1964.

Baker, J. B.: Effects of drugs on the foetus, Pharmacol Rev 12:37-90, 1960.

Balint, M.: The Doctor, His Patient, and the Illness, New York: Internat Univ Press, 1957.

———: Repeat prescription patients: Are they an identifiable group? Psychiat in Med 1:3-14, 1970.

Barker, J. C.: The syndrome of hospital addiction (Münchausen Syndrome): A report on the investigation of seven cases, Brit J Psychiat 108:167-182, 1962.

Behrman, S. J.: Which 'Pill' to choose? Hosp Pract 4:34-39, 1969.

Berczeller, Peter H., and Kupperman, H. S.: The anabolic steroids, Clin Pharmacol Ther 1:464-482, 1962.

Berkman, J. M.: Anorexia nervosa, anorexia, inanition, and low basic metabolic rate, Amer J Med Sci *180:*411-424, 1930.

Bolter, S.: The psychiatrist's role in therapeutic abortion: The unwitting accomplice, Amer J Psychiat *119:*312-316, 1962.

Bradley, J. J.: Severe localized pain associated with the depressive syndrome, Brit J Psychiat *109:*741-745, 1963.

Brandes, J. M.: First-trimester nausea and vomiting as related to outcome of pregnancy, Obstet Gynec *30:*427-431, 1967.

Bratfos, O., and Haug, J. O.: Puerperal mental disorders in manic-depressive females, Acta Psychiat Scand *42:*285-294, 1966.

Bruch, H.: Perceptual and conceptual disturbances in anorexia nervosa, Psychosom Med *24:*187-194, 1962.

———: Anorexia nervosa and its differential diagnosis, J Nerv Ment Dis *141:* 555-566, 1965.

———: Hunger and instinct, J Nerv Ment Dis *149:*91-114, 1969.

Bruhn, J. G., *et al.:* Patients' reactions to death in a coronary care unit, J Psychosom Res *14:*65-70, 1970.

Budnick, I. W., Leikin, S., and Hoeck, L. E.: Effect in the newborn infant of reserpine administered ante partum, J Dis Child *90:*286-289, 1955.

Bursten, B.: On Münchausen's syndrome, Arch Gen Psychiat (Chicago) *13:* 261-268, 1965.

Christy, N. P.: Anorexia nervosa, *in* Beeson, P. B., and McDermott, W. ed.: Cecil-Loeb Textbook of Medicine, Philadelphia and London: Saunders, 1967, pp. 1273-1275.

Clark, M., *et al.:* Sequels of unwanted pregnancy, Lancet *11:*501-503, 1968.

Cleghorn, R. A., and Curtis, C. G.: Psychosomatic accompaniments of latent and manifest depressive affect, Canad Psychiat Ass J *4*(Suppl):S13-S23, 1959.

Cochrane, R.: Neuroticism and the discovery of high blood pressure, J Psychosom Res *13:*21-25, 1969.

Coles, R. B., and Bridger, H.: The consultant and his roles, Brit J Med Psychol *42:*231-241, 1969.

Crisp, A. H.: Clinical and therapeutic aspects of anorexia nervosa—a study of 30 cases, J Psychosom Res *9:*67-78, 1965.

Dally, P. J.: Anorexia nervosa—long-term follow-up and effects of treatment, J Psychosom Res *11:*151-155, 1967.

Dowling, R. H., and Knox, S. J.: Somatic symptoms in depressive illness, Brit J Psychiat *110:*720-722, 1964.

Egbert, L. D., *et al.:* Reduction of postoperative pain by encouragement and instruction of patients. A study of doctor-patient rapport, New Eng J Med *270:* 825-827, 1964.

Ellard, J.: Impending death affects emotions of dying patient, Med J Aust *1:*979-983, 1968.

Elliott, H. W.: Influence of previous therapy on anesthesia, Clin Pharmacol Ther *3:*41-58, 1962.

Farquharson, R. F., and Hyland, H. H.: Anorexia nervosa: Course of 15 patients treated from 20 to 30 years previously, Canad Med Ass J *94:*411-419, 1966.

Fazekas, F.: Anorexigenic agents, New Eng J Med *5:*28-34, 1962.

Fellner, C. H.: Emotional sequelae of minor closed head injury, Psychosomatics *5:*295-300, 1964.

Fras, I., Litin, E. M., and Pearson, J. S.: Comparison of psychiatric symptoms in carcinoma of the pancreas with those in some other intra-abdominal neoplasms, Amer J Psychiat *123:*1553-1562, 1967.

Frazier, S. H.: Anorexia nervosa, Dis Nerv Syst *26:*155-159, 1965.

GAP Publication No. 75: Right to abortion: A psychiatric view, Group Advance Psychiat *7:*203-227, 1969.

Giffin, M. E., *et al.:* Internist's role in the successful treatment of anorexia nervosa, Mayo Clin Proc *32:*171-182, 1957.

Gold, E. M., *et al.:* Therapeutic abortions in New York City: A 20-year review, Amer J Public Health *55:*964-972, 1965.

Graham, D. T., Psychosomatic medicine needs a new start, Hosp Pract *4:*Mar, 1969.

Greene, W. A., and Moss, A. J.: Psychosocial factors in the adjustment of patients with permanently implanted cardiac pacemakers, Ann Intern Med *70:*897-902, 1969.

Gull, W. W.: Anorexia nervosa, Trans Clin Soc London *7:*22-28, 1874.

Hackett, T. P., Cassem, N. H., and Wishnie, H. A.: Coronary-care unit. Appraisal of its psychologic hazards, New Eng J Med *279:*1365-1370, 1968.

Hall, R. E.: Abortion in American hospitals, Amer J Public Health *57:*1933-1936, 1967.

Hill, R. M., and Desmond, M. M.: Management of the narcotic withdrawal syndrome in the neonate, Pediat Clin N Amer *10:*67-86, 1963.

Hill, R. M., Desmond, M. M., and Kay, J. L.: A temporary Parkinson-like syndrome in a newborn infant, Southern Med J *57:*1478, 1964.

————: Extrapyramidal dysfunction in an infant of a schizophrenic mother, J Pediat *69:*589-595, 1966.

Himmelhoch, J. M., et al.: Butting heads—patients who refuse necessary procedures, Psychiatry in Medicine, *1:*241-249, 1970.

Hinkle, L. E., et al.: Occupation, education, and coronary heart disease, Science *161:*238-246, 1968.

Holland, J., Masling, J., and Copley, D.: Mental illness in lower class normal, obese and hyperobese women, Psychosom Med *32:*351-357, 1970.

Impastato, D. J., Gabriel, A. R., and Lardaro, H. H.: Electric and insulin shock therapy during pregnancy, Dis Nerv System *25:*542-546, 1964.

Ireland, P., Sapira, J. D., and Templeton, B.: Münchausen's syndrome, Amer J Med *43:*579-592, 1967.

Janis, I. L.: Emotional inoculation: Theory and research on effects of preparatory communications, in Muensterberger, W., and Axelrad, S., eds.: Psychoanalysis and the Social Sciences, New York: Internat Univ Press, 1958.

Janis, I. L., and Leventhal, H.: Psychological aspects of physical illness and hospital care, in Walman, B., ed.: Handbook of Clinical Psychology, New York: McGraw-Hill, 1964, pp. 1-43.

Kane, F. J., Jr.: Psychiatric reactions to oral contraceptives, Amer J Obstet Gynec *102:*1053-1063, 1968.

Kay, D. W.: Anorexia nervosa: a study in prognosis, Proc Roy Soc Med *46:*669-674, 1953.

Kay, D. W., and Leigh, D.: Natural history, treatment and prognosis of anorexia nervosa, based on a study of 38 patients, J Ment Sci *100:*411-431, 1954.

Kay, D. W. K., Schapira, K., and Brandon, S.: Early factors in anorexia nervosa compared with non-anorexic groups, J Psychosom Res *11:*133-139, 1967.

Kemph, J. P., Bermann, E. A., and Coppolillo, H. P.: Kidney transplant and shifts in family dynamics, Amer J Psychiat *125:*1485-1490, 1969.

Kennedy, J. A., and Bakst, H.: Influence of emotions on the outcome of cardiac surgery: A predictive study, Bull NY Acad Med *42:*811-849, 1966.

Kenyon, F. E.: Hypochondriasis: A clinical study, Brit J Psychiat *110:*478-488, 1964.

————: Hypochondriasis: A survey of some historical, clinical and social aspects, Brit J Med Psychol *38:*117-133, 1965.

Kessel, N., and Munro, A.: Epidemiological studies in psychosomatic medicine, J Psychosom Res *8:*67-81, 1964.

Kimball, C. P.: Psychological responses to the experience of open heart surgery: I., Amer J Psychiat *126:*348-359, 1969.

Kimball, C. P., and Detre, T.: Unpublished data.

King, A.: Primary and secondary anorexia nervosa syndromes, Brit J Psychiat *109:*470-479, 1963.

Klein, R. F., and Brown, W.: Pain descriptions in the medical setting, J Psychosom Res *10:*367-372, 1967.

Knox, S. J.: Severe psychiatric disturbances in the post-operative period—a five-year survey of Belfast hospitals, J Ment Sci *107:*1078-1096, 1961.

Kris, E. B.: Children born to mothers maintained on pharmacotherapy during pregnancy and postpartum, Recent Advances Biol Psychiat *4:*180-187, 1962.

Lascelles, R. G.: Atypical facial pain and depression, Brit J Psychiat *112:*651-659, 1966.

Lesse, S.: Apparent remissions in depressed suicidal patients, J Nerv Ment Dis *144:*291-296, 1967.

————: Multivariant masks of depression, Amer J Psychiat *124*(Suppl):35-40, 1968.

Lewis, A., and Hoghughi, M.: Evaluation of depression as a side effect of oral contraceptives, Brit J Psychiat *115:*697-701, 1969.

Lidz, R. W.: Emotional factors in the success of contraception, Fertil Steril *20:*761-771, 1969.

Lindberg, B. J.: Somatic complaints in the depressive symptomatology, Acta Psychiat Scand *41:*419-427, 1965.

Lipowski, Z. J.: Review of consultation psychiatry and psychosomatic medicine. I. General principles, Psychosom Med *29:*153-171, 1967a.

————: Ibid., II. Clinical aspects, Psychosom Med *29:*201-224, 1967b.

————: Ibid., III. Theoretical issues, Psychosom Med *30:*378-389, 1968.

Lipsitt, D. R.: "Hypochondriasis": Whose responsibility? Psychiat Opinion *6:*26-34, 1969.

London, A. M., and Schreiber, E. D.: Controlled study of the effects of group discussions and an anorexiant in outpatient treatment of obesity. With attention to the psychological aspects of dieting, Ann Intern Med *65*:80-92, 1966.

Matsumoto, S., *et al.:* Electroencephalographic changes during long-term treatment with oral contraceptives, Int J Fertil *11*:195-204, 1966.

Mendeloff, A. I., *et al.:* Illness experience and life stresses in patients with irritable colon and with ulcerative colitis, New Eng J Med *282*:14-17, 1970.

Merskey, H., and Spear, F. G.: Pain: Psychological and Psychiatric Aspects, London: Baillière, Tindall & Cox, 1967.

Mitchell, W. M.: Etiological factors producing neuropsychiatric syndromes in patients with malignant disease, Int J Neuropsychiat *3*:464-468, 1967.

Mozden, P. J.: The management of the patient with advanced cancer, Canad J Clinicians *19*:211-217, 1969.

Murray, R. M., Timbury, G. C., and Linton, A. L.: Analgesic abuse in psychiatric patients, Lancet *1*:1303-1305, 1970.

Nichols, M. M.: Acute alcohol withdrawal syndrome in a newborn, Amer J Dis Child *133*:714-715, 1967.

Nilsson, A., and Almgren, P. E.: Psychiatric symptoms during the postpartum period as related to use of oral contraceptives, Brit Med J *2*:453-455, 1968.

Niswander, K. R., Klein, M., and Randall, C. L.: Changing attitudes toward therapeutic abortion, JAMA *196*:1140-1143, 1966.

O'Connor, J. F., and Stern, L. O.: Symptom alternation, Arch Gen Psychiat (Chicago) *16*:432-436, 1967.

Pasternack, S. A.: When a patient wants to sign himself out, Hosp Physician *5*: 120-127, 1969.

Patt, S. L., Rappaport, R. G., and Barglow, P.: Follow-up of therapeutic abortion, Arch Gen Psychiat (Chicago) *20*: 408-414, 1969.

Patterson, R. M., and Craig, J. B.: Misconceptions concerning the psychological effects of hysterectomy, J Obstet Gynec *84*:104-111, 1963.

Peck, A., and Marcus, H.: Psychiatric sequelae of therapeutic interruption of pregnancy, J Nerv Ment Dis *143*:417-425, 1966.

Pedder, J. R.: Psychosomatic disorder and psychosis, J Psychosom Res *13*:339-346, 1969.

Prugh, D. G.: Toward an understanding of psychosomatic concepts in relation to illness in children, *in* Solnit, A. J., and Provence, S. A., eds.: Modern Perspectives in Child Development, New York: Internat Univ Press, 1963, pp. 246-367.

Ravitch, M. M.: What I say when I have to give a prognosis, Resident Physician *15*:45-47, 1969.

Reiser, M. F.: Models and techniques in psychosomatic research, Comp Psychiat *9:* 406-413, 1968.

Rubinstein, D., and Thomas, J. K.: Psychiatric findings in cardiotomy patients, Amer J Psychiat *126*:360-369, 1969.

Russell, D. H., and Chayet, N. L.: Abortion laws and the physician, I., New Eng J Med *276*:1027-1028, 1967.

Russell, G. F. M.: Nutritional disorder in anorexia nervosa, J Psychosom Res *11:* 141-149, 1967.

Schur, E. M.: Abortion, Ann Amer Acad Polit and Soc Sci *376*:136-147, 1968.

Schwab, J. J., and Brown, J.: Uses and abuses of psychiatric consultation, JAMA *205*:65-68, 1968.

Shipman, W. G., and Plesset, M. R.: Anxiety and depression in obese dieters, Arch Gen Psychiat (Chicago) *8*:530-535, 1963.

Silverstone, J. T., and Solomon, T.: Psychiatric and somatic factors in the treatment of obesity, J Psychosom Res *9:* 249-255, 1965.

Simon, N. M., Senturia, A. G., and Rothman, D.: Psychiatric illness following therapeutic abortion, Amer J Psychiat *124*:59-65, 1967.

Slater, E. T. O., and Glithero, E.: A follow-up of patients diagnosed as suffering from "hysteria," J Psychosom Res *9:* 9-13, 1965.

Sleisenger, M. H.: Malabsorption syndrome, *in* Page, I. H., ed.: Physiology for Physicians, New Eng J Med *281*:1111-1117, 1969.

Sloane, R. B.: Unwanted pregnancy, New Eng J Med *280*:1206-1213, 1969.

Sobel, D. E.: Fetal damage due to ECT, insulin coma, chlorpromazine or reserpine, Arch Gen Psychiat (Chicago) *2*: 606-611, 1960.

Society of Actuaries: Build and Blood Pressure Study, Chicago, Society of Actuaries, 1959.

Solomon, N.: Study and treatment of the obese patient, Hosp Pract *4*:90-94, 1969.

Spargo, J. A., Heald, F., and Peckos, P. S.: Adolescent obesity, Nutr Today *1*:2-9, 1966.

Spear, F. G.: Pain in psychiatric patients, J Psychosom Res *11*:187-193, 1967.

Stavraky, K. M.: Psychological factors in the outcome of human cancer, J Psychosom Res *12*:251-259, 1968.

Stunkard, A., and Burt, J.: Obesity and the body image: II. Age at onset of disturbances in the body image, Amer J Psychiat *123*:1443-1447, 1967.

Stunkard, A., and McLaren-Hume, M.: The results of treatment for obesity: A review of the literature and report of a series, Arch Intern Med (Chicago) *103*: 79-85, 1959.

Szasz, T .S.: The concept of transference, Int J Psychoanal *44*:432-443, 1963.

Taylor, B. W., Litin, E. M., and Litzow, T. J.: Psychiatric considerations in cosmetic surgery, Mayo Clin Proc *41*:608-623, 1966.

Tec, L.: Durabolin in anorexia nervosa, Amer J Psychiat *120*:282, 1963.

Thomä, H.: Anorexia nervosa, Stuttgart: Klett, 1961.

Tumulty, P. A.: Approach to patients with functional disorders, New Eng J Med *263*:123-128, 1960.

VanLeeuwen, G., Guthrie, R., and Stange, F.: Narcotic withdrawal reaction in a newborn infant due to codeine, Pediatrics *36*:635-636, 1965.

Vorster, D. W.: Psychiatric drugs and treatment in pregnancy, Brit J Psychiat *111*:431-438, 1965.

Wagonfeld, S., and Wolowitz, H. M.: Obesity and the self-help group: A look at TOPS, Amer J Psychiat *125*:249-252, 1968.

Walters, A.: Psychogenic regional pain alias hysterical pain, Brain *84*:1-18, 1961.

CHAPTER

THIRTEEN

Psychotherapy

THROUGHOUT HISTORY, people have turned to their fellows for advice and consolation when they felt unable to solve their problems. Family members and friends have generally been most available for such discussions, but when they were unable to help or were a part of the problem, and especially when moral or spiritual matters were involved, the troubled individual turned to whomever his culture had appointed as the legitimate repository of trust— often some representative of the gods. With the advent of the industrial revolution, these sources of help began to seem less effective. Society's increasing mobility, urbanization, and mechanization have loosened the average person's ties to friends, family, and church. Impressed by the technologic advances wrought by science, he has come to believe that the scientifically trained mental health professional has some of the answers he seeks and turns to him increasingly in times of perplexity, most especially when the perplexity is exacerbated by or manifested in interpersonal problems.

Having emerged under these circumstances, the practice of psychotherapy inevitably fulfills many of the needs formerly satisfied by friends or clergymen (Barrett-Lennard 1965, Frank 1961, Schofield 1964). What distinguishes psychotherapy from friendship is that the therapist is paid for his services and committed professionally to do the patient some good, perhaps even a particular kind of good. The transaction is thus not usually so random or give-and-take as that between friends. While the advent of pastoral counseling as a distinct subspecialty has somewhat blurred the clergyman's role, he is generally expected to be more supportive and directive than the professional psychotherapist; less concerned with exploring in depth the individual's reasons for feeling or acting as he does; and more likely to interpret his behavior in the context of a predetermined, stipulated ethical and moral framework. Psychotherapy, friendship, casework, marital or pastoral counseling, it all depends on how the terms are defined.

485

DEFINITION

The term *psychotherapy* is used to describe so wide a variety of activities that it is hard to believe that all who profess to practice it really pursue the same occupation (Mowbray 1966). Wolberg (1954) defines it as

> certain consciously chosen ways in which, within the framework of a deliberately established professional relationship, trained individuals interact with people who seek or need their attention for the purpose of
> *1/* promoting more adaptive behavior patterns;
> *2/* removing, modifying, or retarding symptoms of mental illness or psychological discomfort; and
> *3/* stimulating personality development.

This definition excludes any activity on the part of the therapist that is primarily somatic (such as pharmacotherapy, electroconvulsive treatment (ECT), or psychosurgery) or refers to it only in terms of the effect achieved by the patient's attitude toward the treatment offered and the meaning he ascribes to it.

Many practitioners, and indeed many well-informed laymen, use the term *psychotherapy* only in reference to psychoanalysis or psychoanalytically oriented psychotherapy and consider any other technique supportive therapy, casework, or counseling (Tompkins 1966). Those who adhere to such views would agree with Hollender's (1965) description of definitive psychotherapy as a transaction that

> *1/* involves two persons,
> *2/* depends solely on verbal interchange and nonverbal (or kinesic) cues, and
> *3/* is designed to foster the acquisition of emotionally meaningful self-knowledge for the purpose of changing the patient's feelings and/or behavior; in which
> *4/* the therapist promotes learning by decoding and interpreting what he sees as the patient's unconscious messages,
> *5/* such subtle influences as imitation and identification can also cause the patient to learn something or to change, and
> *6/* the highest premium is placed on the patient's self-determination.

This definition is more specific about goals and techniques than Wolberg's and thus excludes such diverse, widely-practiced activities as group, family, occupational, and recreational therapy, hypnosis, catharsis, conditioning, and giving advice or direction.

The difficulty with both definitions, and indeed with any definition that embodies a specific set of goals, is that it begs the question whether and to what extent these goals are or can be achieved (Fisher 1969). Having seen no evidence that any of the psychotherapeutic techniques currently known are effective in modifying the symptoms of mental illness or stimulating personality development, our definition of the term restricts itself to the most modest, most readily measurable, and most achievable of the listed goals: the maintenance of social skills and the promotion of more adaptive behavior patterns.

THE MATRIX OF TREATMENT

Whatever its goals, psychotherapy can be classified to some extent in terms of its formal characteristics. These characteristics—the number and identities of the participants and the frequency, length, and location of the meetings—can be combined in any one of a large number of ways to form the *matrix* of treatment. The most common treatment matrix, *individual therapy*, entails one patient meeting with one therapist. The number of participants can be expanded, however, to include the patient's "others" (those who form his interpersonal environment), other patients with or without their "others," and the therapist's professional "others" (social workers, nurses, psychologists, psychiatrists, and recreational workers).

Of the possible combinations, the most frequently used are:

> *Couples therapy*, in which the patient and his spouse are always seen together by the same therapist;
> *Concurrent couples therapy*, in which the patient and his spouse are each seen by a different therapist;
> *Conjoint couples therapy*, in which each spouse meets regularly with a therapist of his own and all four meet together at regular intervals;
> *Couples group therapy*, in which two or more couples meet with one or more therapists;
> *Individual group therapy*, in which three or more unrelated individuals meet with one or more therapists.

If children, parents, and numerous therapists are available, such variants as *family therapy, families group therapy, conjoint family therapy* (Curry 1965, Gottlieb 1966, Jackson 1961, Laquer 1964, Satir 1967, Sorrels 1968), and *multiple impact therapy* (MacGregor 1964) are possible. When, in the course of his treatment, the patient participates in several of the above kinds of groups, the program is called *multidimensional group therapy* (Hes 1961).

Therapeutic encounters vary in length and frequency depending on the nature and severity of the patient's pathology, the therapist's goals, and the structural, ideologic, and economic circumstances within which the treatment relationship takes place. Low-income patients in a public hospital's follow-up clinic may meet with a doctor as infrequently as once a month or even once a year, and the sessions may last only a few minutes. "Interesting," well-educated, well-to-do, "well-motivated," or severely ill patients tend to be seen more frequently and for longer periods of time, as do patients who are seeing a private psychiatrist, those who seem to be bene-fiting from intensive treatment, and those whose therapist believes his role demands an intensive involvement. Such patients are usually seen from one to five times a week for periods lasting between 30 and 60 minutes, 50 minutes often being considered optimal. Therapy groups generally meet once or twice weekly for sessions of 60 to 90 minutes' duration. There are also *marathon group* meetings, in which eight to 10 individuals meet with one or two therapists for sessions lasting as long as 48 hours (Bach 1966, Stoller 1968).

The matrix of treatment is merely the stage on which the action takes place and, except tangentially, does not affect what the participants will do. Psychiatrists of quite different theoretical orientations can use identical matrices to pursue quite divergent goals, as the following examples illustrate. Psychoanalysts and psychoanalytically oriented therapists believe that discomfort and maladaptive behavior often stem from unresolved, long-past conflicts that arrested an individual's personality growth at a particular stage of development and thereby caused him to develop inaccurate or distorted feelings and attitudes about himself and his environment. The therapist operates on the assumption that the patient is unaware that his view of the world is at odds with reality and is, in fact, based on earlier, now seemingly irrelevant experiences. For this reason, he encourages the patient to discuss, reexperience, and finally "work through" those earlier conflicts that led to his present difficulties (Freud 1912, Menninger 1958, Novey 1962). Some psychodynamically oriented therapists see the patient together with his spouse, parents, or siblings in order to explore their current and past feelings about each other; others place the patient in a therapy group and, by exploring the feelings and views that the patient develops about the other group members, try to help him understand how this reflects his former reactions to persons close to him (Kadis 1956). Not every psychodynamically oriented therapist insists on exploring the patient's past. Some, considering it futile to add insight to injury, are prepared to step into the shoes of whoever in the patient's past has inadequately played his role.

Other therapists question the whole of psychodynamic theory, consider the patient's distress and dysfunction a result of inadequate social training rather than internal conflicts, and use the therapy meetings to enlarge the individual's repertoire of social skills. In order to motivate the patient to try to behave differently, the therapist may try to show him how ineffective, repetitive, and inflexible his behavior toward his family, fellow group members, or therapist is. If this does not cause the patient to experiment with new ways of behaving, he may be placed into a situation that is so unfamiliar or so paradoxical that it cannot be dealt with in the accustomed ways (Haley 1963).

By amiably satirizing or making light of the patient's difficulties, the therapist may help him see them in a clearer perspective (Coleman 1963). Similar effects are obtained with a technique called *paradoxical intention,* in which the patient is urged to exaggerate rather than combat his symptoms (Frankl 1960, Gerz 1962): the patient who shakes whenever he enters a room full of people is told to stop trying to look calm in such situations but rather to shake as much as he can, saying to himself all the while, "Come now, you can shake more fiercely than that!" When the patient's inadequacy is most pronounced in the presence of a particular person— such as a parent or spouse—that person may be asked to take part in the meetings. Some therapists simply give him direct advice on how to handle disturbing situations. Others, either individually or in *psychodrama,* the kind of group therapy mission introduced by Moreno (1940, 1945, 1952), let him experiment with a number of different ways by *role playing* (Eliasoph 1955).

Still others combine psychodynamics and practical social training. These therapists may teach their patients to deal with others by treating the doctor-patient relationship as a game in which better strategy helps the therapist or (after he learns how) the patient to win (Haley 1963). Used in the group or family treatment matrix, this technique is called *transactional analysis* (Berne 1961) or *reality therapy* (Glasser 1965).

Another approach to changing previous behavior patterns is called *behavior therapy* and consists of such measures as giving the patient an unpleasant stimulus whenever he engages in an act he is supposed to avoid (conditioned aversion), rewarding him whenever he acts in a way he is meant to continue (positive reinforcement), or gradually exposing him to things he could not previously tolerate (desensitization) (Eysenck 1960, 1963, Hain 1966, Paul 1967, Stampfl 1967, Wolpe 1961, 1964). This has also been used in the group therapy matrix, as when apomorphine treatment is given in the presence of other alcoholics (Miller 1960). In fact, the very process of group therapy, almost regardless of its orientation, can be viewed as a type of desensitization for the person afraid of being with others.

THE IMPACT OF SOCIOCULTURAL FACTORS ON THE TREATMENT RELATIONSHIP

The therapist's approach to the patient is also affected by the *professional climate of the community* in which he practices (Sharaf 1964, Stanton 1954). If, for example, most of the therapists in a given community or treatment center are fervent adherents of the analytic or, conversely, the organic approach to psychiatry, departures may be considered heretical and condoned only in the name of research or expediency. Equally or perhaps even more relevant are the *participants' sociocultural backgrounds, personalities, and life philosophies*. The patient's religious affiliation, social class, and ethnic origin will determine in large measure both the ideologic system with which he identifies and the values by which he lives. These factors and his *family's attitude* toward his treatment form an inevitable backdrop for every therapeutic transaction. The patient may find it difficult to discuss topics that his culture considers taboo or to effect behavior changes that his environment disapproves.

The poor, for example, rarely share the middle-class view on which much psychotherapy is based: that action should be preceded by reflection and that personal problems can be solved by discussion. Believing that the doctor should give only advice, medication, and practical assistance (Carlson 1965, White 1964a), they may react to the idea of talking things over with a psychiatrist with the same skepticism and hostility that a nineteenth-century shopkeeper would have exhibited to the recommendation that he discuss his marital problems with the alienist from the local asylum. The issues that emerge may also cause the lower-class patient to retreat from therapy after he has entered it. Discussions of resistance are considered attacks on his truthfulness; inquiries into his sexual fantasies are viewed as naive or prurient or, if they reveal unusual fantasies, can cause him to think of himself as so different or dangerous that he had better keep quiet. Equally problematic is his reaction to the complexity of the concepts used in psychotherapy. Awed by the therapist's apparent erudition, the patient's self-image may erode to the point that he feels stupid or thinks he is being made fun of, or, aping the therapist's language and style in his transactions with his own friends, makes a fool of himself.

The lower-class patient's failure to understand or function in the therapist's world may be matched by the therapist's inability to relate to him without condescension or false friendliness. As a result, the patient may feel so resentful that effective treatment is well-nigh impossible (White 1964b). Despite all good intentions, the doctor may be unable to understand patients whose attitudes and actions do not adhere to the middle-class standards that traditional therapy demands (Gould 1967, Koumans 1969, McMahon 1968). Punctuality is a case in point, as when a patient continually fails to show up at the appointed hour, and drops in when it suits him (Coleman 1965). Should this happen in the treatment of a middle-class patient, the therapist would have to suspect some variety of personality disorder. The lower-class patient, however, may merely be exercising a deeply ingrained life pattern, in which most interpersonal encounters are informal and unscheduled (Rosenthal 1968).

Sociocultural factors thus figure prominently in the difficulties encountered by the poor in obtaining psychiatric treatment and create a gulf between the therapist "haves" and the patient "have-nots" that cannot be spanned by money alone (Lesse 1968). Even when he comes to a free clinic or his treatment is paid for by a health insurance plan or public agency, the lower-class patient is unlikely to be offered intensive psychotherapy (Brown 1964, Hollingshead 1958, Saenger 1970, Schmidt 1968, Weber 1967) or to remain in treatment for long. In recent years, attempts have been made to counter these trends by modifying psychotherapeutic techniques (Nash 1965, Stone 1965). Increasing use is being made of *short-term, problem-oriented psychotherapy* that is restricted to discussion of the issues with which the patient is asking for help and avoids explorations he is likely to find irrelevant (Bernard 1965, Haskell 1969, Yamamoto 1966), *indigenous mental health workers,* and *ghetto mental health facilities* such as storefront or walk-in clinics (Riessman 1964, Rosenbaum 1964).

GUIDELINES FOR A SOCIOADAPTIVE APPROACH TO TREATMENT

The foregoing factors, the availability of treatment facilities, and outright coincidence in the choice of therapist, together determine the kind of treatment the patient will receive. Diagnostic criteria generally play a far smaller role (Levinson 1967), an observation that is not surprising to anyone cognizant of the economic realities of obtaining treatment and the statistical reality that there is no way to predict which kind of psychotherapeutic program will be most effective for a particular patient. Success has been claimed for the most abstruse of therapeutic measures (Borgatta 1959, Poser 1966), and it must be remembered that the practice of psychotherapy rests on certain assumptions that are consistent with common sense but in no way are supported by controlled studies. Among these assumptions are that

> 1/ certain ways of dealing with or behaving in the presence of patients are better for them than other ways would be;
> 2/ individuals trained in psychotherapy are not only familiar with these ways but are able to modify their own behavior to conform to the individual patient's needs; and
> 3/ the favorable changes seen in an individual who has been in therapy can be attributed to his treatment and not to his own decision to change (of which his entering treatment is evidence) or to such extrinsic considerations as maturation, changed circumstances, or the mere passage of time.

Despite certain reservations about the validity of these assumptions, we believe that the kind of relationship offered by psychotherapists is often of benefit for the individual who is impaired in his social or transactional skills, particularly if his impairment is so severe that it causes his environment to respond in a way that reinforces rather than corrects it. These conditions may apply when an individual

> 1/ consistently behaves in a manner so distant or offensive that

he is unable to make friends and consequently has little opportunity to learn how his behavior affects those around him;

   2/ is so defensive, suspicious, or oversensitive that he misunderstands what he is told and, misjudging the feelings and intentions of those who try to correct him, ignores what they say; or

   3/ is so shy that he cannot tolerate any kind of personal intimacy and subjects every relationship into which he enters to such severe and unusual stresses that—whether unintentionally (as he is likely to claim) or by design (as it more often appears)—the relationship ends.

If these problems persist for a time long enough, and especially when they prevail throughout the individual's formative years, his social awkwardness, offensiveness, and shyness will impair his ability to get along with others, and if not offered a corrective relationship, he may become lonely, impulsive, self-damaging, dishonest with himself, or profoundly dissatisfied with his life.

Unable to maintain or benefit from the nonprofessional relationships in which others learn social skills, patients with difficulties of this kind may quite rightly consult a psychotherapist, for among the competent therapist's most obvious attributes are his ability and willingness to establish and engage in a lasting relationship with individuals whom most nonprofessionals would regard as too unpleasant or difficult to tolerate. Although the therapist's willingness to develop a relationship with almost anyone who consults him professionally is somewhat artificial, particularly since he is paid for this willingness, there are decided advantages in such artificiality. The patient who has trouble relating to others because he distorts and distrusts their motives will almost certainly develop similar ideas about the therapist within a brief time (Orr 1954). The experienced therapist differs from the other persons in the patient's environment in having encountered such distortions before and, even more, in understanding himself and his own motives fairly well, so that he is better equipped to gauge the accuracy of the patient's perceptions. Moreover, at least at the outset, the therapist is less personally involved and affected than a friend or a relative might be, has (ideally) less need to appear kind, virtuous, or wise, and is therefore far abler to withstand the patient's and family's blandishments, tolerate their doubts about his competence and the wisdom of his decisions, and take whatever steps the situation requires. Accustomed to contemplating the errors of others, he can permit the patient the luxury of being wrong, hostile, irritable, or affectionate without needing to defend himself, to counterattack, to terminate the relationship, or even (until he considers the time opportune) to acknowledge that he understands the patient's feelings.

The extent to which the relationship with the therapist benefits the patient depends less on the therapist's training than on his personality (Strupp 1969). In our view, most of the patient's learning in psychotherapy derives from his acceptance of the therapist's values plus his observation and imitation of the therapist's behavior. The adolescent who admires and tries to emulate a therapist who interposes discussion and thought between feeling and action may thereby become less impulsive. The patient who glides through life with so little involvement with and understanding of other people that he easily becomes puzzled or hurt by what he views as cruel or incomprehensible behavior may, if treated by a therapist who enjoys conceptualizing human relationships, develop a clearer, more benign view of the motives and behavior of those around him; if such an individual follows the therapist's lead, he can learn to cast aside his feelings of being unfairly attacked in favor of reflecting and theorizing on the possible psychological motives of his critics.

Imitation and identification occur no less in the therapy group. By observing the therapist or the other group members, the individual who feels too shy or too awkward to express or accept feelings of warmth or aggression in public may learn that openness need not cause irreparable offense nor end discussions abruptly (Neighbor 1958, Levine 1969), but, on the contrary, can improve the participants' relationships and enhance the individual's prestige in the group (Fried 1965). A more straightforward communicative style will not necessarily make him more comfortable, but it may well make him feel less devious and in any case teach him something about his own behavior and feelings. His ability to be honest with himself, to express his true feelings to others, and to accept well-meant (and even malevolent) criticism may be limited at first to the therapy sessions, but in time may come to be tested and applied in the wider environment of his daily life (Gergen 1969, Strupp 1969).

CRITERIA FOR SELECTION OF THE OPTIMAL TREATMENT MATRIX

As this Chapter has so far suggested, we consider psychotherapy's primary goal the learning, maintenance, or restoration of the interpersonal skills required for internal comfort and effective social functioning. With this in mind, we generally place the patient into whatever treatment matrix most resembles the area of his life most affected by his deficiencies. The patient who experiences difficulty in developing or maintaining intimate relationships would be offered individual therapy; one who cannot communicate or be at ease with his peers is placed in a therapy group; and one whose difficulties occur in his relationship to his parents or spouse might be advised to participate in family or couples therapy. When the patient's family or spouse is equally isolated or socially awkward, they should participate with him in a families or couples therapy group.

Discomfort and incompetence in particular kinds of situations tend to go hand in hand, so that it is usually easy to identify the area (or areas) in which the patient needs help. Nevertheless, some people are uncomfortable even in situations they handle well, as in the case of a schizophrenic woman who deals with her psychotic mother quite competently, taking her shopping and to the movies, yet becomes extremely disturbed after each encounter. Others are hypersensitive and inept in so many situations that it is hard to say which is most disturbing, or in which they are most incompetent. Finally, some individuals are upset by one kind of transaction but give vent to the difficulty in another, a typical example being the junior executive who handles his boss fairly well despite great feelings of resentment, but then goes home and takes it out on his wife.

It is nevertheless usually possible to make a well-reasoned and effective choice between the available matrices by obtaining a family and social history, a chronological report of the patient's social difficulties and psychological symptoms, a history of the way his current symptoms arose, and a report of the putative precipitating events (Knight 1953). The choice is, of course, subject to modification if the patient's needs become clearer or change, or his rate of improvement proves unsatisfactory. In the following sections, we will review each of the most commonly used matrices, its indications and contraindications, and the considerations involved in switching from one treatment matrix to another.

Individual Psychotherapy

The practice of individual therapy has come under fire in the past few years for its ineffectiveness, for taking more of a specialist's time than the average person can afford, and for costing more per patient than the community could afford if all who needed psychi-

atric attention were to receive it. Its defenders respond that the
latter arguments could as easily be leveled against artificial kidneys
and organ transplants and that the value of any treatment, from a
medical if not from a social standpoint, must be judged in terms of
its effects rather than its cost. Regardless of the justice of these seemingly disparate viewpoints, even those who consider the claims made
for individual psychotherapy excessive generally acknowledge that
there are situations in which it is the treatment of choice.

The distinguishing characteristics of individual psychotherapy
that make it the matrix of choice in a particular case are that it

1/ offers the patient an opportunity to improve his skills in
establishing and maintaining an intimate relationship;

2/ can be geared closely to the patient's particular needs;

3/ is relatively uncomplicated, in that there are fewer variables
to be taken into account in assessing the patient's response to treatment;

4/ enables the therapist to understand the patient's view of his
past and present more rapidly than is possible in any other matrix;
and

5/ can ensure the confidentiality of what the patient reveals and
discovers about himself.

The kind of interpersonal transaction to which the patient responds
best differs in various types and phases of illness and is therefore
discussed at greater length in the chapters describing the treatment
of each disease specifically (see Chap. 3 through 12).

If the patient is lucid enough to communicate, individual meetings are the fastest, most thorough way of gathering information
and therefore desirable whenever the patient's situation is critical
enough to require immediate action or close observation. Individual
therapy is also the treatment of choice for the patient whose discomfort follows an upsetting event like a death in the family, for
he is likely to feel better fairly rapidly and ought not be immersed
in too complex a therapy program. Again, individual meetings are
preferable for the individual who confronts a genuinely difficult
decision, as the discussion can resume at each meeting from the point
at which it left off without being interrupted by the digressions of
other participants.

Individual therapy is particularly valuable for the person whose
problems are related to his difficulty in developing undistorted,
cooperative, one-to-one relationships (Fierman 1965). Since the
average patient deals with the therapist much as he deals with the

rest of the world, the individual psychotherapy matrix can be used as a laboratory in which to observe and perhaps modify the way the patient handles other interpersonal relationships. His competence in such relationships (and thus the urgency of his need for individual therapy) can usually be assessed in a few meetings. From the first meeting on, the therapist tries to determine whether the patient's behavior toward him resembles collaboration between peers, an aggrieved confrontation with an accuser, or a dependent demand for nurturing. Childlike trust in the course of this encounter does not always signal pathologic naiveté or dependence, for the image of doctors as magicians or supermen is so integral a part of what most children are taught that the adult who treats a doctor with undue reverence may be demonstrating only his uncritical acceptance of the cultural myth. This kind of faith is particularly common in individuals who were ill throughout most of their childhood and thus have had a fairly continuous and, almost invariably, dependent relationship with a physician.

In some cases, individual therapy is preferred out of concern about confidentiality, but this advantage ought not be given undue weight. Undeniably, an individual may be disadvantaged by having his secrets disclosed to others (even the secret that he is in treatment at all). In our experience, however, group members rarely embarrass each other outside the therapeutic setting. If the patient referred for group therapy cannot allay his concerns about this matter, the therapist must consider the possibility that his fear of speaking frankly before others is a part of his problem, especially if the secrets in question seem fairly trivial or unlikely to be of interest to anyone else. In many cases, the patient's inordinate concern for secrecy stems from an exaggerated view of his real or imagined misdeeds or a deep distrust of his entire environment. Such an individual may have much to gain from being exposed to a therapy group, but be unable to get involved in its activity until he has been in individual therapy for a long enough period of time to accept his therapist's recommendations with confidence.

The *shortcomings of individual therapy* are also pertinent in making a treatment choice. One commonly encountered problem is that the patient finds his relationship to the therapist so gratifying that he fails to realize that he can develop such relationships with others as well; such a patient may well lose sight of the ultimate goals of treatment and, though constantly singing the praises of psychotherapy and his particular therapist to anyone who will listen, withdraw further and further from traditional social transactions (Lower 1967).

Another patient may view his treatment as an alliance against his intimates, use his therapy time only to berate them, and close his eyes to his own contribution to his difficulties (Gottschalk 1962, Sager 1968). One particularly dangerous reaction to individual therapy is exemplified by what we term "dependency brinkmanship," a form of behavior in which a patient who wants desperately to hold his therapist's interest remains constantly on the verge of a crisis, threatening ever to behave in a self-destructive, socially disruptive, or antisocial manner. Other patients will use their treatment program as a rationale for their passivity and their unwillingness to make any meaningful changes in their lives (Schmideberg 1968). Such patients commonly tell both themselves and those around them that they must postpone making important decisions (particularly uncomfortable ones) until therapy "changes" them, that they cannot, for example, go to work or take on responsibilities until this has been accomplished.

Regressive behavior occurs more frequently in individual therapy than in other treatment matrixes, perhaps because of the emphasis it places on the patient's self-determination (Szasz 1967). Dogmatic adherence to this principle may make the therapist reluctant to counter the patient's regression in the most expedient way, such as telling him that he will view further regression as evidence that the treatment is having so little or so harmful an effect that the patient should be referred to another physician or hospitalized. The longer the therapist postpones taking a firm stand, the further the regression extends, and the greater the danger of decompensation, social disaster, or suicide becomes. Such behavior seems less common among individuals seen in group therapy, partly because the therapy relationship does not become so intimate and partly because fellow-patients are usually less indulgent and more vocal in expressing disapproval than psychotherapists. While peer censure may be more vigorous, it may also be easier for the patient to take, and he may thus listen and conform to the group's demands more easily than he would to the therapist's.

Family and Couples Therapy

In recent years, psychotherapists have become increasingly interested in understanding how marital and familial relationships affect and are affected by the participants' mental health. This interest has culminated in such treatment methods as couples therapy and family therapy, the latter often including children, parents, or other significant relatives as well. The counseling of married couples and other family groups is not a recent psychotherapeutic advance. In the past, it was undertaken, often quite skillfully, by clergymen, family doctors, and in-laws, but their efforts were usually limited to urging kindness, mutual consideration, or a renewal of the vows to love, honor, and obey. Such admonitions have so inconstant an effect, however, that psychotherapists generally try to do something else. What that something else is and what aspect of it, if any, is helpful are among the important questions currently under study. Another important research question is whether patients with a particular mental illness are more likely than others to be involved in a particular kind of marital or family pattern and, if so, what illnesses cluster with what kinds of patterns and why (Gardner 1967, Haley 1959, Jackson 1959).

Although there is no clear-cut relationship between individual and family psychopathology, there is little doubt that the families of psychiatric patients exhibit a remarkably high incidence of psychopathology and that a high correlation exists between the severity of a patient's psychopathology and that of his family (Ackerman 1958, Lidz 1963). Some authors explain these findings in terms of *genetic factors* (Heston 1970); others in terms of *assortative mating* (the tendency of disturbed persons to choose disturbed partners) or as a consequence of the *erosive effect* that long-term contact with a psychologically disturbed person has on his immediate family (Kreitman 1964, 1968, Nielsen 1964, Plansky 1967, Woerner 1968). While none of these hypotheses is generally accepted, it is important to distinguish between the family that has always behaved strangely and the one that seemed fairly unremarkable until the patient became ill, for what looks like family psychopathology may prove to be no more than an unsatisfactory reaction to the patient's disturbed behavior or an uninformed attempt to help him get well (Ellenberger 1961, Lewis 1960).

Relatives' reactions are sometimes so unexpected or even bizarre that it is hard to tell which family member is really the patient. In some cases, they all seem equally disturbed; in others, each seems well and reasonable enough when seen by himself, but as disturbed as the rest when all are seen together. Even when one family member has such obvious symptoms that the label of "patient" is pinned on him, the psychiatrist cannot ignore his relatives' psychopathology and, whether or not they express their desire for help explicitly, should provide them with support and, if needed, with treatment as well (Norton 1963).

Family therapy is unique in that it encourages certain activities that other therapy matrixes seem designed to prevent (Haley 1962). Unlike group and individual therapy, the participants have known each other for a long time. The feelings they experience in the therapy sessions need not be transferred or displaced from family members to others, but can be expressed to and examined with the very persons who provoked them. The objects of their feelings can thus react to what they say during the meeting and may even do so thereafter. As a result, the patient does not enjoy the same immunity from retaliation that he can expect in individual therapy. This will not always be to his disadvantage, though, even if some of his feelings are hostile, for, in this setting, the individual he is angry at may come to understand why and make overtures toward reconciliation (Weakland 1962).

The therapist who sees the whole family together will in any case get a clearer picture of its transactions than the one who hears only one side and must constantly speculate about the possible distortions (Greenberg 1964). In our experience, the problem is not resolved by seeing each family member separately, for this merely provides the therapist with several different descriptions of the same events, and thus serves to compound his confusion. Only when they are all together can each correct or dispute the others' distortions or discrepancies. This, moreover, is the therapist's only way to observe family conflicts in their natural state and, if desirable, help resolve them (Williams 1967). Finally, family therapy is an effective way to combat the resistant patient's reluctance to visit the doctor. No matter how fervently he insists that he does not need, and will not take part in, further treatment, the momentum of his spouse or family getting ready to go usually pulls him along.

That the participants have a prior joint history adds to the setting's therapeutic impetus; many uncomfortable facts that the individual patient might have withheld from the therapist are quickly revealed. Even if the entire family colludes to conceal certain relevant facts, the attempt usually generates so much tension that the therapist begins to suspect that the situation is more involved than it seems. We do not mean to portray the therapist as a latter-day Sherlock Holmes looking for discrepancies in the family's story, nor to suggest that he can invariably tell when he is being duped, but disturbed families are usually as unsuccessful at collusion as they are at other forms of cooperation (Jackson 1965). For all these reasons, the roles of the various family members tend to come into focus more clearly and quickly in family than in individual therapy

(Tharp 1966). It cannot be claimed that such clarification in itself is therapeutic, but there is ample clinical evidence that a significant difference between sick families and healthy ones is not that the former find it more difficult to relate to each other, nor that they take more bizarre roles, but that their conflicts and roles are more likely to be covert and unexpressed (Fleck 1966). For example, a family that freely acknowledges that the husband and father is mentally ill and not to be taken seriously is usually less disturbed than the family that denies his problem and pretends that all the directives the mother issues actually originate with the father.

A family that is otherwise relatively stable may try to protect its mentally ill member from embarrassment and community action by becoming progressively more isolated. A family with several mentally ill members is already isolated from the community, and, when one member's disturbances become more obvious, tends to withdraw even further, may blame or ostracize the disturbed individual, and, worst of all, may prevent him from receiving medical help by pretending that nothing is wrong.

When the family has withdrawn to protect its one deviant member, generally only he is in need of intensive therapy; the others need see the therapist only at a few family meetings in which all are encouraged to live as they did before he fell ill, and he is urged to involve himself once again in their activities. When the family as a whole is disturbed and socially isolated, however, its reintegration into the community may be one of the most important aspects of the patient's treatment, for he may be hard put to flourish if the family's behavior does not change along with his. A convenient way of reintroducing both him and his family to social relationships is to have them join a couples or families group (Kimbro 1967). A group of this kind is also of value when the therapist considers the family unstable and potentially jealous of his role, for he must be sure that his relationship to the patient does not grow more quickly than their ability to accept it. Family therapy can also be used to help the relatives accept the patient's illness and understand and support his treatment (Fleck 1963). The clarification of these issues is especially important when the patient provokes his family into distrusting his doctor or when they are naturally suspicious, for then they may view his therapy as a threat and try to sabotage it.

Even when the family is not expected to be continuously involved in treatment, *three-way meetings* between the patient, family, and doctor may be necessary from time to time. The psychotic patient, for example, may be so fearful when talking to anyone outside his immediate family that no meaningful transaction can take place in their absence. Joint meetings are also essential when the patient is about to enter or leave a hospital or when the situation is so critical that hospitalization can be staved off only if close supervision can be arranged. In the latter case, the purpose of the meeting is to teach the patient's family how to convert their home into a kind of day hospital where he can receive safe and effective treatment. Meetings of this kind are especially important when the therapist is concerned that the family is too primitive or disturbed to undertake his care by themselves. The doctor's efforts in educating and, if necessary, treating them can reap benefits both in improving the home environment and in helping the patient understand that his confusion is caused partly by his family's noncorrective attitudes and behavior.

Family meetings may also be necessary when a patient is psychologically or financially dependent on his family and requires their permission to enter treatment, and they insist on meeting the therapist to evaluate him for themselves. Such meetings are helpful, too, when the patient feels he needs explicit permission to strike out for himself. If the family is reluctant to give such permission on the grounds that the patient is too young or too ill, this need not be taken to mean, as it often is, that they wish him to remain sick or dependent, but may merely reflect their experience that he does poorly on his own. The doctor who believes that the patient will progress more rapidly away from home and advises his family to help him leave is often surprised at the alacrity with which they cooperate (and the suddenness with which the "independence-seeking" patient then discovers a dozen reasons for postponing his departure) (Scherz 1967). If the family's reluctance derives solely from their desire to infantilize or control the patient, their unwillingness to permit him to leave will help the patient understand their motives more clearly and thus permit him a somewhat freer, or at any rate a more honest, choice. Once these difficulties and the issues that underlie them are explored and, when possible, resolved, the family meetings have achieved their purpose and the patient may be placed in individual group and/or individual therapy.

Couples or family therapy is also indicated for the situations known as *folie à deux* or *folie à famille* in which a couple or even a whole family share the delusional patient's ideas. In some cases, the shared delusions are so deeply ingrained that the participants must be separated to prevent their continually reinforcing each other. In others, it is not really a question of delusions but merely that the family, despite finding one member's ideas odd, has decided against actively disputing them, or is even trying to consider the ideas right. Under these circumstances or when the shared ideas are of too little consequence to be called delusional, couples or family therapy may be helpful at some point during treatment. It would be appropriate, for example, if a husband and wife have tacitly agreed never to mention that the husband did not complete college, consciously lie to each other and the rest of the world about it, and then become uncomfortable about the resulting psychological tension. It may be easiest to expose such a troubling, socially embarrassing "secret" (which, since everyone in the family knows about it, is not a secret at all) by initially meeting with each partner separately to get permission to bring the subject out into the open and thereafter holding a joint meeting in which the troubling effects of their conspiracy of silence are discussed.

Group Therapy

When a number of individual patients, couples, or families meet with one or more therapists at the same time, the process is labeled group therapy. When the members are unrelated to each other, it may be subclassified as *individual group therapy;* when the group consists of two or more married couples, as *couples group therapy;* and when the group is composed of several generations of relatives of several families, as *families group therapy.* Combinations of these, such as individuals within couples groups or a couple within an individual group, are of course also possible and are sometimes indicated.

The first reported medical use of group therapy was not to treat patients with psychological disorders but to instruct, advise, and reassure patients suffering from tuberculosis (Pratt 1906). Increasing interest in group processes and in group therapy's value as an arena for social training and retraining has dovetailed in recent years with the scarcity of therapists and the prohibitive cost of individual therapy to produce enthusiastic acceptance and extensive use. It must be emphasized, however, that a patient should never be referred to a therapy group merely for the sake of economy or convenience. The prime purpose is to offer the individual a microcosmic community in which to learn and practice new social skills while examining the sources and manifestations of his difficulties.

The variety of problems and people he may encounter in a therapy group will provide him with a unique opportunity to study his reactions to other people and their reactions to him; to become more sensitive to their problems; and to compare his way of dealing with his world to their ways of dealing with theirs.

The primary indication for group therapy is *difficulty in establishing and maintaining peer relationships.* Such an individual may be so competitive, demanding, or socially awkward that he irritates or repels everyone with whom he comes in contact. Group therapy will also be helpful for the patient whose disorder has developed in the context of an *acculturation* process, such as a student who, after growing up in a small town, enters a large urban university and falls ill; or one who is chronologically an adult but socially and emotionally *dependent* on his parents. *Excessive shyness* is another characteristic indication for group therapy. Whatever its cause—social deprivation, latent schizophrenia, inferior social training, a maturational lag, a noncorrective or paranoid rearing environment, or a protracted illness at the critical period for developing skill in peer relationships—shyness brings in its wake a progressive, self-perpetuating impairment in transactional skills. The shy patient's difficulties in transacting with or becoming interested in others may cause him to object to this recommendation on the grounds that it will make him more uncomfortable, but this need not diminish its benefits: even if he does not enjoy the meetings, he is likely to learn how others react to his social discomfort and how he can manage it somewhat better.

Therapy groups are also indicated for the patient whose previous history or initial presentation leads the clinician to suspect that his own *objectivity will become blurred* in the course of treatment. Typical examples of this include the patient whose passive, regressive, or antisocial behavior exceeds the therapist's tolerance (see p. 253); the patient who induces the therapist to overlook his bad behavior by being "interesting," "seductive," or "earnestly looking for answers"; and the patient who describes his previous therapists in terms that are at once so paranoid and so convincing that the new therapist, even if he momentarily finds the criticism well grounded, sees that he will soon become the target of identical complaints. Here a therapy group can help the therapist in the same way that it can help the patient, or, to put it somewhat differently, as one colleague helps another when countertransference problems arise in individual therapy: it provides the therapist with an arena in which he can get some consensual validation of the real nature of the transactions, and thus helps him avoid such absurd situations as becoming too permissive in order to avoid appearing too strict. Groups are also helpful for treating the *rebellious adolescent* who rejects the individual therapist's help because he views him as a parent surrogate. A therapy group composed of his peers can dilute the hostile feeling he displaces onto the therapist and thus prevent his terminating treatment prematurely. This effect can be further enhanced if from time to time the group meets without the therapist in a *leaderless therapy group* (Astrachan 1967, Kadis 1963).

With the average group, the therapist will try to restrict his advice to a minimum, perhaps suggesting nothing beyond the length, frequency, time, and location of the meetings, and expressing his views concerning the advisability of contact among members outside the group. Nevertheless, his view of the intragroup transactions will inevitably have a major impact on the way the group functions and the topics it chooses to discuss, for the members usually try to do what they think the therapist wants (Harrow 1967). Our own approach is to use the group situation as a model from which each member can learn something about the way groups function and the way he himself functions in groups. For this reason, our comments are generally directed to the activities of the group as a whole, and we tend to avoid interpreting the psychodynamics of any individual member. In our opinion, the *therapist's* most important *functions* as group leaders are to

1/ show the participants that the group's activities and interactions are more than the simple sum of its individual members' personalities and psychopathology, and
2/ explore some of the unspoken basic assumptions and transactional patterns that govern the group's activities (Bion 1961, Whittaker 1964).

In the sense that these assumptions and patterns influence the group's activities without the members' realizing it, they may be thought of as the group's "unconscious," the more so because the group's functioning often improves once these factors become explicit.

While universal *"rules"* for group therapy are impossible, we usually suggest that the meetings take place once or twice weekly, consider it useful for the members to hold one "leaderless" group a week, insist on regular attendance at all scheduled meetings, and accept no "reasons" for absence. These rules must on occasion be drastically modified, however, as in the case of the chronically deprived patient who is so afraid of intimacy that he violates any rigid rule in order to set up a situation in which he will be rejected. Such an individual is more appropriately placed in a group that has a regular meeting time but does not require regular attendance (Jarecki 1964).

The Choice of Group Therapy Matrix

The unmarried adult and the patient whose difficulties seem unrelated to his marital or familial situation are generally placed in an *individual group*. The young person who needs to become independent of his parents may benefit from a *combination of family meetings and individual group therapy,* the former in order to secure parental understanding of the separation and the latter to test his increasing independence. Even the individual whose psychological difficulties seem related to a disturbed marital relationship may profit more from meetings without his spouse. A wife may be so fearful that her husband will consider her foolish or be embarrassed by her that she is unable to talk freely in his presence; a husband who feels guilty about a sexual affair may be reluctant to discuss it in the presence of his wife.

Couples and families therapy groups have certain advantages over other therapeutic matrixes. As in the individual group, the participants generally discover that their problems are not unique, which is especially useful if learned in the presence of the person with whom the problems arose, for even if the discovery does nothing else, it permits them to talk about their differences calmly and objectively. Seeing others caught up in the same dilemmas (the fear of loneliness vs. the discomforts of excessive intimacy, or the feeling of jealousy vs. the guilt associated with too possessive an attitude) helps them broaden their perspectives about their own problems (Papanek 1965). This sharing of experiences and reactions is of particular benefit to the family that has one extremely disturbed member, for it provides a supportive forum in which practical questions of management can be discussed and the disturbed member's relatives can acknowledge how fearful, burdened, guilty, or angry they feel. Couples or family therapy is also advantageous for the family that has little else in common, for the amusements, discomforts, and efforts at insight occurring in the group can provide topics of conversation and shared reflections that may improve the participants' communication even after the therapy session ends.

Families or couples who fight a great deal often learn to restrict their disputes to the therapy sessions. Some report that each time a fight is brewing, one or the other counters by saying, "Save it for the group," and frequently the dispute ends there. Other families report that the group was the first setting in which they behaved civilly to each other, and that after going through the motions of socially appropriate behavior in the group for some months, they were able to behave more congenially outside the group as well. Regardless of how domestic tranquility is achieved, it usually gives such relief that all concerned strive to maintain it. Even if they do not abandon their fights (and this is by no means the only purpose of therapy), they may learn how to use them more productively, less viciously, and possibly with some appreciation of the absurdity of the issues involved.

Notwithstanding their advantages, group and family programs have certain inherent *drawbacks*. For example, some patients accept group therapy enthusiastically only because they are unwilling to subject themselves to the kind of intimate involvement and self-scrutiny required in individual therapy and believe (quite justifiably) that the group setting will make it easier to remain distant. Two typical distancing maneuvers seen in groups are exemplified by

1/ the "group monopolist," whose constant talk prevents other patients from reflecting on either his behavior or their own, and

2/ the "therapist's helper," who agrees with everything the therapist says, explains the therapist's views to the group, and deftly parries all attempts to explore his own psychological difficulties by exploring the motives of the questioner or urging him to get back to the "real topic."

Although a skillful and experienced group therapist can sometimes dampen these practices by pointing out how they paralyze the group, some patients are impervious to such comments and must be seen in individual meetings during which this style and the reasons for adopting it are discussed. These meetings must be additions to, not replacements for, the group meetings, however, for of the many roles the group therapist assumes, one of the most important is that of *guarantor of the group's existence*. No matter how disruptive the patient may be, it is usually more dangerous to the group's continued life to exclude him than to keep him in the group: in any case, the patient's behavior often becomes more bearable after a few individual sessions.

Another abuse of the group therapy matrix is exemplified by the couple who fight constantly, have little or no interest in changing their behavior, come to the meetings only to embarrass each other, and continue to fight even after they understand what they are doing and why. The therapist can sometimes arrange a temporary truce, during which they can explore their behavior without becoming excessively defensive; if no such truce can be arranged, he may well be unable to do anything beyond expressing his amazement at their seeming to enjoy the presence of others during their perverse kind of intimacy while still alleging that they don't like to fight and wish someone could stop them. Problems with such couples are generally short-lived, however, for they usually stop coming as soon as their motives are questioned.

These group transactions are usually conducted outside a hospital, but some patients are so deficient in social skills as to risk serious difficulty unless confined. *Residential treatment* may also be necessary for the patient whose home life is so pathologic or noncorrective that it interferes with his chances of social rehabilitation and for the one without any supportive environment at all. Some psychiatric facilities, especially those that keep patients for an extended period of time, offer the corrective features of 24-hour-a-day group living subsumed under the term *therapeutic community* (Christ 1965, Fleck 1962, Jones 1953, 1968, Marsh 1931), by which is meant a treatment program that

> *1/* emphasizes the importance of extensive communication between all participants, staff and patients alike;
> *2/* deemphasizes the differences between patients and staff; and
> *3/* encourages patients to participate not only in their own treatment program but in that of their fellow residents as well.

For those who stay long enough, such a program can greatly improve the prospects for social rehabilitation (Beckett 1968), particularly when it is combined with vigorous academic and vocational training (Braceland 1966, Wing 1966). Simply by living with others and learning to depend on and be depended on by them, the patient can discover which aspects of his behavior are socially attractive and which offensive. As a result, both he and those around him obtain an unparalleled opportunity to observe his day-to-day strengths and weaknesses and to effect his social reeducation (Almond 1969a,b, Ludwig 1966) (see also pp. 256 and 316).

OTHER FACTORS TO CONSIDER IN MATRIX SELECTION

The proposal that the patient be exposed to whichever therapy matrix most nearly resembles the aspect of his life in which his difficulties originated or became manifest may be hard to implement for the same reasons that it is proposed. The individual may find it so difficult that he threatens to leave treatment altogether. If his condition is too grave to permit him to discontinue and it is considered imperative that he be anchored in therapy as rapidly as possible, it is wisest to place him in a matrix he finds more comfortable and postpone placing him in the more appropriate one until his most acute symptoms have receded and his commitment to treatment seems secure.

Some measure of the difficulties an individual might experience in a given treatment matrix can be obtained by weighing its demands for intimacy against the level of intimacy he can tolerate without becoming anxious; and by weighing the degree of social stimulation it provides against the amount of stimulation he can tolerate without misinterpreting the situation or becoming panicky. If, for example, a patient with an agitated depression is subjected to a series of one-hour individual sessions, he will in all likelihood be hard put to maintain a communicative dialogue throughout. He may indeed come to view his performance as one further proof that he is inadequate, inarticulate, and incurable; and end up feeling worse rather than better (see p. 182). It is therefore preferable to see this patient together with his family first and permit them to carry the burden of explaining things to the doctor. Brief individual interviews devoted to giving him reassurance and support rather than asking him questions or a therapy group in which he can remain silent, if he wishes to, are likely to be of greater benefit for this kind of patient than intensive individual psychotherapy.

Another example would be a schizophrenic patient who is placed in a group while he is so confused and delusional that he finds it hard to follow or comprehend the transactions. If he becomes more confused and starts to weave his faulty observations into the fabric of his delusional interpretations, individual therapy sessions are preferable. Even if he finds such sessions too close for comfort, they are unlikely to add to his confusion. By focusing on immediate issues at first and discouraging the patient's ruminatious about his delusions or his chaotic unconscious, the therapist can maintain enough distance in the relationship to help the patient feel more at ease. Later, as the patient begins to show signs that he can tolerate increased intimacy, a closer and more candid relationship can be achieved.

The patient's intelligence level is another important factor in the choice of treatment matrix. Patients who are unusually intelligent require a matrix that does not seem too simple or dull. The patient who is intellectually limited should either be placed in a group restricted to persons of similar capacities or, if no group is available, seen individually lest, confronted by group transactions too complicated or rapid to grasp, he is relegated to the role of bewildered onlooker.

Although the patient's wishes should be considered in choosing the optimal treatment matrix, they should by no means dictate the choice. Let us say that we see a patient who, despite acting friendly and chatty in the initial interview, shows objective signs of discomfort such as sweating or nervous mannerisms. If his history reveals that he has had problems with teachers ever since childhood, has seen other therapists but felt they became too demanding or "bossy," and gets along well with co-workers but poorly with his immediate supervisor, it is clear that he finds it difficult to relate to authority figures and that the treatment matrix most likely to help him develop competence in this area would be individual therapy. The patient, however, may be so apprehensive about confronting the kind of authority figure he sees in the therapist that he expresses a preference for group therapy. If his discomfort with individual meetings is extreme, group therapy may indeed be indicated as the first step in his treatment, but he should be exposed to individual therapy as soon as his discomfort with the idea abates.

Changes in the patient's environmental situation or psychobiologic needs may also dictate a change in the treatment matrix. The treatment possibilities for a depressed woman torn between loyalties to a possessive, controlling mother and a husband too weak to oppose the matriarch will illustrate the *sequential utilization* of treatment matrices. If she is agitated, anorectic, and unable to sleep, we start with brief, fairly frequent individual meetings, the primary purpose of which is superficial support and the regulation of somatic treatment. As her acute discomfort diminishes and her dissatisfaction with her life emerges, the patient-doctor encounters may be lengthened to the customary 30 to 60 minute individual psychotherapy sessions. Let us suppose that she uses these meetings to express her irritation with the other two protagonists in a way that implies an effort to enlist the doctor as an "ally" against both husband and mother, and then carries this campaign to the home front by making her husband feel left out and vaguely jealous of the therapist. Further individual therapy at this point is in danger of becoming a cul-de-sac: it is time to see the couple together. In the course of subsequent meetings, the husband may come to appreciate his wife's dissatisfaction with his failure to face up to her domineering mother and begin to take a stronger stand. Faced with the husband's new firmness, the mother may release her hold on her daughter; if she does not, it may be advisable to involve her in the therapy sessions. Once this phase is completed, the couple might be placed in a couples group, where they can observe how other couples try to resolve the same kinds of issues and conflicts. After an extended group experience of this nature, the wife may be ready to consolidate the gains made in these several therapeutic matrices by returning to individual psychotherapy, prepared to explore her situation and her contribution to it, rather than merely to complain about her environment without being ready to make any changes.

Such *simultaneous* use of several psychotherapeutic matrices can complicate the situation and make it harder to understand. Nevertheless, it adds certain dimensions for observing and interacting with the patient that improve the therapeutic potential of the encounters. When, for example, a patient being seen in individual therapy is convinced that he has "nothing of interest to say" or is so uncommunicative, depressed, or withdrawn that no meaningful contact can be established, the therapist may find it useful to have him come to a therapy group, and thus provide the two of them together with shared, real-life experiences to discuss in their individual sessions.

The final and perhaps most obvious indication for changing or adding to a therapeutic matrix is that it has been of little or no benefit. This may be assumed when the patient

1/ is regressing not only during the therapy session but in his outside life as well;

2/ over an extended period of time, is unable to translate insight or increased comfort in the therapeutic transaction into improved social behavior; or

3/ is using the fact that he is in treatment to excuse socially inappropriate behavior or to postpone making decisions that will not wait.

Excessive changing around should be avoided, however, as it is confusing to clinician and patient alike: a minimum of eight weeks in a given matrix is usually needed before an informed guess on the patient's ultimate response to it is possible.

MATCHMAKING IN PSYCHOTHERAPY

Since it is generally agreed that much of what happens in treatment depends on the personalities and styles of the participants, the process of referring a patient to a psychotherapist might be expected to entail a careful consideration of the two personalities. Although we know that each therapist's unique interests, attributes, and skills affect the outcome of treatment, there are no scientifically verifiable ways of predicting what that effect will be. In the absence of any such guidelines for matching patients to therapists, or for determining the most effective composition of a group, referrals are based largely on practical and economic considerations and on the referring physician's esteem for the psychotherapist in question. Yet, since different therapists excel in different matrices (some doing their best work in the framework of individual therapy, others with the families of patients, and yet others in the treatment of groups), a patient must not be referred to a particular psychotherapist because he is considered "good," but because he is effective in the matrix the patient requires. The therapist's own life style, and, especially, his mode of relating to others are useful considerations in determining the types of patients for whom his special traits are best adapted. The patient who elects to undergo therapy in order to understand himself better is most likely to be satisfied with a therapist who is himself reflective and can help him fit his ideas and behavior into some kind of conceptual framework. The patient who is disorganized, immature, or lacking in judgment will gain most from a therapist who exhibits a strong sense of decisiveness.

Whether or not the therapist is of a generally optimistic frame of mind should similarly be taken into account. The clinician who believes that almost anyone can markedly change his life and accomplish great deeds if offered the right treatment is likely to have greater success with a poor achiever of high potential than with the patient whose capabilities are clearly limited, who in turn is more suitably referred to a therapist who seeks to change only the patient's attitude, not his abilities, and concentrates on helping him make the most of himself and his limited abilities.

In deciding on the *composition of a therapy group,* the first goal is to ensure that it can function long enough to be of benefit to its members. Since the factors that hold a therapy group together are very like those that influence group formation and stability in the everyday world (Almond 1965), patients are usually matched according to such factors as age, social class, value system, intellectual endowment, and sophistication (Yalom 1966). Severity and length of illness appear to play a surprisingly small role: patients who have never had a psychotic episode and have never been hospitalized may, to be sure, feel peculiar the first time they meet patients who have, but this feeling usually abates quite rapidly if their social backgrounds are similar. While the particular diagnoses are of lesser importance, we avoid placing too many nonverbal patients into the same group. It is also important to avoid combining patients who behave antisocially with patients whose disorders affect primarily their thinking or mood. In our experience, the antisocial patient tends to use the schizophrenic, and especially the manic, patient as a foil in order to attack the therapist or, taking advantage of the other patient's poor judgment, encourages him to behave antisocially also.

Matching group members in terms of their age and social maturation means that the most typical groups are:

1/ the *preadolescent* group;
2/ the *adolescent* group;
3/ the *preadult* group—composed of patients from the midteens to early twenties who have not yet established independence;
4/ the *young adult* group—composed of individuals from their late teens to midtwenties who have achieved or almost achieved independence but not yet married; and
5/ the *adult* group—composed of individuals beyond their midtwenties.

While age similarities are of less importance in married couples groups than in individual groups, it is our experience that couples past the age of 55 generally get bored listening to the growing pains of young marriage.

When persons of very different backgrounds are put into the

same group, they often experience so much discomfort that the cohesiveness and the stability of the group are endangered. *Group heterogeneity* can be of therapeutic value, however, in that the participants are offered a wider range of people with whom to interact and develop transference relationships. As a result, certain issues that might otherwise be ignored may be brought into focus (Furst 1958, Samuels 1964, Slavson 1943). If, for example, a depressed woman who is upset by her husband's domination of their son is placed, together with her husband, in a group that includes a young man whose problems revolve around being dominated by his father, it would not be surprising if the relationship between the two men and the wife's reaction to it illuminated the problems of all three. Transference relationships of various kinds also develop in homogeneous groups. Regardless of the group composition, such relationships can be fostered through the use of psychodramatic and role-playing techniques, which, by temporarily activating the patient's feelings about an important person in his life, enable him to talk about these feelings and, at least for a time, resolve them (Rosenbaum 1965).

The optimal application of the principles outlined above depends on such factors as:

> the availability of a treatment facility that can provide the needed resources;
> the size, extent, and versatility of the therapeutic team; and
> the availability of other patients, families, and therapeutic groups.

These requirements are best fulfilled by a group or clinic practice in which a number of therapists with different skills work with a relatively large number of patients of diverse ages and problems (Freyhan 1963). This kind of practice enables the therapists involved in a given case to pool their ideas, facilitates an ongoing, multidimensional assessment, and makes it easier to transfer a patient to a different treatment program if his response to a particular therapist or treatment matrix appears unsatisfactory. Discussions between the therapists enable each to assess whether the way he feels is a unique or general response to a particular patient. Involving several therapists in the patient's treatment also helps them to understand and perhaps moderate such socially disadvantageous habits as playing different people against each other.

Issues Discussed in Psychotherapy

There is extensive literature about the kind of psychotherapeutic effort it takes to relieve mental distress (Berne 1966, Böszörmenyi-Nagy 1965, Burton 1961, Dicks 1967, Dollard 1950, Ford 1967, Foulkes 1965, Haley 1963, Hollender 1965, Menninger 1958, Rogers 1951, Singer 1965, Slavson 1964, Wolberg 1948, 1967, Wolman 1967, Wolpe 1958). For this reason and because we are skeptical of the common belief that the patient must understand or reexperience his past in order to recover from his current discomfort or be protected from future recurrences (Brady 1967, Marmor 1962), and because we have seen no evidence to suggest that the complicated strategies and measures that go under the name of behavior therapy are any better, we will not recapitulate the views of the various schools of thought. The patient usually starts by ignoring the past and talks about his current situation, about the behavior, symptoms, or feelings that have recently become troublesome and thus prompted him to start treatment. It is generally accepted that, if the patient does not detail his current difficulties in the first interview and explain what it is that has recently gotten worse, he should be asked why he has come (or been sent) at this particular time. Since these questions are, for us, the most obvious points of interest, it is only after we are fully informed about his present situation that we inquire into his past, except to the extent that it provides us with a yardstick to measure his current complaints and a key to understand his reactions to them.

Although the topics discussed will inevitably reflect the interests and personalities of the participants, it is important to avoid nurturing any preconceived notion the patient may have that the therapist is somehow an exalted authority who knows just which topics are "most therapeutic," lest the patient abandon his own line of thought in order to discuss what he thinks will please the therapist. Special attention is paid to those aspects of the patient's thinking that seem erroneous or immoderate and to those aspects of his behavior that seem to be ineffective, harmful, compulsively repetitious, or recapitulations of former earlier experiences. Once the problem has been defined, we consider the meetings an exercise in communication and, depending on the patient's needs, try to

1/ teach him to recognize (and perhaps to avoid) the kinds of situations that interfere with his comfort;

2/ guide him towards an honest and accurate self-assessment of his assets and deficits;

3/ help him to understand what consequences this should and will have on such important decisions as the choice of a job, a friend, or a mate; and

4/ enable him to tolerate the uncertainties of life.

Both to encourage the patient to be absolutely candid in expressing his views about us and to help him acquire a clear picture of his impact on others, we express our thoughts and feelings about him as frankly as the situation permits, giving voice to our disapproval or even disgust as readily as to our fondness and admiration. The technique of psychotherapy, in our view, then, is not to have a "technique" at all, except in regard to making explicit much of what remains covert in the average nontherapeutic relationship.

Therapist and patient spend what to an untrained observer would seem an inordinate amount of time discussing their own relationship: when and how often they will meet and why, what responsibilities each has to the other, what the fee will be and what this means to the patient, what they should talk about, who should decide when the patient is well or needs less treatment, what value psychotherapy has, and so forth. No matter how unrelated to the sources and manifestations of the patient's distress such discussions may appear, they are among the psychotherapist's most important diagnostic and therapeutic tools. They demonstrate the patient's manner of dealing with his environment far better than his subjective descriptions of relationships with people the therapist does not know. From these discussions, the therapist can discover how the patient views the behavior and the motives of those with whom he transacts, what concerns him about starting and maintaining a relationship, and what impact he has on those around him. Discussions of psychodynamics, especially on the theoretical level, seem pretentious and out of place in the consulting room, and tend to degenerate into either (if the patient-therapist relationship is good) a joint agreement that the patient's symptoms do indeed fit the therapist's pet theory about the human condition or (if their relationship is strained) a game of one-upmanship in which the therapist insists that the patient's failure to agree derives from resistance, reaction formation, or some other jargonized vice (Jackson 1963). What the patient needs to know is that the therapist is interested in him and considers it profitable for both of them to understand their own relationship, but this can be accomplished without psychodynamic elaborations (Coleman 1968, Truax 1966).

The matrix and the circumstances of treatment also have a bearing on the topics that are discussed. In individual therapy, a patient might discuss how he reacts to others; in a group, how others react to him, and just what it is about his behavior (and that of others) that gives rise to ostracism, attack, or approbation. Because we believe that psychological measures that change an individual's behavior generally do so by enlarging his repertoire of interpersonal techniques and improving his ability to decide which technique to use when, we encourage the patient to try out techniques he has not previously used and to decide which of them (if any) are more effective in achieving his goals or relieving his distress than his usual coping measures. The timid housewife who is helped to understand her reasons for getting upset and urged to try out a new course of behavior may gather the courage to stand up to her husband; the individual with a low boiling point may learn to postpone blowing up long enough to withdraw from the scene of an impending family altercation.

At the outset, it does not matter whether the patient "feels" the role that he needs to play, for the better he learns his lines, the better his performance will be. For example, patients who stop feeling persecuted while recovering from a paranoid illness usually deny that this proves that their fears sprang from an illness and insist that it proves only that their enemies have desisted. Since the public expression of paranoid views inevitably results in social embarrassment or even disaster, we encourage the patient to refrain from discussing his theories with anyone—even with us—and to conduct his day-to-day affairs *as if* he considered his former beliefs inaccurate (see also p. 213). Similarly, the patient who is manipulative or antisocial is urged—by verbal ultimatums when possible, but by duress if necessary—to act like a social being even if he does not yet feel like one (see p. 256). That the patient may feel he is only "acting" is irrelevant if his family and community view his performance as "real," as they will reward such a performance by considering him "improved" and encouraging him to continue. This positive social feedback often perpetuates more traditional behavior, even though the new way of behaving may not "feel right" until later.

Frequently, it is as important to understand and deal with the psychological and social *consequences* of an illness as it is to deal with its *manifestations* or to explore its *roots*. If the patient's illness has affected his interpersonal relations, it may not be enough to help him improve his social competence; the psychiatrist's assistance may also be needed to moderate the way those nearest him react to his illness (Angrist 1961). Friends or relatives who are unable to distinguish the symptoms of mental illness from mere provocativeness or rudeness should be helped to see the patient's behavior in clearer perspective. If, for example, a depressed woman berates her husband for some long-past misdeed and he counterattacks by reciting all her failings, the exchanges can mount in intensity until they endanger the marriage. Here the therapist's intervention can help hold the marriage together until the wife's depression lifts and their relationship becomes as amicable as in the past. The mere act of labeling the wife's behavior as "illness" can enable the husband to view her accusations more objectively, to moderate his counterattack, and to take part in an exploration of both his feelings and hers.

Since most severe illnesses affect the individual's attitude toward and competence at his work, it is important to review the patient's occupational history and assess the way his job has affected and been affected by his illness. The patient who has never worked or who has long been unemployed may need to be offered vocational counseling, training, or retraining (Chapple 1964, Denber 1960, 1962, Esser 1965, Winick 1963). Once he is fit to work, he may need advice about finding a job, encouragement in accepting it, and emotional support in keeping it. The therapist can also help prevent a patient's quitting his job because he is depressed and believes that he is incompetent or that his recovery hinges on his accepting a less demanding (and usually less rewarding) position. If, on the other hand, the patient is excessively optimistic and confident, he may need to be dissuaded from assuming responsibilities that are too complex or demanding, as failure under these circumstances could endanger not only the individual's record but also his confidence.

Some Reservations About the Socioadaptive Approach

The approach to treatment outlined in the foregoing pages may sometimes be impractical. The patient, family, or community may not be able to afford it; the treatment facilities required may not be available; or the participants it requires—the spouse, the family, children—may be unwilling to participate. Even when the ideal arrangements are possible, treatment may not have the desired effect, as there is no evidence that an individual's transactional skills will necessarily improve when he is placed in a situation that he has previously been unable to master. Even if he were to learn to hold his own in such a setting, the improvement need not extend to other areas of his life or protect him against future episodes of mental illness. If, for example, a therapist notices that each episode of a patient's psychosis is preceded by a family fight, he may initiate family therapy in the hope that this will help them all act in a more civilized way toward each other and thus prevent further episodes. A relationship that is important enough to contribute to decompensation, however, is usually so deeply ingrained that both patient and family find it extremely difficult to change (Zuk 1968). The family's contribution to the chaotic situation suggests, furthermore, that they, too, are disturbed and thus poorly equipped to change their behavior. The patient's illness can recur, of course, even after his family's functioning has improved; and most disheartening in such cases is the rapidity with which the previously established family harmony evaporates.

THE COMBINATION OF SOMATIC AND PSYCHOTHERAPEUTIC TREATMENT PROGRAMS

It is generally recognized today that the decision to give the patient drugs or other somatic treatment should not hinge on whether the illness appears to be of organic origin any more than psychotherapy is indicated only for problems that are clearly psychogenic. It has indeed become almost routine to prescribe drugs for the patient who is too depressed or anxious to develop a meaningful therapeutic relationship or who transacts in a manner that is exclusively symbolic, nonverbal, or otherwise pathologically unconventional. In noting this common practice, however, we do not intend to perpetuate the all-too-prevalent belief that the primary aim of somatic treatment is to make the patient comfortable enough to take part in a psychotherapeutic encounter (Appleton 1967, Linn 1964, Ostow 1962). We would prefer to stress the other side of the coin: that often a principal goal of psychotherapy (especially for the psychotic patient) is to ensure that he is and remains willing to adhere to the prescribed somatic treatment.

When a patient stops taking what his doctor has recommended, it is important to explore his motives, clarify his misconceptions, and reestablish the collaborative relationship. This is by no means a simple process: it may take months or even years of psychotherapy

—perhaps with several intervening relapses—to gain the patient's unqualified collaboration. An individual with a drug-responsive disorder must overcome his suspiciousness and his concern about dependency, weakness, and the effect that medications have on his state of awareness. Only when this has been achieved can he be expected to take faithfully the drugs he needs and to report any changes in mood or thinking that may signal an impending relapse. However difficult this goal may be to reach, its achievement may prevent him from becoming chronically ill and allow him to function as a member of the community.

DOES PSYCHOTHERAPY BENEFIT THE MENTALLY ILL?

We have described certain benefits of the psychotherapeutic relationship and suggested that the most important and enduring of these derive from improving the individual's transactional skills and helping him overcome, accept, or cope with his transactional difficulties. The case for psychotherapy is not usually stated this simply, however. More commonly, it is credited with making people happier or more productive, or with relieving them of mental illnesses. We have made none of these claims, however, nor do we claim to know that current episodes of mental illness can be cured or future episodes averted by helping the individual cope with or resolve some of his life problems. Moreover, it is generally agreed that the transactional skills of an individual who enters a psychotherapeutic relationship in a rational, alert, and untroubled state are more likely to improve than those of a person who is mentally ill (Fiske 1964, Hoehn-Saric 1969, Luborsky 1962, Muench 1965, Roth 1964, Strupp 1963). Despite the curious paradox to which this view leads, that the healthy get more out of psychotherapy than the mentally ill, the establishment of a psychotherapeutic relationship is, for many reasons, even more important for a person who is mentally ill than for one who is not.

In the midst of an acute mental illness, an individual's social and cognitive skills are obviously impaired, and he is unusually sensitive to the stresses of everyday life. If these difficulties persist after the acute illness subsides, the physician must try to determine whether they are residual effects of the illness and thus suggest incomplete recovery or are a part of the patient's premorbid personality. This judgment is not easy, as the patient is usually seen only after the acute illness arises. The therapist must therefore rely on what he is told about the patient's prior condition. Even if he learns that the patient *did have premorbid personality problems*—that he was, for example, socially awkward, unduly sensitive, or odd in his thinking long before he became acutely ill—it may still be difficult to assess the significance of these matters. He may conclude that the symptoms the patient had before becoming acutely ill were a prodromal or subclinical form of the illness. Alternatively, he may decide that the patient's personality problems impaired his ability to cope with stress and thus made him more vulnerable to the precipitating events. Finally, he can dodge the causality question altogether by regarding the premorbid symptoms only as evidence that the individual's nervous system and psychological integration have always been substandard. If he learns that such *symptoms were not seen prior to the acute episode,* several similar explanations are possible. He can interpret the symptoms to represent

a subacute continuation of the disease process;
residual impairments caused by a disease-induced defect state;
consequences of the retardation and distortion of social learning that took place during the illness;
the disturbance in self-image that results from being mentally ill; or
the individual's reaction to the social disadvantages that accrue from the community's knowledge that he has been mentally ill.

This excursion into the questions of cause and effect is relevant from the standpoint of psychotherapeutic decisions only because psychotherapy appears less able to alter the disease process itself than to offer the individual an opportunity for learning that can help remold his premorbid personality and modify the social and transactional consequences of illness. Thus, when the continuing impairments appear secondary to defective equipment, psychotherapy's goals will have to be relatively modest. When the patient's impairments are caused by an ongoing disease process, marked improvement in his transactional skills is likely only if his illness responds to somatic therapy. Psychotherapy alone is likely to be of major benefit only when the impairments originate exclusively in the sociopsychological roots and consequences of the illness.

Whatever their causes, psychological impairments are likely to hinder an individual's further achievements—social, occupational, and educational—and thus isolate him from traditional sources of learning, growth, and development. For this reason, a patient who has had a mental illness should indeed be treated with psychotherapy in the hope that it will restore some of the skills he has lost and help him acquire those he has never learned. The patient whose social skills are already impaired may not be able to afford further deterioration, and the more obvious and disabling his social ineptitude and inappropriateness become, the more disastrous the social consequences will be. By exposing the mentally ill person to a setting wherein he can recoup impaired social and transactional skills and learn and gain confidence in the use of others, psychotherapy may protect him against some of the most damaging consequences of future relapses. Furthermore, it can help the physician in making appropriate decisions concerning treatment and disposition by providing him with an opportunity to observe and assess the patient's competence at regular intervals.

The establishment of a psychotherapeutic relationship can have other advantages for the mentally ill person. The very fact that the patient can talk to someone about his situation may provide him with a source of interest and gratification. The satisfactions inherent in this kind of relationship may encourage him to try to overcome his inadequacies and become more acceptable to others. Such an opportunity for improvement can be of particular value to the patient whose distancing personality or life circumstances—such as abandonment or parental coldness—have previously rendered him unable to form relationships with persons who could offer sympathy and interest. The extent to which he can generalize from his experience in establishing a relationship with a therapist and apply it to other situations is a measure of its long-term benefits. Finally, the successful establishment of a good patient-doctor relationship is especially crucial in recurrent illnesses, for the reservoir of trust that is sustained between episodes of illness may enable the patient, upon the occurrence of a new one, to accept the therapist's recommendations with alacrity, precision, and good will.

REFERENCES

Ackerman, N.: Psychodynamics of Family Life, New York: Basic, 1958.

Almond, R., and Esser, A. H.: Tablemate choices of psychiatric patients: Technique for measuring social contact, J Nerv Ment Dis *141*:68-82, 1965.

Almond, R., Keniston, K., and Boltax, S.: Patient value change in milieu therapy, Arch Gen Psychiat (Chicago) *20*:339-351, 1969a.

——:Milieu therapeutic process, Arch Gen Psychiat (Chicago) *21*:431-442, 1969b.

Angrist, S., *et al.:* Tolerance of deviant behavior, posthospital performance levels, and rehospitalization, Proc III World Cong Psychiat, vol. 1, 1961, pp. 237-241.

Appleton, W. S., and Chien, C. P.: Effect of the doctor's attitude and knowledge on his use of psychiatric drugs, J Nerv Ment Dis *145*:284-291, 1967.

Astrachan, B. M., *et al.:* Unled patient group as a therapeutic tool, Int J Group Psychother *17*:178-191, 1967.

Bach, G. R.: Marathon group: Intensive practice of intimate interaction, Psychol Rep *18*:995-1002, 1966.

Barrett-Lennard, G. T.: Significant aspects of a helping relationship, Canad Ment Health (Suppl 47):1-5, 1965.

Beckett, P. G., Lennox, K., and Grisell, J. L.: Responsibility and reward in treatment. Comparative follow-up study of adolescents, J Nerv Ment Dis *146*:257-263, 1968.

Bernard, V. W.: Some principles of dynamic psychiatry in relation to poverty, Amer J Psychiat *122*:254-267, 1965.

Berne, E.: Transactional Analysis in Psychotherapy: Systematic Individual and Social Psychiatry, New York: Grove, 1961.

——: Principles of Group Treatment, New York: Oxford Univ Press, 1966.

Bion, W. R.: Experiences in Groups, New York: Basic, 1961.

Borgatta, E. F.: New principle of psychotherapy, J Clin Psychol *15*:330-334, 1959.

Böszörmenyi-Nagy, I., and Framo, J. L., eds.: Intensive Family Therapy, New York: Harper, 1965.

Braceland, F. J.: Rehabilitation, *in* Arieti, S., ed.: American Handbook of Psychiatry, vol. 3, New York: Basic, 1966, pp. 643-656.

Brady, J. P.: Psychotherapy, learning theory, and insight, Arch Gen Psychiat (Chicago) *16*:304-311, 1967.

Brown, J. S., and Kosterlitz, N.: Selection and treatment of psychiatric outpatients; determined by their personal and social characteristics, Arch Gen Psychiat (Chicago) *11*:425-438, 1964.

Burton, A., ed.: Psychotherapy of the Psychoses, New York: Basic, 1961.

Carlson, D. A., *et al.:* Problems in treating the lower-class psychotic, Arch Gen Psychiat (Chicago) *13*:269-274, 1965.

Chapple, E. D., and Esser, A. H.: Workshops in state hospitals, Psychiat Quart (Suppl) *38*:317-322, Part 2, 1964.

Christ, J.: Group approaches in the therapeutic community: Discussion, Int J Group Psychother *15*:37-41, 1965.

Coleman, J. V.: Banter as a psychotherapeutic intervention, Amer J Psychoanal *22*:1-6, 1963.

——: Therapy of the "inaccessible" mentally ill patient, Ment Hyg *49*:581-584, 1965.

——: Aims and conduct of psychotherapy, Arch Gen Psychiat (Chicago) *18*: 1-6, 1968.

Curry, A. E.: Therapeutic management of multiple family groups, Int J Group Psychother *15*:90-96, 1965.

Denber, H. C. B.: Industrial workshops for psychiatric patients, Ment Hosp *11*: 16-18, 1960.

Denber, H. C. B., and Rajotte, P.: Problems and theoretical considerations of work therapy for psychiatric patients, Canad Psychiat Ass J *7*:25-33, 1962.

Dicks, H. V.: Marital Tensions, New York: Basic, 1967.

Dollard, J., and Miller, N. E.: Personality and Psychotherapy, New York: McGraw-Hill, 1950.

Eliasoph, E.: Concepts and techniques of role playing and role training utilizing psychodramatic methods in group therapy with adolescent drug addicts, Group Psychother *8*:308-315, 1955.

Ellenberger, H., and Trottier, J.: Impact of a severe, prolonged physical illness of a child upon the family, Proc III World Cong Psychiat, vol. 1, 1961, pp. 465-469.

Esser, A. H., *et al.:* Productivity of chronic schizophrenics in a sheltered workshop. Quantitative evaluation of the effects of drug therapy, Compr Psychiat *6*:41-50, 1965.

Eysenck, H. J.: Behavior Therapy and the Neuroses: Readings in Modern Methods of Treatment Derived from Learning Theory, London: Pergamon, 1960.

——: Behavior therapy, extinction and relapse in neurosis, Brit J Psychiat 109: 12-18, 1963.

Fierman, L. B.: Myths in the practice of psychotherapy, Arch Gen Psychiat (Chicago) 12:408-414, 1965.

Fisher, S.: Primum non nocere: Too much of a good thing? Seminars Psychiat 1:432-442, 1969.

Fiske, D. W., Cartwright, D. S., and Kirtner, W. L.: Are psychotherapeutic changes predictable? J Abnorm Psychol 69:418-426, 1964.

Fleck, S.: Residential treatment of young schizophrenics, Conn Med 26:369-376, 1962.

——: Psychotherapy of families of hospitalized patients, in Masserman, J., ed.: Current Psychiatric Therapies, vol. 3, New York: Grune, 1963, pp. 211-218.

——: Personal communication, 1966.

Ford, D. H., and Urban, H. B.: Systems of Psychotherapy: Comparative Study, New York: Wiley, 1967.

Foulkes, S. H.: Therapeutic Group Analysis, New York: Internat Univ Press, 1965.

Frank, J. D.: Persuasion and Healing: Comparative Study of Psychotherapy, Baltimore: Johns Hopkins Press, 1961.

Frankl, V. E.: Paradoxical intention: Logotherapeutic technique, Amer J Psychother 14:520-535, 1960.

Freud, S.: Dynamics of the transference (1912), in Jones, E., ed.: Collected Papers of Sigmund Freud, vol. 2, London: Hogarth Press, 1953, pp. 312-322.

Freyhan, F. A., and Mayo, J. A.: Concept of a model psychiatric clinic, Amer J Psychiat 120:222-227, 1963.

Fried, E.: Some aspects of group dynamics and the analysis of transference and defenses, Int J Group Psychother 15: 44-56, 1965.

Furst, W.: Homogeneous versus heterogeneous groups, Top Probl Psychother (New York) 2:170-173, 1960.

Gardner, G. G.: Role of maternal psychopathology in male and female schizophrenics, J Consult Psychol 31:411-413, 1967.

Gergen, K. J.: Self theory and the process of self-observation, J Nerv Ment Dis 148:437-448, 1969.

Gerz, H. O.: Treatment of the phobic and the obsessive-compulsive patient using paradoxical intention sec, Viktor E. Frankl, J Neuropsychiat 3:375-387, 1962.

Glasser, W.: Reality Therapy: New Approach to Psychiatry, New York: Harper, 1965.

Gottlieb, A., and Pattison, E. M.: Married couples group psychotherapy, Arch Gen Psychiat (Chicago) 14:143, 1966.

Gottschalk, L. A., and Whitman, R. M.: Some typical complications mobilized by the psycho-analytic procedure, Int J Psychoanal 43:142-150, 1962.

Gould, R. E.: Dr. Strangeclass: Or how I stopped worrying about the theory and began treating the blue-collar worker, Amer J Orthopsychiat 37:78-86, 1967.

Greenberg, L. M., et al.: Family therapy: Indications and rationale, Arch Gen Psychiat (Chicago) 10:7-24, 1964.

Hain, J. D., Butcher, R. H. G., and Stevenson, I.: Systematic desensitization therapy: Analysis of results in twenty-seven patients, Brit J Psychiat 112:295-307, 1966.

Haley, J.: Family of the schizophrenic: A model system, J Nerv Ment Dis 129:357-374, 1959.

——: Whither family therapy? Family Process 1:69-103, 1962.

——: Strategies of Psychotherapy, New York: Grune, 1963.

Harrow, M., et al.: Influence of the psychotherapist on the emotional climate in group therapy, Hum Relations 20:49-64, 1967.

Haskell, D., Pugatch, D., and McNair, D. M.: Time-limited psychotherapy for whom, Arch Gen Psychiat (Chicago) 21: 546-552, 1969.

Hes, J. P., and Handler, S. L.: Multidimensional group therapy, Arch Gen Psychiat (Chicago) 5:70-75, 1961.

Heston, L. L.: Genetics of schizophrenic and schizoid disease, Science 167:249-256, 1970.

Hoehn-Saric, R., et al.: Prognosis in psychoneurotic patients, Amer J Psychother 23:252-259, 1969.

Hollender, M. H.: Practice of Psychoanalytic Psychotherapy, New York: Grune, 1965.

Hollingshead, A. B., and Redlich, F. C.: Social Class and Mental Illness: Community Study, New York: Wiley 1958.

Jackson, D. D.: Family interaction, family homeostasis, and some implications for conjoint family psychotherapy, in Masserman, J. H., ed.: Individual and Familial Dynamics, New York: Grune, 1959.

——: Family rules: Marital quid pro quo, Arch Gen Psychiat (Chicago) 12:589-594, 1965.

Jackson, D. D., and Haley, J.: Transference revisited, J Nerv Ment Dis *137*:363-371, 1963.

Jackson, D. D., and Satir, V.: Review of psychiatric developments in family diagnosis and therapy, *in* Ackerman, N. W., Beatman, F. L., and Sherman, S. N., eds.: Exploring the Base for Family Therapy, New York: Family Service Association of America, 1961, pp. 29-49.

Jarecki, H. G., and Cohen, L.: Group therapy for the regressed, chronically deprived patient. Research Seminar Department of Psychiatry, Yale Univ School of Med, 1964.

Jones, M.: Therapeutic Community: New Treatment Method in Psychiatry, New York: Basic, 1953.

Jones, M., and Polak, P.: Crisis and confrontation, Brit J Psychiat *114*:169-174, 1968.

Kadis, A. L.: Re-experiencing the family constellation in group psychotherapy, J Individ Psychol *12*:63-68, 1956.

——: Coordinated meetings in group psychotherapy, *in* Rosenbaum, M., and Berger, M., eds.: Group Psychotherapy and Group Function, New York: Basic, 1963, pp. 437-448.

Kimbro, E. L., Jr., *et al.*: Multiple family group approach to some problems of adolescence, Int J Group Psychother *17*:18-24, 1967.

Knight, R. P.: Management and psychotherapy of the borderline schizophrenic patient, Bull Menninger Clin *17*:139-150, 1953.

Koumans, A., Jr.: Reaching the unmotivated patient, Ment Hyg *53*:298-300, 1969.

Kreitman, N.: The patient's spouse, Brit J Psychiat *110*:159-173, 1964.

——: Married couples admitted to mental hospital, Brit J Psychiat *114*:699-718, 1968.

Laquer, H. P., Laburt, H. A., and Morong, E.: Multiple family therapy, *in* Masserman, J. H., ed.: Current Psychiatric Therapies, vol. 4, New York: Grune, 1964.

Lesse, S.: Evaluation of the results of the psychotherapies, Springfield (Ill): Thomas, 1968, pp. 239-253.

Levine, S.: Psychotherapy as socialization, Int J Psychiat *8*:645-655, 1969.

Levinson, D. J., Merrifield, J., and Berg, K.: Becoming a patient, Arch Gen Psychiat (Chicago) *17*:385-406, 1967.

Lewis, V. S., and Zeichner, A. M.: Impact of admission to a mental hospital on the patient's family, Ment Hyg *44*:503-509, 1960.

Lidz, T., Fleck, S., and Cornelison, A.: Schizophrenia and the Family, New York: Internat Univ Press, 1963.

Linn, L.: Use of drugs in psychotherapy, Psychiat Quart *38*:138-148, 1964.

Lower, R. B.: Psychotherapy of neurotic dependency, Amer J Psychiat *124*:514-519, 1967.

Luborsky, L.: Patient's personality and psychotherapeutic change, *in* Strupp, H. H., and Luborsky, L., eds.: Research in Psychotherapy, vol. 2, Washington (DC): American Psychological Association, 1962.

Ludwig, A. M., and Farrelly, F.: Code of chronicity, Arch Gen Psychiat (Chicago) *15*:562-568, 1966.

MacGregor, R., *et al.*: Multiple Impact Therapy with Families, New York: Blakiston (division of McGraw-Hill Book Company, Inc.), 1964.

Marmor, J.: Psychoanalytic therapy as an educational process, *in* Masserman, J. H., ed.: Science and Psychoanalysis, vol. 5, New York: Grune, 1962, p. 286.

Marsh, L. C.: Group treatment of the psychoses by the psychological equivalent of the revival, Ment Hyg *15*:328-349, 1931.

McMahon, A. W., and Shore, M. F.: Some psychological reactions to working with the poor, Arch Gen Psychiat (Chicago) *18*:562-568, 1968.

Menninger, K. A.: Theory of Psychoanalytic Technique, New York: Basic, 1958.

Miller, E. C., Dvorak, A., and Turner, D. W.: Methods of creating aversion to alcohol by reflex conditioning in a group setting, Quart J Stud Alcohol *21*:424-431, 1960.

Moreno, J. L.: Psychodramatic treatment of marriage problems, Sociometry *3*:1-23, 1940.

——: Psychodrama and the psychopathology of inter-personal relations, Psychodrama Monogr *16*:3-68, 1945.

——: Sociodrama of a family conflict: Transcript of a session at Psychodramatic Institute March 24, 1944, Group Psychother *5*:20-37, 1952.

Mowbray, R. M., and Timbury, G. C.: Opinions on psychotherapy: Enquiry, Brit J Psychiat *112*:351-361, 1966.

Muench, G. A.: Investigation of the efficacy of time-limited psychotherapy, J Counsel Psychol *12*:294-298, 1965.

Nash, E. H., *et al.*: Systematic preparation of patients for short-term psychotherapy: II. Relation to characteristics of patient, therapist and the psychotherapeutic process, J Nerv Ment Dis *140:*374-383, 1965.

Neighbor, J. E., *et al.:* Approach to the selection of patients for group psychotherapy, Ment Hyg *142:*243-254, 1958.

Nielsen, J.: Mental disorders in married couples (assortative mating), Brit J Psychiat *110:*683-697, 1964.

Norton, N. M., Detre, T. P., and Jarecki, H. G.: Psychiatric services in general hospitals; Family-oriented redefinition, J Nerv Ment Dis *136:*475-484, 1963.

Novey, S.: Principle of "working through" in psychoanalysis, J Amer Psychoanal Ass *10:*658-676, 1962.

Orr, D. W.: Transference and countertransference: Historical survey, J Amer Psychoanal Ass *2:*621-670, 1954.

Ostow, M.: Drugs in Psychoanalysis and Psychotherapy, New York: Basic, 1962.

Papanek, H.: Group psychotherapy with married couples, *in* Current Psychiatric Therapies, vol. 5, New York: Grune, 1965, pp. 157-163.

Paul, G. L.: Insight vs. desensitization in psychotherapy two years after termination, J Consult Psychol *31:*333-348, 1967.

Planansky, K., and Johnston, R.: Mate selection in schizophrenia, Acta Psychiat Scand *43:*397-409, 1967.

Poser, E. G.: Effect of therapists' training on group therapeutic outcome, J Consult Psychol *30:*283-289, 1966.

Pratt, J. H.: "Home sanatorium" treatment of consumption, Boston Med Surg J *154:*210-216 (Feb 22), 1906.

Riessman, F., Cohen, J., and Pearl, A., eds.: Mental Health of the Poor, New York: Free Press, 1964.

Rogers, C. R.: Client-Centered Therapy, Boston: Houghton, 1951.

Rosenbaum, C. P.: Events of early therapy and brief therapy, Arch Gen Psychiat (Chicago) *10:*506-512, 1964.

Rosenbaum, M.: Group psychotherapy and psychodrama, *in* Handbook of Clinical Psychology, New York: McGraw-Hill, 1965.

Rosenthal, A. J., Behrens, M. I., and Chodoff, P.: Communication in lower class families of schizophrenics: Methodological problems, Arch Gen Psychiat (Chicago) *18:*464-470, 1968.

Roth, I., *et al.:* Long-term effects on psychotherapy of initial treatment conditions, J Psychiat Res *2:*283-297, 1964.

Saenger, G.: Patterns of change among "treated" and "untreated" patients seen in psychiatric community mental health clinics, J Nerv Ment Dis *150:*35-50, 1970.

Sager, C. J., *et al.:* The married in treatment: Effects of psychoanalysis on the marital state, Arch Gen Psychiat (Chicago) *19:*205-217, 1968.

Samuels, A. S.: Use of group balance as a therapeutic technique, Arch Gen Psychiat (Chicago) *11:*411-420, 1964.

Satir, V.: Conjoint Family Therapy, rev. ed., Palo Alto (Calif): Science and Behavior, 1967.

Scherz, F. H.: Crisis of adolescence in family life, Soc Casework *48:*209-215, 1967.

Schmideberg, M.: Psychodynamic changes in untreated neurotic patients, Brit J Psychiat *114:*924, 1968.

Schmidt, W., Smart, R. G., and Moss, M. K.: Social class and the treatment of alcoholism, Psychiat Soc Sci Rev *2:*25-27, 1968.

Schofield, W.: Psychotherapy: The Purchase of Friendship, Englewood Cliffs (NJ): Prentice-Hall, 1964.

Sharaf, M. R., and Levinson, D. J.: Quest for omnipotence in professional training: Case of the psychiatric resident, Psychiatry *27:*135-149, 1964.

Sifneos, P. E.: Two different kinds of psychotherapy of short duration, Amer J Psychiat *123:*1069-1074, 1967.

Singer, E.: Key Concepts in Psychotherapy, New York: Random House, 1965.

Slavson, S. R.: Introduction to Group Therapy, New York: Commonwealth Fund, 1943.

——: Textbook in Analytic Group Psychotherapy, New York: Internat Univ Press, 1964.

Sorrells, J. M., and Ford, F. R.: Toward an integrated theory of families and family therapy, Psychother *6:*150-160, 1969.

Stampfl, T. G., and Lewis, D. J.: Essentials of implosive therapy: Learning-theory-based psychodynamic behavioral therapy, J Abnorm Psychol *72:*496-503, 1967.

Stanton, A. H., and Schwartz, M. S.: The Mental Hospital, New York: Basic, 1954.

Stoller, F. H.: Accelerated interaction: Time-limited approach based on the brief, intensive group, Int J Group Psychother *18:*220-235, 1968.

Stone, A. R., *et al.:* Some situational factors associated with response to psychotherapy, Amer J Orthopsychiat *25:*682-687, 1965.

Strupp, H. H., Fox, R. E., and Lessler, K.: Patients View Their Psychotherapy, Baltimore: Johns Hopkins Press, 1969.

Strupp, H. H., *et al.:* Psychotherapists'

assessments of former patients, J Nerv Ment Dis *137*:222-230, 1963.

Szasz, T. S.: Behavior therapy and psychoanalysis, Med Opinion and Rev *3*:24-29, 1967.

Tharp, R. G., and Otis, G. D.: Toward a theory for therapeutic intervention in families, J Consult Psychol *30*:426-434, 1966.

Tompkins, H. J.: Short-term therapy of the neuroses, *in* Usdin, G. L., ed.: Psychoneurosis and Schizophrenia, Philadelphia: Lippincott, 1966.

Truax, C. B.: Therapist empathy, genuineness, and warmth and patient therapeutic outcome, J Consult Psychol *30*:395-401, 1966.

Weakland, J. H.: Family therapy as a research arena, Family Process *1*:63-68, 1962.

Weber, J. J., Elinson, J., and Moss, L. M.: Psychoanalysis and change: Study of psychoanalytic clinic records utilizing electronic data-processing techniques, Arch Gen Psychiat (Chicago) *17*:687-709, 1967.

Whitaker, C. A., Stock, D., and Lieberman, M. A.: Psychotherapy Through the Group Process, Englewood Cliffs (NJ): Prentice-Hall, 1964.

White, A. M., Fichtenbaum, L., and Dollard, J.: Evaluation of silence in initial interviews with psychiatric clinic patients, J Nerv Ment Dis *139*:550-557, 1964a.

———: A measure predicting dropping out of psychotherapy, J Consult Psychol *28*:326-332, 1964b.

Williams, F. S.: Family therapy: Critical assessment, Amer J Orthopsychiat *37*:912-919, 1967.

Wing, J. K.: Social and psychological changes in a rehabilitation unit, Soc Psychiat *1*:21-28, 1966.

Winick, W., Walsh, F. X., and Frost, E. S.: Industrial rehabilitation of the mentally ill, Industr Med Surg *32*:332-336, 1963.

Woerner, P. I., and Guze, S. B.: Family and marital study of hysteria, Brit J Psychiat *114*:161-168, 1968.

Wolberg, L. R.: Medical Hypnosis, vols. 1 and 2, New York: Grune, 1948.

———: Technique of Psychotherapy, New York: Grune, 1954.

———: *Ibid.*, 1967.

Wolman, Benjamin B., ed.: Psychoanalytic Techniques: Handbook for the Practicing Psychoanalyst, New York: Basic, 1967.

Wolpe, J.: Psychotherapy by Reciprocal Inhibition, Stanford: Stanford Univ Press, 1958.

———: Systematic desensitization treatment of neuroses, J Nerv Ment Dis *132*:189-203, 1961.

———: Behavior therapy in complex neurotic states, Brit J Psychiat *110*:28-34, 1964.

Yalom, I. D., and Rand, K.: Compatibility and cohesiveness in therapy groups, Arch Gen Psychiat (Chicago) *15*:267-275, 1966.

Yamamoto, J., and Goin, M. K.: Social class factors relevant for psychiatric treatment, J Nerv Ment Dis *142*:332-339, 1966.

Zuk, G.: Prompting change in family therapy, Arch Gen Psychiat (Chicago) *19*:727-736, 1968.

CHAPTER
FOURTEEN

Psychotropic Agents

Virtually every substance ingested by man can in some circumstances affect his mood and thinking, and can thus be considered psychotropic. However, the term is customarily reserved for those drugs that are given with the specific intent to relieve psychological distress and malfunctioning. Although, as Professor Erik Jacobsen points out in his introductory essay, no single system of classification will be entirely satisfactory, the essentially pragmatic approach of this text has led us to classify drugs in terms of their clinical utility. Accordingly, we distinguish between and discuss separately the "major tranquilizers," used in the treatment of psychotic disorders, especially schizophrenia; the "minor tranquilizers," used in the treatment of anxiety and other neuroses; and the drugs used in the treatment of affective disorders, such as the antidepressants and lithium carbonate. The effects of mental illness and psychotropic drugs on automobile driving are discussed separately at the end of the chapter, as are the consequences of drug overdosage, for the problems involved there are not confined to any particular drug and must be dealt with in general as well as specific terms.

THE PROPERTIES OF PSYCHOTROPIC DRUGS
BY E. JACOBSEN, MD

Desirable as it might be to have a uniform classification system for psychotropic drugs, no single one of the criteria currently proposed for this purpose—whether the drug's chemical composition, neurophysiologic action, action on animal or human behavior, or clinical effect on mental diseases—is wholly satisfactory. A classification system based solely on the drug's chemical composition, for example, would not in itself indicate that the smallest change in a drug's molecular structure can sometimes profoundly alter its effects, nor that compounds belonging to completely dissimilar chemical classes may have almost identical effects. A grouping according to clinical use has obvious practical advantages, but at present can serve only heuristically, both because so little is known about the etiology and pathogenesis of mental diseases and because drugs with different pharmacodynamic properties can be used to relieve the same kinds of symptoms. It is almost certain, moreover, that the clinical pictures to which we so confidently refer as "schizophrenia" or "depression," as if they were discrete entities with a well-defined cause, are in fact merely collections of symptoms that resemble other diseases called by the same name but have several or many different causes. A classification based on neurophysiologic or psychophysiologic properties would have still other limitations, in that two compounds may have the same qualitative effect on one function, yet differ in their effects on other functions. Chlorpromazine and promethazine, for example, are both parasympatholytic, but the former provokes, while the latter antagonizes, extrapyramidal syndromes.

In order to illustrate the problems of classification, a number of diagrams have been prepared, each of which segregates the drugs according to different principles (see Tables 28 to 32). For the sake of clarity, each diagram includes only one or two drugs of each type, omits many clinically important compounds, and includes others that are not used currently but help to illustrate the gradual transition from drug to drug.

Except for producing anesthesia, which if too deep can result in respiratory paralysis, the *gas anesthetics* have no specific effect on cerebral functions. Some of them, such as ether, also have an effect on neuromuscular transmission similar to that of the *curare-like drugs.* For *alcohol,* the ratio between the concentration that produces a slight sedative effect and that that produces unconsciousness is much larger than for gas anesthetics. The cross-tolerance between anesthetics and alcohol suggests that these compounds have a common site of action within the central nervous system. Other aliphatic sedatives, such as *chloral hydrate* or paraldehyde * have properties very similar to alcohol's but have in addition a pronounced hypnotic effect. The same may be said for the group of barbiturates, which, however, vary considerably from one derivative to the next. *Hexo-barbital* and the thiobarbiturates * have a pronounced anesthetic effect, while *amobarbital* and *phenobarbital* are more sedative and hypnotic in relation to their anesthetic effect. Depending on the substitution in the 5,5 position, specific properties can be developed. As a result, while most barbiturates antagonize drug-induced or electrically induced convulsions, some are convulsants. Anticonvul-

---

* The italicized drugs may be found in the diagrams; those marked with an asterisk are not included.

sant activity may also be found in such nonbarbiturate drugs as *diphenylhydantoin* that have neither a specific effect on the sleep centers nor an anesthetic effect. A drug's influence on the sleep centers is not, though, specifically linked to its anesthetic properties: *glutethimide,* which has a chemical structure much like that of the barbiturates, and *thalidomide* (now withdrawn) have almost no anesthetic properties, despite being hypnotic in relatively small doses.

Meprobamate is sedative, but its hypnotic effect is perhaps less pronounced than that of the barbiturates. In contrast to barbiturates, it inhibits internuncial neurons, and overdosage in nonanesthetic doses results in a severe ataxia terminating in a flaccid paralysis. The latter effects can also be produced by certain other compounds, which in the diagram have been placed to the left of meprobamate: *carisoprodol, mephenesin,* and *zoxazolamine.* This last compound has pronounced muscle-relaxing properties but no influence on the higher cerebral functions. Because it has both muscle-relaxing and anesthetic properties, *phenaglycodol* forms a link between the barbiturates and meprobamate. Meprobamate inhibits convulsions induced by pentylenetetrazol, a property it has in common with antiepileptic agents, especially those effective against petit mal.

Like meprobamate, *chlordiazepoxide* and diazepam * are anticonvulsants, but their anesthetic effect is so slight that the dosage required to achieve it is close to that which produces a paralytic or lethal effect. In contrast to alcohol, aliphatic sedatives, barbiturates, and meprobamate (which have no influence on the autonomic nervous system *in vitro,* and only in sublethal concentrations *in vivo*), benzodiazepines act on some autonomic centers and also have antiemetic and appetite-stimulating effects. That benzodiazepines have antiemetic and appetite-stimulating effects in common with the major tranquilizers and have anticonvulsant, sedative, and antianxiety effects in common with meprobamate and other CNS depressants has caused some investigators to consider them a transition between the minor and major tranquilizers. Since, however, the benzodiazepines do not have an antipsychotic effect nor do they produce extrapyramidal symptoms, they cannot be considered fullfledged major tranquilizers.

The term *major tranquilizer* refers to phenothiazines like *chlorpromazine,* thioxanthenes like *chlorprothixene,* butyrophenones like haloperidol,* and rauwolfia alkaloids like *reserpine.* These drugs all have a pronounced effect, in some instances peripherally but especially centrally, on the autonomic nervous system. They are antiemetic, induce hypothermia, increase appetite, and influence endocrine centers in the hypothalamus. While they are not capable of inducing anesthesia, even in sublethal doses, they do effectively potentiate anesthesia induced by other agents. Their effect on the motor system is to diminish spontaneous motor activity and to release an extrapyramidal syndrome, thereby producing catatonia in animals and parkinsonism in man. In large doses, they may facilitate or even produce convulsions. The action of reserpine and its congeners is generally attributed to depletion of biogenic amines in the brain cell. The other major tranquilizers are presumed to interfere with the effect of the amines on the neurons without changing the neuron's catecholamine content. All major tranquilizers have a similar activity spectrum though certain variations can be found from agent to agent that may account for the differences in clinical effect described later in this chapter.

The chlorpromazine group forms a crucial point in the diagram, as its many properties connect many different classes of drugs, each of which has been placed in the diagram as a chain branching out from chlorpromazine.† Phenothiazines with a shorter, sometimes branched side chain, such as promethazine, have a sedative and, especially in man, even a hypnotic effect, but do not share some of the major tranquilizers' principal properties, in particular the specific clinical effect on psychoses. They also potentiate anesthetics without producing anesthesia *per se*. Being antiparkinsonian drugs, their effect on the extrapyramidal system is opposite to that of the major tranquilizers. Moreover, compared with major tranquilizers, they have a more pronounced anticholinergic, and an even more pronounced antihistamine, action. Their sympatholytic action, however, is almost nil. Other antihistamines, such as *diphenhydramine,* have effects quite similar to those of promethazine, despite their different chemical constitution. The *benactyzine* group, which has a structure similar to that of diphenhydramine, has an even greater anticholinergic but a negligible antihistamine effect. This group potentiates the effect of anesthetics more markedly than the antihistamines. Benactyzine forms a link between the centrally acting antihistamines and scopolamine, in that it shares anticholinergic properties with both. Benactyzine, scopolamine, atropine, and certain other strong, centrally acting anticholinergics synchronize the EEG in animals and abolish the electric but not the somatic arousal

† The first registered name of chlorpromazine, "Largactil," was derived from "large action," i.e., the drug of many properties.

response. *Scopolamine, atropine,* and other strong anticholinergics do not potentiate anesthetics, but some potentiate analgesics, and others, such as *meperidine* and methadone,* are strong analgesics per se and form a link beween anticholinergics and *morphine* and similar opium alkaloids.

In close chemical relation to the tricyclic major tranquilizers are *imipramine* and *amitriptyline.* Pharmacodynamically, they have properties in common with the major tranquilizers: they sedate animals, potentiate the effect of anesthetics, lower blood pressure, and are anticholinergic. They do not, however, have a sympatholytic action but on the contrary enhance the peripheral effect of noradrenaline and specifically antagonize the sympatholytic effect of reserpine. As is well known, they form a separate group, entirely different from the major tranquilizers, with a specific clinical action on certain depressive syndromes.

Pretreatment of animals with a *monoamine oxidase inhibitor* (MAOI), such as iproniazid, converts the effect of reserpine from sedation and decreased sympathetic tonus to hyperactivity and increased sympathetic tonus. Biochemically, the MAOI prevents the characteristic reserpine effect, namely, the depletion of serotonin and catecholamines in the central nervous system. Drugs of the imipramine group, on the other hand, do not prevent the reserpine-induced depletion of amines but seem to influence the catecholamines in the brain cells in a different way, especially by preventing the reuptake through the cell membranes, which ordinarily follows their release.

An increased sympathetic tonus is also provoked by the centrally acting sympathomimetics; some of these, such as *amphetamine,* act by releasing norepinephrine from the synaptic nerve endings. The amphetamines have an action directly opposite to that of the major tranquilizers: they produce hyperactivity instead of sedation; antagonize rather than potentiate anesthetics; induce hyperthermia instead of hypothermia; and decrease rather than increase appetite. In addition, amphetamines produce certain specific effects, notably on behavior and mood. Included in the amphetamine groups are drugs like *pipradrol* and methylphenidate,* which have a less pronounced peripheral sympathomimetic effect, as well as certain drugs used to suppress appetite, such as *phenmetrazine.* The stimulant effect of amphetamines and similar drugs is most likely connected with the stimulating action on the cerebral sympathetic centers. Not all stimulant drugs are necessarily sympathomimetic, however; *caffeine* is the prototype of those that are not.

Other drugs with pronounced sympathomimetic properties have actions that differ in some respects from those of amphetamines. *Mescaline,* for example, which is chemically closely related to amphetamine and has a similar stimulating action on the sympathetic system, has as its most striking property a hallucinogenic action with perceptual distortion, an effect that is rarely produced after single, even large, doses of amphetamines. Psilocybin* and *lysergic acid diethylamide* (LSD) have a qualitatively identical effect, although at much smaller doses. L-Δ9-trans *tetra-hydrocannabinol,* the active substance of cannabis (hashish or marijuana), has a behavioral effect very similar to that of the described hallucinogens, although it seems to have a different site of action in the CNS.

The diagrams have been arranged according to the objectively observable effects on normal animals or normal humans. Table 28 displays the effects on the motor system; Table 29 the effects on the sensory system; and Table 30 those on the autonomic nervous system. By indicating only the gross action and omitting differences in the mode of action (e.g., the sympatholytic action of chlorpromazine and reserpine), lines can be drawn on the diagram separating drugs of different actions into larger units with one or a few common properties, such as an anticonvulsant or a sympatholytic effect.

Table 31 illustrates some of the drug's actions on behavior or mood, but the borders here are not always distinct. For instance, a drug may cause hyperactivity at one dosage level and sedation at another, or vary in its effects from one species of laboratory animal to another: morphine causes arousal in the cat and depression in the dog. Only a few examples of behavioral effects are shown. Some drugs specifically enhance conditioned avoidance responses, while others inhibit them. The taming effect is measured in animals by the amount of inhibition occurring in the innate flight-fight reaction that takes place at the approach of an individual of a different species, especially man. The term "conflict-induced behavior" is used to describe what Pavlov called the "experimental neurosis," characterized by restlessness or stupor, lack of cooperation, displacement movements, and failing appetite. It is sometimes accompanied by retching, vomiting, and diarrhea and is the characteristic behavior of animals repeatedly exposed to a given situation and randomly rewarded or punished for their response. Many agents ranging from alcohol to opioids are able to normalize conflict-induced behavior (Jacobsen 1955, Masserman 1946). This effect and the taming effect may be hard to observe when a major tranquilizer is used because they are masked by the abolition of conditioned responses and by the catatonic extrapyramidal syndrome induced; nonetheless, it must be assumed that these effects are a latent property of the major tranquilizers.

Table 32 gives a schematic overview of the clinical indications and uses of the psychotropic agents shown in the five diagrams. Its purpose is to highlight classification problems, not to provide guidelines for treatment, for guidelines are discussed in far greater detail throughout the rest of this book.

Viewed as a whole, the diagrams illustrate that no single property can serve as a satisfactory basis for classifying psychotropic drugs. The placement of the diagram's boundary lines would thus vary according to which property of the drug is being considered; were other properties to be considered, other lines would have to be drawn. To describe a drug adequately, the properties already mentioned and perhaps many others must be considered. The diagrams do suggest, however, that drugs with the same profile of action in animal experiments have similar clinical effects in man. By knowing a drug's effects on animals, it is thus possible to make reasonably well-informed guesses about its potential clinical indications and approximate dose ranges. Drugs that appear to alleviate a particular symptom or syndrome (such as an experimental neurosis) in animals, however, need not be effective in the clinical syndromes of man (which may, of course, mean only that the two types of syndromes, in this case neuroses, are completely unrelated). There is no proof whatsoever, for example, that drugs that have a taming effect on animals relieve anxiety in humans. In short, as long as the etiology of mental diseases remains unknown, any statement linking a drug's clinical effects with information derived from biochemical, physiological, or psychological experiments in animals is at best hypothetical and at worst pure speculation.

MAJOR TRANQUILIZERS

The term *major tranquilizer* refers to agents that

1/ moderate anxiety and psychomotor agitation,
2/ help to restore the disturbed patient's interaction with his environment (Freedman 1960),
3/ do not produce a substantial degree of tolerance, physical dependence, or craving (Battegay 1966),

4/ achieve their effect at doses far lower than those required to produce sleep (Klerman 1960),

5/ have a beneficial effect on the kinds of cognitive disturbances and perceptual changes that are generally considered pathognomonic of schizophrenic illness (Delay 1952, Goldstein 1969, May 1968),

6/ cause little dampening of the arousal response to afferent stimuli (Sedivec 1964, Szatmari 1956), and, in all drugs described to the present as having the above properties,

7/ produce extrapyramidal effects when given in high doses, and

8/ lower the convulsive threshold.

Among the drugs currently marketed in the United States, only phenothiazines, butyrophenones, thioxanthenes, and rauwolfia alkaloids have these properties and could thus be called major tranquilizers (see Table 34).

Phenothiazines

Clinical Pharmacology

The substituted phenothiazines have a wide range of effects: they act in the CNS; produce sedation and endocrine changes; block conditioned avoidance behavior; have antiemetic, antipruritic, and analgesic effects; alter temperature regulation and skeletal muscle tone; facilitate seizure discharge; act in the autonomic nervous system, producing strong adrenergic and weaker peripheral cholinergic blocking, as well as antihistamine and antiserotonin effects; potentiate the action of a number of different drugs; induce local anesthesia; and (depending on the dose) depress or stimulate the reticular activating system (Domino 1962). That each of these effects is not produced in equal strength by every phenothiazine provides the impetus for selective molecular manipulation in the direction of greater specificity. Phenothiazines lend themselves to this sort of selective synthesis relatively easily because side-chain substitutions in positions $2 (R_2) + 10 (R_1)$ of the three-ringed phenothiazine structure change not only the milligram potency and duration of action but may also achieve a partial separation of the various effects.

Efforts to classify the many phenothiazines now available and in this way to match drug and patient and thus maximize therapeutic efficacy while minimizing the risk of side effects have focused either on the chemical composition of the various drugs (and particularly the character of the substituent at position 10) or on their pharmacologic effects on various systems in the normal person and on various systems and syndromes in the mentally ill. Classification in terms of the side chain at position 10 distinguishes between phenothiazines with

1/ an aliphatic side chain: chlorpromazine (Thorazine), promazine (Sparine), and triflupromazine (Vesprin);

2/ a piperidine moiety in the side chain: thioridazine (Mellaril); and

3/ a piperazine (or piperazinyl) group in the side chain: acetophenazine (Tindal), carphenazine (Proketazine), fluphenazine (Prolixin, Permitil) perphenazine (Trilafon), prochlorperazine (Compazine), trifluoperazine (Stelazine) and butaperazine (Repoise). The piperazine group is once more subcategorized into drugs with a CF_3 group in position 2 (like fluphenazine and trifluoperazine) and those without.

Phenothiazines can also be classified in terms of the drowsiness they produce in the first week or two of administration. Given in therapeutic doses, drugs such as chlorpromazine and thioridazine tend to produce the most drowsiness (and are for this reason sometimes called *sedating* phenothiazines); those like fluphenazine and trifluoperazine produce the least amount (and are thus sometimes labeled *alerting*); and drugs like perphenazine, trifluopromazine, acetophenazine, and prochlorperazine lie somewhere between (and may thus be considered *intermediate*). However severe the patient's initial drowsiness may be, he is likely to develop some degree of tolerance to it within a week or ten days and tends thereafter to exhibit only a mild degree of psychomotor retardation. Nevertheless, even after some months of use, those phenothiazines that initially produce the greatest amount of drowsiness tend to produce the greatest amount of dulling and retardation.

Classifying phenothiazines in terms of the drowsiness they produce is akin to classifying them in terms of their *therapeutic potency,* for the sedating ones must be given in higher doses to have an equivalent therapeutic effect. A review of the typical doses employed in psychotic disorders makes it possible to tabulate the most commonly used phenothiazines in the order of their potency (see Table 33). By including the reported incidence of side effects for each drug in this table, the conclusion is reached that a drug's therapeutic potency is related in some way (though not in a directly linear way) to its propensity to cause particular side effects. The figures given on the incidence of side effects are based in large measure on our own observations but are in agreement with a number of large-scale studies (Ayd 1961, Ban 1964, Clark 1968, Galbrecht 1968, Lapolla 1965, Lasky 1962, Prien 1968, 1969). No real consensus concerning their incidence is possible, however, in view of the disparity of criteria used by different investigators for deciding which drug and how much of it is indicated for which patient at which stage of his illness and treatment and for deciding whether to give or withhold antiparkinsonian agents (Avery 1967). There is, moreover, no uniform classification system for side effects (what one investigator calls dyskinesia, another lists as parkinsonism, and a third as hypomotility) and no uniform system for noting and reporting them.

That the incidence of extrapyramidal effects is higher and that of drowsiness and hypotension somewhat lower in the more potent agents does not mean that the more potent agents have entirely different effects from the less potent ones, but rather that, milligram for milligram, the therapeutically more potent agents are far more likely to produce extrapyramidal effects but not equally more likely to produce drowsiness, depression, and hypotension. A 10 mg dose of fluphenazine will cause more drowsiness than an equal amount of chlorpromazine; therapeutic doses of chlorpromazine cause a greater degree of drowsiness or hypotension only because its antipsychotic effect is so low that it is achieved only at dose levels high enough to cause drowsiness. By the same token it is, strictly speaking, an error to call chlorpromazine "sedating," perphenazine "intermediate," or fluphenazine "alerting"—as we do throughout this book—for the last of these, when given in equal doses, is unquestionably the most sedating of the three. The justification for such terminology is strictly pragmatic: *it calls attention to the clinical differences observed when each drug is given in a therapeutic dose.*

From a theoretical standpoint, therefore, fluphenazine might be preferable for the treatment of the agitated patient because it can calm him without putting him to sleep and thus out of contact with an environment into which he needs to be reintegrated. However, the dose required to calm him might well produce such severe extrapyramidal effects that the disadvantages outweigh the advantage of diminished drowsiness and thus a less potent phenothiazine would be more suitable. If the patient is 60 or older or has a history of cardiovascular disease, an intermediate rather than sedating phenothiazine would be chosen, for even though, in doses sufficient to produce sedation, the intermediate agent is more likely to produce extrapyramidal effects, it is less likely to produce hypotension and thus to endanger the patient's cardiac status.

Distribution and Metabolic Fate

Phenothiazines are well absorbed from the gastrointestinal tract and parenteral sites and reach peak concentration in the bloodstream within two hours after oral, and 30 minutes after intramuscular, administration. Approximately 12 to 18 hours after the first dose, the blood level returns to the premedication level (Curry 1970, Huang 1961). When given to pregnant women, approximately 0.5% of the dose crosses the placental barrier within 30 minutes (Behn 1956). Phenothiazines are also excreted in milk but in barely detectable levels (Blacker 1962). The metabolic breakdown proceeds via hydroxylation in the 3 and 7 positions and subsequent conjugation with glucuronic acid to glucuronides, and via sulfoxide formation, metabolic alterations in the side chain, and demethylation (Goldenberg 1961, Huang 1963, 1964, Salzman 1956). Excretion of phenothiazines and their metabolites via urine and feces proceeds fairly slowly; less than 20% appears in the urine within the first five days after a single administration (Hetzel 1961). Given in regular dosage for prolonged periods, 50% of the daily intake is excreted in the urine and the rest in the feces (Forrest 1961). Traces, either as metabolites or as free chlorpromazine, may be found in the urine for six to 12 months after the drug is discontinued (Huang 1961).

Clinical Indications

After two decades of use and clinical trials in almost every psychiatric syndrome, phenothiazines have been found most effective in the treatment of *schizophrenia*. Their merits lie particularly in the management of psychomotor agitation, delusional ideation, auditory hallucinations, blocking, inappropriate affect, and social withdrawal (Goldberg 1965), (see also Chaps. 3 and 5). Indeed, it is now well established that by every criterion of improvement, phenothiazines are more effective than barbiturates, chlordiazepoxide, ECT, psychotherapy, "basic care," or active or inactive placebos in alleviating the symptoms of acute schizophrenic psychosis (Casey 1960, Grinspoon 1968, Hekimian 1967, Kurland 1962, NIMH 1964, 1967) and preventing relapses and rehospitalization (Engelhardt 1967, Gantz 1965, Lutz 1965, Morton 1968, Rosen 1968). Although the results are more dramatic in acute than in chronic schizophrenias, even the patient who has been schizophrenic for many years is likely to experience progressive and sustained reduction of symptoms (Prien 1968, 1969). Even after long-term hospitalization, the patient may show sufficient psychosocial improvement to return to the outside community. In patients over 40 and those hospitalized for more than 10 years, the results are not as impressive; improved adjustment to the institutional setting is usually the most that can be achieved (Honigfeld 1965, Marjerrison 1964).

While phenothiazines produce some measure of improvement in mild hypomanic episodes, the results are disappointing in severe *manic states*. The patient's restlessness and impulsivity may diminish somewhat, but the associated dysphoria, tension, and discomfort tend to be unaffected. Even when massive doses of sedating phenothiazines are used, the patient may be unable to fall or remain asleep and, despite appearing heavily drugged, may seem as driven in his behavior as he was without medication. In *agitated depressions*, phenothiazines can be used to diminish the patient's restlessness and obsessional, self-castigating ruminations and to improve his sleep and appetite (Raskin 1968), but unless he is simultaneously given an antidepressant, he tends to become even more anergic and retarded (Lehmann 1963, Raskin 1970, Simonson 1964). Patients in the depressive phase of *schizo-affective schizophrenia* must also be treated with both phenothiazines and antidepressants, as phenothiazines alone tend to aggravate the depression, and antidepressants the disordered thinking. A combination of phenothiazines and antidepressants may also be of value for the patient with *chronic schizophrenia* who over the years has become increasingly anergic (Hanlon 1964, Hordern 1962).

Behavioral disturbances secondary to *brain damage, seizure disorders,* or other *medical illnesses* may also respond well to small doses of phenothiazines. The choice between a more sedating and a more alerting compound depends in these cases not only on the patient's level of activity, agitation, and alertness but also on the compatibility of the particular phenothiazine with his general medical condition (Blachly 1966). The phenothiazines' appetite-stimulating effect can be of value, furthermore, in *anorexia nervosa,* *"brittle" diabetes,* and other diseases associated with weight loss or appetite disturbance.

Although the effectiveness of phenothiazines is by no means so well documented in neuroses or personality disorders as in schizophrenia, patients with chronic *obsessive-compulsive neurosis* who repeatedly experience bouts of agitation and sleep difficulty may obtain some relief during such episodes if given moderate doses of alerting or intermediate phenothiazines. Recurrent obsessive-compulsive neurosis, in which symptom-free periods alternate with bouts of obsessive-compulsive and sometimes also depressive symptoms, do not respond to phenothiazines alone but require either antidepressants or a combination of phenothiazines and antidepressants. Adolescents with an *emotionally unstable personality,* who alternate between episodes of tenseness and dysphoria accompanied by inactivity and withdrawal and episodes of impulsivity, giddiness, low frustration tolerance, rule-breaking, and shortsighted hedonism, as well as adults with *explosive or antisocial personalities,* may respond to long-term administration of 100 to 200 mg of chlorpromazine (Thorazine) daily (Klein 1969).

Various methods have been used to substantiate the clinical impression that certain types of illness respond better to one phenothiazine than another. In one controlled study, for example, acetophenazine (Tindal) was found to be more effective than perphenazine (Trilafon) for schizophrenics with reasonably well-organized paranoid delusions, but less effective than perphenazine for simple and chronic undifferentiated schizophrenics (Overall 1963). A comparison of individuals according to the drug on which they improved showed that *chlorpromazine improvers* were characterized by auditory hallucinations, retardation, ideas of persecution, confusion, indifference, irritability, poor self-care, poor social participation, feelings of unreality, and agitation, but not guilt feelings, incoherence, disorientation, resistance to treatment, or visual hallucinations. *Fluphenazine* (Prolixin) *improvers* had also exhibited indifference, irritability, poor self-care, poor social participation, and feelings of unreality, but had not manifested incoherence and did experience guilt feelings. *Thioridazine* (Mellaril) *improvers,* finally, had manifested feelings of unreality (like the other two) and agitation (like the chlorpromazine improvers), but had also exhibited pressure of speech and sadness (Goldberg 1967).

Although phenothiazines can be usefully combined with a number of other psychotropic agents (such as CNS depressants during drug withdrawal, antidepressants in depressions, and lithium carbonate during manic episodes), the concurrent use of two or more phenothiazines should be limited to the period of transition from one phenothiazine to another. In our experience, any joint effect that a combination of several phenothiazines might be intended to achieve can be accomplished with a single agent. It is both unnecessary and unjustified, therefore, to compound the risk of allergic reaction that obtains whenever a new drug is administered, especially as it might become necessary then to withdraw both drugs, thus inviting the additional hazard of relapse.

Dosage and Administration

The dosage of phenothiazines required will vary with the particular drug being used, the nature of the illness, and the patient's ability to sleep. Using chlorpromazine as a reference point, the average daily therapeutic dose for psychotic illnesses is 400 to 800 mg; for neurotic disorders, 100 to 200 mg; and for nausea and vomiting, 50 to 100 mg. More potent phenothiazines can of course be used in smaller doses, but the same 8:2:1 ratio holds. In determining the proper initial dosage, it is useful to distinguish between the patient whose psychosis is accompanied by agitation and insomnia and the one who, even if fairly anxious during the day, is able to sleep at night. In the former case, the optimal dosage is determined by viewing the patient's insomnia as the first target symptom and gradually increasing the dose until his sleep is restored. This method of "titrating" the dosage against the patient's sleep is presented on page 173. In the absence of sleep disturbance, one can usually arrive at the optimal dosage by increasing the dose repeatedly until there is no further diminution in his symptoms and no further improvement in his social functioning, or the adverse effects outweigh the therapeutic ones. Further comments on dosage may be found on page 146.

Most phenothiazines are available in tablet or liquid form and, with the exception of thioridazine (Mellaril) and butaperazine (Repoise), in injectable form as well (see Table 34). Patients who are lucid enough to understand and remember what is expected of them will usually take their tablets without serious objection if the recommendation is clear and firm. If, however, the patient is "cheeking" the drug and later spitting it out (particularly common in patient with paranoid delusions) (Wilson 1967), it may be necessary to give the phenothiazine in liquid form. Fluphenazine (Permitil) is especially useful when covert administration is required, for it is available as a fully tasteless and odorless liquid that can be given undetected in coffee, juice, or soup. If this is not feasible, either because the patient is too suspicious to take what he is offered or because his condition requires a different or more rapidly effective drug, parenteral administration may be required. Since a greater amount of the drug is absorbed in parenteral administration, only one third or one fourth of the oral dose need be used. Intramuscular injections should be made in the gluteal region or, if the patient has received too many injections at that site, into the femoral muscle. Subcutaneous administration may cause necrosis and should

be avoided. Intravenous administration is rarely indicated and, especially in the case of promazine (Sparine), can produce both tissue
necrosis and vasculitis if extravasation should occur (Fisher 1966).
Should intravenous administration be necessary, perphenazine
(Trilafon), diluted in 10 cc of saline, can be used. Patients given
phenothiazines parenterally or even in large oral doses should have
their blood pressure taken every half hour for the first two to three
hours. Elderly patients and those given parenteral chlorpromazine
(Thorazine) should remain in a reclining position for at least an
hour after administration. Outpatients who are not reliable enough
to take the medication on their own may be given intramuscular
"depot" injections of 12.5 to 30 mg of fluphenazine enanthate, said
to be effective even when given at weekly or biweekly intervals
(Lowther 1969, Whittier 1967); such injections have so high an
incidence of extrapyramidal side effects, however, that the patient
must routinely be given antiparkinsonian agents and warned of the
consequences of not taking them. While sustained-release capsules
containing phenothiazines may be of some value for the two to
three weeks it usually takes the patient to achieve tolerance to the
drowsiness-producing effect, they are of doubtful value thereafter,
as the typical phenothiazine's half-life is long enough to permit it
to be given as infrequently as once or twice daily with full therapeutic effect (Brophy 1969, DiMascio 1969, Hollister 1970).

Adverse Effects

Adverse effects seen after phenothiazine use may be broadly
classified as hypersensitivity reactions (such as jaundice, blood
dyscrasias, and skin reactions) and toxic effects (such as drowsiness,
hypotension, and extrapyramidal symptoms). While hypersensitivity reactions are unrelated to the drug's pharmacologic effects or
dosage, toxic effects are exaggerations of the pharmacologic effects
and increase in severity and incidence with increasing dosage (see
page 578).

HYPERSENSITIVITY REACTIONS

Hypersensitivity reactions may result from almost any of the
drugs listed in this chapter, but are most frequently produced
by the phenothiazines, especially chlorpromazine. Characteristically,
the majority of these reactions occur within the first two or three
months of treatment; however, if the individual has been sensitized
or is unusually sensitive to start with, symptoms may appear within
a few days. Since patch, scratch, and intradermal tests are of little

predictive value, the individual given such drugs must be told what to look for and carefully examined for the manifestations of hypersensitivity at each visit until the critical period has passed.

JAUNDICE. The *incidence* of chlorpromazine-induced jaundice was once thought to be as high as 4% of all patients who take this drug (Ayd 1963, Hollister 1964), but it seems to have decreased so that jaundice now occurs in appreciably less than 1% of patients (Chalmers 1965). Promazine (Sparine) has also been reported to produce liver damage (Waitzkin 1957), while thioridazine (Mellaril), triflupromazine (Vesprin), and drugs of the piperazine type, such as prochlorperazine (Compazine), fluphenazine (Prolixin), trifluoperazine (Stelazine), and butaperazine (Repoise), produce it only rarely (Barancik 1967, Block 1962, Hollister 1964, McFarland 1963, Solomon 1959). With perphenazine (Trilafon), the reported incidence of jaundice is as low as one in every two million patients (Ayd 1964, Ban 1966).

The *clinical picture* generally develops in the second to fourth week of treatment and is rare after the sixth week. The skin discoloration is often preceded by fever, malaise, and meteorism, followed by nausea, vomiting, and liver tenderness. The patient's urine generally turns dark, and his stool often becomes pale. An increased alkaline phosphatase and an increase in serum glutamic oxaloacetic transaminase (SGOT) to 100 or 200 Karmen units usually precedes other symptoms. While these two tests, especially the former, are the most practical and reliable, increased serum bilubin (direct>indirect) may also be found, as well as bilirubinuria, increased excretion of 5-nucleotidase, increased serum lipids and cholesterol, and eosinophilia. Liver biopsy reveals an intrahepatic cholestasis with bile plugs in dilated bile canaliculi, mononuclear and eosinophile cellular infiltrates in the periportal areas, bile-staining of parenchymal hepatic cells, and minimal centrilobular necrosis of liver cells (Popper 1962). That the disorder is allergic in character is suggested by the observation that *1/* it is unrelated to the daily or even the total dose used; *2/* it is often associated with fever, chills, lymphodenopathy, skin rash, arthralgias, and eosinophilia; and *3/* positive challenge responses may occur for years after the original reaction has subsided (Klatskin 1969).

The *differential diagnosis* includes infectious hepatitis, particularly because it is sometimes endemic in mental hospitals (Siegel 1965). Like most drug-induced side effects, the disorder is more common in women than men (Ayd 1963, Hollister 1961a). Patients with preexisting liver disease do not have a higher incidence of phenothiazine-induced jaundice (Popper 1965), but do have a far more difficult course when they develop an allergic jaundice. Although the eventual *outcome* depends on the extent of the damage (and thus on the rapidity with which the hepatic dysfunction is noted and the drug discontinued), the disorder almost invariably has a benign, self-limiting course. The liver function tests return to normal within a month (though the reversal of the skin discoloration may lag behind), and there have been only 14 deaths reported among the millions of people who have been treated with phenothiazines. In rare instances, when xanthomatous biliary cirrhosis supervenes as a complication, the disorder may last for months (Bolton 1967, Nørredam 1963).

Among the *preventive measures* that have been proposed are weekly urinary bilirubin tests with commercially available reagent kits (The Medical Letter 1968). These provide a very rough screening device that can be performed fairly easily in large mental hospital populations, but are more defensible from the standpoint of expediency than accuracy. Weekly SGOT and alkaline phosphatase measurements are far more reliable, as they make it possible to detect hepatic dysfunctioning fairly early, in any case before the skin discoloration develops (Popper 1959). Minor elevations of SGOT or alkaline phosphatase need not cause alarm, for their values will often return to the baseline without any change in dosage (Wroblewski 1962); if these values continue to rise or the patient becomes jaundiced, the phenothiazine being used must be discontinued immediately. Since with the exception of promazine and chlorpromazine there is no cross-sensitivity, however, it is usually sufficient to change to a different phenothiazine.

BLOOD DYSCRASIAS. Phenothiazines are the leading cause of drug-induced blood dyscrasias. Some patients develop transient leukocytosis, leukopenia, or eosinophilia, but these are usually of no clinical significance (Lomas 1955). Leukocytosis may be due to a wide variety of factors and may even be a result of the anxiety, excitement, and dehydration associated with the disease for which the phenothiazine is being given. If, after the patient is first given a particular drug, his WBC decreases somewhat but reverts to the baseline within a few weeks, this innocuous pattern may repeat itself each time the dosage of that drug is increased. Agranulocytosis, thrombocytopenia, and pancytopenia, on the other hand, are serious complications. A few cases have been reported following the use of thioridazine (Mellaril), trifluoperazine (Stelazine) and others of the piperazine group (Ayd 1961, Dally 1967), but, as with jaundice, the

TABLE 28. *Some Effects of Psychotropic Drugs on the Motor System*

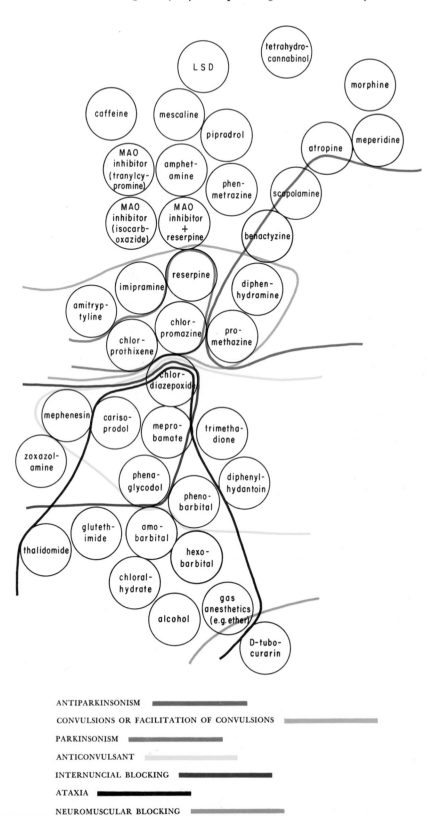

ANTIPARKINSONISM

CONVULSIONS OR FACILITATION OF CONVULSIONS

PARKINSONISM

ANTICONVULSANT

INTERNUNCIAL BLOCKING

ATAXIA

NEUROMUSCULAR BLOCKING

TABLE 29. *Some Effects of Psychotropic Drugs on the Sensory System*

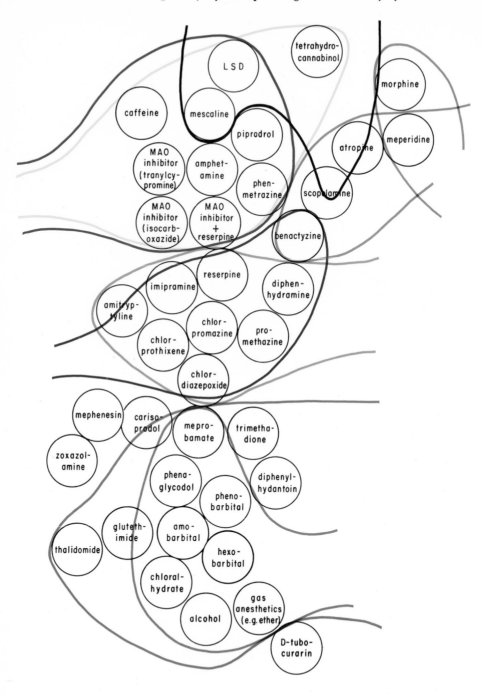

ANTAGONISM TO ANESTHETICS

EEG AROUSAL

HALLUCINOGENIC

ANALGESIC

EEG BLOCKING

POTENTIATION OF ANESTHETICS

PARTIAL BLOCKING OR MIXED EEG EFFECT

EEG SLEEP PATTERN

ANESTHETIC

TABLE 30. *Some Effects of Psychotropic Drugs on the Autonomic Nervous System*

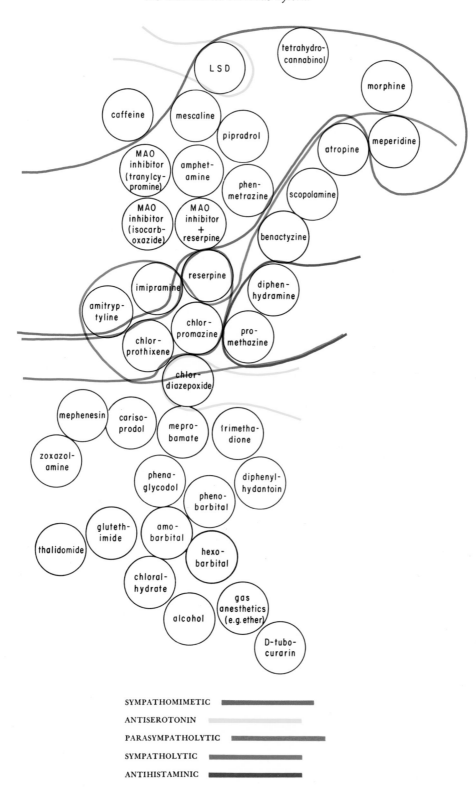

SYMPATHOMIMETIC	▬▬▬▬▬▬
ANTISEROTONIN	▬▬▬▬▬▬
PARASYMPATHOLYTIC	▬▬▬▬▬▬
SYMPATHOLYTIC	▬▬▬▬▬▬
ANTIHISTAMINIC	▬▬▬▬▬▬

TABLE 31. *Some Effects of Psychotropic Drugs on Behavior, Conditioned Reflexes, and Mood*

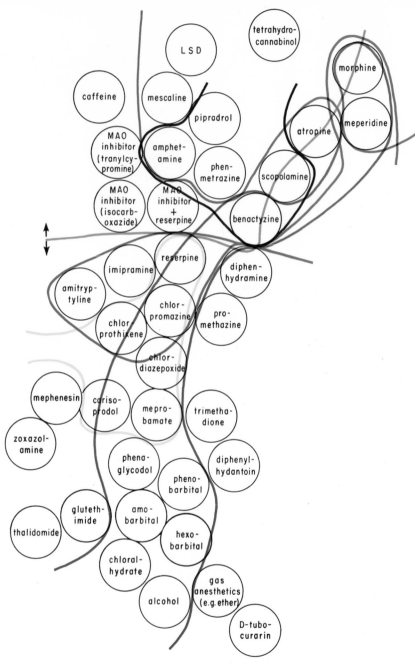

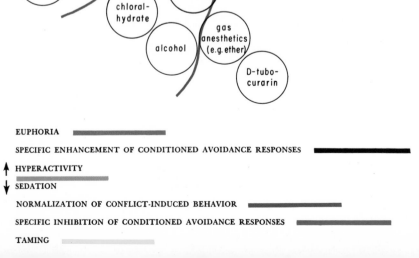

EUPHORIA

SPECIFIC ENHANCEMENT OF CONDITIONED AVOIDANCE RESPONSES

↑ HYPERACTIVITY

↓ SEDATION

NORMALIZATION OF CONFLICT-INDUCED BEHAVIOR

SPECIFIC INHIBITION OF CONDITIONED AVOIDANCE RESPONSES

TAMING

TABLE 32. *Clinical Indications and Uses of Psychotropic Drugs*

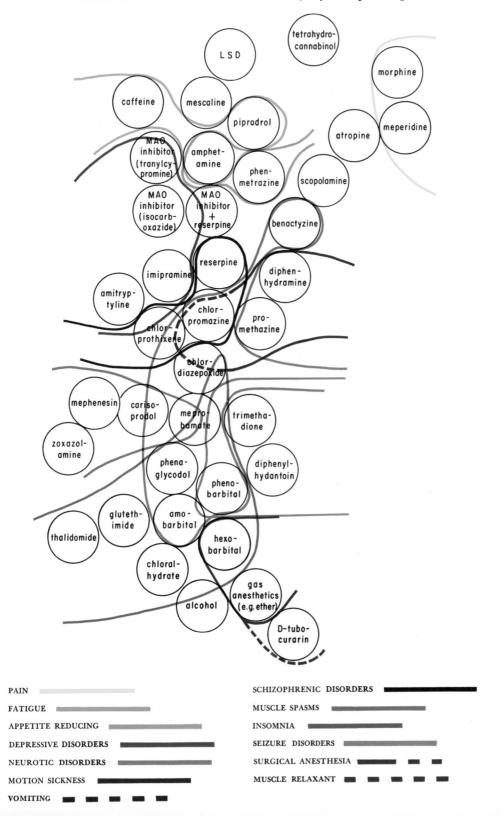

PAIN

FATIGUE

APPETITE REDUCING

DEPRESSIVE DISORDERS

NEUROTIC DISORDERS

MOTION SICKNESS

VOMITING

SCHIZOPHRENIC DISORDERS

MUSCLE SPASMS

INSOMNIA

SEIZURE DISORDERS

SURGICAL ANESTHESIA

MUSCLE RELAXANT

TABLE 33. *Classification of Phenothiazines According to Relative Potency and Frequency of Side Effects*

GENERIC NAME	TRADE NAME	TYPICAL DAILY ORAL DOSE RANGE IN PSYCHOTIC DISORDERS (in mg)	TYPICAL DAILY ORAL DOSE RANGE IN NEUROTIC DISORDERS (in mg)	DYSTONIA IN FIRST WEEK	DROWSINESS IN FIRST WEEK	EXTRAPYRAMIDAL EFFECTS AFTER SOME TIME OF USE	DROWSINESS AFTER SOME WEEKS OF USE	HYPOTENSION
Fluphenazine	Prolixin	5–20	1–4	+++	++	++	+	+
Trifluperazine	Stelazine	15–40	3–8	++	++	+++	+	+
Perphenazine	Trilafon	32–80	8–16	++	+++	++	++	+
Prochlorperazine	Compazine	50–150	15–50	++	++	+++	++	+
Acetophenazine	Tindal	80–160	20–60	++	+	+	++	++
Triflupromazine	Vesprin	150–400	30–60	+	++	+	++	++
Chlorpromazine	Thorazine	400–800	100–200	++	+++	++	+++	++
Thioridazine	Mellaril	400–800	150–200	+	+++	++	+++	+++
				4+ = 6–9% 3+ = 3–6% 2+ = 1½–3% 1+ = <1½%	4+ = 20–25% 3+ = 15–20% 2+ = 10–15% 1+ = 5–10%	4+ = 30–40% 3+ = 20–30% 2+ = 10–20% 1+ = <10%	3+ = 10–15% 2+ = 5–10% 1+ = <5%	3+ = 2–4% 2+ = 1–2% 1+ = <1%

TABLE 34. *Major Tranquilizers* *

GROUP	GENERIC NAME (TRADE NAME-MANUFACTURER)	STRUCTURAL FORMULA	TYPICAL DAILY DOSE RANGE FOR PSYCHOTIC DISORDERS IN ADULTS	HOW SUPPLIED
Phenothiazines	Fluphenazine (*Prolixin*-Squibb) (*Permitil*-White)	$CH_2CH_2CH_2$—N N—CH_2CH_2OH · 2HCl CF_3 N S	5-20 mg	Elixir: 0.5 mg/cc Concentrate: 5 mg/cc Injection: Fluphenazine hydrochloride 2.5 mg/cc Depot injection: Fluphenazine enanthate 25 mg/cc in sesame oil vehicle PROLIXIN: 1 mg, 2.5 mg, 5 mg SRF†: 0.25 mg, 1 mg PERMITIL: 1 mg, 2.5 mg, 5 mg, 10 mg
	Trifluoperazine (*Stelazine*-SKF)	$CH_3CH_2CH_2$—N N—CH_3 · 2HCl CF_3 N S	15-40 mg	Concentrate: 10 mg/cc Injection: 2 mg/cc STELAZINE: 1 mg S03, 2 mg S04, 5 mg S06, 10 mg S07
	Butaperazine (*Repoise*-Robins)	$CH_3CH_2CH_2$—N N—CH_3 2 HCCOOH O CCH_2CH_3 N S	30-80 mg	REPOISE: 5 mg, 10 mg, 25 mg

TABLE 34. *Major Tranquilizers* * (continued)

GROUP	GENERIC NAME (TRADE NAME-MANUFACTURER)	STRUCTURAL FORMULA	TYPICAL DAILY DOSE RANGE FOR PSYCHOTIC DISORDERS IN ADULTS	HOW SUPPLIED
Phenothiazines	Promazine (*Sparine*-Wyeth)	$CH_2CH_2CH_2N(CH_3)_2$ · HCl	100-400 mg	Syrup: 2 mg/cc Concentrate: 30 mg/cc, 100 mg/cc Injection: 25 mg/cc (i.m. or i.v.) 50 mg/cc (i.m. only) 10 mg 25 mg 50 mg 100 mg 200 mg SPARINE
	Triflupromazine (*Vesprin*-Squibb)	CF_3 $CH_2CH_2CH_2N(CH_3)_2$ · HCl	150-400 mg	Suspension: 10 mg/cc Injection: 10 mg/cc, 20 mg/cc 10 mg 25 mg 50 mg VESPRIN
	Chlorpromazine (*Thorazine*-SKF)	Cl $CH_2CH_2CH_2N(CH_3)_2$	400-800 mg	Syrup: 2 mg/cc Concentrate: 30 mg/cc, 100 mg/cc Suppositories: 25 mg, 100 mg Injection: 25 mg/cc 30 mg (1 dot) T63, 75 mg (2 dots) T64, 150 mg (3 dots) T66, 200 mg (4 dots) T67, 300 mg (5 dots, monogram with bars) T69 SRF † 10 mg T73, 25 mg T74, 50 mg T76, 100 mg T77, 200 mg T79 THORAZINE

TABLE 34. Major Tranquilizers * (continued)

GROUP	GENERIC NAME (TRADE NAME-MANUFACTURER)	STRUCTURAL FORMULA	TYPICAL DAILY DOSE RANGE FOR PSYCHOTIC DISORDERS IN ADULTS	HOW SUPPLIED
Phenothiazines	Perphenazine (*Trilafon*-Schering)		32-80 mg	Syrup: 0.4 mg/cc Concentrate: 3.2 mg/cc Injection: 5 mg/cc 2 mg 4 mg 8 mg 16 mg **TRILAFON** 8 mg **SRF** †
	Prochlorperazine (*Compazine*-SKF)		50-150 mg	Syrup: 1 mg/cc Concentrate: 10 mg/cc Suppositories: 2½ mg, 5 mg, 25 mg Injection: 5 mg/cc 10 mg (1 dot) C44, 15 mg (2 dots) C46 30 mg (3 dots) C47, 75 mg (4 dots) C49 **SRF** † **COMPAZINE** 5 mg C66 10 mg C67, 25 mg C69
	Acetophenazine (*Tindal*-Schering)		80-160 mg	20 mg **TINDAL**
	Carphenazine (*Proketazine*-Wyeth)		100-300 mg	Concentrate: 50 mg/cc 12.5 mg 25 mg 50 mg **PROKETAZINE**

TABLE 34. Major Tranquilizers * (continued)

GROUP	GENERIC NAME (TRADE NAME-MANUFACTURER)	STRUCTURAL FORMULA	TYPICAL DAILY DOSE RANGE FOR PSYCHOTIC DISORDERS IN ADULTS	HOW SUPPLIED
Phenothiazines	Thioridazine (*Mellaril*-Sandoz)		400-800 mg	Concentrate: 30 mg/cc MELLARIL — 10 mg, 25 mg, 50 mg, 100 mg, 150 mg, 200 mg
Thioxanthenes	Chlorprothixene (*Taractan*-Roche)		150-400 mg	Concentrate: 20 mg/cc Injection: 12.5 mg/cc TARACTAN — 10 mg, 25 mg, 50 mg, 100 mg
Thioxanthenes	Thiothixene (*Navane*-Roerig)		30-60 mg	NAVANE — 1 mg, 2 mg, 5 mg, 10 mg
Butyro-phenones	Haloperidol (*Haldol*-McNeil)		4-10 mg	Concentrate: 2 mg/cc HALDOL — 0.5 mg, 1 mg, 2 mg, 5 mg

TABLE 34. *Major Tranquilizers* * (continued)

GROUP	GENERIC NAME (TRADE NAME-MANUFACTURER)	STRUCTURAL FORMULA	TYPICAL DAILY DOSE RANGE FOR PSYCHOTIC DISORDERS IN ADULTS	HOW SUPPLIED
Rauwolfia Alkaloids	Reserpine (*Serpasil*-Ciba) Also available in generic form.		4-10 mg	Elixir: .05 mg/cc Injection: 2.5 mg/cc 0.1 mg 0.25 mg 1 mg SERPASIL

* MOST COMMON ADVERSE EFFECTS OF

Major Tranquilizers: drowsiness, hypotension, extrapyramidal actions, increases in weight and appetite, depression, dry mouth, blurred vision, amenorrhea; allergic reactions especially affecting liver, skin and blood are most common with chlorpromazine (additional details on pp. 542-544 also 577-578).

Butyrophenones may produce unusually severe extrapyramidal effects but are less likely to have an effect on weight and appetite than other major tranquilizers.

Rauwolfia alkaloids may produce nasal stuffiness, abdominal cramps, diarrhea, nausea, and aggravation of peptic ulcer; are more likely than phenothiazines to produce depression; but rarely produce allergic reactions.

† SRF = SUSTAINED RELEASE FORM

TABLE 35. *General Depressants of the* CNS: *Minor Tranquilizers* *

GROUP	GENERIC NAME (TRADE NAME-MANUFACTURER)	STRUCTURAL FORMULA	TYPICAL DAILY DOSE RANGE FOR ADULTS	HOW SUPPLIED
Propanediols	Meprobamate (*Equanil*-Wyeth) (*Miltown*-Wallace) Also available in generic form.	$NH_2COOCH_2\overset{\underset{\displaystyle CH_2CH_2CH_3}{}}{\underset{}{C}}CH_2OCONH_2$ with CH_3	400-1,200 mg	Suspension: 40 mg/cc 200 mg 400 mg 400 mg coated EQUANIL 200 mg 400 mg MILTOWN 200 mg MEPROSPAN SRF † 400 mg MEPROTABS 400 mg SRF †
	Tybamate (*Solacen*-Wallace) (*Tybatran*-Robins)	$H_2NCOCH_2\overset{\underset{\displaystyle CH_2CH_2CH_3}{}}{\underset{}{C}}CH_2OCNHCH_2CH_2CH_2CH_3$ with CH_3 and O	500-1,500 mg	AHR 125 125 mg AHR 250 250 mg TYBATRAN AHR 350 350 mg 250 mg 350 mg SOLACEN

TABLE 35. *General Depressants of the* CNS: *Minor Tranquilizers* * (continued)

GROUP	GENERIC NAME (TRADE NAME-MANUFACTURER)	STRUCTURAL FORMULA	TYPICAL DAILY DOSE RANGE FOR ADULTS	HOW SUPPLIED
Benzodiazepines	Chlordiazepoxide (*Librium*-Roche)		20-60 mg	Injection: 20 mg/cc LIBRIUM: 5 mg, 10 mg, 25 mg LIBRITABS: 5 mg, 10 mg, 25 mg
	Diazepam (*Valium*-Roche)		5-15 mg	Injection: 5 mg/cc VALIUM: 2 mg, 5 mg, 10 mg
	Oxazepam (*Serax*-Wyeth)		30-90 mg	SERAX: 10 mg, 15 mg, 30 mg, 15 mg

TABLE 35. *General Depressants of the CNS: Minor Tranquilizers* * (continued)

GROUP	GENERIC NAME (TRADE NAME-MANUFACTURER)	STRUCTURAL FORMULA	TYPICAL DAILY DOSE RANGE FOR ADULTS	HOW SUPPLIED
Diphenylmethane Derivatives	Hydroxyzine (*Atarax*-Roerig, as the dihydrochloride) (*Vistaril*-Pfizer, as the pamoate)		50-150 mg	Syrup (Atarax): 2 mg/cc Suspension (Vistaril): 5 mg/cc Injection: (i.m. only) 25 mg/cc, 50 mg/cc

* MOST COMMON ADVERSE EFFECTS OF

Propanediols and Benzodiazepines: drowsiness, lethargy, slurred speech, paradoxical excitement, ataxia, physical dependence, compulsive use, *Hydroxyzine:* drowsiness, dryness of mouth, involuntary motor activity, tremor and convulsions with high doses; potentiation of CNS depressants and meperidine (Demerol).

† SRF = SUSTAINED RELEASE FORM.

TABLE 36. *General Depressants of the* CNS: *Sedatives and Hypnotics* *

GROUP	GENERIC NAME (TRADE NAME-MANUFACTURER)	STRUCTURAL FORMULA	TYPICAL DOSE RANGE FOR ADULTS	HOW SUPPLIED
Barbiturates	Amobarbital (*Amytal*-Lilly) Also available in generic form.		Sedative: 30-50 mg, 2-3 times a day Hypnotic: 100-200 mg	Pulvules: 65 mg, 200 mg Suppositories: 200 mg Injection: Ampoules of 65 mg, 125 mg, 250 mg, 500 mg 15 mg 30 mg 50 mg 100 mg **AMYTAL**
	Butabarbital (*Butisol*-McNeil) Also available in generic form.		Sedative: 15-30 mg, 3-4 times a day Hypnotic: 50-100 mg	15 gm 30 mg **BUTISOL SODIUM** Tablets: also available in 50 mg, 100 mg 15 mg 30 mg **BUTICAPS** Capsules: also available in 50 mg, 100 mg SRF †: 30 mg, 60 mg Elixir: 6 mg/cc
	Heptabarbital (*Medomin*-Geigy)		Sedative: 50-100 mg, 2-3 times a day Hypnotic: 200-400 mg	200 mg **MEDOMIN**
	Methohexital (*Brevital*-Lilly)		Intravenous hypnotic: 50-100 mg in 1% solution at rate of 10 mg/5 seconds	Ampoules of various sizes to be made into 10% solution (10 mg/cc)

TABLE 36. *General Depressants of the* CNS: *Sedatives and Hypnotics* * (continued)

GROUP	GENERIC NAME (TRADE NAME-MANUFACTURER)	STRUCTURAL FORMULA	TYPICAL DOSE RANGE FOR ADULTS	HOW SUPPLIED
Barbiturates	Pentobarbital (*Nembutal*-Abbott) Also available in generic form.		Sedative: 20-30 mg, 3-4 times a day Hypnotic: 100-200 mg	Elixir: 4 mg/cc Suppositories: 30 mg, 60 mg, 120 mg, 200 mg Injection: 50 mg/cc 30 mg 50 mg 100 mg NEMBUTAL
	Phenobarbital (*Eskaphen*-SKF) (*Eskabarb*-SKF) (*Luminal*-Winthrop) Also available in generic form.		Sedative: 15-30 mg, 2-3 times a day	Elixir (Eskaphen): 3.2 mg/cc Injection: Ampoules of 130 mg, 160 mg, 320 mg 15 mg 60 mg H74 (1 dot) 16 mg J20 100 mg H76 (2 dots) † ESKAPHEN B ESKABARB SRF † 32 mg 100 mg LUMINAL
	Secobarbital (*Seconal*-Lilly) Also available in generic form.		Hypnotic: 100-200 mg	Elixir: 0.4 mg/cc Suppositories: 30 mg, 60 mg, 120 mg, 200 mg Injection: 50 mg/cc 30 mg 50 mg 100 mg SECONAL SODIUM
	Talbutal (*Lotusate*-Winthrop)		Sedative: 30-50 mg, 2-3 times a day Hypnotic: 120-240 mg	30 mg 50 mg 120 mg LOTUSATE

TABLE 36. *General Depressants of the* CNS: *Sedatives and Hypnotics* * (continued)

GROUP	GENERIC NAME (TRADE NAME-MANUFACTURER)	STRUCTURAL FORMULA	TYPICAL DOSE RANGE FOR ADULTS	HOW SUPPLIED
Nonbarbiturates	Ethchlorvynol (*Placidyl*-Abbott)	$CH_3CH_2\underset{OH}{\underset{|}{C}}-CH=CHCl$ with $C\equiv CH$	Sedative: 100-200 mg, 2-3 times a day Hypnotic: 0.5-1.0 gm	100 mg, 200 mg, 500 mg — PLACIDYL
	Ethinamate (*Valmid*-Lilly)	cyclohexane with $O\cdot CO\cdot NH_2$ and $C\equiv CH$	Hypnotic: 0.5-1.0 gm	500 mg VALMID
	Glutethimide (*Doriden*-Ciba)	C_6H_5 phenyl glutarimide structure with N–H	Hypnotic: 0.5-1.0 gm	125 mg, 250 mg, 500 mg — DORIDEN
	Methyprylon (*Noludar*-Roche)	CH_3, C_2H_5 piperidinedione structure with N–H	Hypnotic: 200-400 mg	50 mg, 200 mg, 300 mg — NOLUDAR
	Chloral hydrate (*Felsules*-Fellows) (*Rectules*-Fellows) (*Noctec*-Squibb) (*Somnos*-Merck) Also available in generic form.	$Cl_3C\cdot\underset{OH}{\underset{|}{C}}H\cdot OH$	Hypnotic: 1-2 gm	Syrup (Noctec): 100 mg/cc Suppositories (Rectules): 650 mg, 1300 mg 250 mg #623, 500 mg #626 — NOCTEC 250 mg, 500 mg SQUIBB — FELSULES

TABLE 36. *General Depressants of the* CNS: *Sedatives and Hypnotics* * (continued)

GROUP	GENERIC NAME (TRADE NAME-MANUFACTURER)	STRUCTURAL FORMULA	TYPICAL DOSE RANGE FOR ADULTS	HOW SUPPLIED
Nonbarbiturates	Paraldehyde Available in generic form.		Hypnotic: 3-8 gm	Usually dispensed as 1 gm/cc pure liquid; also available as capsules, ampoules, and rectal suppositories
	Methaqualone (*Quāalude*-Rorer)		Hypnotic: 150-300 mg	

* MOST COMMON ADVERSE EFFECTS :

Drowsiness, lethargy, slurred speech, paradoxical excitement, ataxia, physical dependence, compulsive use.

† SRF = SUSTAINED RELEASE FORM.

TABLE 37. Antidepressants *

GROUP	GENERIC NAME (TRADE NAME-MANUFACTURER)	STRUCTURAL FORMULA	TYPICAL DAILY DOSE RANGE FOR ADULTS WITH DEPRESSIVE DISORDERS	HOW SUPPLIED
Dibenzazepines	Amitriptyline (*Elavil*-Merck)		100-300 mg	Injection: 10 mg/cc — 10 mg, 25 mg, 50 mg ELAVIL
	Desipramine (*Norpramin*-Lakeside) (*Pertofrane*-Geigy)		100-300 mg	25 mg, 50 mg NORPRAMIN — 10 mg, 25 mg, 50 mg PERTOFRANE
	Doxepin (*Sinequan*-Pfizer)		75-150 mg	10 mg, 25 mg, 50 mg SINEQUAN
	Imipramine (*Tofranil*-Geigy)		100-300 mg	Injection: 12.5 mg/cc — 10 mg, 25 mg, 50 mg TOFRANIL
	Nortriptyline (*Aventyl*-Lilly)		20-100 mg	Liquid: 2 mg/cc — 10 mg, 25 mg AVENTYL
	Protriptyline (*Vivactil*-Merck)		20-60 mg	5 mg, 10 mg VIVACTIL

TABLE 37. *Antidepressants* *   (continued)

GROUP	GENERIC NAME (TRADE NAME-MANUFACTURER)	STRUCTURAL FORMULA	TYPICAL DAILY DOSE RANGE FOR ADULTS WITH DEPRESSIVE DISORDERS	HOW SUPPLIED
Monoamine Oxidase Inhibitors	Isocarboxazid (*Marplan*-Roche)		20-40 mg	10 mg MARPLAN
	Nialamide (*Niamid*-Pfizer)		50-200 mg	25 mg / 100 mg NIAMID
	Phenelzine (*Nardil*-Warner)		20-60 mg	15 mg NARDIL
	Tranylcypromine (*Parnate*-SKF)		20-40 mg	10 mg PARNATE
Lithium	Lithium Carbonate (*Eskalith*-SKF) (*Lithonate*-Rowell) (*Lithane*-Roerig)		900-1,500 mg	300 mg ESKALITH / 300 mg LITHONATE / 300 mg LITHANE

* MOST COMMON ADVERSE EFFECTS OF

Dibenzazepines: orthostatic hypotension, syncope, dry mouth, nose and throat, urinary retention, blurred vision, increased intraocular tension, constipation, nausea, drowsiness, weakness, dizziness, weight gain, sweating, ataxia, overstimulation, hypomania, mania, tremors, hyperreflexia, impotence, delayed ejaculation, headache, confusion.

Monoamine Oxidase Inhibitors: orthostatic hypotension, syncope, drowsiness, weakness, dizziness, sweating, dry mouth, nose and throat, constipation, peripheral edema, suppression of anginal pain, overstimulation, hypomania, mania, tremors, hyperreflexia, headache, confusion, insomnia, impotence, delayed ejaculation, hypertensive crises (especially after eating tyramine-containing foods like aged cheeses and the administration of certain drugs).

TABLE 38. *Stimulants* *

GENERIC NAME (TRADE NAME-MANUFACTURER)	STRUCTURAL FORMULA	TYPICAL DAILY DOSE RANGE ‡	HOW SUPPLIED
Amphetamine (*Benzedrine*-SKF) Also available in generic form.	$CH_2-CH-NH_2 \cdot H_2SO_4$ CH_3	10-30 mg	A91 5 mg; A92 10 mg BENZEDRINE; A90 15 mg SRF †
Dextroamphetamine (*Dexedrine*-SKF) Also available in generic form.	CH_3 CH_2CH $\frac{1}{2}H_2SO_4$ NH_2	5-15 mg	Elixir: 1 mg/cc. E19 5 mg; E12 5 mg (no dots); DEXEDRINE; E13 10 mg (1 dot) SRF †; E14 15 mg (2 dots) SRF †
Methamphetamine (*Methedrine*-Burroughs) (*Desoxyn*-Abbott) Also available in generic form.	$CH_2-CH-NH-CH_3 \cdot HCl$ CH_3	7.5-22.5 mg	Elixir: 0.66 mg/cc. Injection: 20 mg/cc. 5 mg METHEDRINE; 2.5 mg SRF †; 5 mg; 10 mg SRF † DESOXYN; 15 mg SRF †
Methylphenidate (*Ritalin*-Ciba)	$CHCOOCH_3 \cdot HCl$ N H	20-40 mg	Injection: 10 mg/cc. 5 mg; 10 mg RITALIN; 20 mg

* MOST COMMON ADVERSE EFFECTS:

Overstimulation, restlessness, insomnia, diarrhea, tremor, sweating, palpitations, tachycardia, elevated blood pressure, headache, psychologic dependence.

‡ In mild depressions, hyperkinetic syndromes of childhood, and drowsiness induced by tranquilizers or anticonvulsants. Dose ranges in narcolepsy are 2-3 times higher.

† SRF = SUSTAINED RELEASE FORM.

TABLE 39. *Anticonvulsants* *

GROUP	GENERIC NAME (TRADE NAME-MANUFACTURER)	STRUCTURAL FORMULA	AVERAGE EFFECTIVE DOSE — CHILDREN	AVERAGE EFFECTIVE DOSE — ADULTS	HOW SUPPLIED
Hydantoin derivatives	Ethotoin (*Peganone-* Abbott)	*(structural formula)*	500 mg, twice a day	500 mg, 3 or 4 times a day	250 mg, 500 mg PEGANONE
Hydantoin derivatives	Mephenytoin (*Mesantoin-* Sandoz)	*(structural formula)*	100 mg, 2 or 3 times a day	100-200 mg, 2 or 3 times a day	100 mg MESANTOIN
Hydantoin derivatives	Diphenyl-hydantoin (*Dilantin-* Parke-Davis) Also available in generic form.	*(structural formula)*	50-100 mg, 2 or 3 times a day	100-200 mg, 2 times a day	50 mg P-D 007; 30 mg P-D 365; 100 mg P-D 362; 100 mg P-D 385 SRF † DILANTIN. Injection: 50 mg/cc
Oxazolidine derivatives	Paramethadione (*Paradione-* Abbott)	*(structural formula)*	150-300 mg, 2 times a day	300 mg, 3 times a day	150 mg, 300 mg PARADIONE. Solution: 300 mg/cc
Oxazolidine derivatives	Trimethadione (*Tridione-Abbott*)	*(structural formula)*	300 mg, 2 times a day	300 mg, 3 times a day	150 mg, 300 mg TRIDIONE. Solution: 40 mg/cc

TABLE 39. *Anticonvulsants* * (continued)

GROUP	GENERIC NAME (TRADE NAME-MANUFACTURER)	STRUCTURAL FORMULA	AVERAGE EFFECTIVE DOSE		HOW SUPPLIED
			CHILDREN	ADULTS	
Acetylureas	Phenacemide (*Phenurone*-Abbott)		250 mg, 2 or 3 times a day	250-500 mg, 3 times a day	 500 mg PHENURONE
Succinimide derivatives	Ethosuximide (*Zarontin*-Parke-Davis)		250 mg, 2 times a day	250 mg, 3 or 4 times a day	 250 mg P-D 237 ZARONTIN
	Methsuximide (*Celontin*-Parke-Davis)		300 mg, 2 times a day	300 mg, 3 or 4 times a day	 300 mg P-D 525 150 mg P-D 537 CELONTIN
	Phensuximide (*Milontin*-Parke-Davis)		250-500 mg, 3 times a day	500-1,000 mg, 3 times a day	 500 mg P-D 393 250 mg P-D 399 MILONTIN Suspension: 60 mg/cc

TABLE 39. *Anticonvulsants* * (continued)

GROUP	GENERIC NAME (TRADE NAME-MANUFACTURER)	STRUCTURAL FORMULA	AVERAGE EFFECTIVE DOSE		HOW SUPPLIED
			CHILDREN	ADULTS	
Barbiturates	Metharbital (*Gemonil*-Abbott)		50-100 mg, 2 or 3 times a day	100-200 mg, 2 to 4 times a day	100 mg GEMONIL
	Mephobarbital (*Mebaral*-Winthrop) Also available in generic form.		32-100 mg, 2 or 3 times a day	Anticonvulsant: 100-200 mg, 2 to 4 times a day Sedative: 32-100 mg, 3 or 4 times a day	32 mg 50 mg 100 mg 200 mg MEBARAL
	Phenobarbital (*Eskaphen*-SKF) (*Eskabarb*-SKF) (*Luminal*-Winthrop) Also available in generic form.		16-32 mg, 3 or 4 times a day	32-100 mg, 3 or 4 times a day	Tablets: 16 mg, 32 mg, 100 mg Elixir (Eskaphen): 3.2 mg/cc Injection: Ampoules of 130 mg, 160 mg, 320 mg 16 mg J20 ESKAPHEN B 60 mg H74 (1 dot) 100 mg H76 (2 dots) ESKABARB SRF†

TABLE 39. *Anticonvulsants* * (continued)

GROUP	GENERIC NAME (TRADE NAME-MANUFACTURER)	STRUCTURAL FORMULA	AVERAGE EFFECTIVE DOSE		HOW SUPPLIED
			CHILDREN	ADULTS	
Barbiturate congener	Primidone (*Mysoline*-Ayerst)		125 mg, 2 or 3 times a day	250-500 mg, 2 or 3 times a day	Suspension: 50 mg/cc 50 mg 250 mg MYSOLINE
Adjuvants	Acetazolamide (*Diamox*-Lederle)		250 mg, 3 or 4 times a day	250-375 mg, 3 or 4 times a day	Tablet: 125 mg Injection: 500 mg vials 250 mg 500 mg SRF † DIAMOX

* MOST COMMON ADVERSE EFFECTS OF

Hydantoin Derivatives: rash, fever, gum hypertrophy, gastric distress, diplopia, ataxia, hirsutism (young females), drowsiness, megaloblastic anemia (due to secondary folic acid deficiency), lymphadenopathy, neutropenia, agranulocytosis.

Oxazolidine Derivatives: rash, gastric distress, visual symptoms (glare, photophobia), neutropenia, agranulocytosis, nephrosis.

Acetylureas: highly toxic: liver damage, agranulocytosis, organic brain syndrome, rash.

Succinimide Derivatives: dermatitis, anorexia, nausea, drowsiness, dizziness, ataxia, hematuria (may be nephrotoxic), blood dyscrasias unusual (pancytopenia, leukopenia).

Barbiturates: drowsiness, gastrointestinal upset, paradoxical excitement, hangover, ataxia, vertigo, respiratory depression, withdrawal symptoms, compulsive use.

Acetazolamide: anorexia, acidosis, drowsiness, numbness of extremities, blood dyscrasias (rare).

† SRF = SUSTAINED RELEASE FORM.

TABLE 40. *Antiparkinsonian Agents* *

GROUP	GENERIC NAME (TRADE NAME- MANUFACTURER)	STRUCTURAL FORMULA	TYPICAL INDIVIDUAL DOSE FOR ADULTS †	HOW SUPPLIED
Atropine-like agents	Benztropine (*Cogentin*-Merck)	CH$_2$—CH$_2$—CH$_2$—N—CH$_2$—CH$_2$—O—CH$_2$—CH$_2$—CH$_2$ · CH$_3$SO$_3$H	1-2 mg	Injection: 0.5 mg/cc 0.5 mg 1 mg 2 mg COGENTIN
	Biperiden (*Akineton*-Knoll)		1-2 mg	Injection: 5 mg/cc 2 mg AKINETON
	Cycrimine (*Pagitane*-Lilly)	· HCl	1.25-2.5 mg	1.25 mg PAGITANE 2.5 mg
	Procyclidine (*Kemadrin*-Burroughs)	· HCl ·	2.5-5 mg	5 mg KEMADRIN
	Trihexyphenidyl (*Artane*-Lederle) (*Tremin*-Schering)	· HCl	2.5-5 mg	Elixir: 0.4 mg/cc 2 mg TREMIN 5 mg 5 mg SRF† ARTANE

TABLE 40. *Antiparkinsonian Agents* * (continued)

GROUP	GENERIC NAME (TRADE NAME-MANUFACTURER)	STRUCTURAL FORMULA	TYPICAL INDIVIDUAL DOSE FOR ADULTS ‡	HOW SUPPLIED
Antihistamines	Diphenhydramine (*Benadryl*-Parke-Davis) Also available in generic form.		25-50 mg, 50 mg i.v.	Elixir: 3 mg/cc Injection: 10 mg/cc, 50 mg/cc 25 mg P-D 471 50 mg P-D 373 BENADRYL
	Orphenadrine (*Disipal*-Riker)		50-100 mg	50 mg DISIPAL

* MOST COMMON ADVERSE EFFECTS OF

Atropine-like agents: dry mouth, nose and throat, blurred vision, diplopia, increased intraocular tension, urinary retention, constipation, gastric irritation, vomiting, nausea, tachycardia, palpitation, hypotension, muscular weakness, euphoria, confusion.

Antihistamines: drowsiness, confusion, nervousness, restlessness, nausea, diarrhea, blurring of vision, diplopia, difficulty in urination, constipation, nasal stuffiness, headache.

† SRF = SUSTAINED RELEASE FORM.

‡ Frequency usually same as that of tranquilizer with which taken.

TABLE 41. *Agents Used in the Treatment of Drug Addiction and Abuse* *

GENERIC NAME (TRADE NAME-MANUFACTURER)	STRUCTURAL FORMULA	TYPICAL DOSE RANGE FOR ADULTS	HOW SUPPLIED
Methadone (*Dolophine*-Lilly)	$(C_6H_5)_2C-CO-C_2H_5$ $CH_2-CH-N(CH_3)_2 \cdot HCl$ CH_3	In confirmed narcotic addicts, 60-100 mg daily is said to "block" effects of other opiates and opioids and thus to enable user to abstain from illegally obtained narcotics	Syrup: 0.33 mg/cc Injection: 10 mg/cc 5 mg 10 mg DOLOPHINE
Levallorphan (*Lorfan*-Roche)	[structural formula] $N-CH_2CH=CH_2$ HO COOH HCOH HOCH COOH	0.5 mg i.v. with additional doses at 3-minute intervals if necessary will usually produce an abstinence syndrome in the narcotics addict or reverse symptoms of narcotics overdosage	Injection: 0.05 mg/cc, 1 mg/cc
Nalorphine (*Nalline*-Merck)	[structural formula] $\cdot HCl$ HO O HO NCH₂CH=CH₂	5-10 mg i.v. with 1-2 additional doses if necessary of 5 mg at 10-15 minute intervals will usually produce an abstinence syndrome in the narcotics addict or reverse symptoms of narcotics overdosage	Injection: 0.2 mg/cc
Disulfiram (*Antabuse*-Ayerst)	C_2H_5 S S C_2H_5 NC—SS—CN C_2H_5 C_2H_5	The individual who takes 250-500 mg daily will usually experience severe discomfort upon ingesting alcohol and may thus be dissuaded from drinking	500 mg ANTABUSE

* MOST COMMON ADVERSE EFFECTS OF

Methadone: nausea, vomiting, dry mouth, dizziness, physical dependence, compulsive use.

Levallorphan: anxiety, visual hallucinations, blurred vision, sweating, nausea, drowsiness.

Disulfiram: confusional psychosis, acneform eruptions, garlic-like or metallic taste in mouth, discoloration of tongue, gastrointestinal dis-

TABLE 42. *Combined Ingestion of* MAO *Inhibitors and Other Pharmacologic Agents*

MAO INHIBITOR		OTHER MEDICATION INGESTED		SYMPTOMS
Type	*Amount*	*Type*	*Amount*	
Tranylcypromine	10 mg t.i.d.	Amobarbital	250 mg	Ataxia, semicoma, vomiting, recent memory loss—3 days, hypotension, survived (Domino 1962).
Tranylcypromine *	175 mg	Imipramine	275 mg	Coma, decerebrate rigidity, fixed dilated pupils, myoclonic seizures, hyperpyrexia, hyperreflexia, bilateral Babinski, recent memory loss—10 days, survived (Luby 1961).
Phenelzine	Unknown	Imipramine	625 mg	Coma, hyperpyrexia (109°), dilated fixed pupils, decerebrate rigidity, bilateral Babinski, died (Lee 1961).
Phenelzine	180 mg	Amitriptyline	800 mg	Urinary retention, bilateral Babinski, somnolence, hypertension and hypotension, survived (Jarecki 1963).

*Patient had been receiving tranylcypromine, 25 mg, t.i.d., until one week prior to admission and imipramine, 25 mg, q.i.d., for one week prior to admission.

TABLE 43. *Forrest tests for Color Readings of Psychoactive Drugs in Urine*

DRUG	TEST SOLUTION	PERFORMANCE OF TEST	RESULTING TEST COLORS					BIBLIOGRAPHY
① Chlorpromazine (*Thorazine*)	20 parts 5% Ferric chloride 80 parts 10% Sulfuric acid	Mix 1 ml urine with 1 ml test solution. Read within 20 seconds	Daily Dose mg	+ 100-300	++ 300-600	+++ 600-900	++++ 900 & over	Forrest, F. M., and Forrest, I. S.: Amer J Psychiat *113*:931, 1957. Forrest, F. M., Forrest, I. S., and Mason, A. S.: *Ibid. 114*:931, 1958.
② Promazine (*Sparine*) and Mepazine (*Pacatal*)	Same as above	Same as above	Daily Dose mg	+ 100-300	++ 300-600	+++ 600-900	++++ 900 & over	*Ibid.*
③ Thioridazine (*Mellaril*)	2 parts 5% Ferric chloride 98 parts 30% Sulfuric acid	Mix 1 ml urine with 1 ml test solution. Read within 30 seconds	Daily Dose mg	+ 75-150	++ 150-450	+++ 450-800	++++ 800 & over	Forrest, I. S., Forrest, F. M., and Mason, A. S.: Amer J Psychiat *116*:928, 1960.
④ Imipramine (*Tofranil*)	25 parts 0.2% Potassium dichromate 25 parts 30% Sulfuric acid 25 parts 20% Perchloric acid 25 parts 50% Nitric acid	Mix 0.5 ml urine with 1 ml test solution. Read within 20 seconds	Daily Dose mg	+ 25-50	++ 50-75	+++ 75-150	++++ 150-250	Forrest, I. S., and Forrest, F. M.: *Ibid.*, p. 840. Forrest, I. S., Forrest, F. M., and Mason, A. S.: *Ibid.*, p. 1021.

TABLE 43. Continued: *Forrest tests for Color Readings of Psychoactive Drugs in Urine*

DRUG	TEST SOLUTION	PERFORMANCE OF TEST	RESULTING TEST COLORS			BIBLIOGRAPHY
⑤ Most phenothi-azines Vesprin Prolixin Trilafon Compazine Stelazine Dartal Tindal Mellaril Pacatal Phenergan Sparine Thorazine etc.	FPN—Universal Test * 5 parts 5% Ferric chloride 45 parts 20% Perchloric acid 50 parts 50% Nitric acid	Mix 1 ml urine with 1 ml test solution Read immediately Disregard all colors appearing after delay of 10 seconds or more	Daily Dose mg 1+ 20-70 4+ 200-400 mg	2+ 70-120 5+ 400-800	3+ 120-200 6+ 800-2000	Forrest, I. S., and Forrest, F. M.: Clin Chem *6*:11, 1960, and *Ibid.*, p. 362.

* For specific directions, see p. 576.

Reprinted with permission from the Amer J Psychiat *118*:300-307, 1961.

SPECIFIC DIRECTIONS FOR UNIVERSAL TEST ⑤

For best results the following should be kept in mind: Because of its sensitivity, it allows detection of small amounts of drug in urine. The colors resulting from the mixture of urine and reagent, as represented in the chart, are compromise colors. Individual phenothiazine drugs, especially in the high dosage ranges (four to six plus), may deviate somewhat towards bluer shades (Thorazine, Mellaril) or towards more reddish tones (Vesprin, Sparine, Pacatal). 2-methoxy-substituted drugs (Veractil or Tentone) do not conform well to the colors of the chart, showing distinctly bluish-green shades. The compromise colors of the chart for test ⑤ were selected to allow demonstration of the various drugs listed, either singly or in combinations, by means of a single reagent. Hospitals or physicians in private practice without a laboratory furnishing the individual test reagents yielding optimal colors for each individual drug, might also prefer a single test solution permitting detection of most phenothiazine drugs.

To avoid *false negatives:* Use concentrated early morning urine specimens, or, when testing for the minimal dosage drugs (Prolixin, Stelazine, Permitil), use urines obtained 1½ to 3 hours after drug administration. During this optimum excretion period, drug levels of 5 to 10 mg per day will conform to the one plus intensity of the chart, in continuous drug administration. In single dose administration the color intensity produced by less than 10 mg of drug will appear somewhat lighter than the one plus level, but readily distinguishable from the urine specimen as such.

To avoid *false positives:* As a rule, these are limited to the lowest level of the color chart. They most frequently are seen at impaired liver function or as a result of drug therapy with conjugated estrogens or paraaminosalicylic acid. Some normal and abnormal catabolic compounds also give rise to color development ranging from pink to brown, olive and grey. Most of these interfering colors appear with a delay of 10 seconds or more. Hence, color development *after 10 seconds should be disregarded.* Most phenothiazine colors appear immediately, and all within 10 seconds. Therefore, it is imperative that the tests be evaluated *immediately.* For some of the factors causing interfering color development see Clinical Chemistry 6, 362 (1960). Note that the urine of phenylketonuric patients may yield low level false positives. On the other hand, color reactions of phenothiazine drugs in the urine of phenylketonurics appear with some delay. Interfering color reactions, including those due to intense urine color and indican, may be eliminated or substantially reduced by the following pretreatment of the urine specimens: Add 100 mg of Dowex AG 3-X4, Analytical Grade Anion Exchange Resin, Chloride Form, 200-400 mesh, (obtainable from California Corp. for Biochemical Research, 3625 Medford Street, Los Angeles 63, Calif.), to 3 ml of mildly acid or acidified urine in a test tube, shake vigorously for 30 to 60 seconds and filter. Use the clear, light colored filtrate for the test, exactly as an untreated urine. This selective adsorption eliminates some undesirable endogenous urinary constituents or e.g. aspirin. Some of the unspecific darkening and brownish color development seen in tests performed with highly concentrated urines is also avoided by this procedure, and the resulting test colors are clearer and more closely conforming to those of the chart.

The same procedure is applicable to test ③ for Mellaril, but unnecessary in tests ① and ② for Thorazine, Sparine and Pacatal and in test ④ for Tofranil, since no false positives have been reported for these tests.

most common offenders are the aliphatic phenothiazines, chlorpromazine (Thorazine) and promazine (Sparine) (Hollister 1960, Huguley 1966, McKinney 1967, Shawver 1960, Shelton 1960). The incidence of chlorpromazine-induced agranulocytosis is difficult to ascertain. In one series, weekly leukocyte counts during the first three months of treatment with phenothiazines led to the identification of only five patients with agranulocytosis out of 28,000 white counts in six years (Pisciotta 1968).

While not strictly dose-related, agranulocytosis is exceedingly rare unless the patient has been taking at least 150 mg of chlorpromazine daily for a period of 10 days (Pisciotta 1969). It is more common in women than in men, in whites than in blacks, in the elderly than in the young, and in the debilitated or physically ill than in the physically healthy (Beutler 1965, Mandel 1968). Almost all drug-induced blood dyscrasias develop within the first three months; most indeed during the sixth to eighth week. The *onset* of agranulocytosis is usually very rapid. Within days of apparent good health, the patient's white count falls to less than 500 with 2% polymorphonuclear leukocytes, and he develops extreme weakness, high fever, chills, and a sore throat. Within 5 days, no neutrophils can be found in the peripheral blood and bone marrow, and signs of bacterial invasion such as septicemia or ulcerations of the mouth, rectum, and vagina are likely to be in evidence (Pisciotta 1968). The development of agranulocytosis is the gravest adverse effect encountered with psychotropic agents. The *outcome* depends on the rapidity with which the diagnosis is made and the drug is discontinued. If this occurs promptly, the agranulocytosis usually remits spontaneously and recovery occurs within five to 10 days. If, however, massive bacterial invasion has set in, there is a 20% to 50% fatality risk (Erslev 1962, Huguley 1964).

Treatment should be directed by the hematologist and includes isolation, scrupulous oral hygiene, and antibiotics when necessary. Once the patient has had agranulocytosis, he must permanently avoid using the drug in question and, given the gravity of the dangers, should probably avoid all phenothiazines, tricyclic agents, or diphenylmethane derivatives (d'Anglejan 1965, Pisciotta 1965a,b, Rosenthal 1967).

Whether regular blood tests are an efficient *preventive measure* in patients taking phenothiazines is a subject of controversy. Considering that the overwhelming majority of cases occur in the first six to 12 weeks, that the full-blown picture of agranulocytosis develops over a period of three to five days, and that the rapidity with which the drug is stopped is directly proportional to the likelihood of recovery, it is our practice to obtain a CBC prior to treatment and at weekly intervals thereafter for the first three months, monthly for the next six months, and at intervals of three months thereafter.

SKIN REACTIONS. Hypersensitivity reactions of the skin are either *systemic* or *topical*. The systemic reactions may be a direct consequence of drug use or an indirect one (in the sense that the drug causes an increased sensitivity to sunlight and the skin reaction occurs only when the individual is exposed to the sun). Systemic reactions include *urticaria, maculopapular rashes, petechiae,* or *edema*. The most common offenders are chlorpromazine (reported to cause a skin reaction in one of every 20 persons who use it), followed by triflupromazine, trifluoperazine, and thioridazine. The symptoms usually develop during the first to fifth week of drug use (earlier if the patient has previously been sensitized), clear up after discontinuation of the drug, and sometimes do not recur even if the drug is taken again. If the reaction is severe, another drug must be substituted. In milder cases, an antihistamine like diphenhydramine (Benadryl), 25 mg tid, should be given and, if the patient has edema, a diuretic may be tried (Wagensommer 1964). *Contact dermatitis,* manifested by itching, burning, erythema, vesiculation, and edema, followed by weeping and crusting, occurs in individuals, like nurses or pharmacists, who must handle these drugs, particularly chlorpromazine. By avoiding contact with the drug, one's lesions heal rapidly, but chronic exposure may lead to lichenification.

Drug-induced photosensitivity is manifested either as photoxicity characterized by abnormal tanning, exaggerated sunburn, or even acute bullous erythema; or photoallergy characterized by an eczematous lesion. The most common offenders are chlorpromazine, prochlorperazine, promazine, promethazine, and trifluoperazine. Treatment consists of discontinuing the drug, but if this seems clinically inadvisable, exposure to the sun should be minimized either by staying indoors or by covering the exposed portions of the skin with red veterinary petrolatum or Uval, a benzophenone lotion that increases the minimal erythema dose 120-fold (Knox 1963, Korenyi 1969).

TOXIC EFFECTS

EFFECTS ON THE CENTRAL NERVOUS SYSTEM. *Drowsiness.* As stated earlier, the degree to which a given phenothiazine produces drowsiness, both in the initial phase of treatment and after some weeks of use, is inversely related to its therapeutic potency (Table 33). Most patients given enough thioridazine (Mellaril) or chlorpromazine (Thorazine) to calm them down feel sluggish, unmotivated, somnolent, and "drugged," at least for the first few weeks, and indefinitely on high doses. Even when the patient appears to have become tolerant to the hypnotic effect, he may from time to time yawn, feel drowsy, or take a nap during the day. Similar effects can occur with more potent phenothiazines, such as triflupromazine (Vesprin), acetophenazine (Tindal), and fluphenazine (Prolixin), but are milder and usually subside after a week or ten days of use. Indeed the sluggishness and anergia experienced by patients on alerting phenothiazines is often caused not by drowsiness but by extrapyramidal hypokinesia, which responds well to an anti-parkinsonian agent. If for any reason phenothiazines are discontinued for a few days, the patient may experience a great sense of relief and increased energy, report that he feels better rather than worse, and ignore the physician's warning that the newly gained comfort may not be lasting.

Whether and to what extent these symptoms can be averted by using alerting phenothiazines or by giving a small dose of amphetamine (2.5 mg p.o. at morning and noon) is an open question. In any event, the physician should try to determine the dosage or drug combination that produces the least possible amount of anergia or drowsiness. This may require a reduction in the dose or, if this is not tolerated, a change to a different phenothiazine or even to a different class of major tranquilizer.

Extrapyramidal Effects. Drug-induced extrapyramidal symptoms fall into one of three basic categories: dystonia (generally occurring sometime between the first hour and fifth day after the drug is first used or the dosage is increased), akathisia (which usually occurs sometime between the fifth and fourteenth day), and pseudoparkinsonism (which usually takes three weeks or more to develop fully). *Dystonia* is manifested by sudden, intermittent, but often persistent spasms of individual muscle groups, particularly those of the head, neck, lips, and tongue. The most common symptoms are torticollis, retrocollis, opisthothonus, oculogyric crisis (fixed forward stare followed by upward and lateral rotation of the eyes with impairment of vision), trismus (sometimes severe enough to cause dislocation of the mandible or damage and even fracture of teeth), dyslalia (slurred speech often aggravated by the protrusion of the tongue), dysphagia (difficulty and pain in swallowing), and laryngospasm, in some cases so severe as to cause acute, life-threatening respiratory distress (Ayd 1961, Christian 1958, Waugh 1960). Generalized or localized pain in the joints and muscles is a common by-product of all dystonias. *Akathisia*, literally the inability to sit down, is characterized by constant pacing and moving of the hands or feet. When standing, the akathisic patient may continually rock back and forth, shifting his weight from one foot to the other; seated, he may keep swinging his legs beneath him until, unable to tolerate what he describes as a creeping sensation relieved only by moving about, he gets up to pace once again. *Pseudoparkinsonism* includes diminished drive, lassitude, hypokinesia, micrographia, and muscular rigidity manifested by a mask-like facial expression, a monotonous and expressionless voice, and a characteristic *marche à petit pas* or festinant (shuffling) gait. As in true parkinsonism, the patient may exhibit pill-rolling movements of the hands, a waxy skin, and excessive salivation. All drug-induced extrapyramidal disorders (especially akathisia and pseudoparkinsonism) are accompanied by some degree of coarse rhythmic *tremor*.

All phenothiazines and all other major tranquilizers produce one or another of these effects when given in high enough doses, but the *incidence* varies with the drug, dose, and route of administration and with the patient's sex and age. The most common extrapyramidal effect is hypokinesia, which, even if it is not obvious on superficial observation, is found in all patients taking phenothiazines (Bishop 1965, Haase 1965). Akathisia occurs in 21%, pseudoparkinsonism in 15%, and dystonia in 2% of patients taking therapeutic doses of chlorpromazine (Ayd 1961). As a rule, the less potent the phenothiazine, the more likely it is to produce pseudoparkinsonism; the more potent the drug, the larger the initial dose, and the more rapidly it is increased, the more likely the patient is to develop dystonia and akathisia. Both intravenous and intramuscular administration therefore tend to increase their incidence. Intramuscular fluphenazine enanthate in doses of 15 to 20 mg, for example, causes extrapyramidal symptoms (primarily akathisia) in 60% of all patients using it, unless it is initiated in gradually increasing doses (Cole 1969). Men develop dystonias twice as often and akathisia and pseudoparkinsonism only half as often as women. As in other extrapyramidal disorders, the symptoms depend in part on the patient's age. Children and young adults are most likely to develop dystonias, middle-aged people akathisia, and older people pseudoparkinsonism. All drug-induced extrapyramidal symptoms are more common in children, young adults, the aged, and the brain-damaged than in physically healthy, middle-aged adults (Cohlan 1960, Kurland 1966, Shaw 1960, Siede 1967, Simpson 1964). Drug-induced dystonias occur frequently in patients with hypoparathyroidism (Schaaf 1966). There is also a familial predisposition to such symptoms, as they are particularly common in families with a high incidence of idiopathic parkinsonism (Freedman 1961, Myrianthopoulos 1962).

An appreciation of the *differential diagnosis* is important, because extrapyramidal symptoms come in so many disguises that they are not always recognized. Dystonia and akathisia may be mistaken for *conversion hysteria* both because they can be controlled voluntarily to some extent and because they may diminish temporarily in response to a forceful command or placebo (Simpson 1970). They may also be confused with *encephalitis* and other acute CNS disorders, especially if the patient is disoriented as well (Hollister 1961a). The akathisic patient's pacing and complaints of restlessness may well suggest *anxiety* and *agitation*. The rigid, expressionless face seen in pseudoparkinsonism may be mistaken for *depression* and when dystonic symptoms are also present, for *catatonia*. Akathisia may also occur in individuals not taking major tranquilizers, as during the recovery phase of *alcoholic neuritis,* in *diabetic neuropathy,* or as part of a CNS *depressant withdrawal syndrome* (Callaghan 1966).

The *treatment* of extrapyramidal symptoms is much like that of parkinsonism. It entails the use of anticholinergics like benztropine mesylate (Cogentin), 1 to 2 mg, 3 to 4 times daily p.o., or trihexyphenidyl (Artane, Tremin), 2 to 5 mg, 3 to 4 times daily p.o. (see Table 40 for other drugs and doses). If a rapid effect is desirable, either because the patient is acutely uncomfortable or the diagnosis is in doubt, however, intravenous administration of 50 mg of diphenhydramine (Benadryl) or 1 to 2 mg of benztropine mesylate (each diluted in 10 cc of saline) produces dramatic improvement in 10 to 15 minutes. The symptoms also subside fairly rapidly if the drug is discontinued. Dystonias generally subside without treatment within 24 hours following discontinuation of the drug and within 45 to 60 minutes with treatment; akathisia and pseudoparkinsonism four to five days without and within a day or two with. Because antiparkinsonian agents are effective in over 97% of cases (Sheppard 1967) even if the patient continues to take the offending agent, it is not generally necessary to discontinue the tranquilizer. Antiparkinsonian drugs can usually be decreased or discontinued after six or eight weeks, as many patients by that time have become tolerant to the extrapyramidal effects.

Among the antiparkinsonian drugs, milligram per milligram, benztropine mesylate is the most effective and possibly the longest acting. In the process of relieving extrapyramidal symptoms, however, the drug's strong anticholinergic properties cause certain side effects of their own (see p. 583), and these may become so severe that a different antiparkinsonian agent is indicated. Since drugs with a weaker anticholinergic effect usually have a weaker antiparkinsonian effect as well (Brumlik 1964), the alternative in the case of uncontrollable extrapyramidal symptoms is to substitute another phenothiazine that is less likely to produce parkinsonian symptoms. In rare instances, benztropine causes a toxic atropine-like psychosis with flushing, dry skin, and delirium, in which case, it must be discontinued and the symptoms will recede within four or five days.

Whether and to what extent it is feasible or advisable to prevent extrapyramidal symptoms by administering antiparkinsonian agents prophylactically is a subject of some controversy. Since extrapyramidal symptoms can be relieved easily, we prefer to avoid the routine use of antiparkinsonian agents, especially when the patient is an adult, in good physical health, ambulatory, and receiving only small to moderate doses of the tranquilizer. Instead, we give him a small supply of one of the antiparkinsonian drugs to keep at home in case of emergency and urge him to call immediately should such side effects develop. Prophylactic use of antiparkinsonian drugs is recommended, however, for the patient who is receiving phenothiazines in high or parenteral doses (especially fluphenazine enanthate). Prophylactic administration of antiparkinsonian drugs is also indicated for the very young, the aged, and the brain-damaged, all of whom have a greater susceptibility to the extrapyramidal symptoms and can become severely frightened if they develop dystonic effects.

Seizures. Phenothiazines have been shown to lower the convulsive threshold in animals and to produce both partial and grand mal seizures in humans. Such seizures generally occur within the first days or weeks of phenothiazine use or soon after an increase in the dose. They are most common in individuals with a prior history of seizures or some other CNS disorder (Logothetis 1967) and in chronic users of CNS depressants during the period of withdrawal. Their overall incidence is less than 1%, being highest with

promazine (Sparine), chlorpromazine (Thorazine), and thioridazine (Mellaril), and lowest with trifluoperazine (Stelazine) and
fluphenazine (Prolixin). The high incidence of seizures following
the use of promazine (Sparine), variously reported as between 6%
and 16% has been caused not by some special ictogenic property
of this drug but (for no good reason that we have been able to discover other than the manufacturer's advertising program) by its
rather frequent use in the management of alcohol withdrawal, a
syndrome in which there is a 4% incidence of seizures even without phenothiazine use (see p. 299). Phenothiazines are therefore
contraindicated in CNS depressant withdrawal syndromes unless, despite reintoxication with a CNS depressant, the patient continues to
be unmanageable, and then only in low doses and in combination
with a CNS depressant (see p. 301).

AUTONOMIC EFFECTS. The autonomic effects of phenothiazine
use include dry mouth and throat (20%), blurred vision (15%),
weakness (about 10%), orthostatic hypotension (up to 4%), and,
far less frequently, diarrhea, dizziness, urinary retention, nasal congestion, nausea, vomiting, and a disturbance in sexual functions.
Dryness of the mouth and throat is most frequent after chlorpromazine and thioridazine use, and in some instances may even be the
substrate of a monilia infection (Kane 1964, Pollack 1964). Visual
disturbances and constipation occur most frequently with the least
potent phenothiazines and are more common in older than in
younger patients. Impotence, frigidity, and decline of sexual interest are fairly rare consequences of phenothiazine use, occurring
primarily in middle-aged patients. Delayed ejaculation is also rare,
except after thioridazine use (Greenberg 1968, Taubel 1962, Zuckerman 1962), which has led to the suggestion that the drug be tried
in the treatment of premature ejaculation (see p. 266), but controlled studies are not available. Autonomic effects produced by
the phenothiazines are rarely severe enough to consider changing
the drug, unless the patient is also taking an antiparkinsonian drug
that produces similar effects and is thus exposed to the atropinizing
effect of the combination. Palliative measures are available, however,
and will usually suffice. Urinary retention or constipation can be
relieved with bethanechol (Urecholine), 2.5 to 5 mg s.c. or, if the
patient is meant to continue with the same drug regimen, 10 to
20 mg p.o., 3 to 4 times daily. Senna syrup and other mildly irritating or bulk-producing agents (such as Agar) may also be helpful
for constipation. Blurred vision and adaptational disturbances can

be managed by +½ to +1½ diopter glasses or clip-ons. Dryness of the mouth can be alleviated with hard candy or chewing gum, and one or two tablespoons of Coca-Cola syrup should be given to patients who feel nauseated.

CARDIOVASCULAR EFFECTS.   Phenothiazines seem to have both direct effects on the myocardium and blood vessels and indirect ones through actions on the CNS and the autonomic reflexes. Clinically, the most relevant of these effects are hypotension, ECG changes, and arrhythmias. *Hypotension* is more frequent and more severe following parenteral administration and with the less potent phenothiazines. Intramuscular injection of 20 to 50 mg of chlorpromazine, for example, may cause a 15% fall in systolic blood pressure, often with compensatory tachycardia (Foster 1954, Korol 1965). Though some degree of tolerance develops, so that after a period of a few weeks the drug's effects on supine blood pressure is negligible, orthostatic hypotension may persist indefinitely (Sletten 1965). ECG *changes,* such as blunting and notching of the T-wave with or without prolongation of the Q-T interval, occur in fewer than 1% of patients taking alerting or intermediate phenothiazines, but in as many as 2.5 to 3.5% of patients taking sedating phenothiazines, particularly thioridazine, even in doses as moderate as 300 mg daily (Ban 1965, Graupner 1964, Huston 1966, Kelly 1963). Ventricular *arrhythmias* have also been reported after large doses of thioridazine (Giles 1968) and are attributed to a direct toxic effect on the myocardium. ECG changes generally appear within the first week of treatment and are believed to represent a benign repolarization disturbance. Since such ECG findings may be mistaken for cardiovascular pathology, all patients who are over 40 or have a previous history of cardiac disease should have an ECG before being given phenothiazines.

Apart from the obvious hazards of hypotension in individuals with cardiovascular disease, blood pressure changes accompanied by faintness and lightheadedness may cause the patient to fall and injure himself when he gets up suddenly from a seated or recumbent position and attempts to walk down a staircase or across a busy street. Postural hypotension may be especially marked when the patient receives an antidepressant concomitantly. Especially during the first few weeks before tolerance to the hypotensive effect develops, therefore, the patient should be carefully instructed to arise slowly and to avoid going up or down stairs until he has been up and about for a few minutes.

ENDOCRINE EFFECTS. *Weight Gain.* One of the most striking, most troublesome, and least mentioned effects of phenothiazines is weight gain (Waitzkin 1966, 1969). Three to six weeks after the patient starts taking these drugs, he may develop an intense craving for sweets and, sometimes despite previously Spartan dietary habits, start to buy chocolates during the day and raid his icebox late at night. The weight gain may amount to 1 to 2 pounds per week for many months (Caffey 1961) and not taper off until it has reached 30 or 40 pounds. At the beginning it is usually restricted to the patient's abdomen, and may in time produce a bulge not unlike that of pregnancy. It is not known whether such weight gain results chiefly from increased appetite and food intake or represents other metabolic changes involving increased utilization of foodstuffs. Phenothiazine use has been shown to produce hyperglycemia and glycosuria, especially in obese patients over 50 years of age and in those with a family history of diabetes, polyuria, and polydipsia (Amdisen 1968, Schwarz 1968, Thonnard-Neumann 1968). It must be remembered, however, that substantial weight gains are extremely common in chronic schizophrenia and that acute schizophrenics tend to lose weight at the height of their illness and to gain much of it back during the recovery phase. Furthermore, if the patient is also taking a tricyclic antidepressant, it cannot be ascertained whether the phenothiazine, the antidepressant, or the combination is causing the weight gain, for such combinations appear to have an even greater effect on weight.

The weight gain will often have a profound effect on the patient's self-esteem and contribute to his social isolation, because of the way he feels about his looks and because of the way others react to his obesity. Not infrequently, the patient finds his impending or accomplished obesity so disturbing that he wants to stop taking the drug or asks for diet pills to keep his weight in check. The patient will indeed stop gaining weight once he stops taking the drug, but this is not always the ideal solution because his psychological well-being may well depend on continuing the drug, and even after he stops taking it, he may find it extremely difficult to return to his former weight. Rigid adherence to a low-calorie diet and, if this is impossible or ineffective, involvement with a group such as Weight Watchers or a change to a different tranquilizer may be indicated. Haloperidol (Haldol) should be considered in such cases, for this drug does not seem to stimulate appetite and may even have a mildly anorectic effect (see p. 592).

Effects on Menstruation and Lactation. With the exception of amenorrhea, drug-induced changes in menstruation or lactation are quite rare. They include menorrhagia, oligomenorrhea, gynecomastia in males (Hooper 1961, Klein 1964, Shader 1968, Sulman 1961, Zuckerman 1962), nonpuerperal galactorrhea, amenorrhea, and a combination of the latter two symptoms (Barnes 1966, Gold 1967). The clinical picture of the *galactorrhea-amenorrhea syndrome* is fairly characteristic. The patient reports that she has not had a menstrual period for a number of months and may complain of diminished libido, vaginal dryness, and dyspareunia. On physical examination, she is found to have well-developed breasts with good turgor and tonus. There is no loss of axillary or pubic hair. The vagina often looks atrophic and, in long-standing cases, even the external genitalia show signs of regression. The cervix and the uterus are usually small, and there is little if any mucus present in the cervix. Often the patient is unaware of the galactorrhea until milk is expressed from her breasts in the course of the physical examination. Urinary assay usually shows a normal level of follicle stimulating hormone (FSH), but urinary assay, vaginal smear, and endometrial biopsy show diminished estrogen activity. 17-ketosteroids, PBI, and serum corticoid values are all within normal limits.

Since the syndrome usually recedes when the medications are stopped, hormonal treatment is indicated only when the patient's psychiatric condition requires continuous use of psychotropic drugs. Replacement therapy with cyclic administration of estrogens (such as Premarin, 1.25 mg daily for three weeks and one week off) may be indicated or, if the patient wishes to have regular menstrual periods, a sequential estrogen-progesterone therapy may be preferred. In those rare instances in which amenorrhea and infertility persist even after the drugs are discontinued, the patient should be referred to a gynecologist for threatment with human menopausal gonadotropin (Pergonal), human chorionic gonadotropin (APL), or clomiphene (Clomid) (Van de Wiele 1965). Other endocrine effects noted after phenothiazine use include false positives on biologic (though less on immunologic) pregnancy tests (Hilbert 1958, Marks 1966) and an elevated I^{131} (Blumberg 1969).

PSYCHOTOXIC EFFECTS. The most common psychotoxic effects to follow the use of phenothiazines are depression, depersonalization, dysphoria, confusion, and somatic delusions. *Depressive symptoms* occurring during phenothiazine administration have a number of different causes. A patient who was severely anxious, agitated, or delusional before being given phenothiazines, but exhibits the symptoms of a full-blown depression as soon as his other symptoms have subsided, has probably had depressive symptoms throughout the course of his illness and should be given an antidepressant. Under these circumstances, the phenothiazine may seem to be the "cause" of the depression, when in reality it is serving only to reveal the mood disorder by stripping away those symptoms that have tended to eclipse it. If, on the other hand, the depression emerges gradually and is characterized more by apathy than by sadness, the mood change may simply be part of the illness' natural course, in the sense that it is the next stage or even a part of the recovery phase, and will usually recede without additional treatment. In either case, it may be useful to give the patient an antiparkinsonian agent for a few days (or to increase the dose if he is already taking one), as what appears to be a depression may be merely the psychomotor retardation and dulling characteristic of pseudoparkinsonism (Simonson 1964).

Depersonalization and *dysphoria* after phenothiazine use usually occur in individuals who have a tendency to such symptoms even when not taking drugs (Brauer 1970) and have responded similarly to a wide variety of other drugs. Within one or two days, and often after the first dose, the patient complains of feeling increasingly foggy, unreal, and so unhappy that the drug must be discontinued. Should it become obvious that the only drugs to which the patient does not respond with depersonalization are barbiturates or alcohol, and especially if he exhibits some degree of tremor, reports feeling tremulous, asks for barbiturates, or finds relief by drinking, it is likely that he was taking CNS depressants before being given the phenothiazines and that the depersonalization and dysphoria are in fact withdrawal rather than side effects.

Confusional episodes with or without somatic delusions also may follow phenothiazine use. Although the emergence of confusional symptoms should alert the clinician to the possibility of hitherto undiscovered organic disease, it is more likely, especially in patients with an organic brain syndrome or schizophrenia, that they represent inadequate control of the original illness, and will recede if the patient's drug dosage is increased. Since such symptoms can also be caused by phenothiazines, antiparkinsonian agents, or antidepressants, and since it may be difficult to distinguish between these various possibilities, it may be soundest in such cases to discontinue or at least lower the dosage of all drugs for a few days (by which time any phenothiazine-induced confusion will have subsided), to try in the interim to control the patient's symptoms with traditional sedatives, and thereafter to reintroduce one drug at a time.

Somatic delusions are not usually caused by phenothiazine use, but the patient may well integrate phenothiazine-induced side effects into whatever delusions he already has. The schizophrenic's body-image changes may thus be aggravated by extrapyramidal symptoms; similarly, the delusion of being "controlled" by outside forces may be augmented by drug-induced retardation and dulling. Delusional elaboration may make the patient's report of his discomfort difficult to understand. The physician must therefore pay close attention to somatic complaints even if they sound bizarre, for they may reflect a side effect he would recognize and be able to treat if it were described differently.

WITHDRAWAL EFFECTS.   Patients who abruptly discontinue taking phenothiazines after eight or more weeks of use may develop such symptoms as nausea, vomiting, diarrhea, headache, and anxiety (Kramer 1961). If anxiety is the most striking of these, it is possible that the symptoms are, at least in part, manifestations of a relapse; if, however, the gastrointestinal symptoms are the most prominent, the patient is probably having a withdrawal reaction that is likely to subside within four or five days without treatment and will subside even more rapidly if he is given a phenothiazine (Gallant 1964, Haden 1964). Abrupt withdrawal of both phenothiazines and anti-parkinsonian agents from a patient who has previously had extra-pyramidal symptoms may cause the symptoms to recur, for the effect of the phenothiazines outlasts that of the antiparkinsonian agents (Simpson 1965).

SUDDEN DEATH.   Whether and to what extent the sudden and otherwise unexplained deaths of patients taking phenothiazines that have been reported are caused by these agents is unclear (Johnson 1964, von Brauchitsch 1968). On the one hand, the incidence of sudden deaths among psychiatric patients has not increased since the introduction of phenothiazines (Claghorn 1967, Hussar 1962); on the other, deaths attributed to phenothiazine use appear to have certain features in common. In some, the autopsy shows multiple myocardial infarcts; in others, the intramyocardial arterioles, arteriolar capillary beds, and interstitial spaces between degenerating myocardial muscles are found to contain acid mucopolysaccharides (Hollister 1965a, Richardson 1966). Most characteristic, however, are those deaths that occur shortly after a meal: the patient exhibits weakness, malaise, marked dyspnea, sudden loss of consciousness, convulsions, vomiting, and aspiration. On autopsy, the trachea is found to contain gastric contents, and death is ascribed to asphyxia. Since such episodes are more frequent in patients who have been taking phenothiazines for some time, it has been conjectured that prolonged tranquilizer therapy interferes with the protective mechanisms that prevent esophageal reflux and thus permits aspiration of vomitus and subsequent asphyxia (Plachta 1965), but abnormalities in the swallowing mechanisms have also been found in schizophrenics not taking chlorpromazine (Hussar 1969).

ADVERSE EFFECTS FOLLOWING LONG-TERM USE

Many patients, particularly those with chronic schizophrenia, must be given phenothiazines for many years (many, indeed, for the rest of their lives) if their symptoms are to remain quiescent. Clinicians are therefore paying increasing attention to reports of potentially deleterious effects caused by the long-term use of phenothiazines (particularly chlorpromazine). What has been reported thus far does not seem to provide grounds for withholding phenothiazines from those who need them; such effects have been connected almost exclusively with the use of chlorpromazine and, even with this drug, are rarely of clinical significance. There are three types of such effects:

1/ Pigmentary changes affecting primarily the skin and eyes occur in approximately 90% of patients taking 2,500 mg and 30% of patients taking 500 mg of chlorpromazine daily for more than two years, but these changes rarely cause an appreciable diminution in visual acuity, and may be reversible upon substitution of a different phenothiazine.

2/ Persistent dyskinesia, a very rare but often irreversible disorder of the extrapyramidal system.

3/ Hepatic changes such as periportal cellular infiltration and fatty infiltration occur in 20% of patients receiving chlorpromazine for more than five years, and are usually asymptomatic, discovered only after percutaneous liver biopsy or autopsy (Bloom 1965), and also found (apparently with the same frequency) in institutionalized patients not taking phenothiazines (Bartholomew 1958, Hollister 1966).

The characteristic *pigment deposits in the eye* may occur simultaneously with or independently of skin pigment changes, and involve the lens, cornea, and conjunctiva. Lens changes consist of the bilateral deposit of fine yellow-brown particles in the anterior subcapsular and capsular portion of the lens, which progress to a stel-late formation of coherent brown and whitish specks (visible only on slit-lamp examination) and thence either to a white-pearled formation on the anterior part of the lens or to anterior cararacts. Only in the most advanced stages of this disorder is the patient likely to show any diminution of visual acuity, however (DeLong 1968, Prier 1970, Siddall 1965, 1968, Wetterholm 1965). Corneal opacities may also occur (especially in patients showing skin pigmen-tation and lens changes), as may a brownish conjunctival discoloration in the palpebral aperture (Dencker 1967, Gombos 1967, Johnson 1966, Mathalone 1965). *Pigmentary skin changes* are characterized by a violet-hued discoloration of the exposed areas of the body (Greiner 1964, Perrot 1962, Zelickson 1966). Discontinuation of chlorproma-zine tends to cause gradual diminution of the skin and eye changes over a 6 to 12 month period. D-penicillamine (Cuprimine), low copper diet, and the avoidance of sunlight have been recommended to reverse the pigmentary changes (Gibbard 1966), but the value of these measures has not been confirmed (Mathalone 1968). The foregoing kinds of pigment deposits should not be confused with *pigmentary retinopathies,* which have been reported after high (though not necessarily long-term) doses of thioridazine (Appel-baum 1963, Connell 1964, Hagopian 1966, Kirk 1970, May 1960) and may cause blurred vision, a brownish hue of the visual field, and night blindness.

Persistent dyskinesias are manifested primarily in choreiform, coordinated, involuntary, stereotyped, rhythmic movements gener-ally limited to the facial, mandibular, and lingual muscle groups. Rhythmic forward, backward, and at times lateral movements of the tongue, occurring every five to eight seconds, and detectable only when the patient opens his mouth, have been described and are said to be similar to the "fly-catcher tongue" seen in Von Eco-nomo's epidemic encephalitis. Although speech, mastication, and swallowing are not usually affected, stereotyped and incessant suck-ing, lip-pursing, and chewing movements have been described, as have jerky movements of the extremities, particularly the fingers, ankles, and toes. These symptoms are controllable voluntarily for only a few minutes at a time, usually disappear during sleep, are aggravated by emotional tension, and occur more frequently in women. It is also reported that advanced age and prior brain damage predispose the patient to these symptoms, but this is still a subject of debate (Crane 1968, Demars 1966, Druckman 1962, Faurbye 1964, Hunter 1964, Pryce 1966, Uhrbrand 1960). It is not yet established whether the more potent phenothiazines are more likely than the less potent to produce persistent dyskinesias.

The symptoms arise almost imperceptibly. Only rarely do they develop to the point of clinical recognition in less than six months of phenothiazine administration. Most cases are identified approximately two years after phenothiazine treatment is initiated, and in some patients symptoms occur for the first time only after the phenothiazine is withdrawn (Degkwitz 1969). While persistent dyskinesias are unresponsive to antiparkinsonian agents, high doses of phenothiazines may relieve them in some cases; in others, symptoms gradually recede several months after the phenothiazine is discontinued (Schmidt 1966). However, with many patients, there is no choice but to continue the phenothiazines, and it would seem that this side effect may have to "be accepted as an unfortunate but at present inevitable price for the benefits of this therapy" (Gilder 1964).

Thioxanthenes

The thioxanthenes are a form of major tranquilizer that differs structurally from the phenothiazines, in that the nitrogen in the central ring is replaced by a carbon. The agents most frequently used in psychiatric practice are the chlorpromazine analog, chlorprothixene (Taractan), and the thioproperazine analog, thiothixene (Navane). There is also a perphenazine analog, clopenthixol (Petersen 1964), but this is not yet marketed in the United States. The thioxanthenes share many of the *pharmacologic properties* of phenothiazines and are indicated for the same types of disorders, especially acute and chronic schizophrenias (Bishop 1966, Karn 1961, Scanlan 1963, Wolpert 1968). Interestingly, chlorprothixene has a definite uricosuric effect (Healey 1965). The daily *therapeutic dose range* is from 200 to 400 mg for chlorprothixene and 40 to 80 mg for thiothixene. Although there are no comparative studies, both clinical experience and the fact that thiothixene is an analog of an alerting phenothiazine, thioproperazine, suggest that it produces more extrapyramidal symptoms but less drowsiness than chlorprothixene.

Orthostatic hypotension with syncopal attacks has been reported with considerable frequency following the use of chlorprothixene (Cornu 1961, Gross 1961), as have tachycardia, lethargy, dryness of the mouth, dizziness, gastrointestinal disturbances, agranulocytosis (Mandel 1968), and jaundice (Hollister 1961a). Like chlorpromazine, thiothixene may cause lenticular pigmentation (Bishop 1968).

Butyrophenones

Developed in Belgium by Janssen (1959), butyrophenones, of which only haloperidol (Haldol) is currently marketed in the US, have been in clinical use as major tranquilizers for the past decade. Their *pharmacologic properties* are much like those of the phenothiazines in that they have antiemetic, hypothermic, and local anesthetic properties; prolong barbiturate sleeping time; and in other ways potentiate the effects of CNS depressants. Their adrenolytic effect is, however, far weaker than that of the phenothiazines. As a result, they are less likely to produce orthostatic hypotension, a feature that makes them particularly valuable for elderly patients (Beaulnes 1964). In addition, they seem less prone than the other major tranquilizers to produce appetite stimulation and weight gain (Gerle 1964) and, for this reason, may be a worthwhile substitute when the patient's weight gain endangers his health, social adjustment, or commitment to treatment.

The *initial dose* of haloperidol should not exceed 2 mg daily, but can be gradually increased to 10 or 12 mg over a period of several weeks. Doses of 0.05 mg/Kg have proved effective in moderating hyperactive and aggressive behavior in children (Faretra 1970) and, like the alerting phenothiazines, are also effective in Gilles de la Tourette's syndrome (see p. 375). Earlier claims that butyrophenones were superior to phenothiazines from the standpoint of antipsychotic activity or the calming of manic excitement (Ban 1964, Divry 1959, Entwistle 1962, Rees 1965) have not been confirmed in controlled studies (Kurland 1964, Stewart 1969).

Since haloperidol, like other major tranquilizers, may aggravate or perhaps even produce depressive symptoms, patients with a prior or family history of depressive disorders must be observed especially carefully as a safeguard against suicide (Gerle 1964, Luckey 1967). Because butyrophenones have a far stronger extrapyramidal effect (Delay 1960, Reitano 1966), an antiparkinsonian agent should be administered concomitantly. Haloperidol has also been found to interfere with the anticoagulant effects of phenindione (Hedulin) (Oakley 1963) and may also cause jaundice (Crause 1963).

Rauwolfia Alkaloids

Clinical Pharmacology

Rauwolfia alkaloids, in the form of the medicinal herb known as snakeroot, have been used for centuries in India, Java, and Africa as a remedy against nervousness and insomnia (Gupta 1943, Rumpf 1755), and were widely hailed in the early 1950s as a major contribution to psychiatric therapy (Kline 1954, Weber 1954). They were soon overshadowed by the advent of phenothiazines, however, and are today more widely used in the treatment of hypertension than in that of mental disorders. Although more than 20 such alkaloids have been extracted or synthesized, the most important is reserpine. Rescinnamine (Moderil) is much like reserpine, but less potent; syrosingopine (Singoserp), less antihypertensive; deserpidine (Harmonyl), equally antihypertensive but with less central depressant action. Synthetic analogs such as tetrabenazine (Nitoman; not marketed in the United States) seem to be shorter-acting and less potent.

In man, the effects of reserpine include hypotension, bradycardia, decreased peripheral vascular resistance, and increased skin blood flow without changes in muscle or cerebral blood flow or cardiac output. Like chlorpromazine, it lowers the convulsive threshold in some animals, but produces no specific effects on the EEG of man (Rinaldi 1955, Steiner 1965). Readily absorbed from the gastrointestinal tract and parenteral sites, reserpine is rapidly taken up by lipid-containing tissues. It is excreted primarily as methyl reserpate at the rate of about 6.5% of a daily dose of 0.5 mg (Maronde 1963). Reserpine crosses the placental barrier with the consequence that newborn infants whose mothers have received it frequently exhibit nasal discharge, lethargy, anorexia, and cutaneous vasodilatation (Budnick 1955).

Dosage, Administration, and Clinical Indications

While the use of phenothiazines and even more modern major tranquilizers has nipped reserpine's once very promising career in the bud, its value should not be underestimated. *Acute schizophrenias* in which the patient exhibits impulsivity, severe agitation, or catatonic excitement, as well as those that develop in early adolescence, sometimes respond better to reserpine than to phenothiazines. The usual starting dose is 2 to 4 mg, 3 to 4 times daily, which is raised gradually to the point at which nighttime sleep is achieved. Although doses as large as 240 mg daily have been used in acute schizophrenias (Kline 1957), we have not found it useful to give more than 20 mg daily.

For the first four to 10 days, the patient will exhibit a good deal of drowsiness and, in most cases, a gradual diminution of symptoms. Some patients remain symptom-free from then on, in which case whatever dose was required to achieve this level of improvement is left unchanged for four to six weeks, then gradually decreased until a maintenance dose of as little as 2 mg daily is reached (Barsa 1955). In other patients, the initial quiescence is replaced by a turbulent phase with nightmares, agitation, and a widely fluctuating blood pressure. The patient may be so disturbed that he must be hospitalized, but in most cases can be afforded some relief with chlorpromazine (Thorazine), 25 to 50 mg, 3 to 4 times daily, or chlordiazepoxide (Librium), 5 to 10 mg, 4 times daily. The turbulent phase rarely lasts longer than eight to 10 days and cannot be shortened by lowering the dose of reserpine.

Certain types or phases of *chronic schizophrenia* may also be more responsive to reserpine than to phenothiazines, particularly those marked by low-grade paranoid irritability (Maggs 1960). A patient who has improved with phenothiazines but continues to lack insight, be mildly delusional or episodically irritable, and verge on being querulant, may become more sociable when 1 to 2 mg of reserpine daily is added to his phenothiazine regimen. That reserpine has a long half-life is an additional advantage, for this renders it particularly suitable as a maintenance medication for the patient who occasionally stops taking his pills for four or five days at a time.

Reserpine may also help in a number of other psychiatric disorders. In *anxiety neuroses,* doses of 0.25 to 1.0 mg, 3 to 4 times daily may be helpful; patients with *anorexia nervosa,* as well as children who are not "truly" anorectic but merely refuse to eat, often develop an enormous increase in appetite when given 0.5 mg, 3 to 4 times daily, for five to 10 days; *thyrotoxic crises* (Dillon 1970), psychomotor excitement, and *acute manic episodes* often subside within 24 to 72 hours on doses of 1.0 to 2.5 mg, 4 times daily. Good results have also been achieved in chronic *obsessive compulsive neuroses* when 0.5 to 1.0 mg of reserpine was given in combination with 25 to 75 mg of imipramine (Tofranil), 4 times daily. The patient with a *depression* whose symptoms are or have become refractory to imipramine sometimes improves when 3 to 5 mg of intramuscular reserpine twice daily is added to his drug regimen for two days (Haskovec 1967, Pöldinger 1963).

Adverse Effects

Like other major tranquilizers, rauwolfia alkaloids can produce drowsiness, extrapyramidal symptoms, seizures, weight gain, amenorrhea, galactorrhea, gynecomastia, loss of libido, and impotence

(Hollister 1961a, Somlyo 1960), all of which are managed as described in the section on phenothiazines. They can also produce bradycardia, hypotension, flushing, severe nasal congestion, diarrhea, and episodic generalized tremors, resembling chills. As long as the pulse rate is not below 60 nor the fall in systolic pressure above 30 mm, these effects are of little concern. While the flushing itself is also of little significance, the thyrotoxic patient with diarrhea and palpitations who is given reserpine may erroneously be considered to have a carcinoid syndrome (Blumenthal 1965). The nasal congestion can be very uncomfortable, but tends to diminish somewhat with the passage of time and can be mitigated with diphenhydramine (Benadryl) 25 mg p.o., 2 to 3 times daily, or a vasoconstrictor such as phenylephrine (Neosynephrine). The chills can usually be somewhat alleviated with antiparkinsonian agents. Increased gastric secretion and intestinal motility leading to diarrhea, as well as the production or reactivation of peptic ulcers with hemorrhage and perforation, have also been described (Kirsner 1957, Roth 1964). A weekly stool examination with testing for occult blood is indicated when abdominal discomfort is reported. A bleeding episode could easily be missed, however, in uncommunicative psychotic patients. Several sudden and otherwise unexplained deaths of psychotic patients who had taken high doses of reserpine for many months have indeed been attributed to perforated viscera caused by the administration of reserpine (Zlotlow 1958). This is one of the reasons why the use of reserpine has been abandoned in most mental hospitals. Migraine attacks are also reported to have been precipitated or aggravated by reserpine (Curzon 1969, Kimball 1966, Tandon 1969). Fluid retention and edema may also occur and be partly responsible for the weight gain, but can usually be managed with diuretics. While allergic or hypersensitivity reactions and agranulocytoses are rare, thrombocytopenic purpura has been reported.

Reserpine can also precipitate depressive episodes with insomnia, nightmares, and anhedonia, and is therefore contraindicated for patients with a prior or a family history of depression. That the schizophrenic given reserpine may not only develop the symptoms of turbulence described earlier but also become depressed as his psychotic symptoms subside (Bernstein 1957, 1960, Bunney 1965, Ferguson 1959, Goslin 1955, Schroeder 1955) gives substance to Kline's (1957) aphoristic comment that, after the patient has recovered from the disease, he must then recover from the treatment. If the patient's response to reserpine has otherwise been satisfactory, he can be given imipramine (Tofranil), 25 to 50 mg, 3 times daily (Freyhan 1960), but if depressive symptoms persist, the reserpine must be withdrawn.

MINOR TRANQUILIZERS

Clinical Pharmacology

In the past few decades, a large number of "minor" tranquilizers (also known as "antianxiety" agents) has been developed and marketed, each purporting to be safer and more effective than the last (see Table 35). The most commonly used types are

1/ propanediols like meprobamate (Miltown) (Berger 1954, Ludwig 1951), a dicarbamate derivative of the muscle relaxant mephenesin (Tolserol), and the recently introduced tybamate (Solacen, Tybatran) (Berger 1964, Raab 1964); and

2/ benzodiazepines like chlordiazepoxide (Librium) (Sternbach 1961), diazepam (Valium), and oxazepam (Serax) (General Practitioner Research Group 1967, Jacobs 1966, Janacek 1966, Jenner 1967, Le Gassicke 1965a).

These drugs are absorbed rapidly, start to take effect within 30 to 40 minutes after oral administration, reach peak blood levels within two hours, and are then excreted slowly over a 48-hour period (Hollister 1961b, Walkenstein 1958).

It is hard to say whether and to what extent it is legitimate to distinguish between the clinical effects of these agents and those of other general depressants of the CNS, such as barbiturates, chloral hydrate, paraldehyde, and even bromides. The similarities in any case are far more striking then any supposed differences (The Medical Letter 1969). What calming effect either group may have is achieved at the cost of making the patient drowsy; and what appetite-stimulating and muscle-relaxant effect minor tranquilizers may have is shared by the rest. The similarity between propanediol or benzodiazepine tranquilizers and other CNS depressants is further supported by the observations that they all

1/ produce the same kind of immediate "lift";

2/ cause a diminished arousal response to afferent stimuli;

3/ have anticonvulsant properties (Henry 1958, Schallek 1962, Watson 1964); and

4/ produce slow-wave and low-voltage fast (beta) activity on the EEG (Brazier 1964).

Furthermore,

5/ like CNS depressants and unlike major tranquilizers (which cause tolerance to their hypnotic but not to their tranquilizing effect), minor tranquilizers cause the individual who takes them to become tolerant to their hypnotic and tranquilizing effect simultaneously;

6/ abrupt withdrawal of minor tranquilizers after protracted use produces the same kinds of symptoms as are seen after withdrawal from other CNS depressants (see p. 296);

7/ minor tranquilizers exhibit cross-tolerance and cross-dependence with other CNS depressants (see p. 290); and

8/ they are often used to excess by individuals who have in the past abused other CNS depressants (see p. 292).

The only clinically relevant differences appear to lie with benzodiazepines, which

1/ seem to be superior to the rest in the treatment of chronic anxiety (Wheatley 1966);

2/ produce less severe withdrawal symptoms than the others (and convulsions only in the rarest of instances); and

3/ cause so little respiratory depression, even when used in massive doses, that successful suicide attempts are rare with benzodiazepines alone.

Not all so-called minor tranquilizers have the same effects. Hydroxyzine (Vistaril), for example, has not only a sedative and antiemetic but also an antihistaminic effect; does not exhibit cross-tolerance or cross-dependence with the groups mentioned above; and, despite its label, does not have a consistent calming effect (Kellner 1968, Mock 1965). If there is any drug with which it can be compared, it is the sedative antihistamine diphenhydramine (Benadryl), a drug that has long been used as a mild soporific and, like hydroxyzine, does not produce symptoms of discomfort when abruptly withdrawn.

The term *minor (tranquilizer)* refers, then, not to some specific tranquilizing effect, nor to some specific difference from traditional hypnotics, but to a clinical pattern of use in which these drugs, after having been found beneficial for anxiety, were used for major psychoses and found wanting, in the sense that they had little immediate and almost no lasting effect on delusions, hallucinations, or mood disturbances.

Clinical Indications and Dosage

Therapeutic doses of propanediols and benzodiazepines (see Table 35) generally relieve both *acute and chronic anxiety* and the associated physical symptoms (Jenner 1967, Kelly 1969, Lorr 1963). However, most patients develop tolerance to this effect, and some then elect to increase the dosage on their own. Since the long-term use of constantly increasing amounts appears to aggravate rather than relieve depressed mood, these drugs should not be prescribed for more than a few weeks at a time, unless it is certain that the patient will take only the amount prescribed. Within these limits, benzodiazepines can be of substantial benefit; because they have rarely been used successfully in suicide attempts and can temporarily relieve agitation, insomnia, and anorexia, they often make the depressed patient more comfortable for a few weeks, until a concurrently administered antidepressant takes effect, without putting yet another potentially lethal drug into the hands of a potential suicide.

Because benzodiazepines exhibit cross-tolerance and cross-dependence with alcohol, are well tolerated even in relatively high doses, and are available in parenteral form for use with combative, delirious, or uncooperative patients, they have become the drug of choice in the management of *alcohol withdrawal* (Kaim 1969, Sereny 1965). If the patient is predelirious or tremulous, he should be given 50 mg of chlordiazepoxide orally every 45 to 60 minutes until the tremor subsides. Over the next 24 hours, he should receive as much chlordiazepoxide as he requires to remain comfortable (up to 400 mg). Thereafter the dose is reduced by about 10% daily until the drug is completely withdrawn (see also Chap. 9).

Benzodiazepines have also come to be used in certain *neurologic disorders.* Diazepam produces marked diminution of spasticity as well as behavioral improvement in children with athetoid cerebral palsy (Denhoff 1964, Marsh 1965); suppresses sustained ankle clonus in quadriparetics (Carlson 1968); and, when administered intravenously in doses up to 100 mg in 500 ml of saline, is effective in recurrent or prolonged seizures (including status epilepticus), even after other anticonvulsants have failed (Little 1969, Parsonage 1967). Hydroxyzine (Vistaril) and diphenhydramine (Benadryl) produce neither the immediate lift nor the withdrawal symptoms characteristic of general depressants of the CNS and are therefore of value as mild sedatives even for the patient with a history of drug abuse.

Adverse Effects

At the recommended dose levels, and even more so at higher dose levels, propanediols and benzodiazepines may cause drowsiness, vertigo, excessive appetite, and (paradoxically) nausea, as well as headache, lightheadedness, muscular weakness, impaired judgment, poor coordination (The Medical Letter 1969), and, especially in elderly patients, a cerebellar type of ataxia. They can also produce hypotension and potentiate the hypotensive effects of narcotics. As with barbiturates, paradoxical reactions can occur; these include bizarre behavior and episodes of apparently unmotivated violence (Hollister 1965b). Prolonged use of benzodiazepines may diminish sexual drive and cause menstrual irregularities with failure to ovulate (Jarvik 1965).

Withdrawal reactions may occur two to six days after a patient is suddenly withdrawn from high or even moderate doses of propanediol and benzodiazepine tranquilizers. The clinical picture is identical with that called *delirium tremens* when seen after alcohol withdrawal: tremulousness, insomnia, vomiting, muscle twitching, anxiety, anorexia, ataxia, acute confusion (sometimes with visual hallucinations), and psychomotor excitement (Hollister 1961b) (see p. 298). Convulsions are extremely rare, however, in patients taking only benzodiazepines at the time of withdrawal. The patient experiencing such withdrawal symptoms should not be given phenothiazines, which tend to aggravate the symptoms and in some cases may even precipitate them (Miller unpublished data). *Allergic phenomena,* affecting primarily the blood and skin, have also been reported. Meprobamate has been implicated in the development of erythemas, acute nonthrombocytopenic purpura, angioneurotic edema, bronchospasm (Zirkle 1960), aplastic anemia, thrombocytopenia, leukopenia, and agranulocytosis (Crosby 1964), and chlordiazepoxide in the development of erythemas (Kaelbling 1960) and agranulocytosis.

ANTIDEPRESSANTS

Clinical Pharmacology

The term *antidepressant* refers to a number of dibenzazepine derivatives and monoamine oxidase inhibitors (MAOI) that moderate certain syndromes characterized by tearfulness, morbid sadness, self-derogation, pessimism, impaired initiative, psychomotor agitation or retardation, and decreased sleep, appetite, and sexual interest. In contrast to the major tranquilizers, they have little or no beneficial effect on the cognitive disturbances seen in early schizophrenia and may indeed even aggravate them (Barker 1960, Ferreira 1958, Gershon 1962, Heinrich 1960).

The prototype and major representative of the *dibenzazepine* (or tricyclic) antidepressant group is imipramine (Tofranil). It was first synthesized in 1954 (Schindler) and, because of its structural relationship to promazine, tested as a tranquilizer but then found to have antidepressant properties (Kuhn 1957). Although it is available in both oral and injectable form, the oral form is by far the most commonly used, as the drug is absorbed from the gastrointestinal tract. It is so rapidly metabolized that plasma levels are measurable for only a brief time and only 3% of the ingested dose is excreted in unchanged form (Jarvik 1965). Other drugs of this group, listed in the approximate decreasing order of potency include *amitriptyline* (Elavil) (Klerman 1965, Reynolds 1969), *protriptyline* (Vivactil) (Daneman 1965, McConaghy 1965), *doxepin* (Sinequan) (Rickels 1969), *nortriptyline* (Aventyl) (Barron 1964, Mendels 1968) and *desipramine* (Pertofrane, Norpramin) (Hargreaves 1967).

The term *monoamine oxidase inhibitor* (MAOI) is applied to a number of structurally diverse agents with the common property of inhibiting a class of enzymes designated as monoamine oxidases. While it is known that all MAOIs have an antidepressant effect, it is not known how, or even whether, the inhibition of monoamine oxidase is linked to their therapeutic effect (Vernier 1961, Zeller 1961). The first MAOI used for depressions was iproniazid (Marsilid), which, while being used as a tuberculostatic, was found to have an antidepressant effect but subsequently proved to have such grave hepatotoxic effects that its use was abandoned. It was the prototype for such hydrazine MAO inhibitors as *isocarboxazide* (Marplan), *nialamide* (Niamid), and *phenelzine* (Nardil) (Greenblatt 1962, Kurland 1967, Wechsler 1965), but nonhydrazine MAO inhibitors, such as *pargyline* (Eutonyl) and *tranylcypromine* (Parnate), a drug structurally similar to amphetamine, have also been found to have an antidepressant effect. The currently used MAOIs are readily absorbed when given by mouth and are not available in injectable form. MAOIs are generally not as effective against depressions as dibenzazepines, although some clinicians believe that they are the drug of choice in certain types of depressive syndromes. Obviously, much work needs to be done to establish whether there are specific indications for their use and how the efficiency of these two types of antidepressants compares with ECT in the treatment of depressions (see p. 644).

Dosage and Administration

The usual starting dose of imipramine (Tofranil) in depressive syndromes is 25 mg, 3 times daily for two days, and, if well tolerated, 50 mg, 3 to 4 times daily thereafter. Should there be no improvement within three weeks, the drug may be slowly increased to 250 or even 300 mg daily, in divided doses (Kielholz 1958), and the therapeutic trial continued for another two to three weeks. If the patient refuses oral medications, he may be given imipramine intramuscularly in doses of 25 mg, 3 times daily. The initial dose of phenelzine (Nardil) is 15 mg, 3 times daily, which may be increased to 4 or even 5 times daily if the patient does not improve within 10 to 14 days. Whatever drug is used, once improvement has been achieved, the dose is maintained until the patient's symptoms recede, continued for an additional 3 to 6 months, and thereafter reduced by 20% to 30% every 4 to 6 weeks until, perhaps 12 to 18 months after the patient first became depressed, an attempt is made to discontinue the antidepressant entirely (Lehmann 1968). If the depression was mild or the patient's first, a somewhat briefer course may be indicated. The dosage of other antidepressants used is listed in Table 37.

Clinical Indications

The syndrome for which antidepressants are most commonly used is the *typical depression* (see p. 172), characterized by insomnia, anorexia, and retardation. Two out of every three depressed patients with such symptoms who are given antidepressants show noticeable improvement within two to three weeks, some even during the first week (Hordern 1963). That antidepressants may also have a beneficial effect on certain other disorders (though perhaps not with the same frequency) has led to the hypothesis that these syndromes are related to or are "in fact" subtypes of the typical depression. However, the merit of this hypothesis cannot be assessed until more is known either of the causes of psychiatric disorders or the effects of these drugs, so for the present it is possible only to list other clinical pictures in which favorable effects have been observed. For example, antidepressants may be helpful for patients who, in the midst of their menopause or involutional period, show an abundance of otherwise *unexplainable physical complaints* (Evans 1960, Paulson 1962, Webb 1962); and in *anxiety neuroses,* especially those of recent origin (see p. 237); *phobic neuroses* .(see p. 219); *obsessive-compulsive neuroses,* especially when given in such high doses as 400 to 500 mg daily (see p. 239); *enuresis nocturna* (see p. 375); *encopresis* (see p. 377); *narcolepsy* (see p. 446); depressed mood and retardation associated with *organic brain syndromes* (see p. 412); and even in *bronchial asthma* (Sugihara 1965).\

Antidepressants may also be used for patients with *systematized paranoid delusions* (p. 211) or *schizoaffective schizophrenias* (see p. 129) and for schizophrenics who have become depressed after being given phenothiazines (see p. 134). In involutional depressions with paranoid features (see p. 211), a *combination of antidepressants and phenothiazines* is required as antidepressants alone have little or no effect on delusions and may even exacerbate them. The combination of MAOI *and dibenzazepine antidepressants* has been reported to be effective in refractory depressions (Dally 1965), but can cause such serious side effects that it seems too hazardous to use under any but the most closely supervised experimental conditions (Pare 1965).

Adverse Effects

The antidepressants currently in use have been implicated in the production of a wide variety of adverse effects, but it is sometimes hard to determine whether the symptoms are caused by the drug or the disease for which it has been prescribed. Patients taking antidepressants often complain of dryness of the mouth, constipation, anxiety, weakness, and impotence, but these symptoms are so common in depressive syndromes that it would be an error to attribute them routinely to the antidepressant alone (Busfield 1962).

Dibenzazepine (tricyclic) antidepressants like imipramine (Tofranil) produce adverse autonomic, cardiovascular, endocrine, CNS, and psychotoxic effects as well as allergic phenomena and withdrawal reactions. The *autonomic effects* include blurring of vision; dryness of mouth; constipation and (in rare instances) paralytic ileus (Milner 1964); difficulty in micturition, which, particularly in patients with prostatic hypertrophy, can lead to urinary retention (Feaver 1967); palpitations; tachycardia; and profuse sweating (especially of the head and neck (Hollister 1964). In most instances, the discomfort can be relieved by giving the patient +½ to +1½ diopter glasses or clip-ons for the blurring; chewing gum for the dryness of mouth; and neostigmine (Prostigmine), bethanechol (Urecholine), or pilocarpine for the sweating, constipation, and urinary retention. Dibenzazepines can aggravate or precipitate glaucoma, but only the narrow-angle glaucoma caused by inadequate drainage of ocular fluid due to excessive angulation of the iris and cornea, and not the far more common open-angle glaucoma. In any case, before being given a dibenzazepine, the patient should be asked whether he has had episodes of eye pain or halos around lights, and his conjunctivae should be examined for evidence of congestion.

Cardiovascular effects include orthostatic hypotension, tachycardia, flattening of the T-waves on the ECG, and cardiac arrhythmias. Patients must be warned of the hypotensive effect, as the most serious consequences of antidepressant use, particularly in elderly patients, have occurred when they have fainted after suddenly getting up to walk or trying to walk up a flight of stairs. The ECG changes are benign and reversible but—especially in the patient over 40 who has not had a pretreatment ECG—can give rise to unwarranted concern. Congestive heart failure, pulmonary emboli, and myocardial infarction have also been reported, but cannot be ascribed with any certainty to the use of the dibenzazepines, for they have occurred almost exclusively in the age group above 60 that is in any case more vulnerable to cardiovascular disorders (Moorhead 1965, Mosbech 1960, Muller 1961, Schou 1962).

Endocrine effects, including impotence in men; amenorrhea and galactorrhea in women; and loss of libido and excessive weight gain in both sexes have been reported with dibenzazepines (Duguay 1964, Gander 1965, Greenberg 1965, Hordern 1964, Klein 1964, Wheatley 1965), as with phenothiazines, and are managed as described in that section (see p. 585).

Central nervous system effects include drowsiness, dysarthria, ataxia, hyperreflexia, tremor (especially of the upper extremities), and a feeling of tremulousness. While a certain degree of tolerance to these effects develops within seven to 10 days, some measure of tremor and drowsiness may persist as long as the drug is used. Doses of dibenzazepines exceeding 150 mg daily have also been reported to produce seizures, especially in individuals with a prior history of seizure disorder (Kiloh 1961, Lehmann 1958, Sharp 1960), and to exacerbate barbiturate withdrawal reactions. That peripheral neuropathies, especially peroneal palsies, have been reported (Miller 1963) may be of particular relevance in considering the use of antidepressants during the first trimester of pregnancy, for neurotoxicity was among the earliest warnings of thalidomide's possible teratogenic effect. Imipramine has been used extensively during pregnancy, however, without any reports of fetal abnormalities.

Patients who abruptly discontinue using imipramine or amitriptyline after they have been taking more than 150 mg daily for six to eight weeks may, after a lapse of four or five days, develop *withdrawal symptoms*. These include nausea, vomiting, abdominal cramps, diarrhea, chills, insomnia and anxiety. Such symptoms last for three to five days, can be relieved by reinstituting the original dose, and can be avoided by gradually withdrawing the drug over a period of three to four weeks (Kramer 1961, Kuhn 1957).

Two types of *psychotoxic effects* have been reported after dibenzazepine use. The *first* is a shift from depression, withdrawal, and retardation to morbid euphoria, garrulousness, and hyperactivity, sometimes to a clear-cut manic episode (Schorer 1960). Whether this shift is entirely a drug effect that might affect anyone taking the drug is a subject of controversy, for it seems more common in individuals whose personal and family history indicates a predisposition for bipolar mood disorders. What appears to be a drug effect might then be merely a mood shift unrelated to, or at most somewhat accelerated by, the drug use. In any case, if the morbid euphoria persists for more than three or four days, the drug dosage should be reduced; if this does not help, treatment with phenothiazines or lithium carbonate should be initiated. The *second* type of psychotoxic effect takes the form of an organic brain syndrome ranging in severity from a transient defect in recent memory (Hankoff 1960) to a full-blown delirium and occurs with greatest frequency in older patients and during the first few weeks of treatment (Heinrich 1960). It is usually sufficient to sedate the patient with a phenothiazine as these episodes tend to be short-lived. Only when the patient is very confused and agitated and the episode lasts longer than two to three days is it necessary to reduce the dose or discontinue the antidepressant altogether. Interestingly, once the episode has subsided, toxic psychosis does not recur in the majority of patients, even when the antidepressants are readministered in high therapeutic dose ranges (Davies in press).

Among the *allergic phenomena* reported with dibenzazepine use are cholestatic jaundice (Hollister 1964, Morgan 1969); urticaria, a confluent or discrete pruritic maculopapular erythema, and photosensitivity; and agranulocytosis, poikilocytosis, and anisocytosis (Bird 1960, Rothenberg 1960).

MAOIs produce almost all the side effects reported for dibenzazepines with the exception of the endocrine effects and withdrawal reactions. *Autonomic effects,* while less frequent and less pronounced with MAOIS than with dibenzazepines, include dry mouth, blurred vision, nausea, constipation, urinary retention, and sweating. *Hypotension,* too, has been observed and, especially with the stronger MAOIS, can be quite severe. *Edema* of the ankles (often unilateral) and periorbital edema may also occur and usually respond well to diuretics. *Central nervous system effects* consist of tremor, hyperreflexia, nighttime twitches and jerks, and seizures (Pilling 1963). *Psychotoxic effects* include the shift into hypomania or mania, the exacerbation of schizophrenic symptoms, and the development of dysmnesia or deliriform confusion, especially in individuals over 45. Most MAOIS produce a mild degree of drowsiness, with the exception of tranylcypromine (Parnate), a drug structurally similar to amphetamine, which may produce insomnia and should not be given after 5 PM. At least one case of tranylcypromine abuse (300 mg daily) has been reported (Le Gassicke 1965b).

Whether the MAOIS' therapeutic effects are related to their inhibition of monoamine oxidase is not known, but it seems very likely that a number of their side effects are. The amino acid tryptophan (an amine precursor), which under ordinary circumstances is a pharmacologically inactive component of the individual's daily diet, can produce excitation in patients taking MAOI when given in only slightly higher amounts than occur in the usual diet (Oates 1960). The *hypertensive crises* that follow the ingestion of certain foods may have a similar explanation (Blackwell 1967). If, for example, a patient taking tranylcypromine (the most potent of the currently marketed MAOIS) or some other MAOI ingests certain foods, such as particular aged cheeses (Asatoor 1963, Blackwell 1964, Breakstone 1965, Cuthill 1964), broad beans (Hodge 1964), beer, yeast products, Chianti wine, pickled herring, chocolate, or chicken livers (Hedberg 1966), he may develop a sharp elevation in blood pressure, usually associated with a severe throbbing headache, nausea, hyperpyrexia, vomiting, sweating, and nuchal rigidity (Brown 1962). In some cases, the patient may develop a subarachnoid hemorrhage (Dorrell 1963, Goldberg 1964), occasionally with fatal outcome (McClure 1962). The cause seems to be the listed foods' high content of tyramine (a pressor agent that has only 2% to 5% of the activity of epinephrine under normal circumstances but, when not inactivated, increases to the point that the symptoms described are produced) (Pettinger 1968), or in the case of broad beans, dopa. That the causative factor is the combination of foods and drug rather than the drug alone seems supported by the observation that the incidence of such reactions has decreased from 8.4% to 3.3% (Bethune 1964) since physicians have become aware of this danger and have instructed their patients to avoid these foods. The similarity of such episodes, both symptomatically and pathophysiologically, to pheochromocytoma crises (Dally 1962, Plass 1964) has led some clinicians to propose that they be treated with phentolamine (Regitine), 5.0 mg (Bethune 1963, Horwitz 1964). Chlorpromazine (in doses of 50 to 100 mg i.m.) has also been used effectively in a number of cases, as has the rapid-acting sympatholytic drug trimethaphan camsylate (Arfonad) (The Medical Letter 1970). The dangers inherent in the hypertensive crises initially caused tranylcypromine to be withdrawn from the market, but it was found sufficiently useful to be reintroduced after a few months, albeit with the limitation that it be used only for severely depressed patients who have had little or no relief from other antidepressants or ECT (Atkinson 1965).

The MAOIS' interference with enzymatic activity also *potentiates the effects of a host of other agents,* including CNS depressants; antihistamines; ganglion-blocking and anticholinergic agents; sympathomimetics, including amphetamines (Cuthbert 1969, Mason 1962, Zeck 1961); opiates and opioids, especially meperidine (Palmer 1960, Taylor 1962); diuretics, such as chlorthiazine (Diuril) and hydrochlorothiazide (The Medical Letter 1963); chloroquine; sulfonylurea type of hypoglycemic drugs (Brown 1969); corticosteroids; antirheumatic compounds; and dibenzazepine antidepressants (Howarth 1961, Jarecki 1963, Lee 1961, Nymark 1963) (see Table 42).

Skin reactions, including maculopapular rashes, pustules, and dryness, have also been described. *Optic atrophy* with red/green blindness has been attributed to the use of pheniprazine, a hydrazine MAOI, which has now been withdrawn from the market. Although hydrazine MAOIS, isocarboxazid, phenelzine, nialamide, and particularly iproniazid (now withdrawn) have also been implicated in the production of *hepatocellular jaundice,* it is rare with the MAOIS currently in use. However, one should note that once hepatocellular injury has been produced by any of the MAOIS, substitution by another is hazardous as there is marked cross-sensitivity (Klatskin 1969).

LITHIUM CARBONATE

Since 1949, when Cade first reported the beneficial effect of lithium salts on mania, enthusiasm for their use has gathered increasing momentum. Lithium carbonate (Eskalith, Lithonate, Lithane), the most commonly used of these salts, is now considered the drug of choice for the treatment of the acute manic episode. Despite the abundance of favorable clinical reports on the thousands of patients treated with lithium over the past two decades, there have been few well-controlled, double-blind studies (Bunney 1968, Goodwin 1969, Johnson 1968, Maggs 1963, Schou 1954). Nevertheless, there is currently fairly general agreement that nine out of ten acute manic episodes can be brought to remission within 10 days with the use of lithium carbonate, and that maintenance lithium therapy will prevent the recurrence of manic attacks in six out of 10 individuals suffering from manic-depressive disease. Current research is directed toward establishing the efficacy of lithium in the treatment and prevention of the depressive phase of manic-depressive disease, recurrent depressive syndromes, cyclothymic personality disorders, schizoaffective disorders, premenstrual tension, cyclically occurring obsessive-compulsive states, and other disorders that, like manic-depressive disease, are marked by periodicity, especially those in which some of the episodes are characterized by overactivity and others by inactivity or even stupor (Annell 1969, Baastrup 1969, Forssman 1969, Fries 1969, Gershon 1968, Goodwin 1969, Gottfries 1968, Sletten 1966).

Clinical Pharmacology

Being a monovalent cation, lithium is neither metabolized nor bound to plasma tissue proteins (Thomsen 1968). Within eight to 10 hours following administration, a dynamic equilibrium is established between the lithium concentration in the blood and that in the tissues. It is excreted almost exclusively in the urine. The rate at which lithium clearance occurs is remarkably constant in a given individual (until he grows older, at which time it declines by approximately 40%), but may vary between 15 and 50 ml per minute from one individual to the next. The average single dose of 300 mg of lithium carbonate corresponds to about 8 mEq of lithium and raises the serum lithium concentration by approximately 0.3 mEq/l. The exact amount of lithium needed to maintain a given serum concentration depends on the patient's body weight and renal excretory capacity, and the dose required depends on his condition and clinical response. Lithium carbonate, 600 to 1,800 mg daily in 2 to 4 doses, usually maintains the patient's serum lithium concentration at the level between 0.6 and 1.5 mEq/L that is therapeutic and does not produce significant toxicity.

Precautions

The hazards associated with lithium therapy and the all-important balance between serum lithium level and renal excretory capacity make it imperative to assess the patient's renal status before starting lithium treatment and to monitor his serum lithium level at regular intervals thereafter. Urinalysis, BUN, and creatinine clearance values should be obtained before the patient is started on lithium. After he begins taking the drug, serum lithium determinations should be performed three times a week until the desired dose has been determined and the patient's clinical condition stabilized. Thereafter, weekly and eventually monthly lithium determinations are sufficient. More frequent determinations must be resumed if the dose is changed, if toxic symptoms appear, or if the patient develops an illness that might affect his lithium clearance and thus his serum lithium level. Since serum concentrations rise steeply in the first two hours after lithium intake, blood samples should be drawn before the first dose of the day or, if this is inconvenient, six to eight hours after the previous dose (Amdisen 1969). Although these determinations are a fairly reliable safeguard against overdosage, they do not replace careful clinical observation of the patient, especially during febrile or other illnesses that cause a loss of fluids or in some other way affect the kidney's excretory capacity, for, under these circumstances, the correlation between serum lithium values and toxic symptoms becomes far less reliable. Because recent evidence implicates lithium in the production of goiter, it is necessary to obtain PBI and T$_3$ values, to palpate the patient's thyroid gland both before treatment and at monthly intervals thereafter, and to prescribe thyroxine or desiccated thyroid when indicated (Schou 1968).

Clinical Indications and Dosage

Treatment of the *acute manic state* consists of giving the patient enough lithium carbonate to achieve a serum lithium level between 0.9 and 1.5 mEq/l. The initial dose is 900 mg daily; this is increased by 300 mg daily every three days until the patient's symptoms diminish or his lithium level reaches 1.5 mEq/l. This can usually be achieved with 1,200 to 1,500 mg daily; only rarely are doses above 2,100 mg daily required. For elderly or debilitated patients and those suffering from hypomanic states, 600 to 900 mg daily are sufficient.

Although the full effect on mood and ideation is not achieved until about the tenth day, some improvement is usually noted on the third or fourth day following administration of the drug. If the patient is sleepless or agitated, he may in the interim be given phenothiazines or a butyrophenone like haloperidol (Haldol) in doses sufficient to promote nighttime sleep and ease his management. If neither of these drugs is of benefit and his behavior remains uncontrollable, it may be necessary to initiate treatment with a brief course of ECT. Once the manic behavior subsides, the dose should be reduced by approximately 300 mg every four to seven days until a maintenance dose of 900 to 1,200 mg is reached, unless, of course, symptoms recur. If it is the patient's first manic episode, he should be maintained on lithium for at least three months after he becomes symptom-free. If the patient has had a previous manic or depressive episode, maintenance therapy should be considered, particularly if the attacks were severe or the symptom-free interval between them was brief. A daily dose of 600 to 1,200 mg, is usually sufficient to keep the serum level within the therapeutic range, but in periods of exacerbation (even if they are mild), the dosage must be increased to whatever nontoxic level is required to relieve the symptoms.

Among the advantages attributed to lithium is that the patient does not experience the memory disturbances suffered by patients receiving ECT (Schlagenhauf 1966) or the slowed-down feeling or nostalgia for the manic phase reported by patients taking phenothiazines. The patient taking lithium seems to be more faithful in following his physician's instructions and reporting an exacerbation of his disorder promptly than the patient under other treatments (Swartzburg unpublished data), but it is not known whether this is because lithium produces a lesser degree of discomfort and disability or a greater degree of insight and health. The drug's good effects seem to be cumulative, moreover, in the sense that the patient feels even better after six or 12 months of taking it than he did after three or four weeks (Wolpert 1969). Many patients, even ones who have never had an overt manic attack, report feeling far less irritable and keyed-up, and far better able to concentrate, and their families often claim a remarkably favorable personality change.

Relapses may occur in patients taking lithium, but seem to be briefer and less disabling than those experienced by patients not taking lithium. Such "hypomanic alerts" can usually be brought under control fairly rapidly by increasing the dose and administering a major tranquilizer during the period of exacerbation. Lithium has also been reported to make some patients more responsive to antidepressants, especially to those of the imipramine group: the patient who gets depressed despite taking lithium is said to respond to antidepressants more rapidly and more favorably than the one not taking lithium (Fieve 1968, Zall 1968).

While there has been no confirmation of the view that lithium affects some genetically distinct type of affective disorder, we have repeatedly seen a favorable response in patients who, though their symptoms seemed characteristic of a personality disorder, schizophrenia, or neurosis, had a family history of manic-depressive disease.

Adverse Effects

The most common side effect of lithium in the first days of administration is a fine tremor of the hands and a tendency to micrographia. Although this tremor may persist even after the patient no longer requires the high doses used during the acute phase of his illness, it is usually so mild that it causes little or no disability, even to the patient whose work requires manual dexterity. For the first week or two of administration, most patients feel slightly nauseated, and some may vomit or experience mild abdominal pain, fatigue, and thirst. These symptoms tend to coincide with the absorptive peaks and usually can be relieved by giving the drug in smaller but more frequent doses. They may reappear for several days each time the dosage is raised, but, with the exception of the tremor and occasionally the nausea, are usually transient and of little concern. If thirst and nausea recur after having subsided for some time, however, impending intoxication must be suspected and immediate (and repeated) serum lithium determinations obtained.

Serum lithium levels in excess of 2 mEq/1 (and in some cases, above 1.5 mEq/1) produce toxic symptoms much like those observed in tricyclic antidepressant poisoning. Besides thirst, anorexia, vomiting, and diarrhea, the symptoms include confusion, coarse tremor, muscle twitching, and dysarthria. With increasing toxicity, the symptoms become more severe: the patient's water intake and urinary output increase, and he exhibits ataxia, giddiness, muscle fasciculation and twitching, nystagmus, seizures, hyperreflexia, stupor, and eventually coma. One remarkable feature of the neurologic findings is that they are sometimes asymmetric. ECG changes, such as flattening and inversion of T-waves, occur in 20% of patients who receive moderate to high therapeutic doses of lithium for about two weeks (Schou 1969). Serial ECG tracings show potentiation and disorganization of background rhythm, diffuse slowing, and widening of the frequency spectrum with increasing lithium levels. Both ECG and EEG tracings return to the baseline as serum lithium levels fall, but the EEG abnormalities tend to lag behind the serum levels. Skin lesions ranging from generalized maculopapular rashes to leg ulcers, particularly on the exterior tibial region, have been reported also, but are rare and usually remit if the dosage is reduced and do not seem to recur even when the dose is increased again (Callaway 1968).

Lithium intoxication has no specific antidote. Given normal kidney function, serum lithium concentration decreases by one half every 24 to 36 hours, even without treatment. Water loading, large doses of thiazides, mercurials, and other diuretics increase water and sodium diuresis without having an appreciable effect on lithium excretion, but urea-induced diuresis, alkalinization of the urine with sodium lactate, and the administration of aminophylline increase elimination by 100% to 200% (Schou 1969). In any case, fatalities are rare: despite lithium's widespread use, first abroad and now in the United States, only 12 fatalities have been reported since 1949.

Except in cases of severe cardiovascular or renal disease, there are no absolute contraindications to the use of lithium therapy. Although no malformations were observed in the few cases in which lithium was given throughout pregnancy (Johansen 1969), too little is known of its teratogenic effects to warrant such use, particularly since it has been demonstrated to cross the placental barrier. Breast feeding is also to be avoided, as lithium is known to be excreted into the milk (Allgén 1969).

MENTAL ILLNESS, PSYCHOTROPIC AGENTS, AND DRIVING SAFETY

Patients, families, governmental agencies, and employers often ask the physician's advice concerning the effects of mental illness and psychotropic drugs on automobile driving (or for that matter, on the performance of such other potentially dangerous tasks as skiing or operating industrial machinery). It is known that individuals with alcoholism and mental illnesses, as well as those suffering from chronic medical and neurologic disorders, such as diabetes, peptic ulcer, cardiovascular illness, or epilepsy, have twice as many traffic accidents and an even larger proportion of traffic violations than drivers without such history (Crancer 1969, Waller 1963). Since the few statistics available do not differentiate between the accident rate of treated and untreated mental patients (or the effects of various treatments), however, a three-way comparison with drivers not suffering from such disorders is at the moment not feasible.

The decision whether or not a given individual should be permitted to drive can be extrapolated empirically only on the basis of what is known of the effects of particular mental illnesses, particular drugs, and the combination of the two on the skills needed to ensure driving safety: alertness, lucidity, sound judgment, good coordination, unimpaired vision, rapid reaction time, and the ability to remember and follow the rules of the road.

While the effect of a given mental illness on driving performance depends, of course, on the particular disorder's nature and severity, it is obvious that a moving automobile is a powerful weapon for the satisfaction of both aggressive and self-destructive impulses. The physician must therefore discourage driving if he fears that the patient might suddenly decide to use his car to commit suicide, react explosively to the everyday frustrations presented by other drivers who overtake or cut in front of him (MacDonald 1964, Muller 1965, Selzer 1963, 1969), or in some other way act bizarrely while at the wheel. A paranoid patient, for example, might take unnecessary risks to elude imagined pursuers; a patient with a retarded depression might ignore horns, traffic lights, and other vehicles; the hallucinating patient's voices might urge him to drive in some dangerous way; the epileptic, even if his seizures are only partial or last for no more than a moment or two, might lose control of the car, especially if he is sensitive to the flicker effect of oncoming cars; the patient with narcolepsy might fall asleep while speeding (Bartels 1965); the obsessive-compulsive might stop suddenly without prior warning to make sure he has not run over something on the road or lost a bolt on his axle; the manic patient tends to be accident-prone both because he habitually speeds and because he has so much confidence in himself that he takes unwarranted risks. The senile or otherwise organically damaged individual is among the most hazardous of drivers, for his deficiencies in judgment, vision, and coordination may be compounded by having forgotten the rules of the road or a tendency to lose his way and stop for directions anywhere he pleases, whether or not he is thus obstructing the flow of traffic.

The effect of psychotropic agents on driving safety is somewhat less obvious. Sedatives, minor tranquilizers, and, at least when first given, phenothiazines tend to dampen the individual's alertness, retard his reaction time and impair both his judgment and his motor coordination (Loomis 1958, McGuire 1958). Tricyclic antidepressants and some antiparkinsonian drugs cause blurred vision, and almost any of these agents may cause tremor and a diminution of motor coordination. Most psychotropic agents will have an additive, and perhaps even a synergistic, effect on a host of over-the-counter remedies that produce drowsiness, as well as alcohol, the most dangerous drug to take while driving (Braunstein 1968, Forney 1968, Landauer 1969, McCarroll 1962, Milner 1969, Reisby 1969, Waller 1966). Psychotropic agents with a mildly sedative and euphoriant effect may, like alcohol, impair the individual's assessment of his own performance (Hughes 1964, US Public Health Service 1968).

If the patient is intent on driving and his judgment and performance are not so severely impaired as to warrant exercising a forceful prohibition (such as hospitalization or notification of the pertinent regulatory authority), however, the physician must attempt to effect a compromise, because forbidding him to drive might cause him to discontinue drugs or office visits rather than driving. The drug's effect on his performance is spelled out (Tozer 1967), and he is asked to refrain from driving only until his mood, self-control, and thinking are improved and his drug regimen, and with it his blood pressure, alertness, and coordination, are stabilized. By the time this measure of improvement is achieved, most of the side effects that might have affected his driving will in all likelihood have diminished, and his overall driving performance will have improved, compared with what it would be were he not taking medications (Kornetsky 1959, Primac 1957, Rosner 1959).

ACCIDENTAL AND INTENTIONAL OVERDOSAGE WITH PSYCHOTROPIC AGENTS

The psychiatrist is not usually expected to manage acute overdosage, but he must be familiar with its effects in order to know how much medication can be safely prescribed at one time for the potentially suicidal patient and to determine the urgency with which treatment must be instituted for a patient who has taken an overdose. The two major principles of treatment are

1/ elimination of the offending agent by gastric lavage, induced vomiting, forced diuresis, or, if the intoxication is grave and the substance is dialyzable, peritoneal or hemodialysis; and

2/ supportive treatment designed to prevent or relieve such effects of poisoning as hypotension, shock, hyperpyrexia, respiratory depression, urinary retention, pneumonitis, other infections, extrapyramidal effects, or grand mal convulsions.

Tables 44 to 46 compare the doses customarily used with those known to produce intoxication and thereby provide some guidelines to the amount of drug a patient may safely be given to take at one time. This precaution is by no means foolproof, however, for the patient may well "save" his drugs, taking them all at once as part of a suicidal plan or, if he does not take them as prescribed, become so much worse that he then has both the motivation and the tools at hand. The figures given on maximum doses survived, on the number of overdosage fatalities, and on the minimal fatal dose should not be overvalued, however, because

1/ most clinical reports concerning intoxication provide insufficient information;

2/ intoxications that are survived are often not reported;

3/ many if not most intoxications entail the use of more than one drug;

4/ dosage of the ingested drug(s) rarely can be determined with objective accuracy, even with a history obtained directly from the patient or from the family;

5/ even in the very rare instances in which ingested drug(s) dosage actually can be established, there are factors (spontaneous vomiting, induced emesis, gastric lavage) that can lead to a difference between ingested dose and absorbed dose;

6/ the sole method for establishing what kind(s) and amount(s) of drug(s) actually entered the blood stream and tissues lies in competent laboratory determinations for fixation and quantification of drug(s). Too often, when one drug is found thus, no other is looked for, and a mixed intoxication thus escapes proper categorization; and

7/ the outcome of any case is dependent not only upon kind(s) and amount(s) of drug(s) ingested and absorbed, but upon

a/ the interval and environmental circumstances between ingestion and initiation of treatment,

b/ type of treatment,

c/ preexisting or concomitant disease, and

d/ tolerance and hepatic enzymatic activity in relation to "inducers" such as various CNS sedatives (Graeme 1969).

TABLE 44. *Overdosage with Major Tranquilizers*

	TYPICAL DAILY DOSE RANGE	MAXIMUM DOSE SURVIVED		NUMBER OF OVERDOSAGE FATALITIES *	MINIMUM FATAL DOSE REPORTED †	SYMPTOMS OF OVERDOSAGE
		IN ADULT	IN CHILD			
PHENOTHIAZINES: Fluphenazine (*Permitil, Prolixin*)	5-20 mg	1,500 mg in 27-year-old	15 mg in 3¾-year-old	2 deaths reported in patients taking drug seem unrelated to its use	—	Dystonia, akathisia, somnolence, weakness, muscular fasciculations, hyperreflexia, agitation, delirium, confusion, diaphoresis, convulsions. Also seen, but almost exclusively in cases of overdosage with the more "sedating" phenothiazines: tachycardia, hypotension, shock, cardiac arrhythmias, hypothermia, hyporeflexia, respiratory depression, coma.
Trifluoperazine (*Stelazine*)	15-40 mg	200 mg	250 mg in 41 lb. child	2	736 mg	
Perphenazine (*Trilafon*)	32-80 mg	No reports of overdosage	220 mg in 2-year-old	0	—	
Prochlorperazine (*Compazine*)	50-150 mg	1,000 mg	225 mg in 28 lb. child	2	Unknown	
Chlorpromazine (*Thorazine*)	400-800 mg	25,000 mg in 165 lb. person	2,000 mg in 30 lb. child	20-25	2,000 mg	
Thioridazine (*Mellaril*)	400-800 mg	20,000 mg	3,600 mg in 2-year-old	13	2,000 mg	

TABLE 44. *Overdosage with Major Tranquilizers* (continued)

	TYPICAL DAILY DOSE RANGE	MAXIMUM DOSE SURVIVED		NUMBER OF OVERDOSAGE FATALITIES *	MINIMUM FATAL DOSE REPORTED †	SYMPTOMS OF OVERDOSAGE
		IN ADULT	IN CHILD			
OTHERS:						
Chlorprothixene (*Taractan*)	150-400 mg	5,000 mg	1,000-1,500 mg in 1½-year-old	2 alone, 4 in combination with other drugs	1,250 mg in 47-year-old	Similar to above but without symptoms seen only with sedative phenothiazines.
Haloperidol (*Haldol*)	4-10 mg	1,000 mg	188 mg in 3-year-old	0 alone, but 1 in which 180 mg was taken in combination with 1,125 mg of amitriptyline	—	Similar to phenothiazines.
Reserpine (*Serpasil*)	4-10 mg	18,750 mg	10,000 mg in child of unreported age; 260 mg in 20-month-old boy	0	—	Similar to phenothiazines.

* NUMBER OF OVERDOSAGE FATALITIES PUBLISHED OR REPORTED TO US BY MANUFACTURER WHEN DRUG IN QUESTION WAS THE ONLY ONE TAKEN.

† MINIMUM FATAL DOSE REPORTED IN ADULT WHEN DRUG IN QUESTION WAS THE ONLY ONE TAKEN.

TABLE 45. *Overdosage with Minor Tranquilizers*

MINOR TRANQUILIZERS	TYPICAL DAILY DOSE RANGE FOR ADULTS	MAXIMUM DOSE SURVIVED		NUMBER OF OVERDOSAGE FATALITIES *	MINIMUM FATAL DOSE REPORTED †	SYMPTOMS OF OVERDOSAGE
		IN ADULT	IN CHILD			
PROPANEDIOLS:						
Meprobamate (*Equanil, Miltown*)	400-1,200 mg	40 Gm	Unknown	16	12 Gm	Drowsiness, ataxia, dysarthria, coma (up to 3 days), muscular facidity, hyporeflexia, bradycardia, respiratory depression, hypotension, hypothermia, shock (resembles barbiturate poisoning; see page 000).
Tybamate (*Solacen*) (*Tybatran*)	500-1,500 mg	14 Gm	No reports of overdosage	0	—	
BENZODIAZEPINES:						
Chlordiazepoxide (*Librium*)	20-60 mg	2,250 mg, possibly 3,750 mg	500 mg in 32 lb. child	2, perhaps 4; 20-54 additional in combination with other drugs	750 mg	As above but without hypotension or respiratory depression.
Diazepam (*Valium*)	5-15 mg	1,500 mg in 145 lb. person	300 mg in 2-year-old child	1, perhaps 2; 10-18 additional in combination with other drugs	640-940 mg in 186 lb. person	
Oxazepam (*Serax*)	30-90 mg	8-12 Gms.	90 mg in 28 lb., 2-year-old girl	0	—	

* NUMBER OF OVERDOSAGE FATALITIES PUBLISHED OR REPORTED TO US BY MANUFACTURER WHEN DRUG IN QUESTION WAS THE ONLY ONE TAKEN.

† MINIMUM FATAL DOSE REPORTED IN ADULT WHEN DRUG IN QUESTION WAS THE ONLY ONE TAKEN.

Table 46. Overdosage with Antidepressants

	TYPICAL DAILY DOSE RANGE	MAXIMUM DOSE SURVIVED		NUMBER OF OVERDOSAGE FATALITIES *	MINIMUM FATAL DOSE REPORTED †	SYMPTOMS OF OVERDOSAGE
		IN ADULT	IN CHILD			
DIBENZAZEPINES: Amitriptyline (Elavil)	100-300 mg	3,125 mg	1,750 mg in 2-year-old male	49	500 mg in 35-year-old female	Mydriasis, ataxia, dysarthria, confusion, hallucinations, clonic or athetoid movements, muscular fasciculations, convulsions, coma, hyper- or hyporeflexia, hypertension, hyperpyrexia, cardiac arrhythmias, respiratory depression, shock.
Desipramine (Norpramine, Pertofrane)	100-300 mg	3,250 mg in 46-year-old 126 lb. female (with 2,250 mg of chlorpromazine)	1,000 mg in 2½-year-old male	16	1,500 mg in 36-year-old female	
Imipramine (Tofranil)	100-300 mg	5,375 mg in 21-year-old female	1,800 mg in 3-year-old male	203	625 mg in 28-year-old female	
Nortriptyline (Aventyl)	20-100 mg	2,100 mg in female	550 mg in 10-year-old boy	5	1,100 mg (with meprobamate)	
Protriptyline (Vivactil)	20-60 mg	No reports of overdosage	No reports of overdosage	0	—	

TABLE 46. *Overdosage with Antidepressants* (continued)

	TYPICAL DAILY DOSE RANGE	MAXIMUM DOSE SURVIVED		NUMBER OF OVERDOSAGE FATALITIES *	MINIMUM FATAL DOSE REPORTED †	SYMPTOMS OF OVERDOSAGE
		IN ADULT	IN CHILD			
MAO INHIBITORS: Isocarboxazide (*Marplan*)	20-40 mg	350 mg in 40-year-old person	200 mg in 2-year-old child	7, all combined with other drugs	400 mg (with 400 mg of chlordiazepoxide)	Agitation, ataxia, dysarthria, tremor, hypotension and later hypertension, diaphoresis, tachypnea, confusion, hallucinations, hyperreflexia, clonus, hyperpyrexia, convulsions.
Nialamide (*Niamid*)	50-200 mg	1,500 mg	No reports of overdosage	1	5,000 mg in 27-year-old male	
Phenelzine (*Nardil*)	20-60 mg	750 mg	225 mg in child of 30 months; 300 mg in 10-year old child	6	375 mg	
Tranylcypromine (*Parnate*)	20-40 mg	750 mg	150 mg in 25 lb. child	4	170 mg	
MISCELLANEOUS: Lithium carbonate (*Lithonate*)	900-1,500 mg	24.5 Gm in 57-year-old female who had not previously taken drug; serum levels of 5.7 mEq have been survived	Unknown	12	1,600 mg daily for 6 days in 57-year-old man	See text.

* NUMBER OF OVERDOSAGE FATALITIES PUBLISHED OR REPORTED TO US BY MANUFACTURER WHEN DRUG IN QUESTION WAS THE ONLY ONE TAKEN.

† MINIMUM FATAL DOSE REPORTED IN ADULT WHEN DRUG IN QUESTION WAS THE ONLY ONE TAKEN.

In those rare cases in which the psychiatrist is called on to advise, the following general guidelines may be helpful:

1/ Psychotropic agents are relatively safe: of the more than 500 cases of overdosage reported prior to 1962, only 28 were fatal, 19 being due to meprobamate, 5 to antidepressants, and 4 to phenothiazines. Balancing each reported death, however, there was another case of overdosage with a similar drug that had been taken in greater amounts (both in absolute terms and in mg/kg) and had been survived.

2/ Convulsions secondary to phenothiazine overdosage should be managed with repeated small doses of a short-acting barbiturate in order to avoid potentiating CNS depression.

3/ Alerting phenothiazines taken in overdosage are rarely fatal, but may cause severe dystonias, which can be relieved with an antiparkinsonian agent. Nonatropinising antiparkinsonian drugs are to be preferred, especially if the patient has also taken an overdose of a tricyclic antidepressant, lest the combination produce an atropine psychosis.

4/ Emetics may be ineffective after phenothiazine overdosage, because of the strong antiemetic action of this class of tranquilizer.

5/ Neither dialysis nor forced diuresis is effective for phenothiazine and tricyclic antidepressant poisoning (Davis 1968a,b, Sjöqvist 1969).

6/ Pyridostigmine may be useful in counteracting the atropinelike effects on the cardiovascular system in tricyclic antidepressant poisoning (Rasmussen 1966).

7/ Stimulants, sympathomimetics, and sedatives that are potentiated by MAOIs should be used as antidotes for MAOI poisoning only with the greatest caution.

8/ The effects of overdosage with a CNS depressant usually reach their peak within one to two hours, with a phenothiazine within four to six hours, and with an MAOI sometimes not for 24 hours or more. It is unsafe, however, to take the patient's word for what he has taken or to consider the critical period to have passed solely on the information he provides. In any case, most poisonings are mixed, as the patient has probably taken a little or a lot of anything he has around or can get.

9/ Suicide attempts with pills have an unusually high incidence of recidivism. Patients who have made such attempts in the past should not be given renewable prescriptions and should not, especially while their depression remains acute, receive more than a few days' supply at a time. It is also advisable to instruct patients to bring all drugs they are no longer using to the physician's office rather than give them the responsibility for disposing of the drugs.

REFERENCES

Allgén, L. G.: Laboratory experience of lithium toxicity in man, Acta Psychiat Scand Suppl *207*:98-104, 1969.

Amdisen, A.: Changes of oral glucose tolerance test during long-term treatment with neuroleptics, Acta Psychiat Scand Suppl *203*:95-96, 1968.

——: Variation of serum lithium concentration during day in relation to treatment control, absorptive side effects and use of slow-release tablets, Acta Psychiat Scand Suppl *207*:55-58, 1969.

Annell, A.-L.: Lithium in treatment of children and adolescents, Acta Psychiat Scand Suppl *207*:19-33, 1969.

Appelbaum, A.: Opthalmoscopic study of patients under treatment with thioridazine, Arch Ophthal (Chicago) *69*:578-580, 1963.

Asatoor, A. M., Levi, A. J., and Milne, M. D.: Tranylcypromine and cheese, Lancet *2*:733-734, 1963.

Atkinson, R. M., and Ditman, K. S.: Tranylcypromine: a review, Clin Pharmacol Ther *6*:631-655, 1965.

Avery, C. W., *et al.:* Systematic errors in evaluation of side effects, Amer J Psychiat *123*:875-878, 1967.

Ayd, F. J., Jr.: Survey of drug-induced extrapyramidal reactions, JAMA *175*: 1054-1060, 1961.

——: Chlorpromazine: ten. years' experience, JAMA *184*:51-54, 1963.

——: Perphenazine: reappraisal after eight years, Dis Nerv Syst *25*:311-318, 1964.

Baastrup, P. C.: Practical clinical viewpoint regarding treatment with lithium, Acta Psychiat Scand Suppl *207*:12-18, 1969.

Ban, T. A.: Phenothiazines alone and in combination, Appl Ther *8*:530-535, 1966.

Ban, T. A., and St. Jean, A.: Electrocardiographic changes induced by phenothiazine drugs, Amer Heart J *70*:575-576, 1965.

Ban, T. A., and Stonehill, E.: Clinical observations on differential effects of butyrophenone (Haloperidol) and phenothiazine (Fluphenazine) in chronic schizophrenic patients, *in* Lehmann, H. E., and Ban, T. A., eds.: The Butyrophenones in Psychiatry, Quebec: First N Amer Sympos on Butyrophenones, 1964, pp. 113-119.

Barancik, M., Brandborg, L. L., and Albion, M. J.: Thioridazine-induced cholestasis, JAMA *200*:69-70, 1967.

Barker, P. A., Ashcroft, G. W., and Binns, J. K.: Imipramine in chronic depression, J Ment Sci *106*:1447-1451, 1960.

Barnes, A. B.: Diagnosis and treatment of abnormal breast secretions, New Eng J Med *275*:1184-1187, 1966.

Barron, A., Rudy, L. H., and Smith, J. A.: Clinical evaluation of a secondary amine, nortriptyline, Amer J Psychiat *121*: 268-269, 1964.

Barsa, J. A., and Kline, N. S.: Treatment of 200 disturbed psychotics with reserpine, JAMA *158*:110-113, 1955.

Bartels, E. C., and Kusakcioglu, O.: Narcolepsy: Possible cause of automobile accidents, Lahey Clin Found Bull *14*:21-26, 1965.

Bartholomew, L. G., *et al.:* Effect of chlorpromazine on liver, Gastroenterology *34*:1096-1107, 1958.

Battegay, R.: Drug dependence as criterion for differentiation of psychotropic drugs, Compr Psychiat *7*:501-509, 1966.

Beaulnes, A.: Aperçu sur la pharmacologie des butyrophenones, *in* Lehmann, H. E., and Ban, T. A., eds.: The Butyrophenones in Psychiatry, Quebec: First N Amer Sympos on Butyrophenones, 1964, pp. 1-11.

Behn, W., Frahm, M., and Fretwurst, E.: Über den diaplacentaren Übergang von Phenothiazin-Derivaten, Klin Wschr *34*: 872, 1956.

Berger, F. M.: Pharmacological properties of 2-methyl-2-n-propyl-1, 3-propanediol dicarbamate (Miltown), new interneuronal blocking agent, J Pharmacol Exp Ther *112*:413-423, 1954.

Berger, F. M., Kletzkin, M., and Margolin, S.: Pharmacologic properties of a new tranquilizing agent, 2-methyl-2-propyltrimethylene butylcarbamate carbamate (Tybamate), Med Exp (Basel) *10*:327-344, 1964.

Bernstein, S.: Serial observations on physiological and psychological changes in patients reacting with depression to reserpine, J Mount Sinai Hosp NY *24*:89-96, 1957.

Bernstein, S., and Kaufman, M. R.: Psychological analysis of apparent depression following rauwolfia therapy, J Mount Sinai Hosp NY *27*:525-530, 1960.

Bethune, H. C., Burrell, R. H., and Culpan, R. H.: Headache associated with monoamine oxidase inhibitors, Lancet *2*: 1233-1234, 1963.

Bethune, H. C., *et al.:* Vascular crises associated with monoamine oxidase inhibitors, Amer J Psychiat *121:*245-248, 1964.

Beutler, E.: reported in Siegel, I.: Symposium on adverse reactions to psychotropic drugs, Psychopharmacol Bull *3:*3-19, 1965.

Bird, C. E.: Agranulocytosis due to imipramine (Tofranil), Canad Med Ass J *82:*1021-1022, 1960.

Bishop, M. P., Fulmer, T. E., and Gallant, D. M.: Thiothixene versus trifluoperazine in newly-admitted schizophrenic patients, Curr Ther Res *8:*509-514, 1966.

Bishop, M. P., Gallant, D. M., and Steele, C. A.: Extended trial of thiothixene in chronic psychotic patients, Psychiat Dig *29:*15-22, 1968.

Bishop, M. P., Gallant, D. M., and Sykes, T. F.: Extrapyramidal side effects and therapeutic response, Arch Gen Psychiat (Chicago) *13:*155-162, 1965.

Blachly, P. H., and Starr, A.: Treatment of delirium with phenothiazine drugs following open heart surgery, Dis Nerv Syst 27 (Suppl):107-110, 1966.

Blacker, K. H., Weinstein, B. J., and Ellman, G. L.: Mother's milk and chlorpromazine, Amer J Psychiat *119:*178-179, 1962.

Blackwell, B., Marley, E., and Price, J.: Hypertensive interactions between monoamine oxidase inhibitors and foodstuffs, Brit J Psychiat *113:*349-365, 1967.

Blackwell, B., Marley, E., and Ryle, A.: Hypertensive crisis associated with monoamine-oxidase inhibitors, Lancet *1:*722-723, 1964.

Block, S. L.: Jaundice following thioridazine administration, Amer J Psychiat *119:*77, 1962.

Bloom, J. B., Davis, N., and Wecht, C. H.: Effect on liver of long-term tranquilizing medication, Amer J Psychiat *121:*788-797, 1965.

Blumberg, A. G., and Klein, D. F.: Chlorpromazine-procyclidine and imipramine: Effects on thyroid function in psychiatric patients, Clin Pharmacol Ther *10:*350-354, 1969.

Blumenthal, M., Davis, R., and Doe, R. P.: Carcinoid syndrome following reserpine therapy in thyrotoxicosis, Arch Intern Med (Chicago) *116:*819-823, 1965.

Bolton, B. H.: Prolonged chlorpromazine jaundice, Amer J Gastroent *48:*497-503, 1967.

Brauer, R., Harrow, M., and Tucker, G. J.: Depersonalization phenomena in psychiatric patients, Brit J Psychiat, 1970, to be published.

Braunstein, P. W., Weinberg, S. B., and Cortivo, L. D.: Drunk and drugged driver versus law, J Trauma *8:*83-90, 1968.

Brazier, M. A. B.: Effect of drugs on the electroencephalogram of man, Clin Pharmacol Ther *5:*102-116, 1964.

Breakstone, I. L.: Hypertensive reaction to two monoamine oxidase inhibitors, Amer J Psychiat *122:*104, 1965.

Brophy, J. J.: Single daily doses of neuroleptic drugs, Dis Nerv Syst *30:*120-123, 1969.

Brown, D. D., and Waldron, D. H.: Unusual reaction to tranylcypromine, Practitioner *189:*83-86, 1962.

Brown, J. D., and Stone, D. B.: IV. Oral hypoglycemic drugs, Curr Med Dig *36:*669-682, 1969.

Brumlik, J., *et al.:* Critical analysis of effects of trihexyphenidyl (Artane) on components of Parkinsonian syndrome, J Nerv Ment Dis *138:*424-431, 1964.

Budnick, I. S., Leikin, S., and Hoeck, L. E.: Effect in the new-born infant of reserpine administered ante partum, Amer J Dis Child *90:*286-289, 1955.

Bunney, W. E., Jr., and Davis, J. M.: Norepinephrine in depressive reactions: A review, Arch Gen Psychiat (Chicago) *13:*483-494, 1965.

Bunney, W. E., Jr., *et al.:* Behavioral-biochemical study of lithium treatment, Amer J Psychiat *125:*499-512, 1968.

Busfield, B. L., Jr., Schneller, P., and Capra, D.: Depressive symptom or side effect: Comparative study of symptoms during pretreatment and treatment periods of patients on three antidepressant medications, J Nerv Ment Dis *134:*339-352, 1962.

Cade, J. F. J.: Lithium salts in the treatment of psychotic excitement, Med J Aust *2:*349-352, 1949.

Caffey, E. M., Jr.: Experiences with large scale inter-hospital cooperative research in chemotherapy, Amer J Psychiat *177:*713-719, 1961.

Callaghan, N.: Restless legs syndrome in uremic neuropathy, Neurology *16:*359-361, 1966.

Callaway, C. L., Hendrie, H. C., and Luby, E. D.: Cutaneous conditions observed in patients during treatment with lithium, Amer J Psychiat *124:*1124-1125, 1968.

Carlson, K. E., and Alston, W.: Measurement of duration of effect of long-acting diazepam in spastic disorders, Arch Phys Med *49*:36-38, 1968.

Casey, J. F., *et al.*: Drug therapy in schizophrenia: Controlled study of relative effectiveness of chlorpromazine, promazine phenobarbital, and placebo, Arch Gen Psychiat (Chicago) *2*:210-220, 1960.

Chalmers, T. C.: reported in Siegel, I.: Symposium on adverse reactions to psychotropic drugs, Psychopharmacol Serv Bull *3*:3-19, 1965.

Christian, C. D., and Paulson, G.: Severe motility disturbance after small doses of prochlorperazine, New Eng J Med *259*: 828-830, 1958.

Claghorn, J. L., and Kinross-Wright, J.: Death rates in psychiatric outpatients, J Nerv Ment Dis *145*:163-167, 1967.

Clark, M. L., *et al.*: Evaluation of butaperazine in chronic schizophrenia, Clin Pharmacol Ther *9*:757-764, 1968.

Cohlan, S. Q.: Convulsive seizures caused by phenothiazine tranquilizers, Practitioner *21*:136-137, 1960.

Cole, J. O.: Symposium on long-acting injectable fluphenazine preparations—report, Psychopharmacol Bull *5*:16-18, 1969.

Connell, M. M., Polley, B. G., and McFarlane, J. R.: Chorioretinopathy associated with thioridazine therapy, Arch Ophthal (Chicago) *71*:816-821, 1964.

Cornu, F., and Hoffet, H.: Clinical experience with Taractan, Dis Nerv Syst *22*:40-44, 1961.

Crancer, A., Jr., and Quiring, D. L.: Mentally ill as motor vehicle operators, Amer J Psychiat *126*:807-813, 1969.

Crane, G. E.: Dyskinesia and neuroleptics, Arch Gen Psychiat (Chicago) *19*: 700-703, 1968.

Crause, J.: Jaundice associated with haloperidol, Lancet *2*:890-891, 1963.

Crosby, W. H., and Kaufman, R. M.: Drug-induced blood dyscrasias: IV. Thrombocytopenia, JAMA *189*:417-418, 1964.

Curry, S. H., *et al.*: Factors affecting chlorpromazine plasma levels in psychiatric patients, Arch Gen Psychiat (Chicago) *22*:209-215, 1970.

Curzon, G., Barrie, M., and Wilkinson, M. I. P.: Relationships between headache and amine changes after administration of reserpine to migrainous patients, J Neurol Neurosurg Psychiat *32*:555-561, 1969.

Cuthbert, M. F., Greenberg, M. P., and Morley, S. W.: Cough and cold remedies: Potential danger to patients on monoamine oxidase inhibitors, Brit Med J *1*: 404-406, 1969.

Cuthill, J. M., Griffiths, A. B., and Powell, D. E. B.: Death associated with tranylcypromine and cheese, Lancet *1:* 1076-1077, 1964.

Dally, P. J.: Fatal reaction associated with tranylcypromine and methylamphetamine, Lancet *1*:1235-1236, 1962.

——: Combining the antidepressant drugs, Brit Med J *1*:384, 1965.

——: Chemotherapy of Psychiatric Disorders, Great Britain: Logos Press Ltd, 1967.

Daneman, E. A.: Clinical experience and double-blind study of new antidepressant, Vivactil Hydrochloride, Psychosomatics *6*: 342-346, 1965.

d'Angeljan, G., Dausset, J., and Bernard, J.: Accidents sanguins provoqués par les phenothiazines, Bull Soc Med Hop Paris *116*:507-518, 1965.

Davies, R. K., *et al.*: Confusional episodes and antidepressant medication, Amer J Psychiat, in press.

Davis, J. M., Bartlett, E., and Termini, B. A.: Overdosage of psychotropic drugs: Review, 1: Major and minor tranquilizers, Dis Nerv Syst *29*:157-164, 1968a.

——: Overdosage of psychotropic drugs: Review, 2. Antidepressants and other psychotropic agents, Dis Nerv Syst *29*:246-256, 1968b.

Degkwitz, R.: Extrapyramidal motor disorders following long-term treatment with neuroleptic drugs, *in* Psychotropic Drugs and Dysfunctions of the Basal Ganglia. A Multidisciplinary Workshop, publication No. 1938, US Public Health Service, 1969.

Delay, J., and Deniker, P.: Trente-huit cas de psychoses traitées par la cure prolongée et continuée de 4560 RF, Le Congrès des Al et Neurol de Langue Fr in Compte rendu du Congrès, Paris: Masson et Cie, 1952.

Delay, J., *et al.*: L'action du halopéridol dans les psychoses, Acta Neurol Belg *60:* 21-38, 1960.

DeLong, S. L.: Incidence and significance of chlorpromazine-induced eye changes, Dis Nerv Syst *29*(Suppl):19-22, 1968.

Demars, J. P.: Neuromuscular effects of long-term phenothiazine medication, electroconvulsive therapy and leucotomy, J Nerv Ment Dis *143*:73-79, 1966.

Dencker, S. J., Enoksson, P., and Persson, P. S.: Pigment deposits in various organs during phenothiazine treatment, Acta Psychiat Scand *43*:21-31, 1967.

Denhoff, E.: Cerebral palsy: pharmacologic approach, Clin Pharmacol Ther *5:* 947-954, 1964.

Dillon, P. T., *et al.:* Reserpine in thyrotoxic crisis, New Eng J Med *283:*1020-1023, 1970.

DiMascio, A., and Shader, R. I.: Drug administration schedules, Amer J Psychiat *126:*796-901, 1969.

Divry, P., *et al.:* Expérimentation Psychopharmacologique d'un nouveau neuroleptique: le R. 1647, Acta Neurol Belg *59:* 1033-1044, 1959.

Domino, E. F.: Human pharmacology of tranquilizing drugs, Clin Pharmacol Ther *3:*599-664, 1962.

Dorrell, W.: Tranylcypromine and intracranial bleeding, Lancet *2:*300, 1963.

Druckman, R., Seelinger, D., and Thulin, B.: Chronic involuntary movements induced by phenothiazines, J Nerv Ment Dis *135:*69-76, 1962.

Duguay, R., and Flach, F. F.: Experimental study of weight changes in depressions, Acta Psychiat Scand *40:*1-9, 1964.

Engelhardt, D. M., *et al.:* Phenothiazines in prevention of psychiatric hospitalization, Arch Gen Psychiat (Chicago) *16:* 98-101, 1967.

Entwistle, C., Taylor, R. M., and MacDonald, I. A.: Treatment of mania with haloperidol (Serenace), J Ment Sci *108:* 373-375, 1962.

Erslev, A. J., and Wintrobe, M. M.: Detection and prevention of drug-induced blood dyscrasias, JAMA *181:*114-119, 1962.

Evans, W. L.: Effect of phenelzine in psychosomatic and psychophysiologic illnesses (final report), Psychosomatics *1:* 263-269, 1960.

Faretra, G., Dooher, L., and Dowling, J.: Comparison of haloperidol and fluphenazine in disturbed children, Amer J Psychiat *126:*1670-1673, 1970.

Faurbye, A., *et al.:* Neurological symptoms in pharmacotherapy of psychoses, Acta Psychiat Scand *40:*10-27, 1964.

Feaver, B. D., and MacEwan, D. W.: Effect of antidepressant drugs on urinary tract. Clinical and animal studies, J Canad Ass Radiol *18:*442-447, 1967.

Ferguson, R. S.: Reserpine and chronic psychosis: Two-year outcome in a treatment group, J Ment Sci *105:*251-255, 1959.

Ferreira, A. J., and Freeman, H.: Clinical trial of Marsilid in psychotic depressed patients, Amer J Psychiat *114:*933-934, 1958.

Fieve, R. R., Platman, S. R., and Plutchik, R. R.: Use of lithium in affective disorders: 1. Acute endogenous depression, 2. Prophylaxis of depression in chronic recurrent affective disorders, Amer J Psychiat *125:*487-498, 1968.

Fisher, T. L.: Intravenous promazine: Cautionary note, Canad Med Ass J *95:* 367, 1966.

Forney, R. B., and Hughes, F. W.: Alcohol with other depressants, *in* Combined Effects of Alcohol and Other Drugs, Springfield (Ill): Thomas, 1968, pp. 42-81.

Forrest, F. M., Forrest, I. S., and Mason, A. S.: Review of rapid urine tests for phenothiazine and related drugs, Amer J Psychiat *118:*300-307, 1961.

Forssman, H., and Walender, J.: Lithium treatment on atypical indication, Acta Psychiat Scand Suppl *207:*34-40, 1969.

Foster, C. A., *et al.:* Chlorpromazine: Study of its action in man, Lancet *2:*614-617, 1954.

Freedman, D. X.: Tranquilizer (definition), McGraw-Hill Encyclopedia of Science and Technology, New York: McGraw-Hill, 1960.

Freedman, D. X., and DeJong, J.: Factors that determine drug-induced akathisia, Dis Nerv Syst *22* (Suppl):69-76, 1961.

Freyhan, F. A.: Psychopharmacology and the controversial clinician, *in* Uhr, L., and Miller, J. G., eds.: Drugs and Behavior, New York: Wiley, 1960, pp. 184-198.

Fries, H.: Experience with lithium carbonate treatment at psychiatric department in period 1964-1967, Acta Psychiat Scand Suppl *207:*41-48, 1969.

Galbrecht, C. R., and Klett, C. J.: Predicting response to phenothiazines: The right drug for the right patient, J Nerv Ment Dis *147:*173-183, 1968.

Gallant, D. M., *et al.:* Withdrawal symptoms after abrupt cessation of antipsychotic compounds: Clinical confirmation in chronic schizophrenics, Amer J Psychiat *121:*491-493, 1964.

Gander, D. R.: Treatment of depressive illnesses with combined antidepressants, Lancet *2:*107-109, 1965.

Gantz, R. S., and Birkett, P.: Phenothiazine reduction as cause of rehospitalization, Arch Gen Psychiat (Chicago) *12:* 586-588, 1965.

General Practitioner Research Group: Oxazepam in anxiety (Report No. 112, General Practitioner Clinical Trials), Practitioner *199:*356-362, 1967.

Gerle, B.: Clinical observations of side effects of haloperidol, Acta Psychiat Scand *40:*65-76, 1964.

Gershon, S.: Possible thymoleptic effect of the lithium ion, Amer J Psychiat *124:* 1452-1456, 1968.

Gershon, S., *et al.*: Imipramine hydrochloride, Arch Gen Psychiat (Chicago) *6:* 96-101, 1962.

Gibbard, B. A., and Lehmann, H. E.: Therapy of phenothiazine-produced skin pigmentation: Preliminary report, Amer J Psychiat *123:*351-352, 1966.

Gilder, S. S. B.: The London letter: side effect of phenothiazines, Canad Med Ass J *91:*1081, 1964.

Giles, T. D., and Modlin, R. K.: Death associated with ventricular arrhythmia and thioridazine hydrochloride, JAMA *205:*108-110, 1968.

Gold, E. M., and Ganong, W. F.: Neuroendocrinology, *in* Martini, L., and Ganong, W. F., eds.: Effects of Drugs on Neuroendocrine Processes, vol 1, New York: Acad Press, 1967, pp 377-437.

Goldberg, L. I.: Monamine oxidase inhibitors: Adverse reactions and possible mechanisms JAMA *190:*456-462, 1964.

Goldberg, S. C., Klerman, G. L., and Cole, J. O.: Changes in schizophrenic psychopathology and ward behaviour as a function of phenothiazine treatment, Brit J Psychiat *111:*120-133, 1965.

Goldberg, S. C., *et al.*: Prediction of improvement in schizophrenia under four phenothiazines, Arch Gen Psychiat (Chicago) *16:*107-117, 1967.

Goldenberg, H., and Fishman, V.: Species dependence of chlorpromazine metabolism, Proc Soc Exp Biol Med *108:*178-182, 1961.

Goldstein, J. J., *et al.*: Psychophysiological and behavioral effects of phenothiazine administration in acute schizophrenics as function of premorbid status, J Psychiat Res *6:*271-287, 1969.

Gombos, G. M., and Yarden, P. E.: Ocular and cutaneous side effects after prolonged chlorpromazine treatment, Amer J Psychiat *123:*872-874, 1967.

Goodwin, F. K., Murphy, D. L., and Bunney, W. E., Jr.: Lithium-carbonate treatment in depression and mania, Arch Gen Psychiat (Chicago) *21:*486-469, 1969.

Goslin, E., and Kline, N. S.: Use of reserpine on admission service, Psychiat Res Rep *#1:*112-121, 1955.

Gottfries, C. G.: Effect of lithium salts on various kinds of psychiatric disorders, Acta Psychiat Scand Suppl *203:*157-167, 1968.

Graeme, J. L.: Personal communication, December, 1969.

Graupner, K. I., Murphree, O. D., and Meduna, L. J.: Electrocardiographic changes associated with use of thioridazine, J Neuropsychiat *5:*344-350, 1964.

Greenberg, H. R.: Erectile impotence during the course of Tofranil therapy, Amer J Psychiat *121:*1021, 1965.

Greenberg, H. R., and Carillo, C.: Thioridazine-induced inhibition of masturbatory ejaculation in adolescents, Amer J Psychiat *124:*991-993, 1968.

Greenblatt, M., Grosser, G. H., and Wechsler, H.: Comparative study of selected antidepressant medications and EST, Amer J Psychiat *119:*144-153, 1962.

Greiner, A. C., and Nicolson, G. A.: Pigment deposition in viscera associated with prolonged chlorpromazine therapy, Canad Med Ass J *91:*627-635, 1964.

Grinspoon, L., Ewalt, J. R., and Shader, R.: Psychotherapy and pharmacotherapy in chronic schizophrenia, Amer J Psychiat *124:*1645-1652, 1968.

Gross, H., and Kaltenbaeck, E.: Taractan (chlorprothixene) as neuroleptic drug in clinical psychiatry, Dis Nerv Syst *22:* 502-507, 1961.

Gupta, J. C., Deb, A. K., and Kahali, B. S.: Preliminary observations on use of rauwolfia serpentina benth. in treatment of mental disorders, Ind Med Gaz *78:*547, 1943.

Haase, H.-J., and Janssen, P. A. J.: The Action of Neuroleptic Drugs, a Psychiatric, Neurologic and Pharmacological Investigation, Amsterdam: North-Holland, 1965.

Haden, P.: Gastrointestinal disturbances associated with withdrawal of ataractic drugs, Canad Med Ass *91:*974-975, 1964.

Hagopian, V., Stratton, D. B., and Busiek, R. D.: Five cases of pigmentary retinopathy associated with thioridazine administration, Amer J Psychiat *123:*97-100, 1966.

Hankoff, L. D., and Heller, B.: Memory changes with MAO inhibitor therapy, Amer J Psychiat *117:*151-152, 1960.

Hanlon, T. E., *et al.*: Comparative effectiveness of amitriptyline, perphenazine, and combination in treatment of chronic psychotic female patients, J New Drugs *4:*52-60, 1964.

Hargreaves, M. A., and Maxwell, C.: Speed of action of desipramine: Controlled trial, Int J Neuropsychiat *3:*140-141, 1967.

Haškovec, L., and Ryšánek, K.: Action of reserpine in imipramine-resistant depressive patients, Psychopharmacologia (Berlin) *11:*18-30, 1967.

Healey, L. A., Harrison, M., and Decker, J. L.: Uricosuric effect of chlorprothixene, New Eng J Med *272:*526-527, 1965.

Hedberg, D. L., Gordon, M. W., and

Glueck, B. C.: Six cases of hypertensive crisis in patients on tranylcypromine after eating chicken livers, Amer J Psychiat 122: 933-937, 1966.

Heinrich, K., and Petrolowitsch, N.: Klinische Ergebnisse und psychopathologische Wirkungsformen der Therapie mit Monoaminoxydaseinhibitoren, Psychopharmacologia (Berlin) 1:506-522, 1960.

Hekimian, L. J., and Friedhoff, A. J.: Controlled study of placebo, chlordiazepoxide and chlorpromazine with thirty male schizophrenic patients, Dis Nerv Syst 28:675-678, 1967.

Henry, C. E., and Obrist, W. D.: Effect of meprobamate on electroencephalogram, J Nerv Ment Dis 126:268-271, 1958.

Hetzel, C. A.: Method for estimation of phenothiazine derivatives in urine and blood, Clin Chem 7:130-135, 1961.

Hilbert, G. H.: False-positive pregnancy tests caused by Sparine and Thorazine, J Florida Med Ass 45:655-657, 1958.

Hodge, J. V., Nye, E. R., and Emerson, G. W.: Monoamine-oxidase inhibitors, broad beans and hypertension, Lancet 1: 1108, 1964.

Hollister, L. E.: Complications from psychotherapeutic drugs I, II, III, New Eng J Med 264:291-293, 345-347, 399-400, 1961a.

———: Complications from psychotherapeutic drugs—1964, Clin Pharmacol Ther 5:322-333, 1964.

———: Toxicity of psychotherapeutic drugs, Practitioner 194:72-84, 1965b.

Hollister, L. E., Caffey, E. M., Jr., and Klett, C. J.: Abnormal symptoms, signs and laboratory tests during treatment with phenothiazine derivatives, Clin Pharmacol Ther 1:284-293, 1960.

Hollister, L. E., et al.: Studies of delayed action medication: V. Plasma levels and urinary excretion of four different dosage forms of chlorpromazine, Clin Pharmacol Ther 11:49-59, 1970.

Hollister, L. E., and Hall, R. A.: Phenothiazine derivatives and morphologic changes in the liver, Amer J Psychiat 123: 211-212, 1966.

Hollister, L. E., and Kosek, J. C.: Sudden death during treatment with phenothiazine derivatives, JAMA 192:1035-1038, 1965a.

Hollister, L. E., Motzenbecker, F. P., and Degan, R. O.: Withdrawal reactions from chlordiazepoxide (Librium), Psychopharmacologia (Berlin) 2:63-68, 1961b.

Honigfeld, G., et al.: Behavioral improvement in the older schizophrenic patient. Drug and social therapies, J Amer Geriat Soc 13:57-72, 1965.

Hooper, J. H., Jr., Welch, V. C., and Shackelford, R. T.: Abnormal lactation associated with tranquilizing drug therapy, JAMA 178:506-507, 1961.

Hordern, A., et al.: Amitriptyline in depressive states: Phenomenology and prognostic considerations, Brit J Psychiat 109: 815-825, 1963.

———: Amitriptyline in depressive states: Six month treatment results, Brit J Psychiat 110:641-647, 1964.

Hordern, A., Somerville, don M., and Krupinski, J.: Does chronic schizophrenia respond to combination of neuroleptic and antidepressant?, J Nerv Ment Dis 134:361-376, 1962.

Howarth, E.: Possible synergistic effects of new thymoleptics in connection with poisoning, J Ment Sci 107:100-103, 1961.

Horwitz, D., et al.: Monoamine oxidase inhibitors, tyramine and cheese, JAMA 188:1108-1110, 1964.

Huang, C. L., and Kurland, A. A.: Quantitative study of chlorpromazine and its sulfoxides in urine of psychotic patients, Amer J Psychiat 118:428-437, 1961.

———: Perphenazine (Trilafon) metabolism in psychotic patients, Arch Gen Psychiat (Chicago) 10:639-646, 1964.

Huang, C. L., Sands, F. L., and Kurland, A. A.: Urinary thorazine metabolites in psychotic patients, Amer Gen Psychiat (Chicago) 8:301-307, 1963.

Hughes, F. W., and Forney, R. B.: Comparative effect of three antihistaminics and ethanol on mental and motor performance, Clin Pharmacol Ther 5:414-421, 1964.

Huguley, C. M., Jr.: Drug induced blood dyscrasias II. Agranulocytosis, JAMA 188: 817-818, 1964.

Huguley, C. M., Jr., Lea, J. W., Jr., and Butts, J. A.: Adverse hematologic reactions to drugs, Progr Hemat 5:105-136, 1966.

Hunter, R., Earl, C. J., and Janz, D.: Syndrome of abnormal movements and dementia in leucotomized patients treated with phenothiazines, J Neurol Neurosurg Psychiat 27:219-223, 1964.

Hussar, A. E.: Effect of tranquilizers on medical morbidity and mortality in mental hospital, JAMA 179:682-686, 1962.

Hussar, A. E., and Bragg, D. G.: Effect of chlorpromazine on swallowing function in chronic schizophrenic patients, Amer J Psychiat 126:570-573, 1969.

Huston, J. R., and Bell, G. E.: Effect of thioridazine hydrochloride and chlorpromazine on electrocardiogram, JAMA *198:* 134-138, 1966.

Jacobs, M. A., Globus, G., and Heim, E.: Reduction in symptomatology in ambulatory patients. The combined effects of a tranquilizer and psychotherapy, Arch Gen Psychiat (Chicago) *15:*45-53, 1966.

Jacobsen, E., and Skaarup, Y.: Experimental induction of conflict-behavior in cat: its use in pharmacological investigations, Acta Pharmacol et Toxicol *11:*117-124, 1955.

Janacek, J., et al.: Oxazepam in the treatment of anxiety states: A controlled study, J Psychiat Res *4:*199-206, 1966.

Janssen, P. A. J., et al.: Chemistry and pharmacology of CNS depressants related to 4-(4-Hydroxy-4-phenylpiperidino) butyrophenone, Part I: Synthesis and screening data in mice, J Med Chem *1:*281-297, 1959.

Jarecki, H. G.: Combined amitriptyline and phenelzine poisoning, Amer J Psychiat *120:*189, 1963.

Jarvik, M. E.: Drugs used in the treatment of psychiatric disorders, *in* Goodman, L. S., and Gilman, A., eds.: The Pharmacological Basis of Therapeutics, ed. 3, New York: Macmillan, 1965, pp. 159-214.

Jenner, F. A., and Kerry, R. J.: Comparison of diazepam, chlordiazepoxide and amylobarbitone (a multidose double-blind crossover study), Dis Nerv Syst *28:*245-249, 1967.

Johansen, K. T., and Ulrich, K.: Preliminary studies of possible teratogenic effect of lithium, Acta Psychiat Scand Suppl *207:*91-97, 1969.

Johnson, A. W., and Buffaloe, W. J.: Chlorpromazine epithelial keratopathy, Arch Ophthal (Chicago) *76:*664-667, 1966.

Johnson, F. P., et al.: Sudden death of catatonic patient receiving phenothiazine, Amer J Psychiat *121:*504-507, 1964.

Johnson, G., Gershon, S., and Hekimian, L. G.: Controlled evaluation of lithium and chlorpromazine in treatment of manic states, Interim Rep Compr Psychiat *9:*563-573, 1968.

Kaelbling, R.: Agranulocytosis due to chlordiazepoxide hydrochloride, JAMA *174:*1863-1865, 1960.

Kaim, S. C., Klett, C. J., and Rothfeld, B.: Treatment of the acute alcohol withdrawal state: Comparison of four drugs, Amer J Psychiat *125:*1640-1646, 1969.

Kane, F. J., Jr., and Anderson, W. B.: Fourth occurrence of oral moniliasis during tranquilizer therapy, Amer J Psychiat *120:*1199-1200, 1964.

Karn, W. N., Mead, B. T., and Fishman, J. J.: Double-blind study of chlorprothixene (Taractan), panpsychotropic agent, J New Drugs *1:*72-79, 1961.

Kelly, D., Brown, C. C., and Shaffer, J. W.: Controlled physiological, clinical and psychological evaluation of chlordiazepoxide, Brit J Psychiat *115:*1387-1392, 1969.

Kelly, H. G., Fay, J. E., and Laverty, S. G.: Thioridazine hydrochloride (Mellaril): Its effect on electrocardiogram and report of two fatalities with electrocardiographic abnormalities, Canad Med Asso J *89:*546-554, 1963.

Kellner, R., Kelly, A. V., and Sheffield, B. F.: Assessment of changes in anxiety in drug trial: Comparison of methods, Brit J Psychiat *114:*863-869, 1968.

Kielholz, P., and Battegay, R.: Behandlung depressiver Zustandsbilder: Unter spezieller Berücksichtigung von Tofranil, einem neuen Antidepressivum, Schweiz Med Wschr *88:*763-767, 1958.

Kiloh, L. G., Davidson, K., and Osselton, J. W.: Electroencephalographic study of analeptic effects of imipramine, Electroenceph Clin Neurophysiol *13:*216-223, 1961.

Kimball, R. W., and Goodman, M. A.: Effects of reserpine on amino-acid excretion in patients with migraine, J Neurol Neurosurg Psychiat *29:*190-191, 1966.

Kirk, L., Rasmussen, K. B., and Faurbye, A.: Retinopathy following thioridazine treatment, Acta Psychiat Scand, Suppl 217, p. 56, 1970.

Kirsner, J. B.: Drug-induced peptic ulcers, Ann Int Med *47:*666-699, 1957.

Klatskin, G.: Toxic and drug-induced hepatitis, *in* Schiff, L., ed.: Diseases of the Liver, ed. 3, Philadelphia: Lippincott, 1969, pp. 498-601.

Klein, D. F., and Davis, J. M.: Diagnosis and Drug Treatment of Psychiatric Disorders, Baltimore: Williams & Wilkins, 1969.

Klein, J. J., Segal, R. L., and Warner, R. R. P.: Galactorrhea due to imipramine, New Eng J Med *271:*510-512, 1964.

Klerman, G. L., et al.: Sedation and tranquilization: Comparison of effects of number of psychopharmacologic agents upon normal human subjects, Arch Gen Psychiat (Chicago) *3:*4-13, 1960.

Klerman, G. L., and Cole, J. O.: Clinical pharmacology of imipramine and related antidepressant compounds, Pharmacol Rev 17:101-141, 1965.

Kline, N. S.: Use of Rauwolfia serpentina Bentham in neuropsychiatric conditions, Ann NY Acad Sci 59:107-132, 1954.

Kline, N. S., and Saunders, J. C.: Reserpine in psychiatric and neurologic disorders, Med Clin N Amer 41:307-326, 1957.

Knox, J. M.: Photosensitivity reactions in various diseases, Postgrad Med 33:564-570, 1963.

Korenyi, C.: Effect of benzophenone sunscreen lotion on chlorpromazine-treated patients, Amer J Psychiat 125:971-974, 1969.

Kornetsky, C., et al.: Comparison of psychological effects of acute and chronic administration of chlorpromazine and secobarbital (Quinalbarbitone) in schizophrenic patients, J Ment Sci 105:190-198, 1959.

Korol, B., et al.: Effects of chronic chlorpromazine administration on systemic arterial pressure in schizophrenic patients: Relationship of body position to blood pressure, Clin Pharmacol Ther 6:587-591, 1965.

Kramer, J. C., Klein, D. F., and Fink, M.: Withdrawal symptoms following discontinuation of imipramine therapy, Amer J Psychiat 118:549-550, 1961.

Kuhn, R.: Über die Behandlung depressiver Zustände mit einem Iminodibenzylderivat (G 22355), Schweiz Med Wschr 87: 1135-1140, 1957.

Kurland, A. A., et al.: Comparative effectiveness of six phenothiazine compounds phenobarbital and inert placebo in treatment of acutely ill patients: Personality dimensions, J Nerv Ment Dis 134:48-61, 1962.

Kurland, A. A., et al.: Critical study of isocarboxazid (Marplan) in treatment of depressed patients, J Nerv Ment Dis 145:292-305, 1967.

Kurland, A. A., Ferro-Diaz, P., and Mc-Cusker, K.: Butyrophenones in the treatment of the psychotic patient, Compr Psychiat 5:179-190, 1964.

Kurland, A. A., Michaux, M. H., and Hanlon, T. E.: Methodological considerations in combined psychotropic drug research, Excerpta Med Internat Congr, Series 129, 1966, pp. 489-495.

Landauer, A. A., Milner, G., and Patman, J.: Alcohol and amitriptyline effects on skills related to driving behavior, Science 163:1467-1468, 1969.

Lapolla, A., and Nash, L. R.: Comparative clinical study of prochlorperazine, SKF 4579, perphenazine, triflupromazine, chlorpromazine and reserpine, Clin Med 72:495-503, 1965.

Lasky, J. J., et al.: Drug treatment of schizophrenic patients: A comparative evaluation of chlorpromazine, chloroprothixene, fluphenazine, reserpine, thioridazine and triflupromazine, Dis Nerv Syst 23:1-8, 1962.

Lee, F. I.: Imipramine overdosage—report of fatal case, Brit Med J 1:338-339, 1961.

Le Gassicke, J., and McPherson, F. M.: Sequential trial of WY 3498 (Oxazepam), Brit J Psychiat 3:521-525, 1965a.

Le Gassicke, J., et al.: Clinical state, sleep and amine metabolism of tranylcypromine ("Parnate") addict, Brit J Psychiat 3:357-364, 1965b.

Lehmann, H. E.: Use and abuse of phenothiazines, Appl Ther 5:1057-1069, 1963.

———: Clinical perspectives on antidepressant therapy, Amer J Psychiat 124: 12-21, 1968.

Lehmann, H. E., Cahn, C. H., and de Verteuil, R. L.: Treatment of depressive conditions with imipramine (G 22355), Canad Psychiat Ass J 3:155-164, 1958.

Little, S. C., and Green, J.: Intravenous use of diazepam in focal status epilepticus, Southern Med J 62:381-385, 1969.

Logothetis, J.: Spontaneous epileptic seizures and electroencephalographic changes in course of phenothiazine therapy, Neurology 17:869-877, 1967.

Lomas, J., Boardman, R. H., and Markowe, M.: Complications of chlorpromazine therapy in 800 mental-hospital patients, Lancet 1:1144-1147, 1955.

Loomis, T. A., and West, T. C.: Influence of alcohol on automobile driving ability: experimental study for evaluation of certain medicological aspects, Quart J Stud Alcohol 19:30-46, 1958.

Lorr, M., McNair, D. M., and Weinstein, G. J.: Early effects of chloridazepoxide (Librium) used with psychotherapy, J Psychiat Res 1:257-270, 1963.

Lowther, J.: Effect of fluphenazine enanthate on chronic and relapsing schizophrenia, Brit J Psychiat 115:691-692, 1969.

Luby, E. D., and Domino, E. F.: Toxicity from large doses of imipramine and an MAO inhibitor in suicidal intent, JAMA 177:68-69, 1961.

Luckey, W. T., and Schiele, B. C.: Comparison of haloperidol and trifluoperazine (double-blind controlled study on chronic schizophrenic outpatients), Dis Nerv Syst *28:*181-186, 1967.

Ludwig, B. J., and Piech, E. C.: Some anticonvulsant agents derived from 1,3-propanediols, J Amer Chem Soc *73:*5779-5781, 1951.

Lutz, E. G.: Dissipation of phenothiazine effect and recurrence of schizophrenic psychoses, Dis Nerv Syst *26:*355-357, 1965.

Macdonald, J. M.: Suicide and homicide by automobile, Amer J Psychiat *121:*366-370, 1964.

Maggs, R.: Treatment of manic illness with lithium carbonate, Brit J Psychiat *109:*56-65, 1963.

Maggs, R., and Ellison, R. M.: Five-year follow-up of results of reserpine therapy in mental hospital practice, J Ment Sci *106:*590-598, 1960.

Mandel, A., and Gross, M.: Agranulocytosis and phenothiazines, Dis Nerv Syst *29:*32-36, 1968.

Marjerrison, G., *et al.:* Withdrawal of long-term phenothiazines from chronically hospitalized psychiatric patients, Canad Psychiat Ass J *9:*290-298, 1964.

Marks, V., and Shackcloth, P.: Diagnostic pregnancy tests in patients treated with tranquillizers, Brit Med J *1:*517-519, 1966.

Maronde, R. F., *et al.:* Monoamine oxidase inhibitor, pargyline hydrochloride, and reserpine. Their evaluation as antihypertensive drugs, JAMA *184:*7-10, 1963.

Marsh, H. O.: Diazepam in incapacitated cerebral-palsied children, JAMA *191:*797-800, 1965.

Mason, A.: Fatal reaction associated with tranylcypromine and methylamphetamine, Lancet *1:*1073, 1962.

Masserman, J. H., and Yum, K. S.: Analysis of influence of alcohol on experimental neurosis in cats, Psychosom Med *8:*36-52, 1946.

Mathalone, M. B. R.: Oculocutaneous effects of chlorpromazine, Lancet *2:*111-112, 1965.

——: Ocular effects of phenothiazine derivatives and reversibility, Dis Nerv Syst *29:*29-35, 1968.

May, P. R. A.: Treatment of Schizophrenia: Comparative Study of Five Treatment Methods, New York: Science House, 1968.

May, R. H., *et al.:* Thioridazine therapy: Results and complications, J Nerv Ment Dis *130:*230-234, 1960.

McCarroll, J. R., and Haddon, W., Jr.: Controlled study of fatal automobile accidents in New York City, J Chronic Dis *15:*811-826, 1962.

McClure, J. L.: Reactions associated with tranylcypromine, Lancet *1:*1351, 1962.

McConaghy, N., *et al.:* Controlled trial comparing amitriptyline and protriptyline in treatment of out-patient depressives, Med J Aust *2:*403-405, 1965.

McFarland, R. B.: Fatal drug reaction associated with prochlorperazine (compazine), Amer J Clin Path *40:*284-290, 1963.

McGuire, T. F., and Leary, F. J.: Tranquilizing drugs and stress tolerance, Amer J Public Health *48:*578-584, 1958.

McKinney, W. T., and Kane, F. J.: Pancytopenia due to chlorpromazine, Amer J Psychiat *123:*879-880, 1967.

The Medical Letter *5:*(May 24), 1963.

Ibid. 10:(October 18), 1968.

Ibid. 11:(October 3), 1969.

Ibid. 12:(April 3), 1970.

Meduna, L. G., Abood, L. G., and Biel, J. H.: N(γ-methylaminopropyl) iminodibenzyl: New antidepressant, preliminary report, J Neuropsychiat *2:*232-237, 1961.

Mendels, J.: Comparative trial of nortriptyline and amitriptyline in 100 depressed patients, Amer J Psychiat *124:*59-62, 1968.

Miller, M.: Neuropathy, agranulocytosis, and hepato-toxicity following imipramine therapy, Amer J Psychiat *120:*185-186, 1963.

Miller, M., and Detre, T. P.: Unpublished data.

Milner, G.: Drinking and driving in 753 general practice and psychiatric patients on psychotropic drugs, Brit J Psychiat *115:*99-100, 1969.

Milner, G., and Buckler, E. G.: Adynamic ileus and amitriptyline: Three case reports, Med J Aust *1:*921-922, 1964.

Mock, J. E., Rickels, K., and Yee, R.: Clinical evaluation of hydroxyzine and placebo in anxious psychiatric outpatients, Int J Neuropsychiat *1:*168-172, 1965.

Moorhead, C. N., and Knox, S. J.: Imipramine-induced auricular fibrillation, Amer J Psychiat *122:*216-217, 1965.

Morgan, D. H.: Jaundice associated with amitriptyline, Brit J Psychiat *115:*105-106, 1969.

Morton, M. R.: Study of withdrawal of chlorpromazine or trifluoperazine in chronic schizophrenia, Amer J Psychiat *124:*1585-1588, 1968.

Mosbech, J.: EKG changes under Tofranil (imipramine) treatment, Nord Psychiat T *14:*326-328, 1960.

Müller, E.: Verkehrsunfall und Selbstmord, Arch fur Kriminologie *135*:61-69, 1965.

Muller, O. F., Goodman, N. and Bellet, S.: Hypotensive effect of imipramine hydrochloride in patients with cardiovascular disease, Clin Pharmacol Ther *2*:300-307, 1961.

Myrianthopoulos, N. C., Kurland, A. A., and Kurland, L. T.: Hereditary predisposition in drug-induced parkinsonism, Arch Neurol (Chicago) *6*:5-9, 1962.

National Institute Mental Health (Collaborative Study Group): Phenothiazine treatment in acute schizophrenia: Effectiveness, Arch Gen Psychiat (Chicago) *10*:246-261, 1964.

———: Difference in clinical effects of three phenothiazines in "acute" schizophrenia, Dis Nerv Syst *28*:369-383, 1967.

Nørredam, K.: Chlorpromazine jaundice of long duration, Acta Med Scand *174*:163-170, 1963.

Nymark, M., and Nielsen, I. M.: Reactions due to combination of monoamineoxidase inhibitors with thymoleptics, pethidine, or methylamphetamine, Lancet *2*:524-525, 1963.

Oakley, D. P., and Lautch, H.: Haloperidol and anticoagulant treatment, Lancet *2*:1231, 1963.

Oates, J. A., and Sjoerdsma, A.: Neurologic effects of tryptophan in patients receiving monoamine oxidase inhibitor, Neurology *10*:1076-1078, 1960.

Overall, J. E. *et al.*: Comparison of acetophenazine with perphenazine in schizophrenics: Demonstration of differential effects based on computer-derived diagnostic models, Clin Pharmacol Ther *4*:200-208, 1963.

Palmer, H.: Potentiation of pethidine, Brit Med J *2*:944, 1960.

Pare, C. M. B.: Treatment of depression, Lancet *1*:923-925, 1965.

Parsonage, M. J., and Norris, J. W.: Use of diazepam in treatment of severe convulsive status epilepticus, Brit Med J *3*:85-88, 1967.

Paulson, G.: Treatment of posttraumatic headache with imipramine, Amer J Psychiat *119*:368, 1962.

Perrot, P., and Bourjala, J.: Cas pour diagnostic "un visage mauve," Bull Soc Franc Derm Syph *69*:631, 1962.

Petersen, P. V., and Nielsen, I. M.: Thioxanthene derivatives *in* Gordon, M., ed.: Psychopharmacological Agents, vol. 1, New York: Acad Press, 1964, p. 301.

Pettinger, W. A., and Oates, J. A.: Supersensitivity to tyramine during monoamine oxidase inhibition in man. Mechanism at the level of the adrenergic neuron, Clin Pharmacol Ther *9*:341-344, 1968.

Pilling, H. H.: Tranylcypromine and convulsions, Brit Med J *2*:1130, 1963.

Pisciotta, A. V.: Studies on agranulocytosis. VII. Limited proliferative potential of CPZ-sensitive patients, J Lab Clin Med *65*:240-247, 1965a.

———: Mechanisms of phenothiazine induced agranulocytosis, *in* Efron, D. H., *et al.*, eds.: Psychopharmacology: A Review of Progress 1957-1967, US Pub Health Serv Pub #1836, 1968, pp. 597-605.

———: Agranulocytosis induced by certain phenothiazine derivatives, JAMA *208*:1862-1868, 1969.

Pisciotta, A. V., and Santos, A. S.: Studies on agranulocytosis VI. Effect of clinical treatment with chlorpromazine on nucleic-acid synthesis of granulocyte precursors in normal persons, J Lab Clin Med *65*:228-239, 1965b.

Plachta, A.: Asphyxia relatively inherent to tranquilization, Arch Gen Psychiat (Chicago) *12*:152-158, 1965.

Plass, H. F. R.: Monoamine-oxidase inhibitor reactions simulating phenochromocytoma attacks, Ann Intern Med *61*:924-927, 1964.

Pöldinger, W.: Combined administration of desipramine and reserpine or tetrabenzine in depressive patients, Psychopharmacologia (Berlin) *4*:308-310, 1963.

Pollack, B., Buck, I. F., and Kalnins, L.: Oral syndrome complicating psychopharmocotherapy: Study II, Amer J Psychiat *121*:384-386, 1964.

Popper, H.: Symposium on clinical drug evaluation and human pharmocology. VIII: Potential drug toxicity to the liver, Clin Pharmacol Ther *3*:385-388, 1962.

Popper, H., *et al.*: Drug-induced liver disease, Arch Intern Med (Chicago) *115*:128-136, 1965.

Popper, H., and Schaffner, F.: Drug-induced hepatic injury, Ann Intern Med *51*:1230-1252, 1959.

Prien, R. F., and Cole, J. O.: High dose chlorpromazine therapy in chronic schizophrenia, Arch Gen Psychiat (Chicago) *18*:482-495, 1968.

Prien, R. F., Levine, J., and Cole, J. O.: High dose trifluoperazine therapy in chronic schizophrenia, Amer J Psychiat *126*:305-313, 1969.

Prien, R. F., *et al.*: Ocular changes occurring with prolonged high dose chlorpromazine therapy. Results from a collaborative study, Arch Gen Psychiat (Chicago) 23:464-468, 1970.

Primac, D. W., Mirsky, A. F., and Rosvold, H. E.: Effects of centrally acting drugs on two tests of brain damage, Arch Neurol Psychiat 77:328-332, 1957.

Pryce, I. G., and Edwards, H.: Persistent oral dyskinesia in female mental hospital patients, Brit J Psychiat 112:983-987, 1966.

Raab, E., Rickels, K., and Moore, E.: Double blind evaluation of tybamate in anxious neurotic medical clinic patients, Amer J Psychiat 120:1005-1007, 1964.

Raskin, A.: High dosage chlorpromazine alone and in combination with an antiparkinsonian agent (procyclidine) in the treatment of hospitalized depressions, J Nerv Ment Dis 147:184-195, 1968.

Raskin, A., et al.: Differential response to chlorpromazine, imipramine, and placebo. A study of subgroups of hospitalized depressed patients, Arch Gen Psychiat (Chicago) 23:164-173, 1970.

Rasmussen, J.: Poisoning by amitriptyline, imipramine and nortriptyline, Danish Med Bull 13:201-203, 1966.

Rees, L., and Davies, B.: Study of value of haloperidol in management and treatment of schizophrenic and manic patients, Int J Neuropsychiat 1:263-266, 1965.

Reisby, N., and Theilgaard, A.: Interaction of alcohol and meprobamate in man, Acta Psychiat Scand Suppl 208, 1969.

Reitano, S., and Mase G.: Experimental observations and physiopathological considerations on some unusual aspects of dysleptic attacks caused by haloperidol, Rass Neuropsychiat 20:589-605, 1966.

Reynolds, E., et al.: Physicians' preferences in a blind trial of imipramine and amitriptyline, Brit J Psychiat 115:1175-1179, 1969.

Richardson, H. L., and Graupner, K. I. and Richardson, M. E.: Intramyocardial lesions in patients dying suddenly and unexpectedly, JAMA 195:254-260, 1966.

Rickels, K., et al.: Doxepin and diazepam in general practice and hospital clinic neurotic patients: A collaborative controlled study, Psychopharmacologia (Berlin) 15:265-279, 1969.

Rinaldi, F., and Himwich, H. E.: Comparison of effects of reserpine and some barbiturates on electrical activity of cortical and subcortical structures of brain of rabbits, Ann NY Acad Sci 61:27-35, 1955.

Rosen, B., et al.: Hospitalization proneness scale as predictor of response to phenothiazine treatment, J Nerv Ment Dis 146:476-480, 1968.

Rosenthal, D. S., Stein, G. F., and Santos, J. C.: Thioridazine agranulocytosis, JAMA 200:81-82, 1967.

Rosner, B. S., Ameen, L., and Kolers, P. A.: Effects of Thorazine and Mebaral on alertness in psychotic patients, Curr Ther Res 1:55-58, 1959.

Roth, J. L. A.: Role of drugs in production of gastroduodenal ulcer, JAMA 187:418-422, 1964.

Rothenberg, P. A., and Hall, C.: Agranulocytosis following use of imipramine hydrochloride (Tofranil), Amer J Psychiat 116:847, 1960.

Rumpf, G. E. (1755): Herbari amboinensis auctuarium, in Schlittler, E., and Plummer, A. J.: Tranquilizing Drugs from Rauwolfia, in Gordon, M., ed.: Psychopharmacological Agents, New York: Acad Press, 1964.

Salzman, N. P., and Brodie, B. B.: Physiological disposition and fate of chlorpromazine and method for its estimation in biological material, J Pharmacol Exp Ther 118:46-54, 1956.

Scanlan, E. P., and May, A. E.: Controlled trial of Taractan in chronic schizophrenia, Brit J Psychiat 109:418-421, 1963.

Schaaf, M., and Payne, C. A.: Dystonic reactions to prochlorperazine in hypoparathyroidism, New Eng J Med 275:991-995, 1966.

Schallek, W., Kuehn, A., and Jew, N.: Effects of chlordiazepoxide (Librium) and other psychotropic agents on the limbic system of the brain, Ann NY Acad Sci 96:303-314, 1962.

Schindler, W., and Häfliger, F.: Über Derivate des Iminodibenzyls, Helv Chim Acta 37:472-483, 1954.

Schlagenhauf, G., Tupin, J., and White, R. B.: Use of lithium carbonate in treatment of manic psychoses, Amer J Psychiat 123:201-205, 1966.

Schmidt, W. R., and Jarcho, L. W.: Persistent dyskinesias following phenothiazine therapy, Arch Neurol (Chicago) 14:369-377, 1966.

Schorer, C. E.: Report of hypomanic excitement with imipramine treatment of depression, Amer J Psychiat 116:844-845, 1960.

Schou, M.: Electrocardiographic changes during treatment with lithium and with drugs of the imipramine-type, Acta Psychiat Scand 38:331-336, 1962.

————: Occurrence of goitre during lithium treatment, Brit Med J *3:*710-713, 1968.

————: Lithium: Elimination rate, dosage, control, poisoning, goiter, mode of action, Acta Psychiat Scand Suppl *207:*49-54, 1969.

Schou, M., *et al.:* Treatment of manic psychoses by administration of lithium salts, J Neurol Neurosurg Psychiat *17:* 250-260, 1954.

Schroeder, H. A., and Perry, H. M.: Psychoses apparently produced by reserpine, JAMA *159:*839-840, 1955.

Schwarz, L., and Munoz, R.: Blood sugar levels in patients treated with chlorpromazine, Amer J Psychiat *125:*253-255, 1968.

Sedivec, V.: Effect of psychotropic drugs on electrical brain activity, Activ Nerv Sup (Praha) *6:*204-205, 1964.

Selzer, M. L., *et al.:* Alcoholism, mental illness and the "drunk driver," Amer J Psychiat *120:*326-331, 1963.

————: Alcoholism, mental illness, and stress in 96 drivers causing fatal accidents, Behav Sci *14:*1-10, 1969.

Sereny, G., and Kalant, H.: Comparative clinical evaluation of chlordiazepoxide and promazine in treatment of alcohol-withdrawal syndrome, Brit Med J *1:* 92-97, 1965.

Shader, R. I., and DiMascio, A.: Endocrine effects of psychotropic drugs: I. Galactorrhea and gynecomastia, Conn Med *32:*106-108, 1968.

Sharp, W. L.: Convulsions associated with antidepressant drugs, Amer J Psychiat *117:*458-459, 1960.

Shaw, E. B.: Side reactions from tranquilizing drugs, Pediat Clin N Amer *7:* 257-267, 1960.

Shawver, J. R., and Tarnowski, S. M.: Thrombocytopenia in prolonged chlorpromazine therapy, Amer J Psychiat *116:*845-846, 1960.

Shelton, J. G., Kingston, W. R., and McRae, C.: Aplastic anaemia and agranulocytosis following chlorpromazine therapy, Med J Aust *1:*130-131, 1960.

Sheppard, C., and Merlis, S.: Drug-induced extrapyramidal symptoms: Their incidence and treatment, Amer J Psychiat *123:*886-889, 1967.

Siddall, J. R.: Ocular toxic findings with prolonged and high dosage chlorpromazine intake, Arch Ophthal (Chicago) *74:* 460-464, 1965.

————: Ocular complications related to phenothiazines, Dis Nerv Syst *29:*10-13, 1968.

Siede, H., and Müller, H. F.: Choreiform movements as side effects of phenothiazine medication in geriatric patients, J Amer Geriat Soc *15:*517-522, 1967.

Siegel, I.: Symposium on adverse reactions to psychotropic drugs, Psychopharmacol Bull *3:*3-23, 1965.

Simonson, M.: Phenothiazine depressive reaction, J Neuropsychiat *5:*259-265, 1964.

Simpson, G. M., Amin, M., and Kunz, E.: Withdrawal effects of phenothiazines, Compr Psychiat *6:*347-351, 1965.

Simpson, G. M., and Angus, J. W. S.: Drug induced extrapyramidal disorders, Acta Psychiat Scand Suppl 212, 1970.

Simpson, G. M., *et al.:* Phenothiazine-produced extra-pyramidal system disturbance, Arch Gen Psychiat (Chicago) *10:*199-208, 1964.

Sjöqvist, F., *et al.:* pH-dependent excretion of monomethylated tricyclic antidepressants—In dog and man, Clin Pharmacol Ther *10:*826-833, 1969.

Sletten, I. W., *et al.:* Chronic chlorpromazine administration: Some pharmacological and psychological effects in man, Clin Pharm Ther *6:*575-586, 1965.

Sletten, I. W., and Gershon, S.: Premenstrual syndrome, discussion of its pathophysiology and treatment with lithium ion, Compr Psychiat *7:*197-206, 1966.

Solomon, F. A., and Campagna, F. A.: Jaundice due to prochlorperazine (Compazine), Amer J Med *27:*840-843, 1959.

Somlyo, A. P., and Waye, J. D.: Abnormal lactation: Report of case induced by reserpine and brief review of subject, J Mount Sinai Hosp NY *27:*5-9, 1960.

Steiner, W. G., and Pollack, S. L.: Limited usefulness of EEG as a diagnostic aid in psychiatric cases receiving tranquilizing drug therapy, *in* Himwich, W. A., and Schade, J. P., eds.: Progress in Brain Research, vol. 16, Amsterdam: Elsevier, 1965.

Sternbach, L. H., and Reeder, E.: Quinazolines and 1,4-benzodiazepines II. Rearrangement of 6-chloro-2-chloromethyl-4-phenylquinazoline 3-oxide into 2-amino derivatives of 7-chloro-5-phenyl-3h-1, 4-benzodiazepine 4-oxide, J Org Chem *26:* 1111-1118, 1961.

Stewart, A., Lafave, H. G., and Segovia, G.: Haloperidol—New addition to the drug treatment of schizophrenia, Behav Neuropsychiat *1:*23-28 (No. 7), 1969.

Sugihara, H., Ishihara, K., and Noguchi, H.: Clinical experience with amitriptyline (Tryptanol) in treatment of bronchial asthma, Ann Allergy *23:*422-429, 1965.

Sulman, F. G.: Mammotropic effect of ataractic drugs, Biochem Pharmacol *8:*101-102, 1961.

Swartzburg, M.: Unpublished data.

Szatmari, A.: Clinical and electroencephalogram investigation on Largactil in psychoses (preliminary study), Amer J Psychiat *112*:788-794, 1956.

Tandon, R. N., Sur, B. K., and Nath, K.: Effect of reserpine injections in migrainous and normal control subjects, with estimations of urinary 5-hydroxyindoleacetic acid, Neurology *19*:1073-1079, 1969.

Taubel, D. E.: Mellaril: Ejaculation disorders, Amer J Psychiat *119*:87, 1962.

Taylor, D. C.: Alarming reaction to pethidine in patients on phenelzine, Lancet *2*:401-402, 1962.

Thomsen, K., and Schou, M.: Renal lithium excretion in man, Amer J Physiol *215*:823-827, 1968.

Thonnard-Neumann, E.: Phenothiazines and diabetes in hospitalized women, Amer J Psychiat *124*:978-982, 1968.

Tozer, F. L., and Kasik, J. E.: Medical-legal aspects of adverse drug reactions, Clin Pharmacol Ther *8*:637-646, 1967.

Uhrbrand, L., Faurbye, A.: Reversible and irreversible dyskinesia after treatment with perphenazine, chlorpromazine, reserpine and electroconvulsive therapy, Psychopharmacologia (Berlin) *1*:408-418, 1960.

US Pub Health Serv Pub No. 1640: Alcohol and Alcoholism, Washington, DC: Government Printing Office, 1968.

Van de Wiele, R. L., and Turksoy, R. N.: Treatment of amenorrhea and anovulation with human menopausal and chorionic gonadotropins, J Clin Endocr *25*:369-384, 1965.

Vernier, V. G.: Pharmacology of antidepressant agents, Dis Nerv Syst *22* (5) Pt 2:7-13, 1961.

von Brauchitsch, H.: Deaths from aspiration and asphyxiation in a mental hospital, Arch Gen Psychiat (Chicago) *18*:129-136, 1968.

Wagensommer, J.: Therapeutisch unerwünschte Wirkungen der Thymoleptika, Fortschr Neurol Psychiat *32*:497-512, 1964.

Waitzkin, L.: Hepatic dysfunction during promazine therapy, New Eng J Med *257*:276-277, 1957.

———: Weight gain among hospitalized mentally ill men, Behav Neuropsychiat *1*:15-18, 1969.

Waitzkin, L., and Carbonell, F.: Overweight among hospitalized psychotic men, Psychiat Quart Suppl *40*: (Part 1), 91-96, 1966.

Walkenstein, D. D., *et al.*: Excretion and distribution of meprobamate and its metabolites, J Pharmacol Exp Ther *123*:254-258, 1958.

Waller, J. A., and Thuneu, R. V.: Medical handicaps to driving: Physician's dilemma in evaluation, Calif Med *98*:275-278, 1963.

Waller, J. A., and Turkel, H. W.: Alcoholism and traffic deaths, New Eng J Med *275*:532-536, 1966.

Watson, C. W., Bowker, R., and Calish, C.: Effect of chlordiazepoxide on epileptic seizures, JAMA *188*:212-216, 1964.

Waugh, W. H., and Metts, J. C., Jr.: Severe extrapyramidal motor activity induced by prochlorperazine: Its relief by intravenous injection of diphenhydramine, New Eng J Med *262*:353-354, 1960.

Webb, H. E., and Lascelles, R. G.: Treatment of facial and head pain associated with depression, Lancet *1*:355-356, 1962.

Weber, E.: Ein Rauwolfiaalkaloid in der Psychiatrie: seine Wirkungsähnlichkeit mit Chlorpromazin, Schweiz med Wschr *84*:968-970, 1954.

Wechsler, H., Grosser, G. H., and Greenblatt, M.: Research evaluating antidepressant medications on hospitalized mental patients: Survey of published reports during five-year period, J Nerv Ment Dis *141*:231-239, 1965.

Wetterholm, D. H., Snow, H. L., and Winter, F. C.: Clinical study of pigmentary change in cornea and lens in chronic chlorpromazine therapy, Arch Ophthal (Chicago) *74*:55-56, 1965.

Wheatley, D.: Report from British General Practitioner research group on Mebanazine in treatment of depression, J New Drugs *5*:348-357, 1965.

———: Chlordiazepoxide in the treatment of the domiciliary case of anxiety neurosis, Excerpta Med Internat Congr Series No. 150 (Proceedings of the IV World Congr of Psychiat, Madrid, 1966), pp. 2034-2037.

Whittier, J. R., *et al.*: Effect of long-acting injectable Prolixin in 23 psychotic patients, Dis Nerv Syst *28*:459-461, 1967.

Wilson, J. D., and Enoch, M. D.: Estimation of drug rejection by schizophrenic in-patients with analysis of clinical factors, Brit J Psychiat *113*:209-211, 1967.

Wolpert, A., Sheppard, C., and Merlis, S.: Thiothixene, thioridazine, and placebo in male chronic schizophrenic patients, Clin Pharmacol Ther *9*:456-464, 1968.

Wolpert, E. A., and Mueller, P.: Lithium carbonate in the treatment of manic-depressive disorders, Arch Gen Psychiat (Chicago) *21*:155-159, 1969.

Wroblewski, F.: Follow-up of thioridazine administration, Amer J Psychiat *119:*589-590, 1962.

Zall, H., Therman, P-O. G., and Meyers, J. M.: Lithium Carbonate—clinical study, Amer J Psychiat *125:*549-555, 1968.

Zeck, P.: Dangers of some antidepressant drugs, Med J Aust *2:*607-608, 1961.

Zelickson, A. S.: Skin changes and chlorpromazine, JAMA *198:*341-344, 1966.

Zeller, E. A.: Some remarks about monoamine oxidase and monoamine oxidase inhibitors, J Neuropsychiat 2 (Suppl 1): 125-130, 1961.

Zirkle, G. A., *et al.:* Meprobamate and small amounts of alcohol: Effect on human ability, coordination, and judgment, JAMA *173:*1823-1825, 1960.

Zlotlow, M., and Paganini, A. E.: Fatalities in patients receiving chlorpromazine and reserpine during 1956-1957 at Pilgrim State Hospital, Amer J Psychiat *115:*154-156, 1958.

Zuckerman, F.: Amenorrhea occurring during Mellaril treatment, Amer J Psychiat *118:*947, 1962.

CHAPTER
FIFTEEN

Convulsive Therapies

A CENTURY AND A HALF after Oliver (1785) first reported that convulsions induced by camphor had a therapeutic effect on psychiatric patients, Meduna (1933) revived the technique, using a 25% solution of camphor in oil intramuscularly. This method of treatment had many drawbacks: sometimes it produced no convulsion at all and sometimes several convulsions; and the time lapse from the administration of the drug to the onset of convulsions was unpredictable, ranging from only 15 minutes to several hours. The subsequent use of intravenous pentylenetetrazol (Metrazole), a soluble synthetic camphor compound, in doses of 0.5 to 1.0 gm proved far more reliable but, as with the camphor in oil, many patients experienced an overwhelming sense of panic just before the convulsion. Shortly after the introduction of Metrazol, Cerletti and Bini (1938) conceived the idea of inducing convulsions by passing an electric current through the patient's brain. This treatment technique, now called electroconvulsive therapy (ECT), was easier to administer and more predictable in its effects, and did not provoke a preconvulsion panic; it thus soon made the use of Metrazol obsolete.

In recent years, other drugs that induce convulsions have been introduced, the most notable of which is the anesthetic flurothyl (Indoklon) (Krantz 1957), which is generally administered by inhalation but is also under study for intravenous use. While it appears to equal ECT in therapeutic effectiveness, claims that it produces less discomfort, postconvulsive confusion, or dysmnesia have not been documented, and it has not gained wide acceptance. Its one indisputable advantage is psychological: it permits the clinician to avoid the odious and somewhat terrifying word *shock* (Fazio 1967, Laurell 1970).

Despite general agreement that ECT is effective and that, at the time it was introduced, it was one of the few treatment procedures of any kind that helped the gravely ill psychiatric patient, neither the procedure nor those who administered it ever enjoyed much esteem within the medical community. Many psychiatrists believe shock therapy should be used only when all else has failed or the patient is too poor, uneducated, or psychologically unenlightened to be treated by psychotherapy. Those who administer ECT are likely to be derogated as "psychiatric electricians" and relegated to the lowest rung on the profession's status ladder (Hollingshead 1958, MacIver 1959). Questions concerning the advisability of the use of ECT have gathered even greater momentum, of course, since the introduction of antidepressants and phenothiazines. These drugs have considerably narrowed ECT's range of indications, but, in our opinion, have not made its use obsolete. To this day, there are many patients for whom ECT, either alone or in combination with other measures, is still the safest, fastest, least expensive, and most effective form of treatment.

TECHNIQUE OF ADMINISTRATION

The decision to use ECT and, especially, the selection of the most suitable technique require a careful assessment of the patient's health. If the individual suffers from some medical condition that poses special hazards, the psychiatrist may wish to consult with the family doctor or other specialist. As the absolute contraindications are very few (see p. 640), it is ultimately the psychiatrist alone who must weigh the risks involved in giving ECT against those of withholding it, and make the final decision. Having made the decision, he should convey his findings and recommendations candidly to the patient and his family, advise them about the potential benefits, hazards, and aftereffects, and thus enable them to give or withhold consent. If the patient is ambulatory, the psychiatrist may at this juncture decide to hospitalize him; ECT can, however, be administered on an outpatient basis (see p. 651).

If the patient is unduly anxious about treatment or has difficulty in falling asleep the evening before, he may be given a sedative or a minor tranquilizer. While a heavy meal is not an absolute contraindication to treatment in an emergency, the patient should be advised not to eat for at least four hours, and not to drink for at least two hours, before treatment. This will diminish the possibility of vomiting and aspiration pneumonia, which, in succinylcholine-modified ECT, can result from the temporary abolition of the gag reflex and, in unmodified ECT, from the sudden expulsion of stomach contents.

Atropine, 0.6 mg, should be given subcutaneously or intramuscularly 30 to 60 minutes before treatment, both to prevent cardiac arrhythmias produced by vagal stimulation and to diminish the secretion and thus the potential aspiration of saliva during or after a seizure. Since 0.6 to 1.2 mg of atropine given intravenously immediately before treatment has an adequate vagal blocking effect even if it has little antisialogogue effect (Parry-Jones 1964) and since the only complication saliva causes is a noisy stridor, atropine given intravenously together with barbiturate is equally satisfactory.

The patient should be requested to empty his bladder and bowels prior to lying down on the treatment table; he should be dressed in loose-fitting clothes or pajamas without shoes. It is no longer considered necessary to place him in a hyperextended position by putting one or two pillows beneath his middorsal spine, for this does not diminish the incidence of vertebral fractures, even when ECT is administered without a muscle relaxant. Artificial dentures should be removed in order to prevent their being damaged during the tonic phase, unless the patient's remaining teeth are so irregularly spaced that they would be in greater danger of breaking without the protection of the dentures. In questionable cases, it is useful to have a dentist see the patient before treatment both to determine the degree of dental risk and to ascertain how best to protect the patient's teeth during the convulsion (Durrant 1966). In order to prevent the patient's biting his tongue or lips during the convulsion, a gauze-covered tongue depressor or other mouth gag should be inserted between the upper and lower molars.

The electrodes are placed on the anterior portion of the temples, not because this improves the results, but because more posterior placement tends to give rise to headaches after treatment. Metal electrodes coated with conductive jelly can be used, but these are unnecessarily messy, and cloth-covered electrodes wetted with saline are preferable. As cutaneous sebum can adhere to electrodes of this kind and, by increasing the electrode's own resistance, cause an inadequate response or even skin burns, the patient's temples should be cleansed with an alcohol sponge before treatment, and the electrodes washed against each other before and after each use.

It was formerly believed that the voltage and character of the current required depended on, and had to be adjusted for, the particular illness involved, but today it is recognized that these factors are irrelevant to the therapeutic effect as long as a grand mal seizure is evoked. However, since the duration and intensity of the current applied seem to correlate with the severity of the postconvulsive memory disturbances (Ottoson 1960), it is necessary to determine the lowest amount of current that will evoke a seizure in a given patient. In most instances, the desired response can be achieved by delivering 80 to 140 volts of alternating current across the electrodes for 0.1 to 0.8 second (Davies 1970). The amount of current that passes through the brain is estimated to be between 200 to 1,600 milliamperes (Kalinowsky 1967).

Within a few seconds of receiving unmodified treatment, the patient will exhibit a strong tonic contraction of the extensor muscles throughout his body, which lasts for approximately 10 seconds and is followed by generalized clonic movements that last for another 30 to 40 seconds. If the amount of current is insufficient, the patient will exhibit only the tonic contraction, a response described by the original Italian experimenters as "shock man-cato." This response has little therapeutic effect, can cause the patient to feel uncomfortable for several hours, and is therefore an indication to readminister the treatment immediately, perhaps using higher voltage or applying the current for a longer period of time.

The strength of the muscular contractions in the tonic phase of the unmodified convulsion and, to a limited extent, in the clonic and flailing movements that follow can cause fractures, disloca-tions, muscle pain, and exhaustion. Moreover, the physical exertion and stress to which the procedure subjects the entire organism may themselves be hazardous, especially for patients who are ad-vanced in years or in poor physical condition. Accordingly, it is now common practice to give patients 20 to 40 mg (0.5 mg/kg) of a short-acting muscle relaxant like *succinylcholine* (Anectine) prior to treatment (Pitts 1968). If the patient suffers from a medical or surgical condition that makes it imperative to avoid muscular or other physical strain, doses as high as 60 mg or more should be used in order to eliminate the contraction almost completely. The use of succinylcholine has the further advantage of facilitating arti-ficial respiration immediately before and after treatment, thus re-ducing the danger of anoxia, a potential cause of brain damage and a contributing factor to cardiac arrest. Some clinicians prefer to administer 100% oxygen starting immediately after the succinyl-choline is injected until the ECT is given (McAndrew 1967), as an additional safeguard against anoxia.

Since the generalized paralysis caused by succinylcholine can pro-duce an intensely uncomfortable feeling of suffocation, the patient is first put to sleep with an *intravenous barbiturate*. Giving the barbiturate and the muscle relaxant simultaneously does not seem to prevent this feeling, as the paralysis may set in before the patient falls asleep, and he may remember his discomfort and fear even after he awakes. For this reason, we first inject an ultrashort-acting barbiturate like thiopental (Pentothal) or metho-hexital (Brevital), 70 to 100 mg, in 7 to 10 cc of saline. Metho-hexital is said to be especially suited for ambulatory ECT, in that patients awaken and become alert more rapidly and are able to walk from the treatment room to the recovery area within 10 minutes (Osborne 1963, Pitts 1965). As soon as the patient has been given the barbiturate, he is asked to count backwards from 100; when his speech starts to slur (which occurs after about 30 seconds), 20 to 40 mg of succinylcholine (Anectine) are injected through the same needle via a T-shaped stopcock. Small muscular fascicula-tions, starting in the patient's trunk and most visible around his neck, usually appear 45 to 60 seconds after the injection, and shortly thereafter spread to the patient's feet. As soon as these movements subside, the shock is administered (Whitwam 1963).

The succinylcholine-modified convulsion, like the unmodified, is marked by a tonic and a clonic phase, but may be so attenuated that there is only a mild grimace or blepharospasm at the time the current is applied, a slow plantar flexion during the tonic phase, and tiny movements in the toes, arms, or facial musculature during the clonic phase. Close attention to the appearance of these phenomena is extremely important, for they may constitute the only evidence that the patient has in fact had a seizure and not merely a brief clouding of consciousness, as such an abortive response is often accompanied by severe nausea and vertigo. A reliable clue is the slow downward movement of the patient's toes that can usually be detected 10 to 15 seconds before the clonic phase begins. When this fails to occur within 45 seconds after the current was applied, a grand mal seizure is unlikely, and the patient should be reshocked quickly before the succinylcholine wears off. Another way of determining whether the patient has had an adequate seizure is to apply a small tourniquet to his forearm or thigh before in-jecting the succinylcholine, thereby excluding this extremity from the generalized muscle paralysis and permitting it to exhibit typical tonic and clonic movements (Adderley 1953).

Whether or not succinylcholine is used, the patient should be held gently by the shoulders and upper extremities during the con-vulsion. Two assistants are required for this purpose. They should be instructed to moderate rather than prevent the patient's movements, as the exertion of too firm a counterpressure can cause the fracture it is intended to prevent.

As soon as the clonic phase ends, a patent airway must be assured: the patient's head should be extended, his tongue and lower jaw pulled forward, and excessive saliva removed by suction. The patient given succinylcholine may be apneic for as long as five minutes after treatment, and must be ventilated mechanically with room air until his cyanosis diminishes and he is breathing independently. If he does not start to breathe spontaneously within seven to 10 minutes, he may be considered to have *prolonged apnea,* a complication described in more detail further on. Once his respiration has returned, the patient should be kept recumbent for five to 10 minutes, after which he should be asked to sit up and given something to drink. If he appears weak or pale, his blood pressure should be taken before he is permitted to stand. Upon returning to his hospital room or to his home, the patient should be permitted to sleep as long as he wishes. Since he may be confused when he awakens, he should not be left unattended until he is lucid and alert.

RISKS, COMPLICATIONS, AND CONTRAINDICATIONS

Statistics show that complications occur in only one out of every 2,600 ECT treatments and fatalities in one out of every 28,000 (Barker 1959, Gaitz 1956). Most large-scale studies concerning the risks associated with the use of ECT fail to distinguish between succinylcholine-modified and unmodified treatment, and controversy continues over which is safer for the patient in good health. While the incidence of morbidity and mortality in either case depends greatly on the patient's physical condition, there is general agreement that the introduction of modified ECT has made treatment fairly safe even for patients with disorders in which unmodified ECT would be dangerous (such as thrombophlebitis, aortic aneurysm, advanced coronary or myocardial disease, hypertension, acute or chronic endocarditis, Paget's disease, and advanced osteoporosis). Modified ECT has also been given during pregnancy without precipitating labor (as late as the eighth month) or producing any deleterious effect on the fetus (Forssman 1955, Sobel 1960, Smith 1956). Moreover, while the hazards of ECT increase with the patient's age (patients over 45 being 10 times as likely as younger ones to suffer some complication), treatment has been successfully administered to patients in their 90s. Only for patients suffering from brain tumors or other conditions associated with increased intracranial pressure does ECT seem to be absolutely contraindicated.

Fractures and subluxations, the most common hazards of unmodified ECT, result largely from the vigor and abruptness of the muscular contraction. These complications are thus more likely to occur in individuals who are unusually muscular, such as laborers, or in those who have a weakened skeletal system because of advanced age or such illnesses as osteoporosis or Paget's disease. Especially common are compression fractures of the lumbar vertebrae, which, while they rarely give rise to long-term neurologic sequelae, can cause severe and disabling back pain of many weeks' duration (Polatin 1949). Such complications are relatively rare, however, since the introduction of succinylcholine (Anectine), occurring only when the dosage of the muscle-relaxant is too low or the current is applied before the drug has had a chance to work. *Cardiovascular complications* are even less frequent, but are potentially far more serious and include cardiac arrhythmia, cardiac arrest, and myocardial infarction. Since the two latter complications occur almost exclusively in individuals with preexisting cardiac disease, it is important to assess the patient's cardiovascular status before treatment, especially if he is over 45.

Another possible complication of ECT is *prolonged apnea.* While this can occur in the patient who did not receive succinylcholine, its most common cause is an undue prolongation of succinylcholine's muscle-relaxant effect, generally as a result of a recessive inherited disorder called *pseudocholinesterase deficiency.* In this disorder, the enzyme needed to hydrolyze and thus inactivate succinylcholine is not only deficient but also abnormal, in that it is less active against all substrates and more resistant to most esterase inhibitors (Kalow 1958, Lehmann 1964). Since prolonged apnea occurs in only one of every 2,500 individuals (Foldes 1960, Kalow 1959, Sabawala 1959) and is invariably reversible, it does not seem practical (as suggested) to test every patient's serum for atypical esterase activity or to give a small test dose of succinylcholine prior to the first treatment (Porter 1964). Treatment is supportive and consists of mechanical ventilation until spontaneous respiration returns. Nevertheless, any patient who is apneic longer than seven minutes after ECT should be seen by an anesthesiologist as soon as possible.

Among the most disturbing—if least life-threatening—of ECT's deleterious effects are *dysmnesia* and *confusion*. Even after the first treatment, the patient may be confused for several hours, but the more treatments he receives, the longer and the more severe the confusional episodes become. After four or five treatments, his disorientation may persist for several days at a time; if he is receiving ECT three times a week, he may remain confused almost continuously until several weeks after his treatment has been completed. The more treatments he receives, the further back his memory disturbance extends and the more globally disoriented he becomes. Initially, only his time orientation and ability to recall recent events are impaired. With additional treatments, he may also forget events of the past and be confused about where he is or where he lives. Finally, after 12 to 15 treatments (fewer if he is of advanced age or has been taking phenothiazines), he will be unable to remember the names or faces of those around him, and, in extreme cases, will not even remember his own occupation. Attempts have been made to mitigate this effect by spacing the treatments further apart or by giving unilateral ECT on the nondominant hemisphere's side of the scalp (Cannicott 1963, Lancaster 1958). That the right-handed patient given ECT on the left shows a greater decrement in verbal skills than the one given ECT on the right is consistent with what is known of the functional asymmetry of the brain and of great benefit in reducing post-ECT dysmnesia (Cohen 1968, Gottlieb 1965, Martin 1965, Zamora 1965, Zinkin 1968).

The patient who is grossly confused tends to be fairly placid about his state, perhaps sitting and staring or repetitively performing some useless task. Only in rare instances will he become more delusional or agitated after ECT; but when he does, it is important to decide whether his condition is a product of the treatment or a manifestation of his original illness, in short, whether additional treatments will lessen or increase the agitation. Although no sure guidelines exist, the more severe the memory impairment and confusion are, the less likely they are to diminish with additional treatments. The combination of confusion and agitation that sometimes occurs immediately after the patient awakens from treatment is called *postconvulsive excitement* and is identical with the delirious states seen following clinically occurring seizures. The patient may be assaultive, unreasonable, and aimlessly hyperactive, but can usually be calmed down fairly rapidly with perphenazine (Trilafon), 5 mg intramuscularly, or even (if the situation is urgent enough) intravenously.

The grossest symptoms of disorientation and dysmnesia usually recede within a few weeks of the final treatment; the more treatments the patient has had and the older he is, the longer this will take (Janis 1951). Some memory gaps and difficulty in retaining new material may persist for six months or longer; a few details may not be recalled for as long as 12 to 18 months; and some memories, especially of events that took place during the weeks of treatment, may be lost altogether (Janis 1968). Since some degree of impaired or retarded intellectual functioning is common in all depressions, an attempt must be made to determine whether the patient's complaints of dysmnesia or difficulty in concentrating are wholly the result of treatment or whether they are, at least in part, symptoms of the original illness. Studies performed one week after the administration of three or four shock treatments have shown that patients whose mood was improved by ECT tend to have fewer complaints of impairment than those whose mood was unchanged (Cronholm 1963), which means either that patients who are euphoric after ECT tend to ignore their memory deficits or that such patients also experience an improvement in memory functions.

Since the patient's placidity about his dysmnesia and confusion will disappear as his critical faculties return, it is important that his family help him mitigate the consequences of his memory disturbance by arranging his life in as uncomplicated a way as possible and by explaining things to him as often as necessary. The more responsible the patient's position, the more he will suffer from not remembering facts that he ought to have at his command, and the more important it is for him to pursue a well-planned program of reorientation.

Although most clinicians consider ECT's effect on mental functioning reversible, we know of no systematic, long-term studies that demonstrate this conclusively, and almost every experienced clinician knows of a number of patients whose memory functions have in some measure remained impaired indefinitely. Efforts to find permanent morphologic changes have been inconclusive. Hartelius (1952) performed one of the most thorough experimental studies of this question. Examining the brains of cats sacrificed at various intervals after electrically induced convulsions, he found glial reactions, changes in the vessel walls, and various stages of chromophobia and nuclear hyperchromatisms in the nerve cells, but concluded that the majority of such changes were reversible. Similarly, multiple petechiae have been found in the cerebral cortex, white matter, and brainstem of some ECT-treated patients (Alpers 1942), but such changes have also been described in patients who have never had ECT and in individuals whose mental functioning was intact at the time of their death. EEG changes have also been found to occur after ECT, but seem largely transient in character and cannot be clearly related to the extent of intellectual disturbance. After about 12 treatments, 3-6 cps moderately high-voltage slow waves appear, first in the frontal area and thereafter throughout the entire cortex. These waves usually disappear within three months (Klotz 1955), but an unusual high-voltage alpha rhythm may persist (Kalinowsky 1961).

INDICATIONS

The Choice Between ECT and Drugs

Since most illnesses that respond to ECT are also likely to respond to drugs, the choice between these modalities cannot be based on diagnostic considerations alone. Unfortunately, most attempts to compare their effectiveness, like studies comparing one drug with another, are weakened by the lack of sufficient data concerning the nature of treatments administered, the criteria used for assessing improvement, and the duration of the remissions achieved (Riddell 1963). The comparative efficacy of the two has been most widely studied in depressive syndromes. The results seen immediately on completion of treatment seem to favor ECT (77% to 94% versus 66%) (Ball 1959, Greenblatt 1964, Kiloh 1960, Nyström 1964, Robin 1962); the results six or 12 months later show no such superiority, as only half remain well with either treatment (Kiloh 1960, Oltman 1962).

Undoubtedly, some patients respond better to ECT than to drugs, but unless the patient's response to treatment in the past provides some clues, there is currently no way of singling them out in advance. Attempts to predict ECT responsiveness on the basis of biologic tests or psychological examinations (Feldman 1958, Pearson 1950) or on the basis of the patient's age, premorbid personality, or symptoms have turned up a number of factors that correlate with a favorable post-ECT course. The value of many of the tests proposed, however, cannot be confirmed (Bannister 1961, Sloane 1956); and many of the clinical criteria that seem to be predictors are in fact merely prognostic indexes that suggest a favorable outcome regardless of treatment. For example, in a study of 400 patients given ECT, Nyström (1964) found a good response in patients who

1/ were depressed,
2/ had early morning awakening,
3/ showed psychomotor retardation,
4/ had been sick for less than six months or for more than a year, or
5/ had previously had a good response to ECT.

A poor response to ECT was found in patients who

1/ were withdrawn,
2/ had ideas of reference,
3/ had obsessive-compulsive symptoms,
4/ were under 35, or
5/ were hysteroid and unstable.

The finding that ECT was helpful for patients one or both of whose parents had died suddenly at 65 or older was as unequivocal as puzzling.

Given that there are no reliable predictors of therapeutic response, the choice between ECT and drugs can be made only in terms of their respective advantages and disadvantages for the patient under consideration. Among the *advantages of* ECT are

1/ the rapidity with which it can relieve many of the symptoms seen in acute psychoses;
2/ the assurance that the patient is actually receiving the treatment prescribed because a physician is always present and that it need not depend, as it does in giving drugs, on the intelligence and cooperation of the patient and his relatives or on the astuteness with which they (or the hospital nursing staff) detect surreptitious disposal of unwanted medications; and
3/ excepting confusion and dysmnesia, the rarity of complications (such as prolonged apnea, fractures, and dislocations) and their occurrence, if at all, during and immediately after the treatment, when the patient is still under medical observation and the appropriate countermeasures can be taken.

The *advantages of drug therapy* include

1/ greater patient acceptance;

2/ easier administration, since no trained personnel or specialized facilities are needed;

3/ less, and in most instances, no impairment in intellectual functioning; and

4/ the rapid diminution of most of the drug's adverse effects when it is discontinued and the tendency to diminution even on continued administration.

The effect of ECT on the patient's intellectual functioning is very different: some degree of dysmnesia and confusion develops in almost all instances; it may last for weeks or months after treatment is discontinued and can be so severe that the patient requires hospitalization or close supervision. That drug therapy leaves the patient's intellectual functioning more or less intact has the further advantages of promoting, right from the beginning, a doctor-patient relationship that is conducive to the patient's learning to accept future medical recommendations, cope with his illness and its consequences, and participate in a psychotherapeutic exploration of his total life situation. The ECT-treated patient, on the other hand, is likely to be too confused to participate in a meaningful discussion or to develop a lasting relationship with the doctor. The entire episode, moreover, may be blanketed by a memory disturbance that causes an unsettling discontinuity in his life experience and makes him view his illness and treatment as a disturbing mystery rather than a phase of his life that he can accept with any kind of understanding.

Certain other claims that have been advanced in favor of one form of treatment or the other do not appear to have equal validity. Some clinicians believe that depressed patients treated with drugs have a lower relapse rate than those treated with ECT because drug dosage, unlike ECT, can be adjusted upward should the patient's condition deteriorate. Others, citing the necessity of giving drugs to depressed patients over extended periods of time, believe that patients who repeatedly fail to take their drugs can be better protected against relapse by being given a course of ECT (Robin 1962). Both these positions—one favorable to the use of ECT and one to the use of drugs—imply an unproved view: that ECT's effect on a patient's depression continues long after treatment is discontinued, while that of drugs does not. This view, taken to its logical conclusion, would mean that, in order to be considered effective, ECT would have to relieve the patient's symptoms not only while it is being given, but for a prolonged period thereafter, whereas drugs would have to provide relief only during the period in which they are being administered. That this view is fairly widespread is shown by the fact that illnesses that respond well initially to ECT but relapse some months later are termed "ECT-refractory," while those that respond well initially to drugs are considered "drug-responsive," even if (and especially when) the patient relapses after the drug is withdrawn.

The fallacies of this reasoning become obvious when the results of treatment are examined. As already pointed out, the relapse rate six months after treatment ends is almost identical for both drug and shock therapy; therefore it is reasonable to assume that both forms treat symptoms only and that neither has a lasting effect on the underlying mechanism or the illness's natural history. Viewed in this light, the patient whom treatment has seemed to cure (in the sense that he remains symptom-free after the treatment is stopped) might be someone who by that time would have felt better in any case; the depressive syndrome that worsens after ECT need not be thought (as it often is) to have been aggravated by treatment, but to have deteriorated in spite of it; the patient who improves after receiving ECT and then relapses might be in much the same state as the one who relapses after he withdraws himself from drugs; the latter need not be viewed as someone who would have remained well if only he had received ECT; and, until the underlying illness recedes, the repeatedly relapsing patient might receive as much benefit from maintenance ECT as from maintenance medications. In other words, the argument that drugs are preferable to ECT because drug dosage can be adjusted upward if the patient's condition deteriorates should be rephrased: maintenance drug treatment is preferable to maintenance ECT, perhaps on the ground that it entails fewer disadvantages.

SPECIFIC INDICATIONS FOR ECT

Accessibility, convenience of administration, and the avoidance of dysmnesia are undeniable advantages of drug treatment over ECT. Other considerations being equal, then, it would follow that shock therapy is indicated only after an attempt to treat the patient with drugs has failed. However, ECT should be the physician's initial preference when

1/ previous episodes of the same illness have not responded to drug treatment;

2/ the patient's medical condition (first trimester of pregnancy, history of multiple drug idiosyncrasies) makes drug use inadvisable;

3/ the patient's illness is severe and progressing so rapidly that no time is available for even a brief trial on drugs; or

4/ the available treatment facilities are inadequate or the responsible family members cannot be relied on to supervise his medication.

Shock therapy, for example, will be indicated for the patient in an *acute catatonic state* whose behavior is dangerous to himself and those around him and cannot be controlled with drugs, or whose sleep does not improve within a day or two of being given phenothiazines (see p. 128). ECT is also indicated for the catatonic patient who exhibits such typical precursors of impulsivity and sudden violence as immobilization, religious or sexual preoccupations, and delusions that the world is about to end, or who is plagued by voices ordering him to become assaultive, to mutilate or kill himself, or, in some other way, act bizarrely (see p. 118). A patient of this kind should be given as many treatments (even several in a day) as needed to restore some element of reasonableness, but the total number of ECT treatments required rarely exceeds four.

ECT should also be given to any seriously *depressed patient* whose illness does not respond to a three or four week course, first with a tricyclic antidepressant like imipramine (Tofranil), and then, if this has been unsuccessful, with a monoamine oxidase inhibitor (MAOI) like isocarboxazide (Marplan). The decision to give the depressed patient ECT should be made even sooner if he is suicidal, severely withdrawn, profoundly anorectic, or if his sleep disorder is getting worse. In the majority of cases, six to 12 treatments will relieve the most distressing symptoms, but followup drug treatment may be needed to maintain the remission (see p. 178). Patients with *manic states* who do not improve following two weeks of treatment with either lithium carbonate or massive doses of phenothiazines are also candidates for ECT, and, in most cases, will behave in a far less disruptive manner after two or three treatments a day for three or four consecutive days (see p. 193).

ECT has also been used in many other syndromes, albeit with variable results. Patients suffering from *chronic schizophrenia* whose behavior is extremely disruptive and who cannot be controlled with drugs may become calmer and easier to manage after receiving ECT. The calming effect does not usually last more than a few days or weeks, however, which means that the chronic schizophrenic who responds favorably to ECT and poorly to drugs must usually be given ECT regularly in order to maintain his improvement (see p. 147). Results in the so-called *symptomatic neuroses* are generally poor. Patients with chronic obsessive-compulsive or depersonalization neuroses (see p. 239), for example, usually feel worse after ECT unless their symptoms first appeared in the midst of a depression (see p. 239), in which case they are likely to subside when the patient's mood improves (Ackner 1960). Patients with an *acute delirium* or a *prolonged twilight state associated with a seizure disorder* may also respond fairly well to ECT, sometimes even after the first few treatments (Lieser 1957, Roth 1953); patients with *dementiform brain syndromes,* on the other hand, tend to become more confused and often more agitated. ECT has also been reported of value in syndromes as far afield as *psychogenic pain* (Boyd 1956, Krantz 1956, Von Hagen 1957) or *chronic neurodermatitis* (Valdivia-Ponce 1957), but one cannot, in such cases, discount a possible placebo effect. Indeed, patients with a variety of disorders including schizophrenic and depressive syndromes occasionally benefit just as much from "placebo shock" (being prepared for ECT in the traditional manner but then given only the barbiturate) as from shock treatment itself (Brill 1959, Miller 1953).

FREQUENCY AND DURATION OF TREATMENT

Shock treatment is usually given two or three times weekly, but clinicians differ in their views regarding the total number of treatments needed in particular illnesses. Although no magic number can be assigned to any syndrome, a fairly useful general rule is that the briefer the patient's illness has been and the more excited he is at the outset, the fewer treatments he will require. The patient with an acute catatonic excitement of but a few days' duration usually responds after fewer treatments than the one who has had a psychotic depression for a number of months. A patient with paranoid schizophrenia (which may have been in progress a year or two before the patient was ill enough to be seen) often requires 20 treatments before any improvement is noticeable. In acute schizophrenic episodes, we usually discontinue ECT as soon as the patient's excitement diminishes; in psychotic depressions, soon after his sleep improves and his mood lifts; and in paranoid schizophrenias, two or three treatments after the intensity of his delusional ideas starts to diminish.

Some physicians use confusion to gauge the end of treatment, and give the patient 2-3 treatments beyond the point at which he becomes confused. Others induce confusion deliberately, seeking to help the patient to forget or repress unpleasant events. In this technique, the confusional effect of ECT is maximized through very frequent treatments over a long period of time. In effect, the patient develops a reversible organic psychosis, he becomes incontinent, is oblivious to his environment and totally dependent on those around him. From this "depatterned" state the attempt is made to effect a fresh start on the road to rehabilitation (Cameron 1958, 1962, Glueck 1957). Also used are *Page-Russell treatments,* in which, for a period of 3-4 weeks, the patient is given six tonic convulsions twice daily in such rapid succession that no clonic phase develops until after the final stimulation (Page 1948, Russell 1953). Although polydiurnal treatment may, in some cases, be used to diminish excitement (Jacobs 1946, Sogliani 1939), the effectiveness of this technique as a rehabilitative measure has never been documented in controlled studies and it seems unnecessarily heroic. In any case, it is rare that severe excitement does not diminish after two treatments a day, and if given tranquilizers concomitantly, even the most excited patient does not require more than four treatments in a single day.

As the patient gets better, it is usually advisable to discontinue treatments gradually rather than abruptly. The patient who relapses after a successful course of thrice weekly ECT should start over on three treatments weekly; when he again improves, the schedule should be reduced to one ECT weekly for four to six weeks. Then intervals between treatments should gradually be increased to two, three, and finally four weeks. After a period of monthly treatments, an attempt should be made once more to discontinue the program altogether. In some illnesses, however, the patient may need to continue indefinitely with monthly ECT. Such an extended treatment course may be required in some cases of cyclical psychoses or recurring depressions (especially those occurring in the 50s and 60s) that do not respond to drugs and in patients with longstanding paranoid schizophrenias who refuse to take medications (Geohegan 1949, Karliner 1965).

SIMULTANEOUS USE OF ECT AND DRUGS

As most patients nowadays will have been taking drugs for some time prior to shock treatment, the question of whether the patient should be treated with ECT *or* with drugs is largely academic. The really relevant decision is usually whether to continue administering drugs during and after the ECT program, particularly since some authors claim pretreatment or aftercare with drugs can reduce the number of shock treatments required for depressed patients (Kielholz 1959) and help to maintain an ECT-induced remission (Oltman 1961, Seager 1962).

Giving ECT to a patient who has been taking drugs, however, can cause some problems. Continued administration of tranquilizers throughout a course of ECT tends to augment the patient's confusion and is reported to lengthen the postconvulsive apnea (Ferguson 1956, Foster 1956). Some clinicians will not administer ECT to patients who are receiving reserpine, as this drug allegedly increases the incidence of post-ECT arrhythmias and cardiac arrest (Bracha 1956, Foster 1955). Such caution is probably excessive (Gonzales 1964), however, and the patient whose condition is severe enough to require both high-dosage phenothiazine (or reserpine) treatment and subsequent ECT would be exposed in all likelihood to even greater hazards if his psychosis were permitted to go unchecked.

Our practice is to continue the administration of phenothiazines both during and after the course of ECT for patients with manic or schizophrenic illnesses. We do not give phenothiazines (or other major tranquilizers) to the nondelusional depressed patient, however, as the concomitant administration seems to increase both the number of treatments required and the incidence of post-ECT relapse (Perris 1966). The situation is somewhat different with antidepressants: the patient who has obtained some (even if minimal) benefit from one of the dibenzazepine derivates like imipramine, prior to shock treatment, should continue to receive it during and after ECT. Drugs of the MAOI group, however, should be discontinued, especially in the patient over 45, for they can potentiate a number of other drugs, among them the pressor amines, that might have to be administered should the patient develop cardiovascular complications in the process of receiving ECT.

OUTPATIENT ECT

If the patient's general health is good and his illness not sufficiently dangerous to warrant hospitalization, and if his relatives are able to bring him for treatment and to remain with him for six to 12 hours thereafter, he may be given shock therapy as an outpatient. The psychiatrist who does not have the necessary equipment and nursing personnel available in his office may be able to use the outpatient clinic of his local hospital, a practice that has the added advantages of providing easy access to an anesthesiologist should need for his services arise, and of having sufficient personnel available should the patient develop a post-convulsive excitement and become unmanageable. Since the family must assume many of the supervisory functions otherwise delegated to the hospital, it is even more important to warn them about the memory disturbances that may cause confusion so that they do not become unduly concerned that "something has gone wrong" should the patient's confusion become so severe that he has to be hospitalized.

Among the advantages of outpatient shock therapy are that it is less expensive, avoids the unnecessary use of hospital bed space, and does not further isolate the patient from his family. Some patients may be able to continue working or at least to do some chores around the house. Its principal disadvantage is that the patient may become too difficult to manage at home, though he can, of course, be hospitalized at this juncture and his treatment continued on an inpatient basis. Moreover, since ECT-treated patients tend to forget how ill they have been and to be too intellectually impaired to reason with, those receiving outpatient ECT may simply stop coming as soon as they feel better (while the hospitalized patients can usually be kept until they have recovered sufficiently to understand the importance of medications and aftercare). Obviously this factor is of more relevance for the highly independent person, such as the family breadwinner, who is not inclined to listen to his family, than for the person who is likely to take his family's advice even if he does not yet quite understand why he should. In general, patients with depressive, chronic schizophrenic and relapsing manic illnesses are best suited for outpatient ECT, while paranoid patients are least suited, for they may incorporate the treatment into their delusional systems, accuse the physician of trying to hurt them, and refuse to return.

REFERENCES

Ackner, B., and Grant, Q. A. F. R.: Prognostic significance of depersonalization in depressive illnesses treated with electro-convulsive therapy, J Neurol Neurosurg Psychiat 23:242-246, 1960.

Adderley, D. J., and Hamilton, M.: Use of succinylcholine in ECT, with particular reference to its effect on blood pressure, Brit Med J 1:195-197, 1953.

Alpers, B. J., and Hughes, J.: Brain

changes in electrically induced convulsions in the human, J Neuropath Exp Neurol 1:173-180, 1942.

Ball, J. R. B., and Kiloh, L. G.: Controlled trial of imipramine in treatment of depressive states, Brit Med J 2:1052-1055, 1959.

Bannister, D., and Beech, H. R.: Evaluation of the Feldman prognosis scale for shock therapy, J Ment Sci 107:503-508, 1961.

Barker, J. C., and Baker, A. A.: Deaths associated with electroplexy, J Ment Sci 105:339-348, 1959.

Boyd, D. A., Jr.: Electroshock therapy in atypical pain syndromes, Lancet 76:22-25, 1956.

Bracha, S., and Hes, J. P.: Death occuring during combined reserpine-electroshock treatment, Amer J Psychiat 113:257, 1956.

Brill, N. Q., et al.: Relative effectiveness of various components of electroconvulsive therapy: Experimental study, Arch Neurol Psychiat 81:627-635, 1959.

Cameron, D. E., and Pande, S. K.: Treatment of the chronic paranoid schizophrenic patient, Canad Med Ass J 78:92-96, 1958.

Cameron, D. E., Lohrenz, J. G., and Handcock, K. A.: Depatterning treatment of schizophrenia, Compr Psychiat 3:65-76, 1962.

Cannicott, S. M.: Technique of unilateral electroconvulsive therapy, Amer J Psychiat 120:477-480, 1963.

Cerletti, U., and Bini, L.: L'elettroshock, Arch Gen Neurol Psichiat 19:266-268, 1938.

Cohen, B. D., Noblin, C. D., and Silverman, A. J.: Functional asymmetry of the human brain, Science 162:475-477, 1968.

Cronholm, B., and Ottosson, J. O.: Experience of memory function after electroconvulsive therapy, Brit J Psychiat 109:251-258, 1963.

Davies, R., et al.: Personal communication to the authors, 1970.

Durrant, B. W.: Dental care in electroplexy, Brit J Psychiat 112:1173-1176, 1966.

Fazio, C., et al.: La Terapia Chemioconvulsivante con Flurotil in Psichiatria, Sist Nerv 19:367-373, 1967.

Feldman, M. J.: Evaluation scale for shock therapy, J Clin Psychol 14:41-45, 1958.

Ferguson, R. S.: Influences of reserpine on ECT: Preliminary observations, J Ment Sci 102:826-829, 1956.

Foldes, F. F.: Pharmacology of neuromuscular blocking agents in man, Clin Pharmacol Ther 1:345-395, 1960.

Forssman, H.: Follow-up study of sixteen children whose mothers were given electric convulsive therapy during gestation, Acta Psychiat Scand 30:437-441, 1955.

Foster, M. W., Jr., and Gayle, R. F.: Dangers in combining reserpine (Serpasil) with electronconvulsive therapy, JAMA 159:1520-1522, 1955.

———: Chlorpromazine and reserpine as adjuncts in electroshock treatment, Southern Med J 49:731-735, 1956.

Gaitz, C. M., Pokorny, A. D., and Mills, M., Jr.: Death following electroconvulsive therapy: Report of three cases, Arch Neurol Psychiat 75:493-499, 1956.

Geohegan, J. J., and Stevenson, G.: Prophylactic electroshock, Amer J Psychiat 105:494-496, 1949.

Glueck, B. C., Reiss, H., and Bernard, L. E.: Regressive electric shock therapy: Preliminary report on 100 cases, Psychiat Quart 31:117-136, 1957.

Gonzalez, J. R., and Imahara, J. K.: Electroshock therapy with the phenothiazines and reserpine: Survey and report, Amer J Psychiat 121:253-256, 1964.

Greenblatt, M., Grossner, G. H., and Weschsler, H.: Differential response of hospitalized depressed patients to somatic therapy, Amer J Psychiat 120:935-943, 1964.

Hartelius, H.: Cerebral changes following electrically induced convulsions: Experimental study on cats, Acta Psychiat Scand (Suppl 77):3-128, 1952.

Hollingshead, A., and Redlich, F.: Social Class and Mental Illness: A Community Study, New York: Wiley, 1958.

Jacobs, J. S. L., and Gilson, W. E.: Treatment of schizophrenia with intensive electric convulsive therapy, Wisconsin Med J 45:395-397, 1946.

Janis, I. L.: Personal communication to the authors, 1968.

Janis, I. L., and Astrachan, M.: Effects of electroconvulsive treatments on memory efficiency, J Abnorm Psychol 46:501-511, 1951.

Kalinowsky, L.: Convulsive therapies, in Freedman, A. M., and Kaplan, H. I., eds.: Comprehensive Textbook of Psychiatry, Baltimore: Williams & Wilkins, 1967, pp. 1279-1285.

Kalinowsky, L. B., and Hippius, H.: Pharmacological, Convulsive and Other Somatic Treatments in Psychiatry, New York: Grune, 1969.

Kalow, W., and Davis, R. O.: Activity of various esterase inhibitors towards atypical human serum cholinesterase, Biochem Pharmacol 1:183-192, 1958.

Kalow, W., and Gunn, D. R.: Some statistical data on atypical cholinesterase of human serum, Ann Hum Genet 23:239-250, 1959.

Karliner, W., and Wehrheim, H. K.: Maintenance convulsive treatments, Amer J Psychiat 121:1113-1115, 1965.

Kielholz, P.: Drug treatment of depressive states, Canad Psychiat Ass J 4:S129-S137, 1959.

Kiloh, L. G., Child, J. P., and Latner, G.: Controlled trial of iproniazid in treatment of endogenous depression, J Ment Sci 106:1139-1144, 1960.

Klotz, M.: Serial electroencephalographic changes due to electrotherapy, Dis Nerv Syst 16:120-121, 1955.

Krantz, J. C., et al.: Pharmacologic response to hexafluorodiethyl ether, J Pharmacol Exp Ther 121:362-368, 1957.

Krantz, L.: Douleurs rebelles du membre fantome avec toxicomanie guéries spectaculairment par quatre electrochocs, Concours Med 78:4215, 1956.

Lancaster, N. P., Steinert, R. R., and Frost, I.: Unilateral electro-convulsive therapy, J Ment Sci 104:221-227, 1958.

Laurell, B.: Flurothyl convulsive therapy, Acta Psychiat Scand, Suppl 213, 1970.

Lehmann, H., and Liddell, J.: Suxamethonium sensitivity, Brit Med J 2:501, 1964.

Lieser, H.: Heilkrämpfe als lebensrettende Therapie, Med Mschr 11:350-352, 1957.

MacIver, J., and Redlich, F.: Patterns of psychiatric practice, Amer J Psychiat 115:692-697, 1959.

Martin, W. L., et al.: Clinical evaluation of unilateral E.S.T., Amer J Psychiat 121:1087-1090, 1965.

McAndrew, J., and Hauser, G.: Preventilation of oxygen in electroconvulsive treatment: Suggested modification of technique, Amer J Psychiat 124:251-252, 1967.

Meduna, L. J.: General discussion of the cardiazol therapy, Amer J Psychiat 94 (Suppl):40-50, 1938.

Miller, D. H., Clancy, J., and Cumming E.: Comparison between unidirectional current nonconvulsive electrical stimulation given with Reiter's machine, standard alternating current electroshock (Cerletti method), and pentothal in chronic schizophrenia, Amer J Psychiat 109:617-620, 1953.

Nyström, S.: On relation between clinical factors and efficacy of ECT in depression, Acta Psychiat Scand 40 (Suppl 181): 5-140, 1964.

Oliver, W.: Account of the effects of camphor in a case of insanity, London Med J 6:120-130, 1785.

Oltman, J. E., and Friedman, S.: Comparison of EST and antidepressant drugs in affective disorders, Amer J Psychiat 118:355-357, 1961.

———: Comparison of temporal factors in depressive psychoses treated by EST and antidepressant drugs, Amer J Psychiat 119:579-580, 1962.

Osborne, R. G., Tunakan, B., and Barmore, J.: Anesthetic agent in electroconvulsive therapy: Controlled comparison, J Nerv Ment Dis 137:297-300, 1963.

Ottosson, J. O.: Experimental studies of memory impairment after electroconvulsive therapy: Role of the electrical stimulation and of the seizure studied by variation of stimulus intensity and modification by lidocaine of seizure discharge, Acta Psychiat Scand 35:103-124, 1960.

Page, L. G. M., and Russell, R. J.: Intensified electrical convulsion therapy in the treatment of mental disorders, Lancet 254:597-598, 1948.

Parry-Jones, W., Ll.: Oral atropine in premedication for electroconvulsive therapy, Lancet 1:1067-1068, 1964.

Pearson, J. S.: Prediction of the response of schizophrenic patients to electro-convulsive therapy, J Clin Psychol 6:285-287, 1950.

Perris, C.: Study of bipolar (manic-depressive) and unipolar recurrent depressive psychoses, Acta Psychiat Scand 42 (Suppl 194):7-189, 1966.

Pitts, F. N., Jr., et al.: Induction of anesthesia with methohexital and thiopental in electroconvulsive therapy: Effect on the electrocardiogram and clinical observations in 500 consecutive treatments with each agent, New Eng J Med 273: 353-360, 1965.

———: Drug modification of ECT: II. Succinylcholine dosage, Arch Gen Psychiat (Chicago) 19:595-598, 1968.

Polatin, P., and Linn, L.: Orthopedic and neurological follow-up study of vertebral fractures in shock therapy, Amer J Psychiat 105:825-828, 1949.

Porter, I. H.: Genetic basis of drug

metabolism in man, Toxic Appl Pharmacol *6:*499-511, 1964.

Riddell, S. A.: Therapeutic efficacy of ECT, Arch Gen Psychiat (Chicago) *8:*546-556, 1963.

Robin, A. A., and Harris, J. A.: Controlled comparison of imipramine and electroplexy, J Ment Sci (Brit J Psychiat) *108:*217-219, 1962.

Roth, M., and Rosie, J. M.: Use of electroplexy in mental disease with clouding of consciousness, J Ment Sci *99:*103-111, 1953.

Russell, R. J., Page, L. G. M., and Jillett, R. L.: Intensified electroconvulsant therapy: Review of five years' experience, Lancet *265:*1177-1179, 1953.

Sabawala, P. B., and Dillon, J. B.: Mode of action of depolarizing agents, Acta Anaesth Scand *3:*83-101, 1959.

Seager, C. P., and Bird, R. L.: Imipramine with electrical treatment in depression: Controlled trial, J Ment Sci (Brit J Psychiat) *108:*704-707, 1962.

Sloane, R. B., and Lewis, D. J.: Prognostic value of adrenaline and mecholyl responses in electroconvulsive therapy, J Psychosom Res *1:*273-286, 1956.

Smith, S.: Use of electroplexy (ECT) in psychiatric syndromes complicating pregnancy, J Ment Sci *102:*796-800, 1956.

Sobel, D. E.: Fetal damage due to ECT, insulin coma, chlorpromazine, or reserpine, Arch Gen Psychiat (Chicago) *2:*606-611, 1960.

Sogliani, G.: Elettroshockterapia e cardiazolterapia, Rass Studi Psichiat *28:*652-661, 1939.

Valdivia-Ponce, O.: Electroshock in neurodermatitis, Foreign letters, JAMA *163:*301, 1957.

Von Hagen, K. O.: Chronic intolerable pain: Discussion of its mechanism and report of eight cases treated with electroshock, JAMA *165:*773-777, 1957.

Whitwam, J. G. Moreton, T., and Norman, J.: Clinical signs with modified electroconvulsive therapy, Brit J Psychiat *109:*399-403, 1963.

Zamora, E. N., and Kaelbling, R.: Memory and electroconvulsive therapy, Amer J Psychiat *122:*546-554, 1965.

Zinkin, S., and Birtchnell, J.: Unilateral electroconvulsive therapy: Its effects on memory and its therapeutic efficacy, Brit J Psychiat *114:*973-988, 1968.

CHAPTER
SIXTEEN

Some Special Techniques

THE DIAGNOSTIC AND THERAPEUTIC USES OF INTRAVENOUS HYPNOTICS AND STIMULANTS

ALTHOUGH THE "TRUTH SERUM" of spy stories and detective fiction has in reality yet to emerge, the physician does have at his disposal a number of agents—amphetamines, barbiturates, hallucinogens—that can promote freer expression of feelings in taciturn, shy, or negativistic individuals. The communication produced in this altered state may provide the clinican with an additional dimension for diagnosis, but the veracity of the information is a different matter. Under the influence of these drugs, a person can engage in willful lying if he wishes (Gottschalk 1960); even when he means to be truthful, the drug may so distort his experience that he will present fantasies as facts (Dession 1953).

Both sedatives and stimulants are of value in such explorations, which are commonly called *narcosynthesis*. The relaxation and diminished alertness effected by *sedatives* tend to promote the flow of fantasy material and the ventilation of repressed feelings and forgotten events. *Stimulants* have a somewhat different effect: they produce a strong almost irresistible urge to talk, but the talk does not have the dreamlike quality induced by sedatives. It consists rather of ideas, emotions, and memories of which the individual is wholly conscious, even if he might be reluctant to discuss them without the aid of drugs.

HYPNOTICS

Amobarbital (Amytal) and thiopental (Pentothal) are the drugs most commonly used in narcosynthesis. The procedure is relatively simple: 20 cc of a 2.5% solution (25 mg/cc) is prepared and drawn up in a syringe. Approximately 2 cc (50 mg) is injected intravenously every minute until the patient is somewhat drowsy but still able to communicate. The required dosage is ascertained by asking the patient to count backwards and watching his eyelids: the injection is stopped or slowed when his speech begins to slur, his counting becomes uneven, or his eyelid tone decreases. The needle is left in the patient's vein, and diagnostic exploration begins. When his drowsiness starts to lift, he is given a few more cc's until he again reaches the desired level, but in no case should the total dosage exceed 500 mg. Another way of achieving the same result is to inject slowly whatever amount of barbiturate is required to induce a light sleep (200 to 500 mg, depending on the person and drug), wait for a few minutes until the patient awakens, and then begin the interview.

The manner in which the interview is conducted depends on its purpose. The interviewer who is trying to help the patient talk about disturbing feelings, embarrassing events, or repressed fantasies will obviously adopt a friendlier tone and present his questions more slowly than the interviewer who is trying to make the subject reveal a consciously concealed secret or looking for contradictions in a story he has told before. In some cases, an inquisitorial manner so upsets the patient that he fabricates new lies to cover the old, but such efforts at subterfuge are fairly transparent in an individual who is slightly obtunded, and he may lie so badly that the flaws in his story stick out. Even when he is not trying to deceive the interviewer, his disclosures must be taken with a grain of salt, for he will be markedly suggestible and thus likely to say what he thinks is expected of him rather than what he really thinks.

Interviews under the influence of hypnotics can clarify symptoms of organic, depressive, or schizophrenic illness that might otherwise elude the examiner. Patients showing confusion, negativism, and mutism are often given intravenous barbiturates in the hope that this will help the clinician decide whether the symptoms are functional or organic in origin. A sudden return of the patient's speech or a lifting of his confusion in response to barbiturates is usually viewed as evidence of functional disease, while a worsening of symptoms (such as an excessive degree of somnolence or the development of denial) is thought to prove that they are organic in origin. The first part of this equation is somewhat too simple, however, for hypnotics may have a normalizing effect on brain rhythms: a patient whose confusion is caused by some kind of cerebral dysrrhythmia may improve rather than deteriorate when given a hypnotic.

The deleterious effect of barbiturates on the organically damaged patient's condition is usually limited to an aggravation of current symptoms, such as dysphasia, confusion, or anosognosia. In some cases, however, the patient exhibits new symptoms or a resurgence of symptoms previously overcome. For example, intravenous barbiturates given to patients recovering from brain lesions tend to evoke disorientation and denial of illness whether or not they had had such symptoms at an earlier stage of their illness (Weinstein 1955). The patient who at one time denied but thereafter came to accept the incapacitation of a stroke-paralyzed arm may once more deny his loss on being given intravenous barbiturates. If some weeks later, after again being given an intravenous barbiturate, such denial is no longer shown, it may be assumed that his impairment is diminishing even though his manifest symptoms have shown no change.

Narcosynthesis may also be of value in demonstrating the presence of a suspected depressive or schizophrenic disease. When given a hypnotic, the depressed patient may at first show no signs of his illness or only such nonspecific signs as lethargy, easy fatigability, or somatic complaints, but then, as the interview progresses, become increasingly gloomy and self-castigating, and perhaps even break into tears. Similarly, the patient with an incipient or underlying schizophrenia may reveal delusional and hallucinatory material for the first time. If the patient is mute, withdrawn, and perhaps suffering from catatonic schizophrenia, an intravenous hypnotic may temporarily restore his speech and thus permit the interviewer to determine whether his thinking is bizarre enough to confirm the diagnosis.

Intravenous hypnotics have also been used for individuals who report that they are amnesic concerning specific events, both to aid recollection and to determine the validity of their claim of amnesia (Kiersch 1962, Lipton 1950). Individuals accused of a crime may ask to be interviewed while under the influence of hypnotics in the hope that this will corroborate their allegation of innocence. Such techniques, however, will not prevent a psychologically well-integrated person from lying or pretending to be amnesic in order to protect himself from a criminal conviction. The results with psychologically disturbed patients may be even more unreliable, for their memories may include "events" that are partially or wholly imaginary; they may confess all kinds of things, even crimes that they never committed. The situation becomes especially complex when the patient has both a reason to lie and an organic injury. For example, the individual may have committed a crime under the influence of alcohol or some other drug, or he may have become involved in a fight and subsequently been charged with assault and sustained a head injury. That he does not remember the actions with which he is charged, even under a hypnotic, is often viewed as evidence for his innocence. This view, however, is unequivocally inaccurate, for head traumas and alcoholic bouts can both affect an individual's ability to remember the past and leave him unable to recall what has happened under any conditions. In some cases, the psychiatrist will be told that the individual "can remember what he wants to," that his memory loss is out of proportion to the trauma he experienced, or that his memory has improved since the incident and that this proves he is shamming. This assessment may be unfounded, however, for it is well established that posttraumatic memory loss can initially extend well into the period prior to the accident but, in the course of recovery, progressively diminishes (Benson 1967, Fisher 1964, Zangwill 1961).

The hazards of narcosynthesis are the same as those encountered in anesthesia. The procedure, therefore, should be used with great caution, especially with patients who are debilitated, over 60, or suffering from some kind of organic brain syndrome. In such cases, it will be useful to have an experienced anesthiologist on hand and, at least for the first session, to limit the dose to 200 mg.

STIMULANTS

Intravenous methamphetamine (Methedrine) and methylphenidate (Ritalin) are the stimulants most commonly used for diagnostic exploration and abreaction (Blair 1959, Kerenyi 1960, Schein 1951). Doses of 20 to 30 mg in 10 cc of saline are injected slowly over a five-minute period. Within five or ten minutes, most patients will show dilated pupils, circumocular twitching, facial pallor, dryness of the mouth, cold, clammy hands, and dryness of the skin. The systolic blood pressure may rise as much as 40 or 50 mm; the pulse rate accelerates, and, in many cases, the patient feels tense and uncomfortable. Headaches, shortness of breath, paresthesias, and cardiac arrhythmias, especially supraventricular tachycardia (Chernoff 1962), have also been noted, but are extremely rare. Within 10 to 15 minutes, the initial symptoms and discomfort abate, the blood pressure returns to normal, and the patient seems more alert. At this time, he will generally start talking, whether or not he has been asked to do so. As his inhibitions fade, he pours forth his thoughts, sometimes with such feeling and suddenness that the narrative assumes explosive proportions. The loquaciousness may persist for as long as eight hours, during which time he may experience increased psychomotor activity, diminished appetite, and inability to sleep.

The intravenous administration of stimulants, in general, has the same diagnostic indications as that of hypnotics. It is particularly effective in uncovering masked depressions and delusional ideation. Even when there is no discussion of emotionally laden material, spontaneous sobbing can occur within 30 minutes after the administration of the drug and is often accompanied by a vivid reliving and recounting of certain unpleasant past experiences. When stimulants are given to borderline patients (those whom we might call latent schizophrenics) or to schizophrenics in a period of partial remission, erotic and hostile material with a somewhat delusional flavor may emerge. With the upsurge of hostile material, the patient may become increasingly excited and even combative, thus revealing the depth of the impulse-control disturbance that lurks behind his placid social facade.

Choice between Stimulants and Depressants for Exploratory Interviews

The choice of drugs depends to some extent on the diagnostic questions. Their range of usefulness overlaps in so many areas, however that it may make little difference which drug is used (Smith 1970), and it is often best to administer them sequentially (Abenson 1964, Ehrentheil 1963, Gottlieb 1945). The primary *advantage of stimulants* over hypnotics is that they preserve, or even heighten, the individual's alertness. Thus, the events that occur under the influence of a stimulant can be remembered even after the drug effect wears off. Their *disadvantage* is that they mobilize more affect than the hypnotics. The discharge of affect can be massive and the individual's behavior grossly disturbed. Stimulants are therefore to be avoided in patients suspected of being catatonic (Pennes 1954), unless enough nursing assistance is available to restrain the patient if the need should arise.

Hypnotics are preferable when it is necessary to explore certain dynamic issues, for they enable patients to discuss problems that they would normally be loath to acknowledge. Such discussions, however, tend to wander from one topic to the next by the most abstruse connections that are much like free association. The patient who has taken hypnotics, moreover, finds it difficult to retain the content of the proceedings, so much so that he may be unable to follow his own thread (Osborn 1967) or may forget what he has talked about. To some extent such memory lapses can hinder the desired effect of helping the patient face up to certain unpleasant issues, and they may evoke concern in paranoid patients, who often become frightened when they cannot remember what they have disclosed. The *sequential administration of both types of drugs* makes it possible to study the patient from both perspectives, in which case the barbiturate is usually administered first and, after the exploration under this drug is concluded (without removing the needle from the patient's arm), the stimulant is administered.

THERAPEUTIC USE OF INTRAVENOUS HYPNOTICS AND STIMULANTS

Difficult as it may be to explain why these drugs can temporarily relieve amnesia, mutism, or conversions, it is even more difficult to understand why such improvements often endure beyond the interview. Perhaps such cures occur because the patient becomes less negativistic while under their influence and can speak with the therapist, thus promoting a relationship that will continue even after the pharmacologic effects wear off. Perhaps they are effective because of the dramatic nature of the intervention and the conditions under which it takes place. Or perhaps they merely speed up remission in a patient whose symptoms are already easing.

Because these drugs facilitate emotional catharsis or abreaction, some clinicians consider them useful for patients who have an intellectual, but not an emotional, appreciation of their difficulties, for the patient, thus enabled to experience the feelings he has about the issues involved, can reconnect the affective component to the intellectual understanding. A drug-facilitated interview may also be helpful when an individual wants very much to discuss some particular matter but is too embarrassed to broach the topic or fears that doing so would be disloyal to the other persons involved. When given a "truth serum," which ostensibly "forces" him to talk, he may feel absolved of responsibility. As a result, he is able to release without guilt pent-up thoughts and feelings, an experience that can prove rewarding in terms of his sense of relief as well as the greater frankness and clarity in the psychotherapeutic transaction.

The foregoing may be among the reasons why the use of intravenous stimulants and hypnotics can produce a sudden amelioration of symptoms. Rapid results are also seen following other dramatic procedures, such as the use of ether, carbon dioxide abreaction, or intravenous acetylcholine (Meduna 1950, Palmer 1945, Sargant 1945, Sim 1966, Wilcox 1951). Indeed the "cures" resulting from these treatment forms are strikingly similar to those that utilize suggestion more directly, such as directive therapy or hypnoanalysis. In assessing the favorable therapeutic results of these drugs (Scarbrough 1958), their euphorizing or relaxing effects cannot be ignored, as these may well explain why patients are often extremely fond of the procedure and urge their physician to continue using it by telling him how much progress they are making. Herein lies also one of the major disadvantages of repeated narcosynthesis: some patients derive so much satisfaction from these drugs and the truth ceremony surrounding their use that they may, for months or even years, demand that this special state be induced whenever they become upset.

THERAPEUTIC USE OF PSYCHOTOMIMETICS

Psychiatric interest in the psychotomimetics has greatly intensified over the past decades. While these drugs are undoubtedly additions to the researcher's armamentarium (and to the headaches of the psychiatrist who deals with adolescents), it has not been established that they are of value in the treatment of mental illnesses (Faillace 1966). It is hard to say whether it is accurate to describe as "mind-expansion" the drug-induced distortions of perceptual and affective experience and the temporarily heightened sensitivity to areas of perceptual experience that would otherwise be ignored.

There are many reports that a hallucinogen-induced delirious state can enhance the individual's insight and thereby improve the way he thinks, feels, and behaves (Unger 1963). Most of these reports come from users, but the possibility must not be discounted that the dramatic character of the experience and the meaning the individual ascribes to it could enable him to use it as a starting point from which to change or even radically restructure his life, though the restructuring may not always be positive, especially from a social standpoint. Such radical changes have most often been described in well-integrated but somewhat withdrawn or affectless individuals who, after hallucinogen use, find new kinds of pleasure in artistic or musical pursuits they had previously considered irrelevant to their lives. The long-term therapeutic effect, however, cannot be separated from the placebo effect, particularly since the cognitive changes induced by these drugs are accompanied by a sense of portentousness. That they have this placebo effect does not, of course, speak against them. On the contrary, therapists using these techniques should consider how best to exploit this effect therapeutically (Jackson 1962).

Lsd and other hallucinogens should not be given to patients who have previously been psychotic, for they can decompensate under their influence. Hallucinogens are also contraindicated during pregnancy and in seizure disorders or other conditions in which marked excitement can be harmful (Hollister 1968).

PSYCHOSURGERY

The considerable attention that clinicians and researchers once paid to psychosurgery (Burckhardt 1890, Freeman 1942, Moniz, 1936) was so abruptly diverted by the introduction of chemotherapy that we may never know what its full potential might have been—whether, for example, the development of more refined techniques, less mutilating operations, or clearer indications would have allayed both the public's and the medical community's fears about such procedures. These fears were justified, to be sure, for the operations performed at that time were often followed by a deterioration of intellectual functioning and undesirable personality changes (Smith 1959). Silliness, lethargy, a lowering of ethical standards (Sykes 1964), and seizures (Logothetis 1968, Miller 1967) were among the more problematic consequences.

Almost all these undesirable effects are said to be preventable in the more recently developed operations (Sargant 1963). Open operative techniques include topectomy, orbitomedial undercutting (Busch 1955, Pool 1949, Scoville 1949, 1960), orbitoventromedial undercutting (Hirose 1965), LeBeau 1954); closed operative techniques include transorbital lobotomy (Freeman 1961), blind rostral leukotomy (McKissock 1959), electrocoagulation of the medial ventral quadrant (Grantham 1951, Thorpe 1960), and stereotactic thermolesions of the frontal white matter (Herner 1961). Ultrasound irradiation of the bimedial and frontal quadrants (Lindstrom 1963) and stereotactic implantation of radioactive yttrium Y [90] in the substantia innominata have also been used (Knight 1969). Choosing from this vast array of techniques is based largely on the psychiatrist's and surgeon's personal preference, for there are no controlled studies demonstrating that a particular operation is best for a particular illness, or indeed that the therapeutic outcome is in any way related to the procedure used. The beneficial effect of these operations, moreover, is little understood, though it seems related to a lessening of the patient's feeling of tenseness. His preoccupation with his symptoms is also diminished, perhaps as a result of his inability to concentrate on any particular thought or action for long. Delusions and hallucinations are reported to diminish in both quantity and perturbation of the patient, but such symptoms as isolation and withdrawal are little affected, and the gains made in the patient's manageability are often temporary.

That psychosurgery has not fallen into the same disfavor in Europe and Japan (Hirose 1965, Tooth 1961) as in the United States is partly due to sociocultural factors. The modern American family is generally unwilling and unable to take care of a member whose competence is much impaired (Vosburg 1962) and is thus not impressed by an operation that results only in increased sociability and manageability. In Europe, and especially in Japan, the family structure remains cohesive, and someone is usually available to stay home with the patient. An operation that diminishes the nursing and security problems enables the patient to go home and is thus considered a worthwhile achievement.

Although surgical intervention may not yet be regarded as totally outmoded, its uses have been largely preempted by other techniques, and there is little likelihood that it will ever assume a major role in psychiatric practice. That surgical interventions, even the smaller ones, are not and will not become "short cuts to mental health" is obvious. First, the effectiveness of psychosurgery has never been demonstrated in controlled studies (McKenzie 1964). Furthermore, the same effects can be achieved in most cases by psychotropic agents without risk of the irreversible changes attending surgery, thus leaving the door open to further trials whenever new drugs become available. For these reasons, psychosurgery is recommended only for those chronic schizophrenics who cannot be managed in any other way and who require constant restraint or isolation even in a hospital setting, for patients with phobic-obsessive tension states (Pippard 1962, Thorpe 1960) who are tortured and crippled by their symptoms and have failed to respond to other treatment measures, and for those with certain intractable seizure disorders (see p. 436).

INSULIN COMA TREATMENT

Insulin coma treatment (Sakel 1933, Steck 1932), which, less than two decades ago, was considered one of the most reliable methods of rehabilitating a schizophrenic patient, has today been almost completely abandoned. Although comparative studies are few and display various methodological weaknesses, it appears that phenothiazines are at least equally effective or superior in the treatment of schizophrenia (Ackner 1957, Fink 1958, Markowe 1967, McNeill 1961). There is growing belief that the results achieved with insulin coma can be attributed, at least partly, to the psychosocial impact of the insulin treatment wards rather than to the drug's biologic effects. In many ways, these wards were forerunners of today's active psychosocial treatment units, in that they were uniquely collaborative, well-structured, and optimistic oases of activity in the midst of an otherwise overcrowded, understaffed, and nihilistic hospital setting.

CONTINUOUS SLEEP TREATMENT

Prolonged sleep treatment, introduced into modern psychiatry by Kläsi in 1922 for the treatment of psychotic patients, has never been extensively used in the United States, and, like many other treatment forms, has been superseded by tranquilizers and antidepressants. However, it does enjoy some popularity in the Soviet Union, perhaps as an outgrowth of the Pavlovian concept that sleep is a state of diffuse inhibition, which exerts a protective influence on nervous function. The method used in the Soviet Union consists of giving the patient amobarbital (Amytal), 100 to 300 mg, every two or three hours, until he falls asleep. Thereafter, he is given enough barbiturate to keep him asleep for 16 to 20 hours a day. If the maximum dose of 1,200 mg of amobarbital daily is not sufficient to keep the patient asleep, he may be given some other hypnotic like chloral hydrate (1,500 to 2,000 mg/day in a single dose), or a combination of amobarbital (200 mg) and chlorpromazine (Thorazine), 75 mg, every four to six hours. Throughout the course of treatment, he is awakened only twice daily for one to three hours to be fed and ambulated.

From the first to the third day, the patient sleeps very deeply and, in the brief periods of waking, may show a somewhat euphoric and intoxicated state (Hartman 1968). From the fourth to the eighth day, the dosage of the hypnotic is gradually decreased until his sleep becomes lighter. From the eighth to the twelfth day, the dosage is further decreased until finally the patient sleeps only at night (Antonelli 1954). In mild cases, briefer courses of treatment may be used, but dosage must be diminished gradually, nonetheless, in order to avoid withdrawal symptoms.

The complications of continuous sleep treatment are identical with those of anesthetic or barbiturate poisoning (see p. 290), and precautionary measures require continuous supervision by a nurse specialized in the procedure. The patient is examined at least twice daily for evidence of neurologic and respiratory complications. Pulse, temperature, respiratory rate, and blood pressure must be measured at least six times daily, especially before each fresh dose of the drug. Fluid intake and output must also be measured and recorded. Approximately 3,500 to 4,000 cc of fluid daily are required to prevent dehydration and intoxication. If the patient is unable to drink this amount, fluids must be administered intravenously.

Pneumonitis, atelectasis, shock, cardiac arrhythmia, venous thrombosis, and intercurrent infections are among the more serious complications. Thus, continuous sleep treatment is contraindicated for any patient whose age, cardiovascular, pulmonary, metabolic, or nutritional status makes him a poor anesthetic risk. The potential hazards of the treatment, the demands made on nursing personnel, and the questionable and often temporary results of its effects have discouraged most clinicians from using sleep therapy except in manic excitement, in cases of severe and intractable anxiety states sometimes seen in young patients, and in certain psychosomatic disorders.

Another form of artificial sleep used in the treatment of neurotic and psychophysiologic disorders is the so-called "electrosleep." Light sleep of between 30 and 120 minutes' duration is induced by devices that put out small modulated electric impulses (usually rectangular waves with a peak voltage of 20 to 40 volts and a duration of 0.4 to 1.2 ms). The electrodes are placed on the patient's forehead above the eye and on the nape of the neck. Treatment is usually given five or six times weekly for a total of 15 to 20 times. During treatment, the patient is also exposed to a "white noise"; and this combination allegedly produces sleep in the majority of patients (Magora 1965, Sergeev 1963). Electrosleep has never gained wide popularity in the United States, and controlled studies have failed to confirm the therapeutic results reported abroad (Miller 1965, Woods 1965).

REFERENCES

Abenson, M. H., and Beattie, R. T.: Comparison of reagents in the abreaction of mute schizophrenics, Acta Psychiat Scand 40:234-239, 1964.

Ackner, B., Harris, A., and Oldham, A. J.: Insulin treatment of schizophrenia: A controlled study, Lancet 1:607-611, 1957.

Antonelli, F.: La narcoterapia nella nervosi reumatica, Reumatismo 6:166-173, 1954.

Benson, D. F., and Geschwind, N.: Shrinking retrograde amnesia, J Neurol Neurosurg Psychiat *30*:539-544, 1967.

Blair, R. A., Shafar, S., and Krawiecki, J. A.: Methylphenidate (Ritalin): An adjunct to psychotherapy, Brit J Psychiat *105*:1032-1034, 1959.

Burckhardt, G.: Über Rindenexcisionen als Beitrag zur operativen Therapie der Psychosen, Allg Ztschr f Psychiat *74*:463-548, 1890.

Busch, E., *et al.*: Orbitomedial frontal undercutting in mental disease: A follow-up examination of 154 patients, Danish Med Bull *2*:10-20, 1955.

Chernoff, R. W., Wallen, M. H., and Muller, O. F.: Cardiac toxicity of methylphenidate: Report of two cases, New Eng J Med *266*:400-401, 1962.

Dession, G. H., *et al.*: Drug-induced revelation and criminal investigation, Yale Law J *62*:315-347, 1953.

Ehrentheil, O. F.: Thought content of mute chronic schizophrenic patients: Interviews after injection of amobarbital sodium (sodium amytal) and methamphetamine hydrochloride (Methedrine), J Nerv Ment Dis *137*:187-197, 1963.

Faillace, L. A.: Clinical use of psychotomimetic drugs, Compr Psychiat *7*:13-20, 1966.

Fink, M., *et al.*: Comparative study of chlorpromazine and insulin coma therapy of psychosis, JAMA *166*:1846-1850, 1958.

Fisher, C. M., and Adams, R. D.: Transient global amnesia, Acta Neurol Scand *40* (Suppl 9):1-83, 1964.

Freeman, W.: Psychosurgery a quarter of a century later, Proc III World Cong Psychiat, vol. 6, 1961, pp. 141-148.

Freeman, W., and Watts, J. W.: Psychosurgery: Intelligence, Emotion and Social Behavior Following Prefrontal Lobotomy for Mental Disorders, Springfield (Ill): Thomas, 1942.

Gottlieb, J. S., Krouse, H., and Freidinger, A. W.: Psychopharmalologic study of schizophrenia and depressions, Arch Neurol Psychiat (Chic) *54*:372-377, 1945.

Gottschalk, L. A.: The use of drugs in information-seeking interviews, *in* Uhr, L. M., and Miller, J. G., eds.: Drugs and Behavior, New York: Wiley, 1960, pp. 515-518.

Grantham, E. C.: Prefrontal lobotomy for the relief of pain, with a report of a new operative technique, J Neurosurg *8*:405-410, 1951.

Hartman, E.: Dauerschlaf: A poly-graphic study, Arch Gen Psychiat (Chicago) *18*:99-111, 1968.

Herner, T.: Treatment of mental disorders with frontal stereotaxic thermolesions, Acta Psychiat Scand *36*(Suppl 158): 8-11 and 132-134, 1961.

Hirose, S.: Orbito-ventromedial undercutting 1957-1963: Follow-up study of 77 cases, Amer J Psychiat *121*:1194-1202, 1965.

Hollister, L. E.: Chemical psychoses: LSD and related drugs, Springfield (Ill): Thomas, 1968.

Jackson, D. D.: LSD and the new beginning, J Nerv Ment Dis *135*:435-439, 1962.

Kerenyi, A. B., Koranyi, E. K., and Sarwer-Foner, G. J.: Depressive states and drugs—III: Use of methylphenidate (Ritalin) in open psychiatric settings and in office practice, Canad Med Ass J *83*:1249-1254, 1960.

Kiersch, T. A.: Amnesia: A clinical study of ninety-eight cases, Amer J Psychiat *119*:57-60, 1962.

Kläsi, J.: Über die therapeutische Anwendung der "Dauernarkose" mittels Somnifen bei Schizophrenen, Z Ges Neurol Psychiat *74*:557-592, 1922.

Knight, G. C.: Bi-frontal stereotactic tractotomy: Atraumatic operation of value in the treatment of intractable psychoneurosis, Brit J Psychiat *115*:257-266, 1969.

Le Beau, J.: Psycho-Chirurgie et Fonctions Mentales: Techniques, Resultats, Applications Physiologiques, Paris: Masson, 1954.

Lindstrom, P. A., Moench, L. G., and Rovnaek, A.: Prefrontal sonic treatment (PST), Amer J Psychiat *120*:487-491, 1963.

Lipton, E.: The amytal interview, Amer Practit *1*:148-163, 1950.

Logothetis, J.: Long-term evaluation of convulsive seizures following prefrontal lobotomy, J Nerv Ment Dis *146*:71-79, 1968.

Magora, F., *et al.*: Observations on electrically induced sleep in man, Brit J Anaesth *37*:480-491, 1965.

Markowe, M., Steinert, J., and Heyworth-Davis, F.: Insulin and chlorpromazine in schizophrenia: Ten year comparative survey, Brit J Psychiat *113*:1101-1106, 1967.

McKenzie, K. G., and Kaczanowski, G.: Prefrontal leukotomy: A five-year controlled study, Canad Med Ass J *91*:1193-1196, 1964.

McKissock, W.: Discussion on psychosurgery, Proc Roy Soc Med *52*:206-209, 1959.

McNeill, D. L. M., and Madgwick, J. R. A.: Comparison of results in schizophrenics treated with (1) insulin, (2) trifluoperazine (Stelazine), J Ment Sci *107*:297-299, 1961.

Meduna, L. J.: Carbon-dioxide Therapy: Neurophysiological Treatment of Nervous Disorders, Springfield (Ill): Thomas, 1950.

Miller, A.: The lobotomy patient—A decade later, Canad Med Ass J *96*:1095-1103, 1967.

Miller, E. C., and Mathas, J. L.: Use and effectiveness of electrosleep in the treatment of some common psychiatric problems, Amer J Psychiat *122*:460-462, 1965.

Moniz, E.: Les possibilitiés de la chirurgie dans le traitement de certaines psychoses, Lisboa Med *13*:141-151, 1936.

Osborn, A. G., et al.: Effects of thiopental sedation on learning and memory, Science *157*:574-576, 1967.

Palmer, H. A.: Abreactive techniques —ether, J Roy Army Med Cps *84*:86-87, 1945.

Pennes, H. H.: Clinical reactions of schizophrenics to sodium amytal, pervitin hydrochloride, mescaline sulfate, and d-lysergic acid diethylamide (LSD25), J Nerv Ment Dis *119*:95-112, 1954.

Pippard, J.: Leucotomy in Britain today, Brit J Psychiat *108*:249-255, 1962.

Pool, J. L., Heath, R. G., and Weber, J. J.: Topectomy: Surgical indications and results, Bull NY Acad Med *25*:335-344, 1949.

Sakel, M.: Neue Behandlung der Morphinsucht (Eine Insulinkur beseitigt die Abstinenzerscheinungen durch Ausgleich des während der Entziehung gestörten Gleichgewichtes im vegetativen Nervensystem), Z Ges Neurol Psychiat *143*:506-534, 1933.

Sargant, W., and Shorvon, H.: Acute war neurosis, Arch Neurol Psychiat (Chic) *54*:231-240, 1945.

Sargant, W., and Slater, E.: An Introduction to Physical Methods of Treatment in Psychiatry, Baltimore: Williams & Wilkins, 1963.

Scarbrough, H. E., and Wheelis, D. E.: Treatment of therapeutic blockades with thiopental (Pentothal) sodium and methamphetamine (Desoxyn), 1948-1957, Psychosom Med *20*:108-116, 1958.

Schein, J., and Goolker, P.: Preliminary report on the use of d-desoxephedrine hydrochloride in the study of psychopathology and psychotherapy, Amer J Psychiat *107*:850-855, 1951.

Scoville, W. B.: Selective cortical undercutting as a means of modifying and studying frontal lobe function in man: Preliminary report of forty-three operative cases, J Neurosurg *6*:65-73, 1949.

———: Late results of orbital undercutting: Report of 76 patients undergoing quantitative selective lobotomies, Amer J Psychiat *117*:525-532, 1960.

Sergeev, G. V.: Electrosleep as a method of neurotropic therapy of patients with hypersensitive disease, Amer Heart J *66*: 138-139, 1963.

Sim, M., and Houghton, H.: Phobic anxiety and its treatment, J Nerv Ment Dis *143*:484-491, 1966.

Smith, A., and Kinder, E. F.: Changes in psychological test performances of brain operated schizophrenics after 8 years, Science *129*:3342-3345, 1959.

Smith, B. M., Hain, J. D., and Stevenson, I.: Controlled interviews using drugs, Arch Gen Psychiat (Chicago) *22*:1-10, 1970.

Steck, H.: Die Behandlung des Delirium tremens mit Insulin, Schweiz Arch Neurol Neurochir Psychiat *29*:173, 1932.

Sykes, M. K., and Tredgold, R. F.: Restricted orbital undercutting: A study of its effects on 350 patients over the ten years 1951-1960, Brit J Psychiat *110*:609-640, 1964.

Thorpe, F. T.: Electrocoagulation of the cerebral orbital projection in the persistent depressive psychoses of the elderly, J Ment Sci *106*:771-779, 1960.

Tooth, G. C., and Newton, M. P.: Leucotomy in England and Wales 1942-1954, Ministry of Health Reports on Public Health and Medical Subjects No. 104, London, Her Majesty's Stationery Office, 1961.

Unger, S. M.: Mescaline, LSD, psilocybin and personality change: A review, Psychiatry *26*:111-125, 1963.

Vosburg, R. L.: Lobotomy in western Pennsylvania: Looking backward over ten years, Amer J Psychiat *119*:503-510, 1962.

Weinstein, E. A., and Kahn, R. L.: Denial of Illness, Springfield (Ill): Thomas, 1955.

Wilcox, P. H.: Psychopenetration, Dis Nerv Syst *12*:35-38, 1951.

Woods, L. W., Tyce, A. J., and Bickford, M. B.: Electric sleep-producing devices: An evaluation using EEG monitoring, Amer J Psychiat *122*:153-158, 1965.

Zangwill, O. L.: Psychological studies of amnesic states, Proc III World Cong Psychiat, vol. 3, 1961, pp. 219-222.

Appendix

TABLE 47. *Agents Used in Psychiatry Listed by Generic Name*

GENERIC NAME	TRADE NAME (MANUFACTURER)	CATEGORY OF AGENT
Acetazolamide	Diamox (Lederle)	Anticonvulsants Adjuvant
Acetophenazine	Tindal (Schering)	Major tranquilizers Phenothiazines
Amitriptyline	Elavil (Merck)	Antidepressants Dibenzazepines
Amobarbital	Amytal (Lilly)	General depressants of the CNS Sedatives and hypnotics
Amphetamine	Benzedrine (SKF)	Stimulants
Benztropine	Cogentin (Merck)	Antiparkinsonian agents Atropine-like agents
Biperiden	Akineton (Knoll)	Antiparkinsonian agents Atropine-like agents
Butabarbital	Butisol (McNeil)	General depressants of the CNS Sedatives and hypnotics
Butaperazine	Repoise (Robins)	Major tranquilizers Phenothiazines
Carphenazine	Proketazine (Wyeth)	Major tranquilizers Phenothiazines
Chloral hydrate	Felsules (Fellows) Noctec (Squibb) Somnos (Merck)	General depressants of the CNS Sedatives and hypnotics
Chlordiazepoxide	Librium (Roche)	General depressants of the CNS Minor tranquilizers
Chlorpromazine	Thorazine (SKF)	Major tranquilizers Phenothiazines
Chlorprothixene	Taractan (Roche)	Major tranquilizers Thioxanthenes
Cycrimine	Pagitane (Lilly)	Antiparkinsonian agents Atropine-like agents
Desipramine	Norpramin (Lakeside) Pertofrane (Geigy)	Antidepressants Dibenzazepines
Dextroamphetamine	Dexedrine (SKF)	Stimulants
Diazepam	Valium (Roche)	General depressants of the CNS Minor tranquilizers
Diphenhydramine	Benadryl (Parke-Davis)	Antiparkinsonian agents Antihistamines
Diphenylhydantoin	Dilantin (Parke-Davis)	Anticonvulsants Hydantoin derivatives
Disulfiram	Antabuse (Ayerst)	Agents used in the treatment of drug addiction and abuse
Doxepin	Sinequan (Pfizer)	Antidepressants Dibenzazepines
Ethchlorvynol	Placidyl (Abbott)	General depressants of the CNS Sedatives and hypnotics
Ethinamate	Valmid (Lilly)	General depressants of the CNS Sedatives and hypnotics
Ethosuximide	Zarontin (Parke-Davis)	Anticonvulsants Succinimide derivatives

TABLE 47 *Agents Used in Psychiatry Listed by Generic Name* (continued)

GENERIC NAME	TRADE NAME (MANUFACTURER)	CATEGORY OF AGENT
Ethotoin	Peganone (Abbott)	Anticonvulsants Hydantoin derivatives
Fluphenazine	Permitil (White) Prolixin (Squibb)	Major tranquilizers Phenothiazines
Glutethimide	Doriden (Ciba)	General depressants of the CNS Sedatives and hypnotics
Haloperidol	Haldol (McNeil)	Major tranquilizers Butyrophenones
Heptabarbital	Medomin (Geigy)	General depressants of the CNS Sedatives and hypnotics
Hydroxyzine	Atarax (Roerig) Vistaril (Pfizer)	General depressants of the CNS Minor tranquilizers
Imipramine	Tofranil (Geigy)	Antidepressants Dibenzazepines
Isocarboxazid	Marplan (Roche)	Antidepressants MAO inhibitors
Levallorphan	Lorfan (Roche)	Agents used in the treatment of drug addiction and abuse
Lithium carbonate	Eskalith (SKF) Lithane (Pfizer) Lithonate (Rowell)	Antidepressants Normothymics
Mephenytoin	Mesantoin (Sandoz)	Anticonvulsants Hydantoin derivatives
Mephobarbital	Mebaral (Winthrop)	Anticonvulsants Barbiturates
Meprobamate	Equanil (Wyeth) Miltown (Wallace)	General depressants of the CNS Minor tranquilizers
Methadone	Dolophine (Lilly)	Agents used in the treatment of drug addiction and abuse
Methamphetamine	Desoxyn (Abbott) Methedrine (Burroughs)	Stimulants
Methaqualone	Quäälude (Rorer)	General depressants of the CNS Sedatives and hypnotics
Metharbital	Gemonil (Abbott)	Anticonvulsants Barbiturates
Methohexital	Brevital (Lilly)	General depressants of the CNS Sedatives and hypnotics
Methsuximide	Celontin (Parke-Davis)	Anticonvulsants Succinimide derivatives
Methylphenidate	Ritalin (Ciba)	Stimulants
Methyprylon	Noludar (Roche)	General depressants of the CNS Sedatives and hypnotics
Nalorphine	Nalline (Merck)	Agents used in the treatment of drug addiction and abuse
Nialamide	Niamid (Pfizer)	Antidepressants MAO inhibitors
Nortriptyline	Aventyl (Lilly)	Antidepressants Dibenzazepines
Orphenadrine	Disipal (Riker)	Antiparkinsonian agents Antihistamines

TABLE 47 *Agents Used in Psychiatry Listed by Generic Name* (continued)

GENERIC NAME	TRADE NAME (MANUFACTURER)	CATEGORY OF AGENT
Oxazepam	Serax (Wyeth)	General depressants of the CNS Minor tranquilizers
Paraldehyde	Paral (Fellows)	General depressants of the CNS Sedatives and hypnotics
Paramethadione	Paradione (Abbott)	Anticonvulsants Oxazolidine derivatives
Pentobarbital	Nembutal (Abbott)	General depressants of the CNS Sedatives and hypnotics
Perphenazine	Trilafon (Schering)	Major tranquilizers Phenothiazines
Phenacemide	Phenurone (Abbott)	Anticonvulsants Acetyl ureas
Phenelzine	Nardil (Warner)	Antidepressants MAO inhibitors
Phenobarbital	Eskabarb (SKF) Eskaphen (SKF) Luminal (Winthrop)	General depressants of the CNS Sedatives and hypnotics Anticonvulsants
Phensuximide	Milontin (Parke-Davis)	Anticonvulsants Succinimide derivatives
Primidone	Mysoline (Ayerst)	Anticonvulsants Barbiturate congener
Prochlorperazine	Compazine (SKF)	Major tranquilizers Phenothiazines
Procyclidine	Kemadrin (Burroughs)	Antiparkinsonian agents Atropine-like agents
Promazine	Sparine (Wyeth)	Major tranquilizers Phenothiazines
Protriptyline	Vivactil (Merck)	Antidepressants Dibenzazepines
Reserpine	Serpasil (Ciba)	Major tranquilizers Rauwolfia alkaloids
Secobarbital	Seconal (Lilly)	General depressants of the CNS Sedatives and hypnotics
Talbutal	Lotusate (Winthrop)	General depressants of the CNS Sedatives and hypnotics
Thioridazine	Mellaril (Sandoz)	Major tranquilizers Phenothiazines
Thiothixene	Navane (Roerig)	Major tranquilizers Thioxanthenes
Tranylcypromine	Parnate (SKF)	Antidepressants MAO inhibitors
Trifluoperazine	Stelazine (SKF)	Major tranquilizers Phenothiazines
Triflupromazine	Vesprin (Squibb)	Major tranquilizers Phenothiazines
Trihexyphenidyl	Artane (Lederle) Tremin (Schering)	Antiparkinsonian agents Atropine-like agents
Trimethadione	Tridione (Abbott)	Anticonvulsants Oxazolidine derivatives
Tybamate	Solacen (Wallace) Tybatran (Robins)	General depressants of the CNS Minor tranquilizers

TABLE 48 *Agents Used in Psychiatry Listed by Trade Name* *

TRADE NAME (MANUFACTURER)	GENERIC NAME	CATEGORY OF AGENT
Akineton (Knoll)	Biperiden	Antiparkinsonian agents Atropine-like agents
Amytal (Lilly)	Amobarbital	General depressants of the CNS Sedatives and hypnotics
Antabuse (Ayerst)	Disulfiram	Agents used in the treatment of drug addiction and abuse
Artane (Lederle)	Trihexyphenidyl	Antiparkinsonian agents Atropine-like agents
Atarax (Roerig)	Hydroxyzine	General depressants of the CNS Minor tranquilizers
Aventyl (Lilly)	Nortriptyline	Antidepressants Dibenzazepines
Benadryl (Parke-Davis)	Diphenhydramine	Antiparkinsonian agents Antihistamines
Benzedrine (SKF)	Amphetamine	Stimulants
Brevital (Lilly)	Methohexital	General depressants of the CNS Sedatives and hypnotics
Butisol (McNeil)	Butabarbital	General depressants of the CNS Sedatives and hypnotics
Celontin (Parke-Davis)	Methsuximide	Anticonvulsants Succinimide derivatives
Cogentin (Merck)	Benztropine	Antiparkinsonian agents Atropine-like agents
Compazine (SKF)	Prochlorperazine	Major tranquilizers Phenothiazines
Desoxyn (Abbott)	Methamphetamine	Stimulants
Dexedrine (SKF)	Dextroamphetamine	Stimulants
Diamox (Lederle)	Acetazolamide	Anticonvulsants Adjuvant
Dilantin (Parke-Davis)	Diphenylhydantoin	Anticonvulsants Hydantoin derivatives
Disipal (Riker)	Orphenadrine	Antiparkinsonian agents Antihistamines
Dolophine (Lilly)	Methadone	Agents used in the treatment of drug addiction and abuse
Doriden (Ciba)	Glutethimide	General depressants of the CNS Sedatives and hypnotics
Elavil (Merck)	Amitriptyline	Antidepressants Dibenzazepines
Equanil (Wyeth)	Meprobamate	General depressants of the CNS Minor tranquilizers
Eskabarb (SKF)	Phenobarbital	General depressants of the CNS Sedatives and hypnotics Anticonvulsants
Eskalith (SKF)	Lithium carbonate	Antidepressants Normothymics
Eskaphen (SKF)	Phenobarbital	General depressants of the CNS Sedatives and hypnotics Anticonvulsants

TABLE 48 *Agents Used in Psychiatry Listed by Trade Name* (continued)

TRADE NAME (MANUFACTURER)	GENERIC NAME	CATEGORY OF AGENT
Felsules (Fellows)	Chloral hydrate	General depressants of the CNS Sedatives and hypnotics
Gemonil (Abbott)	Metharbital	Anticonvulsants Barbiturates
Haldol (McNeil)	Haloperidol	Major tranquilizers Butyrophenones
Kemadrin (Burroughs)	Procyclidine	Antiparkinsonian agents Atropine-like agents
Librium (Roche)	Chlordiazepoxide	General depressants of the CNS Minor tranquilizers
Lithane (Pfizer)	Lithium carbonate	Antidepressants Normothymics
Lithonate (Rowell)	Lithium carbonate	Antidepressants Normothymics
Lorfan (Roche)	Levallorphan	Agents used in the treatment of drug addiction and abuse
Lotusate (Winthrop)	Talbutal	General depressants of the CNS Sedatives and hypnotics
Luminal (Winthrop)	Phenobarbital	General depressants of the CNS Sedatives and hypnotics Anticonvulsants
Marplan (Roche)	Isocarboxazid	Antidepressants MAO inhibitors
Mebaral (Winthrop)	Mephobarbital	Anticonvulsants Barbiturates
Medomin (Geigy)	Heptabarbital	General depressants of the CNS Sedatives and hypnotics
Mellaril (Sandoz)	Thioridazine	Major tranquilizers Phenothiazines
Mesantoin (Sandoz)	Mephenytoin	Anticonvulsants Hydantoin derivatives
Methedrine (Burroughs)	Methamphetamine	Stimulants
Milontin (Parke-Davis)	Phensuximide	Anticonvulsants Succinimide derivatives
Miltown (Wallace)	Meprobamate	General depressants of the CNS Minor tranquilizers
Mysoline (Ayerst)	Primidone	Anticonvulsants Barbiturate congener
Nalline (Merck)	Nalorphine	Agents used in the treatment of drug addiction and abuse
Nardil (Warner)	Phenelzine	Antidepressants MAO inhibitors
Navane (Roerig)	Thiothixene	Major tranquilizers Thioxanthenes
Nembutal (Abbott)	Pentobarbital	General depressants of the CNS Sedatives and hypnotics
Niamid (Pfizer)	Nialamide	Antidepressants MAO inhibitors
Noctec (Squibb)	Chloral hydrate	General depressants of the CNS Sedatives and hypnotics

TABLE 48 *Agents Used in Psychiatry Listed by Trade Name* (continued)

TRADE NAME (MANUFACTURER)	GENERIC NAME	CATEGORY OF AGENT
Noludar (Roche)	Methyprylon	General depressants of the CNS Sedatives and hypnotics
Norpramin (Lakeside)	Desipramine	Antidepressants Dibenzazepines
Pagitane (Lilly)	Cycrimine	Antiparkinsonian agents Atropine-like agents
Paradione (Abbott)	Paramethadione	Anticonvulsants Oxazolidine derivatives
Paral (Fellows)	Paraldehyde	General depressants of the CNS Sedatives and hypnotics
Parnate (SKF)	Tranylcypromine	Antidepressants MAO inhibitors
Peganone (Abbott)	Ethotoin	Anticonvulsants Hydantoin derivatives
Permitil (White)	Fluphenazine	Major tranquilizers Phenothiazines
Pertofrane (Geigy)	Desipramine	Antidepressants Dibenzazepines
Phenurone (Abbott)	Phenacemide	Anticonvulsants Acetyl ureas
Placidyl (Abbott)	Ethchlorvynol	General depressants of the CNS Sedatives and hypnotics
Proketazine (Wyeth)	Carphenazine	Major tranquilizers Phenothiazines
Prolixin (Squibb)	Fluphenazine	Major tranquilizers Phenothiazines
Quäälude (Rorer)	Methaqualone	General depressants of the CNS Sedatives and hypnotics
Repoise (Robins)	Butaperazine	Major tranquilizers Phenothiazines
Ritalin (Ciba)	Methylphenidate	Stimulants
Seconal (Lilly)	Secobarbital	General depressants of the CNS Sedatives and hypnotics
Serax (Wyeth)	Oxazepam	General depressants of the CNS Minor tranquilizers
Serpasil (Ciba)	Reserpine	Major tranquilizers Rauwolfia alkaloids
Sinequan (Pfizer)	Doxepin	Antidepressants Dibenzazepines
Solacen (Wallace)	Tybamate	General depressants of the CNS Minor tranquilizers
Somnos (Merck)	Chloral hydrate	General depressants of the CNS Sedatives and hypnotics
Sparine (Wyeth)	Promazine	Major tranquilizers Phenothiazines
Stelazine (SKF)	Trifluoperazine	Major tranquilizers Phenothiazines
Taractan (Roche)	Chlorprothixene	Major tranquilizers Thioxanthenes

TABLE 48 *Agents Used in Psychiatry Listed by Trade Name* (continued)

TRADE NAME (MANUFACTURER)	GENERIC NAME	CATEGORY OF AGENT
Thorazine (SKF)	Chlorpromazine	Major tranquilizers Phenothiazines
Tindal (Schering)	Acetophenazine	Major tranquilizers Phenothiazines
Tofranil (Geigy)	Imipramine	Antidepressants Dibenzazepines
Tremin (Schering)	Trihexyphenidyl	Antiparkinsonian agents Atropine-like agents
Tridione (Abbott)	Trimethadione	Anticonvulsants Oxazolidine derivatives
Trilafon (Schering)	Perphenazine	Major tranquilizers Phenothiazines
Tybatran (Robins)	Tybamate	General depressants of the CNS Minor tranquilizers
Valium (Roche)	Diazepam	General depressants of the CNS Minor tranquilizers
Valmid (Lilly)	Ethinamate	General depressants of the CNS Sedatives and hypnotics
Vesprin (Squibb)	Triflupromazine	Major tranquilizers Phenothiazines
Vistaril (Pfizer)	Hydroxyzine	General depressants of the CNS Minor tranquilizers
Vivactil (Merck)	Protriptyline	Antidepressants Dibenzazepines
Zarontin (Parke-Davis)	Ethosuximide	Anticonvulsants Succinimide derivatives

* For an international index of trade names see Pöldinger, W., and Schmidlin, P.: Index Psychopharmacorum, 1966, Bern: Huber, 1966.

TABLE 49 *Agents Used in Psychiatry Listed by Category*

CATEGORY OF AGENT	GENERIC NAME	TRADE NAME (MANUFACTURER)
MAJOR TRANQUILIZERS		
Phenothiazines	Fluphenazine	Permitil (White)
		Prolixin (Squibb)
	Trifluoperazine	Stelazine (SKF)
	Butaperazine	Repoise (Robins)
	Perphenazine	Trilafon (Schering)
	Prochlorperazine	Compazine (SKF)
	Acetophenazine	Tindal (Schering)
	Carphenazine	Proketazine (Wyeth)
	Promazine	Sparine (Wyeth)
	Triflupromazine	Vesprin (Squibb)
	Chlorpromazine	Thorazine (SKF)
	Thioridazine	Mellaril (Sandoz)
Thioxanthenes	Chlorprothixene	Taractan (Roche)
	Thiothixene	Navane (Roerig)
Butyrophenones	Haloperidol	Haldol (McNeil)
Rauwolfia Alkaloids	Reserpine	Serpasil (Ciba)
GENERAL DEPRESSANTS OF THE CNS		
Minor Tranquilizers		
Propanediols	Meprobamate	Equanil (Wyeth)
		Miltown (Wallace)
	Tybamate	Solacen (Wallace)
		Tybatran (Robins)
Benzodiazepines	Chlordiazepoxide	Librium (Roche)
	Diazepam	Valium (Roche)
	Oxazepam	Serax (Wyeth)
Diphenylmethane Derivatives	Hydroxyzine	Atarax (Roerig)
		Vistaril (Pfizer)
Sedatives and hypnotics		
Barbiturates	Amobarbital	Amytal (Lilly)
	Butabarbital	Butisol (McNeil)
	Heptabarbital	Medomin (Geigy)
	Methohexital	Brevital (Lilly)
	Pentobarbital	Nembutal (Abbott)
	Phenobarbital	Eskabarb (SKF)
		Eskaphen (SKF)
		Luminal (Winthrop)
	Secobarbital	Seconal (Lilly)
	Talbutal	Lotusate (Winthrop)
Nonbarbiturates	Ethchlorvynol	Placidyl (Abbott)
	Ethinamate	Valmid (Lilly)
	Glutethimide	Doriden (Ciba)
	Methyprylon	Noludar (Roche)
	Chloral hydrate	Felsules (Fellows)
		Noctec (Squibb)
		Somnos (Merck)
	Paraldehyde	Paral (Fellows)
	Methaqualone	Quäälude (Rorer)

TABLE 49 *Agents Used in Psychiatry Listed by Category* (continued)

CATEGORY OF AGENT	GENERIC NAME	TRADE NAME (MANUFACTURER)
ANTIDEPRESSANTS		
Dibenzazepines	Amitriptyline	Elavil (Merck)
	Desipramine	Norpramin (Lakeside)
		Pertofrane (Geigy)
	Doxepin	Sinequan (Pfizer)
	Imipramine	Tofranil (Geigy)
	Nortriptyline	Aventyl (Lilly)
	Protriptyline	Vivactil (Merck)
MAO Inhibitors	Isocarboxazid	Marplan (Roche)
	Nialamide	Niamid (Pfizer)
	Phenelzine	Nardil (Warner)
	Tranylcypromine	Parnate (SKF)
Normothymics	Lithium carbonate	Eskalith (SKF)
		Lithane (SKF)
		Lithonate (Rowell)
STIMULANTS	Amphetamine	Benzedrine (SKF)
	Dextroamphetamine	Dexedrine (SKF)
	Methamphetamine	Desoxyn (Abbott)
		Methedrine (Burroughs)
	Methylphenidate	Ritalin (Ciba)
ANTICONVULSANTS		
Hydantoin derivatives	Ethotoin	Peganone (Abbott)
	Mephenytoin	Mesantoin (Sandoz)
	Diphenylhydantoin	Dilantin (Parke-Davis)
Oxazolidine Derivatives	Paramethadione	Paradione (Abbott)
	Trimethadione	Tridione (Abbott)
Acetyl Ureas	Phenacemide	Phenurone (Abbott)
Succinimide Derivatives	Ethosuximide	Zarontin (Parke-Davis)
	Methsuximide	Celontin (Parke-Davis)
	Phensuximide	Milontin (Parke-Davis)
Barbiturates and barbiturate congeners	Mephobarbital	Mebaral (Winthrop)
	Metharbital	Gemonil (Abbott)
	Primidone	Mysoline (Ayerst)
Adjuvant	Acetazolamide	Diamox (Lederle)
ANTIPARKINSONIAN AGENTS		
Atropine-like agents	Benztropine	Cogentin (Merck)
	Biperiden	Akineton (Knoll)
	Cycrimine	Pagitane (Lilly)
	Procyclidine	Kemadrin (Burroughs)
	Trihexyphenidyl	Artane (Lederle)
		Tremin (Schering)
Antihistamines	Diphenhydramine	Benadryl (Parke-Davis)
	Orphenadrine	Disipal (Riker)
AGENTS USED IN THE TREATMENT OF DRUG ADDICTION AND ABUSE	Methadone	Dolophine (Lilly)
	Levallorphan	Lorfan (Roche)
	Nalorphine	Nalline (Merck)
	Disulfiram	Antabuse (Ayerst)

TABLE 50 *Summary of American Psychiatric Association's Diagnostic and Statistical Manual (DSM-II)*

(Many of the titles here are listed in abbreviated form.)

I. MENTAL RETARDATION

- 310. Borderline
- 311. Mild
- 312. Moderate
- 313. Severe
- 314. Profound
- 315. Unspecified

With each: following or associated with

- .0 Infection or intoxication
- .1 Trauma or physical agent
- .2 Disorders of metabolism, growth, or nutrition
- .3 Gross brain disease (postnatal)
- .4 Unknown prenatal influence
- .5 Chromosomal abnormality
- .6 Prematurity
- .7 Major psychiatric disorder
- .8 Psychosocial (environmental) deprivation
- .9 Other condition

II. ORGANIC BRAIN SYNDROMES (OBS)

A. PSYCHOSES

Senile and presenile dementia
- 290.0 Senile dementia
- 290.1 Presenile dementia

Alcoholic psychosis
- 291.0 Delirium tremens
- 291.1 Korsakov's psychosis
- 291.2 Other alcoholic hallucinosis
- 291.3 Alcohol paranoid state
- 291.4 Acute alcohol intoxication *
- 291.5 Alcoholic deterioration *
- 291.6 Pathological intoxication *
- 291.9 Other alcoholic psychosis

Psychosis associated with intracranial infection
- 292.0 General paralysis
- 292.1 Syphilis of CNS
- 292.2 Epidemic encephalitis
- 292.3 Other and unspecified encephalitis
- 292.9 Other intracranial infection

Psychosis associated with other cerebral condition
- 293.0 Cerebral arteriosclerosis
- 293.1 Other cerebrovascular disturbance
- 293.2 Epilepsy
- 293.3 Intracranial neoplasm
- 293.4 Degenerative disease of the CNS
- 293.5 Brain trauma
- 293.9 Other cerebral condition

Psychosis associated with other physical condition
- 294.0 Endocrine disorder
- 294.1 Metabolic and nutritional disorder
- 294.2 Systemic infection
- 294.3 Drug or poison intoxication (other than alcohol)
- 294.4 Childbirth
- 294.8 Other and unspecified physical condition

TABLE 50 *Summary of American Psychiatric Association's Diagnostic and Statistical Manual (DSM-II)* (continued)

(Many of the titles here are listed in abbreviated form.)

II. ORGANIC BRAIN SYNDROMES (OBS) (continued)

    B. NONPSYCHOTIC OBS

309.0	Intracranial infection
309.13	Alcohol (simple drunkenness) *
309.14	Other drug, poison, or systemic intoxication *
309.2	Brain trauma
309.3	Circulatory disturbance
309.4	Epilepsy
309.5	Disturbance of metabolism, growth, or nutrition
309.6	Senile or presenile brain disease
309.7	Intracranial neoplasm
309.8	Degenerative disease of the CNS
309.9	Other physical condition

III. PSYCHOSES NOT ATTRIBUTED TO PHYSICAL CONDITIONS LISTED PREVIOUSLY

Schizophrenia

295.0	Simple
295.1	Hebephrenic
295.2	Catatonic
295.23	Catatonic type, excited *
295.24	Catatonic type, withdrawn *
295.3	Paranoid
295.4	Acute schizophrenic episode
295.5	Latent
295.6	Residual
295.7	Schizo-affective
295.73	Schizo-affective, excited *
295.74	Schizo-affective, depressed *
295.8	Childhood *
295.90	Chronic undifferentiated *
295.99	Other schizophrenia *

Major affective disorders

296.0	Involutional melancholia
296.1	Manic-depressive illness, manic
296.2	Manic-depressive illness, depressed
296.3	Manic-depressive illness, circular
296.33	Manic-depressive, circular, manic *
296.34	Manic-depressive, circular, depressed *
296.8	Other major affective disorder

Paranoid states

297.0	Paranoia
297.1	Involutional paranoid state
297.9	Other paranoid state

Other psychoses

298.0	Psychotic depressive reaction

IV. NEUROSES

300.0	Anxiety
300.1	Hysterical
300.13	Hysterical, conversion type *
300.14	Hysterical, dissociative type *
300.2	Phobic
300.3	Obsessive compulsive
300.4	Depressive
300.5	Neurasthenic

TABLE 50. *Summary of American Psychiatric Association's Diagnostic and Statistical Manual (DSM-II)* (continued)

(Many of the titles here are listed in abbreviated form.)

IV. NEUROSES (continued)

    300.6   Depersonalization
    300.7   Hypochondriacal
    300.8   Other neurosis

V. PERSONALITY DISORDERS AND CERTAIN OTHER NON-PSYCHOTIC MENTAL DISORDERS

Personality disorders
    301.0   Paranoid
    301.1   Cyclothymic
    301.2   Schizoid
    301.3   Explosive
    301.4   Obsessive compulsive
    301.5   Hysterical
    301.6   Asthenic
    301.7   Antisocial
    301.81 Passive-aggressive *
    301.82 Inadequate *
    301.89 Other specified types *

Sexual deviation
    302.0   Homosexuality
    302.1   Fetishism
    302.2   Pedophilia
    302.3   Transvestitism
    302.4   Exhibitionism
    302.5   Voyeurism *
    302.6   Sadism *
    302.7   Masochism *
    302.8   Other sexual deviation

Alcoholism
    303.0   Episodic excessive drinking
    303.1   Habitual excessive drinking
    303.2   Alcohol addiction
    303.9   Other alcoholism

Drug dependence
    304.0   Opium, opium alkaloids, and their derivatives
    304.1   Synthetic analgesics with morphine-like effects
    304.2   Barbiturates
    304.3   Other hypnotics and sedatives or "tranquilizers"
    304.4   Cocaine
    304.5   Cannabis sativa (hashish, marihuana)
    304.6   Other psychostimulants
    304.7   Hallucinogens
    304.8   Other drug dependence

VI. PSYCHOPHYSIOLOGIC DISORDERS

    305.0   Skin
    305.1   Musculoskeletal
    305.2   Respiratory
    305.3   Cardiovascular
    305.4   Hemic and lymphatic
    305.5   Gastrointestinal
    305.6   Genitourinary
    305.7   Endocrine
    305.8   Organ of special sense
    305.9   Other type

TABLE 50. *Summary of American Psychiatric Association's Diagnostic and Statistical Manual (DSM-II)* (continued)

(Many of the titles here are listed in abbreviated form.)

VII. SPECIAL SYMPTOMS

306.0	Speech disturbance
306.1	Specific learning disturbance
306.2	Tic
306.3	Other psychomotor disorder
306.4	Disorders of sleep
306.5	Feeding disturbance
306.6	Enuresis
306.7	Encopresis
306.8	Cephalalgia
306.9	Other special symptom

VIII. TRANSIENT SITUATIONAL DISTURBANCES

307.0	Adjustment reaction of infancy *
307.1	Adjustment reaction of childhood *
307.2	Adjustment reaction of adolescence *
307.3	Adjustment reaction of adult life *
307.4	Adjustment reaction of late life *

IX. BEHAVIOR DISORDERS OF CHILDHOOD AND ADOLESCENCE

308.0	Hyperkinetic reaction *
308.1	Withdrawing reaction *
308.2	Overanxious reaction *
308.3	Runaway reaction *
308.4	Unsocialized aggressive reaction *
308.5	Group delinquent reaction *
308.9	Other reaction *

X. CONDITIONS WITHOUT MANIFEST PSYCHIATRIC DISORDER AND NON-SPECIFIC CONDITIONS

Social maladjustment without manifest psychiatric disorder

316.0	Marital maladjustment *
316.1	Social maladjustment *
316.2	Occupational maladjustment *
316.3	Dyssocial behavior *
316.9	Other social maladjustment *

Nonpsychiatric conditions

317	Nonspecific conditions *

No mental disorder

318	No mental disorder

* These diagnoses are for use in the US only and do not appear in the international nomenclature (ICD-8).

TABLE 51. *Drug Argot Glossary*

Acid	LSD, LSD-25 (lysergic acid diethylamide)
Acidhead	Frequent user of LSD
Bag	Packet of drugs
Ball	Absorption of stimulants and cocaine via genitalia
Bang	Injection of drugs
Barbs	Barbiturates
Bennies	Benzedrine, an amphetamine
Bindle	Packet of narcotics
Blank	Extremely low-grade narcotics
Blast	Strong effect from a drug
Blue angels	Amytal, a barbiturate
Blue velvet	Paregoric (camphorated tincture of opium) and Pyribenzamine (an antihistamine) mixed and injected
Bombita	Amphetamine injection, sometimes taken with heroin
Bread	Money
Bum trip	Bad experience with psychedelics
Bummer	Bad experience with psychedelics
Busted	Arrested
Buttons	The sections of the peyote cactus
Cap	Capsule
Chipping	Taking narcotics occasionally
Coasting	Under the influence of drugs
Cokie	Cocaine addict
Cold turkey	Sudden withdrawal of narcotics (from the gooseflesh, which resembles the skin of a cold plucked turkey)
Coming down	Recovering from a trip
Connection	Drug supplier
Cop	To obtain heroin
Cop out	Quit, take off, confess, defect, inform
Crash	The effects of stopping the use of amphetamines
Crash pad	Place where the user withdraws from amphetamines
Cubehead	Frequent user of LSD
Cut	Dilute drugs by adding milk sugar or another inert substance
Dealer	Drug supplier
Deck	Packet of narcotics
Dexies	Dexedrine, an amphetamine
Dime bag	$10 package of narcotics
Dirty	Possessing drugs, liable to arrest if searched
Dollies	Dolophine (also known as methadone), a synthetic narcotic
Doper	Person who uses drugs regularly
Downers	Sedatives, alcohol, tranquilizers, and narcotics
Drop	Swallow a drug
Dummy	Purchase which did not contain narcotics
Dynamite	High-grade heroin
Fix	Injection of narcotics
Flash	The initial feeling after injecting
Flip	Become psychotic
Floating	Under the influence of drugs

TABLE 51. *Drug Argot Glossary* (continued)

Freakout	Bad experience with psychedelics; also a chemical high
Fuzz	The police
Gage	Marihuana
Good trip	Happy experience with psychedelics
Goofballs	Sleeping pills
Grass	Marihuana
H	Heroin
Hard narcotics	Opiates, such as heroin and morphine
Hard stuff	Heroin
Hash	Hashish, the resin of Cannabis
Hay	Marihuana
Head	Person dependent on drugs
Hearts	Dexedrine tablets (from the shape)
Heat	The police
High	Under the influence of drugs
Holding	Having drugs in one's possession
Hooked	Addicted
Hophead	Narcotics addict
Horse	Heroin
Hustle	Activities involved in obtaining money to buy heroin
Hustler	Prostitute
Hype	Narcotics addict
Joint	Marihuana cigarette
Jolly beans	Pep pills
Joy-pop	Inject narcotics irregularly
Junkie	Narcotics addict
Kick the habit	Stop using narcotics (from the withdrawal leg muscle twitches)
Layout	Equipment for injecting drug
Lemonade	Poor heroin
M	Morphine
Mainline	Inject drugs into a vein
Maintaining	Keeping at a certain level of drug effect
(The) Man	The police
Manicure	Remove the dirt, seeds, and stems from marihuana
Mesc	Mescaline, the alkaloid in peyote
Meth	Methamphetamine
Methhead	Habitual user of methamphetamine
Mikes	Micrograms (millionths of a gram)
Narc	Narcotics detective
Nickel bag	$5 packet of drugs
O. D.	Overdose of narcotics
On the nod	Sleepy from narcotics
Panic	Shortage of narcotics on the market
Pillhead	Heavy user of pills, barbiturates or amphetamines or both
Pop	Inject drugs
Pot	Marihuana

TABLE 51. *Drug Argot Glossary* (continued)

Pothead	Heavy marihuana user
Purple hearts	Dexamyl, a combination of Dexedrine and Amytal (from the shape and color)
Pusher	Drug peddler
Quill	A matchbook cover for sniffing Methedrine, cocaine, or heroin
Rainbows	Tuinal (Amytal and Seconal), a barbiturate combination in a blue and red capsule
Red devils	Seconal, a barbiturate
Reefer	Marihuana cigarette
Reentry	Return from a trip
Roach	Marihuana butt
Roach holder	Device for holding the butt of a marihuana cigarette
Run	An amphetamine binge
Satch cotton	Cotton used to strain drugs before injection; may be used again if supplies are gone
Scag	Heroin
Score	Make a purchase of drugs
Shooting gallery	Place where addicts inject
Skin popping	Injecting drugs under the skin
Smack	Heroin
Smoke	Wood alcohol
Snorting	Inhaling drugs
Snow	Cocaine
Speed	Methamphetamine
Speedball	An injection of a stimulant and a depressant, originally heroin and cocaine
Speedfreak	Habitual user of speed
Stash	Supply of drugs in a secure place
Stick	Marihuana cigarette
Stoolie	Informer
Strung out	Addicted
Tracks	Scars along veins after many injections
Tripping out	High on psychedelics
Turned on	Under the influence of drugs
Turps	Elixir of Terpin Hydrate with Codeine, a cough syrup
25	LSD (from its original designation, LSD-25)
Uppers	Stimulants, cocaine, and psychedelics
Weed	Marihuana
Works	Equipment for injecting drugs
Yellow jacket	Nembutal, a barbiturate
Yen sleep	A drowsy, restless state during the withdrawal period

From: *A Federal Source Book:* Answers to the Most Frequently Asked Questions About Drug Abuse, US Govt Printing Office, 1970.

Author Index

Subject Index*

* Prepared with the assistance of Mr. Steven Lower.

707